# Legionella

# SPONSORS

# SCIENTIFIC REVIEW COMMITTEE

# Legionella

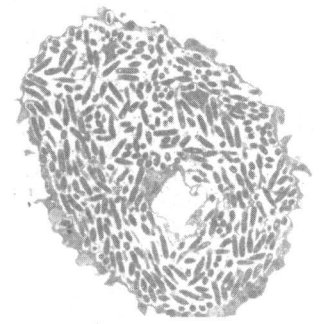

*Edited by*

**Reinhard Marre**
Department of Medical Microbiology and Hygiene
University of Ulm
Ulm, Germany

**Yousef Abu Kwaik**
Department of Microbiology and Immunology
University of Kentucky Medical Center
Lexington, Kentucky

**Christopher Bartlett**
Centre for Infectious Disease Epidemiology
University College London
London, United Kingdom

**Nicholas P. Cianciotto**
Department of Microbiology-Immunology
Northwestern University Medical School
Chicago, Illinois

**Barry S. Fields**
Division of Bacterial and Mycotic Diseases
National Center for Infectious Diseases
Centers for Disease Control and Prevention
Atlanta, Georgia

**Matthias Frosch**
Institute of Hygiene and Microbiology
Julius-Maximilians University
Wuerzburg, Germany

**Jörg Hacker**
Institut für Molekulare Infektionsbiologie
Julius-Maximilians University
Wuerzburg, Germany

**Paul Christian Lück**
Institut für Medizinische Mikrobiologie und Hygiene
Dresden, Germany

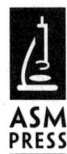

ASM
PRESS

*Washington, DC*

Address editorial correspondence to ASM Press, 1752 N St. NW, Washington, DC 20036-2904, USA

Send orders to ASM Press, P.O. Box 605, Herndon, VA 20172, USA
Phone: (800) 546-2416 or (703) 661-1593
Fax: (703) 661-1501
E-mail: books@asmusa.org
Online: www.asmpress.org

**Library of Congress Cataloging-in-Publication Data**

Legionella / edited by Reinhard Marre . . . [et al.].
    p. cm.
    "5th International Conference on Legionella, September 26–29th, 2000, in Ulm"—Pref.
    ISBN 1-55581-230-9
    1. Legionella pneumophila—Congresses.   2. Legionnaires' disease—Congresses.   I.
Marre, Reinhard.   II. International Conference on Legionella (5th : 2000 : Ulm, Germany)

QR201.L44.L427 2002
616.2′41—dc21

                                                                            2001045740

10 9 8 7 6 5 4 3 2 1

*Cover photo:* Electron micrograph of *Acanthamoeba polyphaga* infected by *Legionella pneumophila* AA100 24 h after initiation of infection. Photo courtesy of Yousef Abu Kwaik.

# CONTENTS

# PREFACE

A quarter of a century after the outbreak of Legionnaires' disease at the 1976 Legionnaires' convention in Philadelphia, Pa., we continue to be fascinated by *Legionella*, a bacterial genus which in a unique way is adapted to the aquatic environment and to the intracellular milieu of phagocytic cells of the human host. Legionellosis is still a disease of public concern. Therefore, an electronic communication network has been set up to facilitate communications between laymen and experts (http://www.q-net.net.au/~legion). In addition, a European surveillance scheme for travel-associated legionellosis (http://ewgli.org) was introduced in the last years.

In order to offer a forum for scientific presentations and discussions and to allow exchange of ideas and formation of personal relationships between representatives of the different groups working on Legionella, we organized the 5th International Conference on Legionella, from 26 to 29 September 2000, in Ulm, Sweden.

The main topics addressed were pathogenesis and immunology, molecular ecology, aspects of clinical microbiology and therapy, epidemiology, surveillance, and prevention. Controversies concerning copper–silver ionization systems were discussed by a panel. The conference thus provided an overview of recent findings, current opinions, matters of debate, and recommendations.

This book summarizes the contributions presented at the meeting and reflects the current state of the art as well as future perspectives. The scientific committee and organizers of the meeting thank everyone who contributed to the success of the meeting and who contributed to this book.

R. MARRE  
Y. ABU KWAIK  
C. BARTLETT  
N. P. CIANCIOTTO  

B. S. FIELDS  
M. FROSCH  
J. HACKER  
P. C. LÜCK  
*April 2001*

# LEGIONNAIRES' DISEASE 25 YEARS LATER: LESSONS LEARNED†

*Joseph E. McDade*

Although most of my chapter will relate to early work on Legionnaires' disease, I will begin with some additional observations, to place those investigations in a somewhat broader perspective.

> "In many ways one can think of the middle of the twentieth century as the end of one of the most important social revolutions in history, the virtual elimination of the infectious disease as a significant factor in social life."
> Nobel Laureate McFarlane Burnet, 1962 (2)

Burnet's prediction reflected the prevailing thinking of that period, particularly with the rapid advance in vaccine development and widespread availability of antibiotics that were effective at the time. But notwithstanding the eradication of smallpox in the 1970s and the current efforts to eliminate polio, infectious diseases remain serious problems, in both developing and industrialized nations. For example, in 1991, epidemic cholera reappeared in South America after a lengthy absence; dur-

ing the next 3 years, the Pan American Health Organization received reports of more than 1 million cases of cholera and 9,000 deaths (3). In 1990, epidemic diphtheria began to emerge in the New Independent States of the former Soviet Union; by 1996, approximately 125,000 cases of diphtheria and 4,000 deaths had been reported (11). Also in the 1990s, the incidence of pertussis increased substantially in The Netherlands, despite active immunization programs (4).

In the United States, deaths caused by infectious diseases increased significantly from 1980 to 1992, even when AIDS-related illnesses were not included. For example, deaths due to respiratory disease increased 32%, and deaths due to septicemia increased 83% (1). Now the widespread prevalence of antimicrobial resistance worldwide is exacerbating many infectious disease problems and complicating treatment of patients.

> "Isolation of a new infectious agent is really an anachronism in this day and time."
> An esteemed colleague, circa 1978

In 1978, while I was attending a meeting of the Infectious Diseases Society of America, I had the opportunity to discuss the Centers for Disease Control's (CDC's) early work on Legionnaires' disease with one of the distin-

*Joseph E. McDade*   National Center for Infectious Diseases, Centers for Disease Control and Prevention, Atlanta, GA 30333.

† Dedicated to the memory of Dr. Charles C. Shepard, former mentor and colleague during the investigation of Legionnaires' disease in 1976.

*Legionella*, Edited by Reinhard Marre et al.
© 2002 ASM Press, Washington, D.C.

guished members of the society. Although he appreciated our studies, he was quite unimpressed with the discovery of a new infectious agent. In his mind, all the important infectious agents had already been discovered. "An anachronism, really," he said. I didn't think I was in a position to argue with him, although I should have mentioned that a new hemorrhagic fever agent, the Ebola virus, had just been identified in Africa. What neither of us could foresee, however, was that these discoveries were just the beginning of a trend that has continued to the present.

Since 1977, at least 30 new infectious agents or diseases have been identified. Table 1 lists some of them, beginning with the discovery of the Ebola virus in 1977 and continuing through the discovery of the Nipah virus in 1999. In some cases, new etiologic agents have been identified as the cause of known diseases or syndromes; for example, Hantaan virus was identified as the cause of hemmorrhagic fever with renal syndrome (HFRS), and *Helicobacter pylori* is now known to be a principal cause of peptic ulcer disease. Some microorganisms, such as *Cryptosporidium parvum*, had been associated with animals, but initially

were not known to be human pathogens. In some instances, both the etiologic agent and disease were completely unknown to science, such as human immunodeficiency virus and AIDS and Nipah and Hendra virus infections. So nearly 25 years after the Philadelphia outbreak of Legionnaires' disease, identification of new infectious diseases is not at all unusual, and the threat of infectious disease reemergence continues throughout the world.

In the early 1990s, the Institute of Medicine (IOM) convened a special panel to study the problem of infectious disease emergence. The panel's report (7), published in 1992, summarized existing problems and provided numerous recommendations for disease prevention. The IOM Report described six basic causes underlying infectious disease emergence: (i) Human demographics and behavior. The tremendous increase in the human population is drastically changing the world's ecology; for example, human encroachment on forested areas causes exposure to infected wildlife. (ii) Technology and industry. New technology is usually associated with improvements in the quality of life, but new technology also creates new problems and challenges.

**TABLE 1**  Selected etiologic agents and infectious diseases identified since 1977

| Year | Agent | Disease(s) |
|------|-------|------------|
| 1977 | Ebola virus | Ebola hemorrhagic fever |
| 1977 | *Legionella pneumophila* | Legionnaires' disease |
| 1977 | Hantaan virus | Hemorrhagic fever with renal syndrome |
| 1977 | *Campylobacter* sp. | Global enteric pathogen |
| 1982 | *Escherichia coli* O157 | Hemorrhagic colitis |
| 1982 | *Borrelia burgdorferi* | Lyme disease |
| 1983 | *Helicobacter pylori* | Gastric ulcers |
| 1983 | Human immunodeficiency virus | Acquired immunodeficiency syndrome |
| 1989 | Hepatitis C | Non-A, non-B hepatitis |
| 1991 | *Ehrlichia chaffeensis* | Human ehrlichiosis |
| 1991 | Guanarito virus | Venezuelan hemorrhagic fever |
| 1993 | Hantavirus | Hantavirus pulmonary syndrome |
| 1993 | *Bartonella henselae* | Cat scratch disease, bacillary angiomatosis |
| 1994 | Human herpes virus-8 | Kaposi's sarcoma |
| 1994 | *Ehrlichia phagocytophilia* | Human granulocytic ehrlichiosis |
| 1995 | Equine morbillivirus | Severe respiratory disease |
| 1995 | Hendra virus | Respiratory illness, meningoencephalitis |
| 1996 | Australian lyssavirus | Human rabies |
| 1997 | H5N1 influenza virus | New human strain |
| 1999 | Nipah virus | Encephalitis, respiratory illness |

A good example is Legionnaires' disease, which is associated with air conditioning systems. (iii) Economic development and land use. Construction of the Aswan Dam in the 1960s was followed by large outbreaks of Rift Valley fever in the 1970s because of an increase in mosquito populations in irrigated lands adjacent to growing population centers. (iv) International travel and commerce. Meningitis outbreaks have been associated with the annual pilgrimage of thousands to Mecca; the dissemination of antibiotic-resistant gonococci has also been accelerated by people's frequent travel. (v) Microbial adaptation and change. For example, a new strain of influenza virus (H5N1) emerged in Hong Kong in the winter of 1997–1998. (vi) Breakdown of public health measures. As one illustration, in the United States in the early 1990s, most states did not have even one person devoted to surveillance of food-borne diseases, despite problems with large outbreaks.

## NEW DISEASES IDENTIFIED BY DIFFERENT APPROACHES

The new diseases and infectious agents in Table 1 were identified in various scenarios and by different investigative approaches. For example, human ehrlichiosis was first detected by a follow-up investigation of a single case report. We now know that ehrlichiosis is prevalent throughout the world. In contrast, *H. pylori* was identified as the cause of peptic ulcers by long-term studies of an obscure bacterium. Surveillance for viral hepatitis in the United States began in the 1960s and over the years, researchers identified large numbers of persons with parenterally transmitted non-A, non-B hepatitis. This information stimulated the search for the etiologic agent, which culminated with the discovery of the hepatitis C virus in 1989.

## FREQUENTLY, PROBLEMS ARE JUST OPPORTUNITIES IN DISGUISE

Disease outbreaks are yet another stimulus to discovery. Certainly no one wishes for large numbers of people to become ill; however, outbreaks usually are investigated in consid-

erable detail, whereas single cases are much less likely to receive such attention. Certainly this rule of thumb held true with the Legionnaires' disease outbreak in Philadelphia in 1976, the toxic shock syndrome outbreak several years later, and the outbreak of hantavirus pulmonary syndrome in the Four Corners area of the United States in 1993. In each of these outbreaks, evaluations of multiple patients facilitated description of the clinical presentation of the new disease, which in turn provided the basis for follow-up epidemiologic studies. Also, each of these outbreak investigations involved scientists from multiple disciplines, including laboratory scientists, which ensured a thorough search for etiologic agents. Finally, large numbers of specimens from well-characterized patients were available for laboratory studies, and characterized archival specimens were also available for follow-up investigations, if needed.

## PARADIGMS, ALGORITHMS, AND SCIENTIFIC DISCOVERY

Few things are as elusive as a formula to ensure successful research. Most discoveries are not made by blind luck; instead, discoveries are more likely to be made by the recognition and pursuit of anomalies that occur during the course of routine experimentation. At least that is the opinion of Thomas Kuhn, who is best known for his book, *The Structure of Scientific Revolutions* (8). Unfortunately, the corollary to Kuhn's hypothesis is that most of us fail to recognize significant anomalies when we see them. As Kuhn notes, scientists formulate basic paradigms to explain a given body of knowledge. Then we develop algorithms, which are analytical approaches, experimental designs, and standard methods to test or validate the basic theory. Anomalies, of course, test the fitness of the paradigm as well as the rigor of our thinking. For example, the germ theory has provided a testable hypothesis for studying disease of unknown etiology since the 19th century. Over the years, microbiologists have developed different algorithms or investigative approaches that have been followed as tools of the trade. For example, virtually every introductory microbiology course has a laboratory exercise in which the students are asked to identify microbial pathogens by following well-known diagnostic schemes. They are instructed to use a blood culture system for specimens from patients with a particular constellation of symptoms or special plating medium for specimens from another group of patients. As a rule, all testing materials are discarded if nothing is recovered after a certain number of days. In the modern clinical laboratory, the entire approach is automated. But what happens when negative results are obtained when performing the standard drill?

## OUTBREAKS OF PONTIAC FEVER AND LEGIONNAIRES' DISEASE

The response to anomalous laboratory results turned out to be a critical factor during the investigations of Legionnaires' disease and Pontiac fever. Pontiac fever was the name given to an outbreak of acute febrile respiratory illness that occurred among 95 of 100 persons who worked in a single building of the Oakland County Health Department in Pontiac, Mich., in 1968 (6). The illness lasted 3 or 4 days but there was no pneumonia nor any fatalities. Epidemiologic investigations quickly established that the disease was airborne, but there was no evidence of person-to-person spread. Conditioned air was incriminated as the source of infection when researchers realized that of all the people who entered the building, the only ones who didn't get sick were those who were there only when the air conditioning was turned off.

Sentinel guinea pigs developed fever and pneumonia 2 to 3 days after they had been placed in the affected building, but guinea pigs left in unaffected buildings remained completely healthy. Histologic examination of lung tissue collected at necropsy revealed definitive evidence of focal bronchopneumonia in ill guinea pigs; but despite intensive efforts, no agent could be recovered consistently from their lungs. An unusual bacterium was occasionally seen in embryonated eggs that had been inoculated with suspensions of guinea pig lung tissue, but it was considered inconsequential because random contamination with various types of bacteria also occurred in some of the same eggs.

The investigation of Legionnaires' disease in 1976 (5) received much more publicity than did the Pontiac fever study. The United States had been sensitized to the possibility of a major influenza epidemic when, earlier that year, reports of swine flu originated from Ft. Dix, N.J. The reports of swine flu turned out to be unfounded, but were still fresh in everyone's mind on August 2 when the CDC received word that three persons in Pittsburgh, Pa., had died from complications following severe bouts of pneumonia. Quick telephone calls to other hospitals in Pennsylvania also revealed unusual numbers of pneumonia patients. By nightfall, three epidemiologists were dispatched from the CDC to Pittsburgh, Harrisburg, and Philadelphia, Pa., to investigate the disease; specimens began to arrive in Atlanta the next day. An estimated 221 cases occurred with 34 deaths, giving a case fatality rate of about 15% (Fig. 1).

Attendance at the American Legion convention at the Bellevue-Stratford Hotel in Philadelphia was a common factor among ill persons. Disease was also associated with time spent in the hotel lobby. By late November, the CDC had devoted more than 73,000 h to the investigation without success. Throughout the investigation, the CDC also sought input from experts throughout the world. In fact, late in 1976, a distinguished panel of pathologists, epidemiologists, and other scientists met for several days in Atlanta to review all available data on the Legionnaires' disease outbreak. They reached one basic conclusion. Although they did not know what caused the epidemic, they were certain the epidemic could not have been caused by a bacterium!

How could such a talented group of scientists fail to see something that now appears so obvious? At that time, Legionnaires' disease and the bacterium that causes it were anomalies that were not part of the standard clinical and microbiologic diagnostic algorithms.

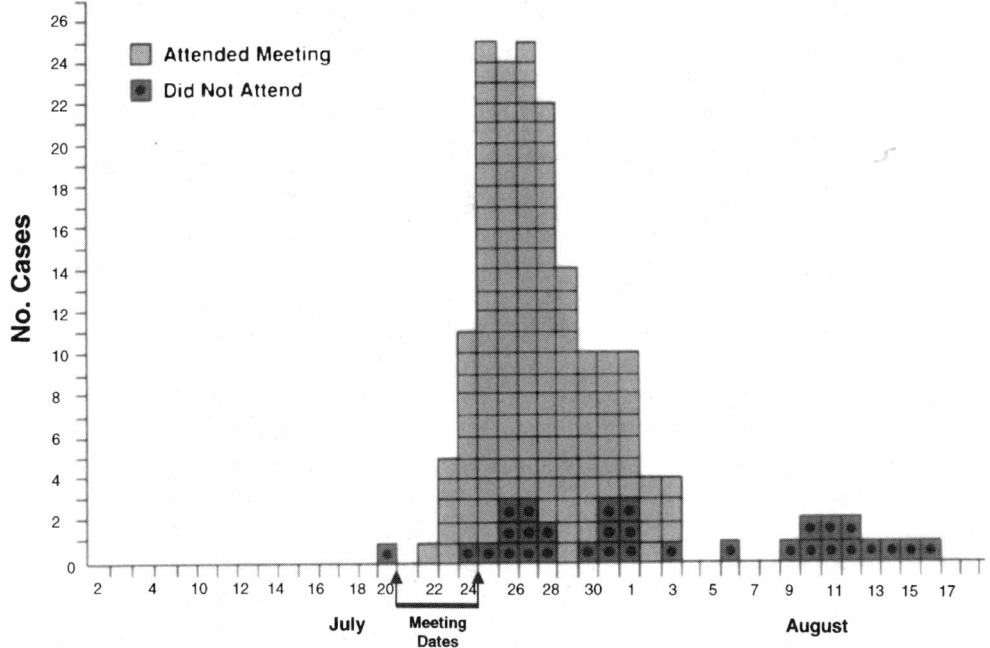

**FIGURE 1** Outbreak of Legionnaires' disease in Philadelphia, 1976, in association with a meeting of the Pennsylvania unit of the American Legion.

The pulmonary manifestations of the Philadelphia patients were considered more typical of viral pneumonia than of bacterial. However, no virus was consistently isolated from tissues collected at autopsy. The first pathologic studies also failed to incriminate bacteria. Patients' lung tissues, obtained at autopsy, were stained by hematoxylin and eosin, Brown-Brenn, Brown-Hopps, and several other standard methods for detecting bacteria in tissues, but, remarkably, the Legionnaires' bacillus is refractory to these stains. Also, no specific reproducible agent was isolated from patient tissues on 14 different bacteriologic and mycologic media. Tests of patient sera against 77 known infectious agents were also negative (9).

## ULTIMATELY, YOU HAVE TO TRUST YOUR OWN INSTINCTS

I, too, became so entrapped in a standard diagnostic algorithm that I couldn't see the proverbial forest for the trees. I was asked to rule out Q fever as a possible cause of Legion-naires' disease. I had an instant bias against performing this drill because Q fever is a relatively mild rickettsial disease, not at all like Legionnaires' disease; it is acquired primarily from exposure to domestic animals and is rarely fatal. Nevertheless, I immediately began to process the autopsy specimens according to the standard algorithm for isolating Q fever rickettsiae.

To test for Q fever, blood or tissue specimens are ground into a suspension and inoculated into guinea pigs. When the guinea pigs become febrile, usually a week or so later, guinea pig blood or tissue specimens are passed into embryonated eggs to enhance growth of the rickettsiae. Typically, one adds combinations of certain antibiotics to the guinea pig tissues before passaging them in eggs, to inhibit the growth of contaminating bacteria.

But when I inoculated the guinea pigs with lung tissue of Legionnaires' disease patients, something unusual happened. They became extremely febrile within 1 to 2 days. I shared my observation with several colleagues, and we agreed that the rapid onset of fever must be due to either a toxic compound or bacteria in the lung tissue. Not quite sure how to proceed, I continued to follow the standard algorithm for rickettsial isolation. First, I inoculated aliquots of guinea pig tissues into embryonated eggs. Next, I obtained a fresh scalpel, cut a clean face on several guinea pig tissues, and made replicate impression smears for staining. I sent several sets of tissue smears to colleagues for their evaluation. I stained my set by the Gimenez technique, which is a standard method for visualizing rickettsiae; my colleagues stained their smears by other methods. Then, I prepared additional suspensions of guinea pig tissues in buffer, without adding antibiotics, and placed a few small drops of those suspensions onto several different bacteriologic growth media. This procedure would allow us to isolate and identify any bacteria that might be present.

Nothing grew in the eggs, but that was expected. Legionnaires' disease was not at all like Q fever and so it was no surprise that rickettsiae were not recovered. I also concluded that if bacteria caused the fever in guinea pigs, they had been inactivated by the antibiotics that I added to the tissue suspensions. Of course, if Legionnaires' disease had been caused by some sort of toxic compound, we would not expect to recover any microorganisms. But there was one discrepant result. I saw an occasional rod-shaped bacterium in smears of guinea pig spleen stained by the Gimenez technique; however, I did not recover rod-shaped bacteria on any of the bacteriologic media. In contrast, my colleagues found absolutely no evidence of rod-shaped bacteria in the tissue smears that they had stained by other methods. When I asked one colleague about the possible significance of my observation, he concluded that the rod-shaped bacterium probably was not recovered on culture media simply because it was a rare, adventitious agent, hardly a suspect in this case. Any remaining qualms I had at the time were allayed a few weeks later, when toxicologic studies showed elevated levels of nickel carbonyl in the lung tissues of deceased Legionnaires' disease patients.

But by December 1976, the nickel carbonyl theory was also invalidated; the elevated levels of metal were traced back to the scalpel blades that had been used to collect human lung tissue at autopsy. The demise of the toxic metal hypothesis was particularly important because now we had no other logical leads to further investigation. Within that vacuum, one thought kept coming to my mind: why had we not been able to cultivate that rod-shaped bacterium?

During the Christmas holidays, I decided to reexamine the stained preparations of guinea pig tissue. After looking at the slides for some time, I saw something I hadn't seen before—a cluster of rod-shaped bacteria! The presence of the cluster suggested that the bacterium I had seen previously was more than a random contaminant. But how could the earlier failure to cultivate this agent be explained? All previous results could be reconciled quite easily, however, if two simple points were true: first, that the bacterium could be visualized with Gimenez but not the other stains, and second, that the bacterium was a fastidious organism that could not be cultivated on standard bacteriologic media.

I knew that embryonated eggs could provide a very permissive environment for cultivating fastidious microorganisms, provided that antibiotics were not added to the inoculum. I retrieved the suspensions of guinea pig tissue from the freezer and once more I inoculated them into embryonated eggs, this time without adding antibiotics. In contrast to my earlier experiments, all embryos died several days later. When I examined smears of yolk sac tissue stained by the Gimenez method, I saw that they were teeming with rod-shaped bacteria! By indirect fluorescent-antibody assay (IFA), we showed that more than 90% of the Philadelphia patients had developed antibodies to the bacterium during the course of their illness (Table 2). Later, we successfully isolated the same bacterium from four of six additional autopsy specimens.

**TABLE 2** Results of IFA tests of sera from Legionnaires' disease patients with isolate

| Serologic status | No. of patients |
|---|---|
| Seroconversions (fourfold increase) ......... | 62 |
| Positive (titer ≥128) ..................... | 39 |
| Negative ............................... | 10 |
| Questionable........................... | 25 |
| Total patients tested..................... | 136 |

## GOOD COLLABORATORS, LIKE GOOD FRIENDS, ARE A REAL TREASURE

We learned a lot about Legionnaires' disease during the next few years, and progress was directly proportional to the number of collaborations. For example, our results with patient sera were only significant when linked with the comprehensive epidemiologic information generated by others. Thanks to David Fraser, Ted Tsai, and others at the CDC, who provided us with paired serum specimens from well-characterized Legionnaires' disease, we were able to study the kinetics of the antibody response following infection and to establish provisional criteria for minimum positive titers by IFA testing (9).

We soon learned that earlier outbreaks of pneumonia had been caused by the Legionnaires' disease bacterium. I refer specifically to the outbreak of pneumonia of unknown etiology that occurred at St. Elizabeth's hospital in Washington, D.C. in August 1965. This outbreak had also been investigated by the CDC. There were 34 cases, with 3 deaths occurring within an 11-day period (10). Retrospective testing of well-characterized archival serum specimens showed that the outbreaks at St. Elizabeth's Hospital in 1965, as well as the outbreak in Pontiac in 1968, were caused by the same agent (Table 3).

Recall that conditioned air was implicated as a possible source of infection in the outbreak of Pontiac fever. Investigators of that outbreak hypothesized that the etiologic agent was either in conditioned air or in water from the cooling tower, or both, and so they collected specimens from guinea pigs exposed to air and water during their investigation in 1968. Arnold Kaufmann provided us with archival specimens from the Pontiac outbreak, and we performed isolation attempts, as was done with the Philadelphia specimens. Positive test results (Table 4) supported their hypothesis, and basic concepts of the epidemiology of the disease began to form. Of course, it would be many years before the scientific community would fully understand the ecology of the bacterium and its association with protozoa in water.

The contributions of several laboratory scientists at the CDC during the early days of the Legionnaires' disease investigation should also be noted. Francis Chandler first showed that the Legionnaires' disease bacillus could be visualized directly in autopsy specimens by the Dieterle silver impregnation technique, and although it was a nonspecific procedure, it proved a convenient technique for establishing a postmortem diagnosis. Vester Lewis showed that erythromycin and rifampin inhibited the growth of the Legionnaires' disease bacterium in embryonated eggs; clinical evaluations were consistent with his findings.

We should also not forget the contributions of Robert Weaver, who first grew the Legionnaires' disease bacterium on an axenic culture medium. Others quickly built on his success. Using cultured bacteria from the Philadelphia outbreak as antigens, Roger McKinney and William Cherry prepared fluorescein-labeled antisera for direct testing of lung tissue from suspect cases. These antisera were quite useful in providing rapid and specific diagnosis in fatal cases. However, my colleague Charles Shepard maintained a more conservative approach, and he insisted that we continue to isolate the agent from patient blood or autopsy tissue. As it turned out, it was quite fortunate that we did. We obtained isolates from several patients when their tests were negative. As a result, the first serotype differences among isolates became apparent.

The late James Feeley and George Gorman performed the painstaking task of identifying optimal growth media and conditions for the

**TABLE 3**  IFA results with isolate on serum specimens from other outbreaks

| Serologic status | No. of patients in outbreak with indicated status | |
|---|---|---|
| | St. Elizabeth's Hospital | Pontiac fever |
| Seroconversions | 17 | 31 |
| Positive only | 4 | 1 |
| Negative | 2 | 5 |
| Total patients tested | 23 | 37 |
| Percentage positive | 91 | 86 |

bacterium, which has greatly facilitated diagnosis and research even today. Don Brenner was another wonderful collaborator. Don had extensive expertise, unusual at the time, in characterizing microorganisms at the DNA level—long before DNA sequencing was commonplace. He also had an enormous database, which allowed interpretation of results with unknown microorganisms. DNA-to-DNA hybridization testing showed that the bacterium was not significantly related to any of the many bacterial species in his collection, indicating that it was indeed a new species.

Another collaborator, Marilyn Bozeman, provided yet another valuable lesson—do not overlook early research. Marilyn had a long-standing interest in rickettsial diseases, including Q fever, while she worked at Walter Reed Institute in Washington, D.C. Over the years, she and her colleague, Elizabeth Jackson, had been asked to determine if Q fever rickettsiae were the cause of illness in many patients. Marilyn isolated some unusual microorganisms from tissues of several patients, using the guinea pig–embryonated egg system. Like rickettsiae, these microorganisms did not grow on the bacteriologic culture media she used. However, she was unable to link the isolates to the respective patient's illness by serologic testing. Marilyn concluded that her colony of guinea pigs was chronically infected with these "rickettsialike" organisms, and that she inadvertently had recovered them while processing human specimens.

At the annual meeting of the American Society for Microbiology in New Orleans in 1977, Marilyn attended our presentation, in which my colleague Charles Shepard and I described our initial findings with Legionnaires' disease. Afterward, Marilyn discussed the similarity of her guinea pig agents to the Legionnaires' disease bacterium and offered to send us four isolates for study: OLDA, WIGA, HEBA, and Tatlock. By IFA testing, we obtained positive titers for each isolate with sera from Legionnaires' disease patients; interestingly, we also observed positive results with sera from several patients with compatible illnesses, whose specimens were negative in tests with the Legionnaires' disease bacterium.

**TABLE 4**  Isolation of Legionnaires' disease bacterium (LDB) from guinea pigs exposed to air or evaporative condenser water aerosols 6 weeks after outbreak in Pontiac, Mich., 1968

| Exposure history of guinea pigs in 1968 | No. cultured in 1977 | No. positive for LDB |
|---|---|---|
| Unfiltered air | 10 | 4 |
| Untreated water | 10 | 6 |
| Filtered water | 7 | 0 |
| None (control animals left at animal shelter) | 9 | 0 |

These results suggested to us that some of these isolates were similar to the Legionnaires' disease bacterium. Importantly, the other isolates might also be additional agents of pneumonia. Results of DNA-to-DNA hybridization studies with OLDA showed it was indistinguishable from the Legionnaires' disease bacterium. Her other isolates were not closely related genetically but were very similar phenotypically to the Legionnaires' disease bacterium. When we saw the aggregate data, we realized for the first time that we could be dealing with a whole group of related pathogens. However, none of us could imagine that one day, more than 40 different species would be discovered.

## NAMING OF AN ORGANISM

Too many people had been involved in the study of this agent to name the bacterium after a single scientist. What seemed more appropriate was honoring the military veterans, members of the American Legion, many of whom had died of the illness in Philadelphia. The bacterium thus came to be named *Legionella pneumophila*—the meaning is self-evident. Pneumophila, "lung loving" or "having an affinity for lungs," still distinguishes *L. pneumophila* from many other *Legionella* species. The guinea pig agents, of course, have also been named as *Legionella* species: OLDA, isolated in 1947, is an early isolate of *L. pneumophila*; WIGA, isolated in 1959, is now *L. bozemanii*; and Tatlock, isolated in 1943, was named *L. micdadei*. HEBA and Tatlock turned out to be the same species.

## BALANCING EGOS AND OBJECTIVITY IN SCIENCE

The late Charles Shepard was my mentor and colleague during the Legionnaires' disease investigation, and we worked very closely together during that period. About a year or so after we had identified the cause of the outbreak, I was finishing a manuscript describing the results of a study we had done. I put a rough draft of the manuscript on his desk; several days later I returned to his office to get

his input. It quickly became obvious that we completely disagreed about the interpretation of the data.

We discussed the matter for quite some time, and eventually the discussion became very spirited. Suddenly, he simply stopped talking. He leaned back in his chair, clasped his hands together behind his head, looked up, and stared quietly at the ceiling for 2 or 3 full minutes. It seemed like an eternity, but I sat there, saying nothing. Finally, he looked at me and said "You know, nothing that you write and nothing that I say can change the truth. The truth just is. It's our job as scientists to find the truth the best way we know how."

## REFERENCES

1. **Armstrong, G. L., L. A. Conn, and R. W. Pinner.** 1999. Trends in infectious disease mortality in the United States during the 20th century. *JAMA* **281:**61–66.
2. **Burnet, M.** 1962. *Natural History of Infectious Disease,* 3rd ed., p. 3. Cambridge University Press, Cambridge, United Kingdom.
3. **Centers for Disease Control and Prevention.** 1995. Update: *Vibrio cholerae* 01-Western Hemisphere, 1991–1994 and *V. cholerae* 0139-Asia, 1994. *Morb. Mortal. Wkly. Rep.* **44:**215–219.
4. **de Melker, H. E., M. A. E. Conyn-van Spaendonck, H. C. Rumke, J. K. Wijngaarden, F. R. Mooi, and J. F. P. Schellekens.** 1977. Pertussis in the Netherlands: an outbreak despite high levels of immunization with whole cell vaccine. *Emerg. Infect. Dis.* **3:**175–178.
5. **Fraser, D. W., T. R. Tsai, W. Orenstein, H. W. Beecham, J. Harris, R. G. Sharrar, W. Parking, G. F. Mallison, S. M. Martin, J. E. McDade, C. C. Shepard, P. S. Brachman, and the Field Investigation Team.** 1977. Legionnaires' disease: description of an epidemic of pneumonia. *N. Engl. J. Med.* **297:** 1189–1197.
6. **Glick, T. H., M. B. Gregg, B. Berman, G. Mallison, W. W. Rhodes, and I. Kassanoff.** 1978. An epidemic of unknown etiology in a health department. I. Clinical and epidemiologic aspects. *Am. J. Epidemiol.* **107:**149–160.
7. **Institute of Medicine.** 1992. *Emerging Infections: Microbial Threats to Health in the United States.* National Academy Press, Washington, D.C.
8. **Kuhn, T. S.** 1996. *The Structure of Scientific Revolutions.* University of Chicago Press, Chicago, Ill.
9. **McDade, J. E., C. C. Shepard, and D. W. Fraser.** Legionnaires' disease: isolation of a bac-

terium and demonstration of its role in other respiratory disease. 1977. *N. Engl. J. Med.* **297:**
1197–1203.

10. **Thacker, S. B., J. V. Bennett, T. F. Tsai,
D. W. Fraser, J. E. McDade, C. C. Shepard,
K. H. Williams, W. H. Stuart, H. B. Dull,
and T. C. Eickhoff.** 1978. An outbreak in 1965
of severe respiratory illness caused by the Legionnaires' disease bacterium. *J. Infect. Dis.* **138:**512–
519.

11. **Vitek, C. R., and M. Wharton.** 1998. Dipth-
eria in the former Soviet Union: reemergence
of a pandemic disease. *Emerg. Infect. Dis.* **4:**539–
550.

# PATHOGENESIS

I

# ROLE OF THE TYPE II PROTEIN SECRETION PATHWAY IN PATHOGENESIS OF *LEGIONELLA PNEUMOPHILA*

*Ombeline Rossier, Paul H. Edelstein, and Nicholas P. Cianciotto*

# 2

In gram-negative bacteria, prepilin peptidases process both the pilin subunits, which assemble into adhesive type IV pili, as well as "pseudopilins." One set of pseudopilins is involved in the assembly of the pilus, and another set is necessary for type II protein secretion (4). Our previous mutational analysis showed that the *Legionella pneumophila* prepilin peptidase, PilD, is required for the production of *Legionella* pili and the secretion of several enzymatic activities (1, 3). Most notably, the *pilD* mutant, unlike a pilin structural mutant (*pilE$_L$*), was 100- to 1,000-fold impaired for intracellular growth in U937 macrophages and *Hartmannella* amoebae (3). To test whether the phenotype of the *pilD* mutant is due to loss of the type II protein secretion system and/or the type IV pilus assembly apparatus, we employed a genetic approach. First, we mutated two loci involved in type II protein secretion. On the one hand, a deletion was generated in the *lspDE* locus, which encodes proteins homologous to the type II outer membrane secretin and ATPase. On the other hand, the *lspGHIJK* locus, encoding the type II secretion pseudopilins, was mutated by a disruption of *lspG* by a kanamycin resistance cassette. Second, we analyzed the phenotypes of two mutants defective in the biogenesis of *L. pneumophila* type IV pilus. In addition to the *pilE$_L$* mutant, kindly provided by Y. Abu Kwaik (5), a pilus mutant was generated by a deletion in the outer membrane secretin gene, *pilQ*. All mutations were introduced into *L. pneumophila* virulent strain 130b (American Type Culture Collection BAA-74, Wadsworth), such that the *lspDE, lspG, pilE$_L$,* and *pilQ* mutants could be directly compared with the strain deficient in *pilD*, permitting distinctions between relative roles of *pilD*, type II protein secretion, and type IV pilus assembly.

## THE SECRETION OF FIVE *pilD*-DEPENDENT ENZYMATIC ACTIVITIES DEPENDS ON *lsp* GENES

Previous analysis of supernatants of the *L. pneumophila* prepilin peptidase mutant showed the absence of protease, acid phosphatase, *p*-nitrophenyl phosphorylcholine (PNPPC) hydrolase, lipase, and phospholipase A activities (1). Aside from the zinc metalloprotease (2), none of these activities had been formally

*Ombeline Rossier and Nicholas P. Cianciotto* Department of Microbiology-Immunology, Northwestern University Medical School, Searle 6-541, 320 E. Superior Street, Chicago, IL 60611. *Paul H. Edelstein* Department of Pathology and Laboratory Medicine and Department of Medicine, University of Pennsylvania School of Medicine, 3400 Spruce Street, Philadelphia, PA 19104.

*Legionella*, Edited by Reinhard Marre et al.
© 2002 ASM Press, Washington, D.C.

linked to the *Legionella* type II secretion pathway. Thus, all strains were grown in buffered yeast extract to late exponential phase, and then filtered supernatants and cell lysates were assayed as described previously (1). The protease, acid phosphatase, and PNPPC hydrolase activities were similarly reduced in the supernatant of the *pilD, lspDE,* and *lspG* mutants compared with the wild type and the *pilE*$_L$ and *pilQ* mutant strains (Fig. 1A to C). As expected for secretion mutants, the enzyme levels were elevated in the cell lysates of *lspDE* and *lspG* mutants (data not shown). In addition, the lipase and phospholipase A activities were also reduced in the supernatants of both *lsp* mutants relative to the wild type and the *pilE*$_L$ mutant (Fig. 1D and E). These results demonstrate that five *pilD*-dependent activities are secreted by the *L. pneumophila* type II protein secretion pathway.

## MUTANTS IN *lspDE* AND *lspG* ARE AS DEFECTIVE AS THE *pilD* MUTANT FOR GROWTH WITHIN *HARTMANNELLA VERMIFORMIS*

To assess the contribution of type II secretion versus PilD to intracellular replication within a natural *Legionella* host, the amoeba *Hartmannella vermiformis* was co-cultured with *lspDE, lspG,* and *pilD* mutants in parallel with the

A
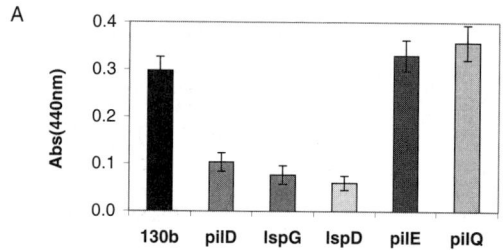

B
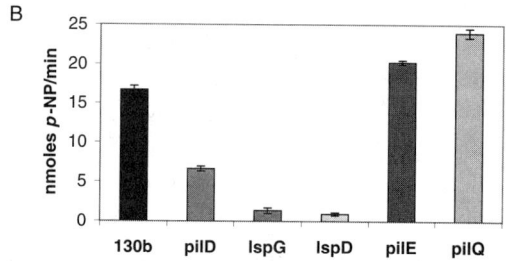

C
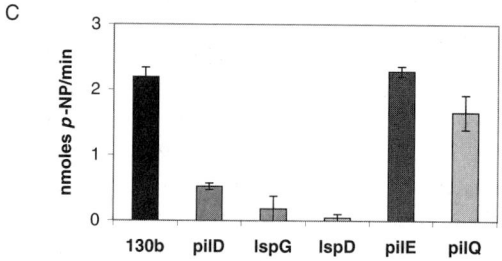

D
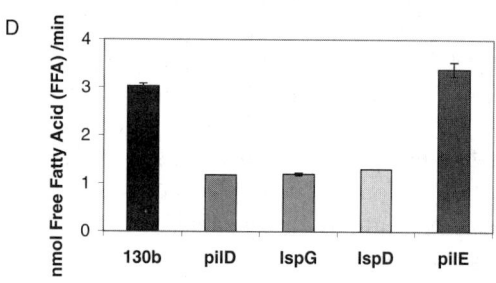

E
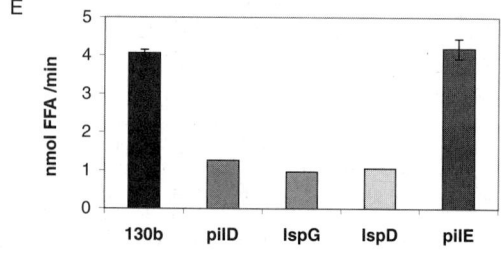

**FIGURE 1** Secreted enzymatic activities of *L. pneumophila* strains. Late logarithmic phase supernatants of wild-type 130b, *pilD, lspG, lspDE, pilE*$_L$, and *pilQ* mutants were tested for (A) protease activity as determined by azocasein hydrolysis; (B) acid phosphatase activity as determined by the release of *p*-nitrophenyl (PNP) from PNP phosphate at pH 5.0; (C) PNPPC hydrolysis; (D) lipase activity as determined by the release of free fatty acid (FFA) from 1-monopalmitoyl glycerol; and (E) phospholipase A activity as determined by phosphatidylcholine hydrolysis. These data represent the mean and standard deviation for duplicate cultures. For all, the difference between the wild type and the *pilD* and *lsp* mutants were significant ($P < 0.01$, Student's *t* test). Note that the *pilQ* mutant was not tested for the lipolytic activities. Comparable results were obtained on at least two other occasions (data not shown).

wild type. The *lsp* and *pilD* mutants exhibited a similar and dramatic intracellular growth defect (Fig. 2). This result shows that type II secretion is important for intramoebal growth. As seen before (3, 5), the $pilE_L$ mutant was not impaired in growth within *H. vermiformis* (Fig. 2), indicating that the intracellular growth defect of the *pilD* negative strain within amoebae can be explained nearly, if not completely, by the loss of the type II secretion system.

## INTRACELLULAR INFECTION OF U937 MACROPHAGE CELLS BY *L. PNEUMOPHILA* STRAINS

To test the role of type II protein secretion in macrophage infection, we determined the relative ability of *lspDE* and *lspG* mutants to in-

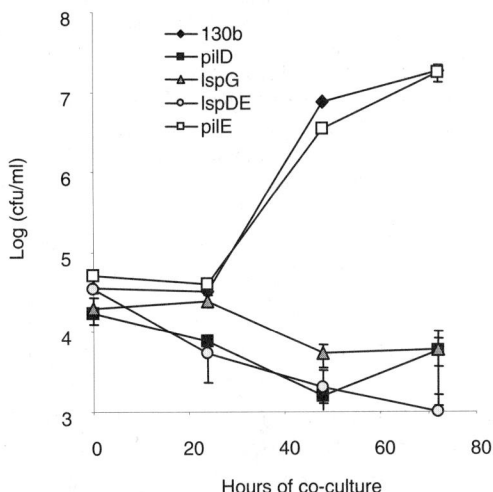

**FIGURE 2** Intracellular infection of amoebae with *L. pneumophila* strains. Wells containing *H. vermiformis* were infected at a multiplicity of infection of 0.1 with wild-type 130b (black diamonds), *pilD* mutant (black squares), *lspDE* mutant (shaded circles), *lspG* mutant (shaded triangles), and $pilE_L$ mutant (white squares). Bacterial CFU per well were determined at 0, 24, 48, and 72 h after inoculation. Each datum point represents the mean and standard deviation of three wells. With the exception of the $pilE_L$ mutant, significant differences in recovery between 130b and its mutant derivatives were evident at 48 h ($P < 0.01$, Student's *t* test). These differences were observed in three additional experiments (data not shown).

fect U937 cells, a human macrophage-like cell line. Both *lsp* mutant strains were reproducibly defective for intracellular growth within U937 macrophages (Fig. 3A). In four independent experiments, the type II secretion mutants showed a 5- to 10-fold reduction in CFU from that of the wild type (Fig. 3A). The growth defect of both types of *lsp* mutants correlated with a reduced cytopathic effect (data not shown). These results indicate that the type II protein secretion pathway does have a role, albeit a modest one, in *L. pneumophila* intracellular growth within U937 macrophages. Perhaps the most intriguing result of our study was the observed difference between the *lsp* and *pilD* mutant strains for intracellular infection of U937 macrophages (Fig. 3A). The growth defect of the *pilD* mutant was consistently 100-fold more than both *lsp* mutants. It is unlikely that this difference is explained by the absence of the type IV pilus in the *pilD* mutant, since the $pilE_L$ mutant shows no defect in growth within U937 cells (Fig. 3A) (3, 5). Taken together, these data indicate that the *L. pneumophila* PilD protein influences an additional pathway that has particular relevance for infection in macrophages. Since bacterial prepilin peptidases process pseudopilins involved in the pilus assembly, it is possible that the assembly apparatus, rather than the pilus organelle, may promote intracellular infection. To test this hypothesis, five independently obtained *pilQ* mutants were tested for their ability to infect U937 cells. Three mutants did not show any intracellular growth defect (Fig. 3B). However, two *pilQ* mutants were slightly defective for growth within U937 macrophages, i.e., they exhibited a 5- to 10-fold reduction in CFU from that of the wild type (Fig. 3B). Hence, although all mutants were confirmed by DNA hybridization, two different phenotypes were observed for the same mutation in *pilQ*. This discrepancy could be explained by a second site mutation(s) linked to the inactivation of *pilQ*. Thus, the role of the pilus assembly apparatus in intracellular growth remains unclear. Clearly, though, loss of the pilus

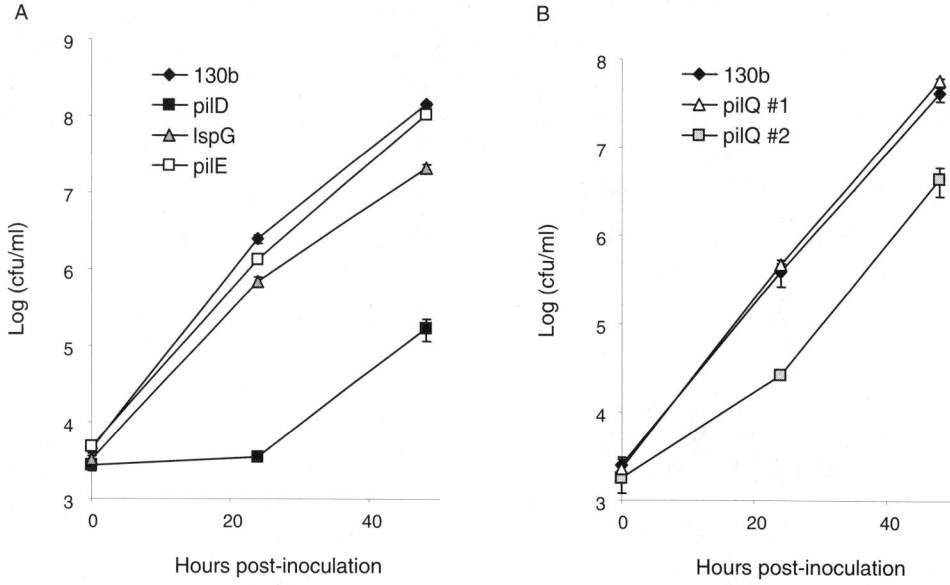

**FIGURE 3** Macrophage infection by *L. pneumophila* strains. (A) U937 cells were infected at a multiplicity of infection of 0.1 with 130b (black diamonds), *pilD* mutant (black squares), *lspG* mutant (gray triangles), and *pilE$_L$* mutant (white squares). (B) U937 cells were infected at a multiplicity of infection of 0.1 with 130b (black diamonds), *pilQ* mutant 1 (white triangles), and *pilQ* mutant 2 (gray squares). Two *pilQ* mutants were comparable to *pilQ* 1, while another was like *pilQ* 2. Bacterial CFU per monolayers were determined at 0, 24, and 48 h after inoculation. Each datum point represents the mean and standard deviation of three wells. Unlike the *pilE$_L$* mutant, significant differences in recovery between 130b and the *lspG* mutant were evident at 48 h (*P* < 0.001, Student's *t* test). Similar results were obtained for the *lspDE* mutant and were observed in three additional experiments (data not shown).

apparatus does not explain the large infectivity defect of the *pilD* mutant.

Our study has provided new insights in the contribution of *pilD*-dependent pathways to *L. pneumophila* intracellular infections and led to the following model (Fig. 4). By its ability to process the pseudopilins LspG-K, the prepilin-like peptidase PilD controls the assembly of a functional type II protein secretion apparatus. Type II secreted proteins first travel across the inner membrane to the periplasm via the Sec pathway. These proteins are then exported to the extracellular medium by the type II secretion pathway and contribute greatly to intra-amoebal growth. The type II exoproteins also influence macrophage infection, albeit modestly. PilD also controls the assembly of the type IV pilus, which promotes

attachment to host cells (5) and may play a role in biofilm formation. Since the *pilD* mutant is more defective for macrophage infection than the type II secretion and type IV pilus mutants, we hypothesize the existence of another *pilD*-dependent pathway promoting growth in human phagocytes. Indeed, the small growth defect exhibited by some *pilQ* mutants in U937 cells could hint at a minor role of the type IV pilus assembly apparatus itself for macrophage infection. This defect, added to the small defect due to the loss of type II secretion, could account for the growth impairment of the *pilD* mutant in macrophages. Alternatively, PilD could control a third unidentified pathway promoting macrophage infection. Thus, continued analysis of *L. pneumophila pilD, lsp,* and pilus

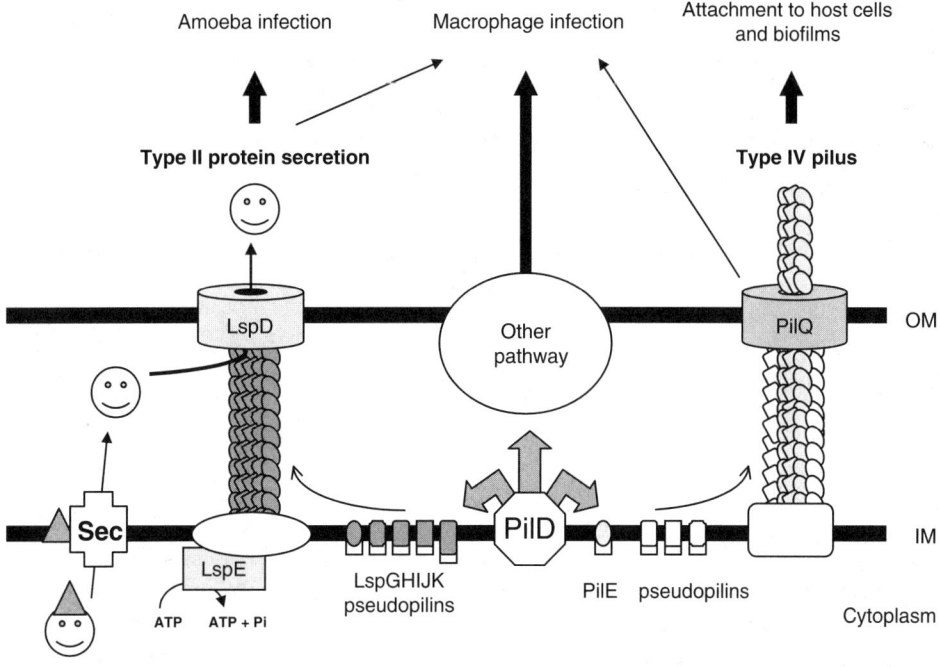

**FIGURE 4** Model for the contributions of *L. pneumophila* type II protein secretion, type IV pilus, and prepilin peptidase PilD to intracellular infection. IM, inner membrane; OM, outer membrane. For more details see text.

mutants should not only expand our understanding of Legionnaires' disease but may provide new paradigms for protein secretion systems.

## REFERENCES

1. **Aragon, V., S. Kurtz, A. Flieger, B. Neumeister, and N. P. Cianciotto.** 2000. Secreted enzymatic activities of wild-type and *pilD*-deficient *Legionella pneumophila*. *Infect. Immun.* **68:** 1855–1863.

2. **Hales, L. M., and H. A. Shuman.** 1999. *Legionella pneumophila* contains a type II general secretion pathway required for growth in amoebae as well as for secretion of the Msp protease. *Infect. Immun.* **67:**3662–3666.

3. **Liles, M. R., P. H. Edelstein, and N. P. Cianciotto.** 1999. The prepilin peptidase is required for protein secretion by and the virulence of the intracellular pathogen *Legionella pneumophila*. *Mol. Microbiol.* **31:**959–970.

4. **Russel, M.** 1998. Macromolecular assembly and secretion across the bacterial cell envelope: type II protein secretion systems. *J. Mol. Biol.* **279:**485–499.

5. **Stone, B. J., and Y. Abu Kwaik.** 1998. Expression of multiple pili by *Legionella pneumophila*: identification and characterization of a type IV pilin gene and its role in adherence to mammalian and protozoan cells. *Infect. Immun.* **66:**1768–1775.

# ANALYSIS OF ACID PHOSPHATASE AND ESTERASE/LIPASE MUTANTS OF *LEGIONELLA PNEUMOPHILA*

*V. Aragon, S. Kurtz, M. McClain,*
*N. C. Engleberg, and N. P. Cianciotto*

# 3

The identification of a *pilD* gene in *Legionella pneumophila* offered new insight into the molecular pathogenesis of legionellosis (7). In a variety of gram-negative bacteria, PilD is a prepilin peptidase and is involved in both type IV pilus biogenesis and type II protein secretion. These two functions of PilD have been confirmed in *L. pneumophila*, since a mutation in *pilD* renders bacteria nonpiliated and deficient for protein secretion. The existence of type IV pili and a *Legionella* type II secretion system in *Legionella* was confirmed by the identification of the pilin subunit and some of the genes encoding components of the secretion apparatus (4, 13). We previously demonstrated that the PilD prepilin peptidase is crucial for intracellular infection by *L. pneumophila*, and that the secreted *pilD*-dependent proteins include a metalloprotease, an acid phosphatase, an esterase/lipase, a phospholipase A, a ribonuclease, and a *p*-nitrophenyl phosphorylcholine (PNPPC) hydrolase (2, 6). Since mutants lacking type IV pili, the pro-tease, or the phosphorylcholine hydrolase are not defective for intracellular growth (2, 13, 14), we sought to determine the significance of the secreted acid phosphatase and lipase/esterase activities through the identification of structural mutants in the corresponding genes.

## MUTANTS DEFICIENT IN THE MAJOR ACID PHOSPHATASE (Map)

A population of mini-Tn*10* mutagenized *L. pneumophila* strain 130b (ATCC BAA-74, Wadsworth) was screened for mutants deficient in the hydrolysis of *p*-nitrophenyl phosphate (PNPP) at pH 5. Three mutants, NU254, NU255, and NU256, were selected from the screening and further studied. Supernatants from these mutants contained minimal acid phosphatase activity, while possessing normal levels of other *pilD*-dependent exoproteins. When the cell lysates were examined, we did not detect an accumulation of the acid phosphatase activity, indicating that NU254, NU255, and NU256 were not secretion mutants. Genetic studies revealed that the gene affected by the transposon insertions encoded a novel bacterial histidine acid phosphatase, which we designated Map for major acid phosphatase. Interestingly, the *Legionella* Map protein showed homology only to eukaryotic acid phosphatases. To fur-

*V. Aragon, S. Kurtz, and N. P. Cianciotto* Department of Microbiology and Immunology, Northwestern University Medical School, Chicago, IL 60611. *M. McClain and N. C. Engleberg* Department of Microbiology, Med Sci II 6643, University of Michigan, Ann Arbor, MI 48109.

*Legionella*, Edited by Reinhard Marre et al.
© 2002 ASM Press, Washington, D.C.

ther characterize the enzyme, the complete *map* gene was cloned and expressed in *Escherichia coli*. Subsequent inhibitor studies indicated that Map, like its eukaryotic homologs, is a tartrate-sensitive acid phosphatase. Also, the cloned Map was examined for its ability to hydrolyze some physiological substrates. Although the best substrates for the enzyme were the artificial substrates methylumbelliferyl phosphate and PNPP, we could also detect hydrolysis of phosphotyrosine, fructose-6-phosphate, and, to a lesser extent, ATP and ADP. We could not detect hydrolysis of phosphothreonine by Map. To determine if the *map* gene was necessary for intracellular replication of *Legionella*, macrophage-like U937 cells and *Hartmannella vermiformis* amoebae were infected at multiplicity of infection of 0.1 and 1, respectively. In these hosts, the *map* mutants grew to the same degree as did wild-type legionellae, indicating that this acid phosphatase is not essential for *L. pneumophila* intracellular infection. However, in the course of characterizing our new mutants, we obtained evidence for a second *pilD*-dependent acid phosphatase activity. The *map* mutants were missing the majority of the acid phosphatase activity in their supernatants, but maintained a small level of activity that, unlike Map, was tartrate resistant. So this second acid phosphatase, or other enzymes, may compensate for the lack of Map. Also, even though Map is not essential for U937 cell infection, it may play a role in *Legionella* survival within other host cells, such as activated macrophages or neutrophils. In support of a role of Map in pathogenesis, two secretory histidine acid phosphatases, with significant homology to Map, have been identified in *Leishmania donovani* and they are believed to have a role in human infection (3, 12). On the other hand, it is possible that the *pilD*-dependent tartrate-resistant acid phosphatase is the enzyme most important for U937 cell or amoebae infection. Indeed, tartrate-resistant acid phosphatases of *Francisella tularensis*, *Coxiella burnetii*, *L. donovani*, and more significantly of *Legionella micdadei* (5, 8–11), have

been implicated in the resistance of these intracellular pathogens to the oxidative burst of phagocytes. In summary, we have demonstrated that *L. pneumophila* has two acid phosphatases that can be differentiated by their different sensitivity to tartrate, and while the tartrate-sensitive Map seems not to be essential for intracellular replication, the role of the tartrate-resistant phosphatase has yet to be determined (1).

## MUTANTS DEFICIENT IN LIPOLYTIC ACTIVITIES

A population of *L. pneumophila* 130b mutagenized with mini-Tn*10-phoA* was screened for insertions in genes encoding secreted pro-

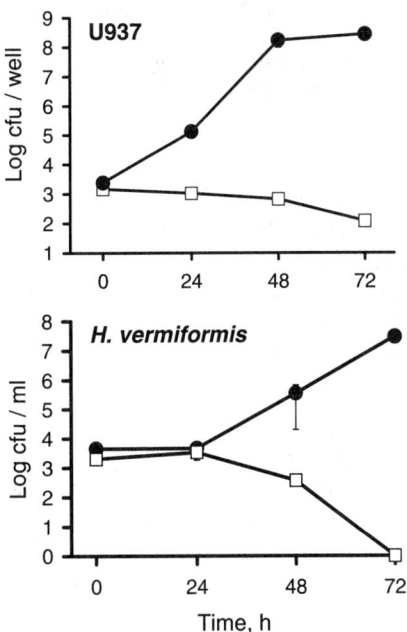

**FIGURE 1** Intracellular infection by wild-type and mutant *L. pneumophila*. U937 cells (top panel) and *H. vermiformis* amoebae (bottom panel) were infected at a multiplicity of infection (MOI) of 0.1 and 1, respectively, with wild-type 130b (●) or lipase/esterase mutant AA407 (□). The number of bacteria in each well was quantitated at 0, 24, 48, and 72 h by plating aliquots on buffered charcoal-yeast extract (BCYE) agar. Results represent the mean (± standard deviation) of triplicate wells and are representative of two independent experiments.

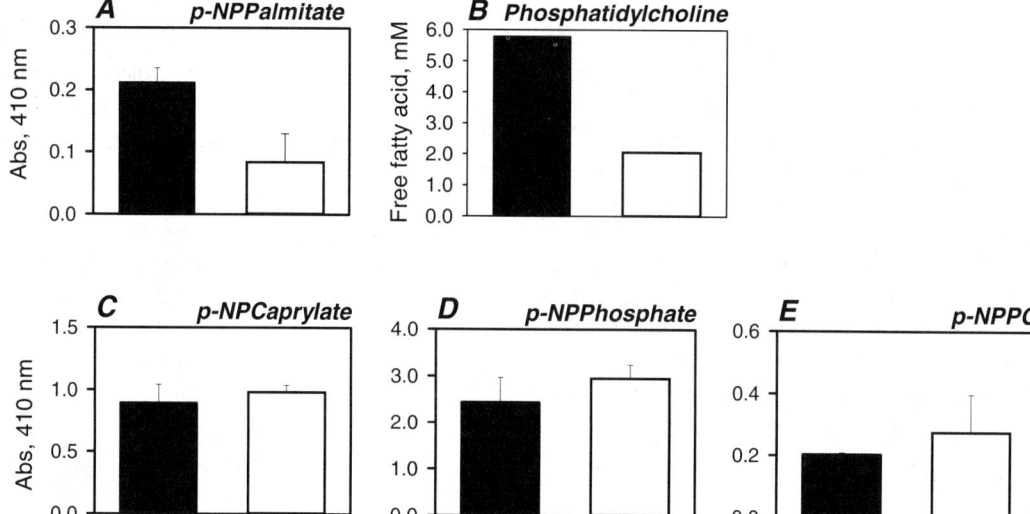

**FIGURE 2** Enzymatic activities secreted by *L. pneumophila* strains. Late-log phase supernatants of wild-type 130b (black bars) and AA407 (white bars) were tested for their ability to hydrolyze PNPpalmitate (A), phosphatidylcholine (B), PNPcaprylate (C), PNPphosphate (D), and PNPphosphorylcholine (E). Bars represent the mean (± standard deviation) of the activity found in three cultures and are representative of the results obtained in two independent experiments.

teins as indicated by PhoA alkaline phosphatase activity. Subsequently, the selected mutants were tested for their ability to infect macrophages and amoebae. One of these mutants, AA407, was impaired more than 1,000-fold in intracellular replication within both U937 cells and *H. vermiformis* (Fig. 1), while presenting an extracellular growth in buffered yeast extract (BYE) similar to wild-type 130b. The gene that was interrupted by the transposon was determined, and a BLAST (basic local alignment search tool) analysis of the sequence showed that the putative protein shared some homology to lipase enzymes. Since we knew that *L. pneumophila* had some lipolytic activities that were secreted in a *pilD*-dependent fashion, we examined the supernatant of the mutant for these and other *pilD*-dependent secreted enzymes (Fig. 2). Supernatants from the mutant presented a defect in its ability to hydrolyze PNPpalmitate (indication of esterase/lipase) and in the liberation of free fatty acid from phosphatidylcholine (indication of phospholipase A) (Fig. 2A and B). When examined

for *pilD*-dependent esterase, acid phosphatase, and PNPPC hydrolase activities, the supernatants showed wild-type levels of the enzymes (Fig. 2C to E), indicating that AA407 is not a secretion mutant. The enzymatic defect found in the supernatant could be explained by the lack of a single lipolytic enzyme responsible for both reactions, or by a defect in a protein necessary for the processing of two independent enzymes. The first possibility seems improbable, since type II secretion mutants lacking lipase/esterase and phospholipase A, among other activities, do not show the level of defective replication in macrophages that AA407 does (see chapter 2). Thus, it is probable that the transposon insertion has a wider effect on the bacterium, interfering with other functions or structures that are essential for the intracellular replication of *Legionella*.

### REFERENCES

1. Aragon, V., S. Kurtz, and N. P. Cianciotto. 2001. *Legionella pneumophila* major acid phosphatase and its role in intracellular infection. *Infect. Immun.* **69:**177–185.

2. **Aragon, V., S. Kurtz, A. Flieger, B. Neumeister, and N. P. Cianciotto.** 2000. Secreted enzymatic activities of wild-type and *pilD*-deficient *Legionella pneumophila*. *Infect. Immun.* **68:** 1855–1863.

3. **Ellis, S. L., A. M. Shakarian, and D. M. Dwyer.** 1998. *Leishmania:* amastigotes synthesize conserved secretory acid phosphatases during human infection. *Exp. Parasitol.* **89:**161–168.

4. **Hales, L. M., and H. A. Shuman.** 1999. *Legionella pneumophila* contains a type II general secretion pathway required for growth in amoebae as well as for secretion of the Msp protease. *Infect. Immun.* **67:**3662–3666.

5. **Li, Y. P., G. Curley, M. Lopez, M. Chavez, R. Glew, A. Aragon, H. Kumar, and O. G. Baca.** 1996. Protein-tyrosine phosphatase activity of *Coxiella burnetii* that inhibits human neutrophils. *Acta Virol.* **40:**263–272.

6. **Liles, M. R., P. H. Edelstein, and N. P. Cianciotto.** 1999. The prepilin peptidase is required for protein secretion by and the virulence of the intracellular pathogen *Legionella pneumophila. Mol. Microbiol.* **31:**959–970.

7. **Liles, M. R., V. K. Viswanathan, and N. P. Cianciotto.** 1998. Identification and temperature regulation of *Legionella pneumophila* genes involved in type IV pilus biogenesis and type II secretion. *Infect. Immun.* **66:**1776–1782.

8. **Reilly, T. J., G. S. Baron, F. E. Nano, and M. S. Kuhlenschmidt.** 1996. Characterization and sequencing of a respiratory burst-inhibiting acid phosphatase from *Francisella tularensis. J. Biol. Chem.* **271:**10973–10983.

9. **Remaley, A. T., D. B. Kubus, R. H. Basford, R. H. Glew, and S. S. Kaplan.** 1984. Leishmanial phosphatase blocks neutrophil $O_2$ production. *J. Biol. Chem.* **259:**11173–11175.

10. **Saha, A. K., J. N. Dowling, K. K. LaMarco, S. Das, A. T. Remaley, N. Olomur, M. T. Pope, and R. H. Glew.** 1985. Properties of an acid phosphatase from *Legionella micdadei* which blocks superoxide anion production by human neutrophils. *Arch. Biochem. Biophys.* **243:**150–160.

11. **Saha, A. K., J. N. Dowling, A. W. Pasculle, and R. H. Glew.** 1988. *Legionella micdadei* phosphatase catalyzes the hydrolysis of phosphatidylinositol 4,5-biphosphate in human neutrophils. *Arch. Biochem. Biophys.* **265:**94–104.

12. **Shakarian, A. M., S. L. Ellis, D. J. Mallinson, R. W. Olafson, and D. M. Dwyer.** 1997. Two tandemly arrayed genes encode the (histidine) secretory acid phosphatases of *Leishmania donovani. Gene* **196:**127–137.

13. **Stone, B. J., and Y. Abu Kwaik.** 1998. Expression of multiple pili by *Legionella pneumophila:* identification and characterization of a type IV pilin gene and its role in adherence to mammalian and protozoan cells. *Infect. Immun.* **66:**1768–1775.

14. **Szeto, L., and H. A. Shuman.** 1990. The *Legionella pneumophila* major secretory protein, a protease, is not required for intracellular growth or cell killing. *Infect. Immun.* **58:**2585–2592.

# *LEGIONELLA PNEUMOPHILA* SECRETES DIFFERENT PHOSPHOLIPASES A

*Antje Flieger, Shimei Gong, Marion Faigle, Stefan Stevanovic, Hinnak Northoff, Nicholas P. Cianciotto, and Birgid Neumeister*

# 4

*Legionella pneumophila* secretes several enzymes, including phospholipase A (PLA), via a *pilD*-dependent type II secretion pathway (1, 6, 13). PLAs, a heterogenous group of enzymes produced by bacteria as well as eukaryotic cells, catalyze the removal of a fatty acid from phospholipids generating cytotoxic lysophospholipids. When fatty acids are liberated from lysophospholipids, the responsible enzyme is named lysophospholipase A (LPLA). Phospholipases possess distinct substrate specificities with respect to both the phospho-head groups and the length and saturation of acyl chains esterified to the glycerol backbone.

Although more frequently described for phospholipases C, PLAs are suspected to be virulence factors of bacteria. As has been found for bacterial infections, phospholipases may be responsible for the bacterial escape from phagosomes and host cells after intracellular multiplication (3), the destruction of macrophages and epithelial cells (2), the generation of signal transducers like lysophosphatidylcholine and derivatives of both arachidonic and linoleic acid (4), the destruction of lung surfactant (7), and the induction of inflammation (9).

We had previously shown that *L. pneumophila* secretes PLA, which acts on phosphatidylcholine (PC) and phosphatidylglycerol (6, 7). Since the destruction of host lipid substrates may be advantageous for *L. pneumophila*, we aimed to identify the range of phospholipid and lipid substrates cleaved by concentrated culture supernatants (CCS) of virulent strain 130b. We now demonstrate that *L. pneumophila* PLA(s) actually cleave a variety of phospholipids, including especially glycerol, inositol, and choline derivatives (Fig. 1). In fact, strain 130b CCS liberated the highest quantity of FFA from dipalmitoylphosphatidylglycerol (DPPG), a finding that might be simply due to the cleavage of both fatty acids from the phospholipid. The ability of CCS to cleave both dipalmitoylphosphatidylcholine (DPPC) and DPPG is compatible with our previous observation that *L. pneumophila* de-

*Antje Flieger and Nicholas P. Cianciotto* Department of Microbiology-Immunology, Northwestern University Medical School, 320 E. Superior St., Searle 6-573, Chicago, IL 60611. *Shimei Gong* Department of Microbiology and Immunology, Chandler Medical Center, University of Kentucky, 800 Rose St., Lexington, KY 40536. *Marion Faigle, Hinnak Northoff, and Birgid Neumeister* Abteilung für Transfusionsmedizin, Universitätsklinikum Tübingen, Otfried-Müller-Str. 4/1, D-72076 Tübingen, Germany. *Stefan Stevanovic* Interfakultäres Institut für Zellbiologie, Abt. Immunologie, Universitätsklinikum Tübingen, Auf der Morgenstelle 15, D-72076 Tübingen, Germany.

*Legionella*, Edited by Reinhard Marre et al.
© 2002 ASM Press, Washington, D.C.

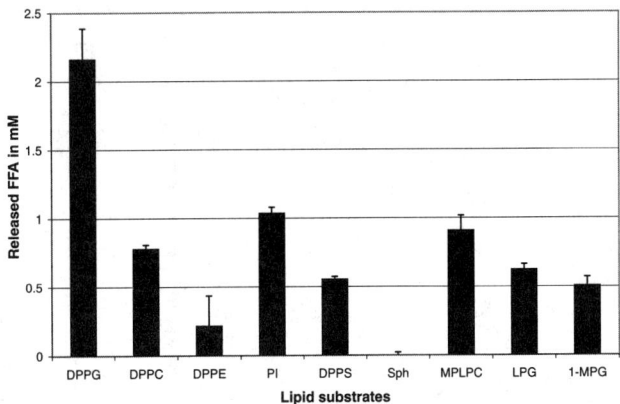

**FIGURE 1** Release of fatty acids by 10-fold concentrated CCS of *L. pneumophila* from different lipids. DPPG, DPPC, DPPE, phosphatidylinositol (PI), dipalmitoylphosphatidylserine (DPPS), sphingomyeline (Sph), MPLPC, LPG, and 1-MPG were incubated with CCS for 5 h. Data are means ± standard deviation of four experiments and are shown as the difference between release of fatty acids by CCS and by negative control (20 mM Tris-HCl, pH 7.2).

grades lung surfactant, a mixture of mainly phosphatidylglycerol (PG) and PC (6, 7). Interestingly, dipalmitoylphosphatidylethanolamine (DPPE), which, unlike DPPC, lacks three methyl groups in the alcoholic part of the molecule, was hydrolyzed by CCS to only a small and not reproducible extent. However, other experiments with lung surfactant, which contains moderate amounts of phosphatidylethanolamine (PE), suggested that this phospholipid can be degraded by *Legionella* enzymes (A. Flieger, unpublished observation). The absence of DPPE-hydrolysis in the present study could be due to the high purity of DPPE (99%) or due to the high gel-to-liquid crystalline phase transition temperature of the palmitoyl derivate used in these experiments, whereas surfactant comprises a mixture of several phospholipids with distinct esterified fatty acids.

In addition to the cleavage of phospholipids containing fatty acids in both the sn1 and sn2 positions, the nonphospholipid 1-monopalmitoylglycerol (1-MPG) and lysophospholipids like monopalmitoyl lysophosphatidylcholine (MPLPC) and lysophosphatidylglycerol (LPG) were also degraded by CCS (Fig. 1). The additional destruction but not complete erasement of lysophosphatidylcholine (LPC) had already been noticed when lung surfactant was incubated with *L. pneumophila* bacteria and was discussed as a possible protection

mechanism of the bacteria from dangerous concentrations of LPC (7).

Since different lipids were hydrolyzed by CCS, we investigated whether distinct lipolytic activities were indeed responsible for the cleavage of phospholipids, lysophospholipids, and monoacylglycerol. Anion exchange chromatography (AEC) was performed on CCS, and the eluted fractions were tested for PLA, LPLA, and lipase activities. For PLA, we identified activities that hydrolyzed phospholipids containing both fatty acids, such as DPPG and DPPC. LPLA activity was present when free fatty acids (FFA) were released from MPLPC. Lipase activities were defined as those that released FFA from 1-MPG. Four major peaks (fractions 7, 10, 13, 15) revealed from AEC were capable of causing DPPG and DPPC hydrolysis (Fig. 2). It remains to be determined whether the PLAs found in the different AEC I-fractions are derivatives of one parental protein. Reducing sodium dodecyl sulfate-polyacrylamide gel electrophoresis (SDS-PAGE) was performed from AEC fractions (Fig. 2). The pattern of protein bands, observed in fractions 7, 10, 13, and 15 did not allow the prediction of molecular weights for PLA. Fraction 17 was distinct from the fractions containing PLA activity, due to their major activity in releasing FFA from MPLPC and, to a lesser extent, from 1-MPG (8). The peak of this lipase activity corresponded to the

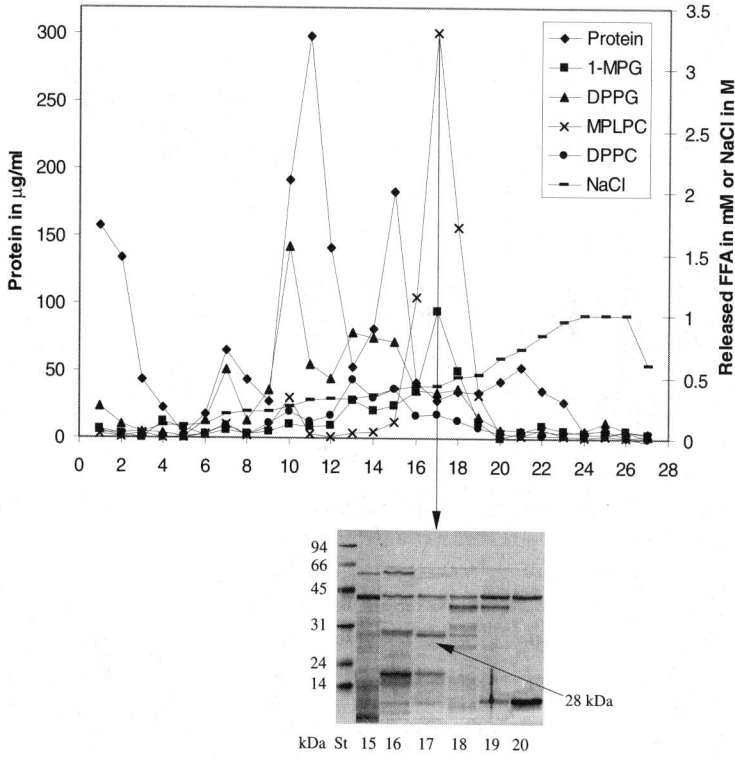

**FIGURE 2** Separation of *L. pneumophila*'s lipolytic activities by AEC. 10-fold concentrated bacterial supernatant from a 5000-ml culture supernatant was subjected to AEC. Fractions (10 ml) eluted from 0 to 1 M sodium chloride were investigated for protein content and FFA release during a 1-h incubation with DPPG, DPPC, MPLPC, and 1-MPG. Reducing SDS-PAGE was performed on fractions 15 to 20, and the separated proteins were visualized by silver staining. St, molecular weight standard; numbers to the left indicate molecular mass (in kilodaltons). The 28-kDa protein band is designated by the arrow. The experiment shown is representative of 10 additional trials. Reprinted from reference 8 with permission.

peak of MPLPC cleavage in fraction 17, implying that the activity responsible for MPLPC cleavage may be able to release FFA also from nonphospholipids. It is known that phospholipases may additionally catalyze the destruction of non-phosphate-containing lipids, and lipases may additionally catalyze the destruction of phospholipids (14). Concentration of protein bands after reducing SDS-PAGE and hydrolytic pattern of proteins in AEC fractions 16 to 18 suggested that a 28-kDa protein is responsible for both MPLPC and 1-MPG hydrolysis (Fig. 2). Subsequently, the 28-kDa

protein was further purified by additional AEC and gel filtration chromatography. During the course of purification, the intensity of the 28-kDa protein band always paralleled the hydrolytic activity of MPLPC and 1-MPG (8), suggesting that this protein cleaves both substrates with a preference to MPLPC. $NH_2$-terminal amino acid sequencing revealed a sequence with homology to enzymes containing the catalytic motif FGDSLS of a recently described new group of lipolytic enzymes (8). The hydrolysis of both MPLPC and 1-MPG by LPLA corresponds to the substrate specificities of the enzyme family to which LPLA may belong, comprising lipases, phospholipases A, esterases, and acyltransferases.

Finally, we investigated a *pilD*-deficient mutant (NU 243) of 130b, formerly described as lacking the ability to secrete factors causing hydrolysis of DPPC and 1-MPG (1), for the loss of capacity to release FFA from DPPG and MPLPC. In fact, the ability to release FFA from DPPG and MPLPC was considerably reduced, i.e., DPPG to 23%, DPPC to 13%, MPLPC to 7%, and 1-MPG to 12%, in comparison with wild-type 130b (Fig. 3). This indicates that LPLA and PLA secretion of *L. pneumophila* is *pilD* dependent and might therefore account for the loss of cytopathicity, intracellular multiplication, and virulence in the *pilD*-deficient mutant (8, 11).

How could PLA and LPLA of *L. pneumophila* contribute to the development of Legionnaires' disease? Phosphatidylethanolamine, PG, cardiolipin, and PC are major constituents of the bacterial membranes of *L. pneumophila* (5). Phospholipases, which cleave these substrates, may fulfill nutritional tasks for the bacterium by acquisition of important bacterial constituents. Due to the localization of the bacterium in the lung, phospholipases may cause damage to alveolar epithelial cells and macrophages. Since PLA and LPLA of *L. pneumophila* are potent in destruction of a variety of phospholipids and the composition of membranes of different cell membranes varies considerably, they might affect many cell types.

DPPG is the preferred substrate for FFA release by CCS of *L. pneumophila*. Since PG and PC are major constituents of lung surfactant and it has been recently shown that *L. pneumophila* is able to degrade these phospholipids and to generate the hemolytic agent LPC, this might be a major mechanism by which bacteria can induce acute respiratory distress syndrome (7). In addition to its hemolytic activity, LPC is known to elicit inflammation (9), and to influence signal transduction in host cells (4). Since cell swelling has been suggested to be essential for bacterial multiplication in host cells (12), and the generation of glycerophosphorylcholine—a reaction product of LPLA, which is able to cause cell swelling (10)—was recently shown (6), LPLA is suspected to contribute to bacterial growth. Furthermore, LPLA could be an important agent for the survival of bacteria since it may protect *L. pneumophila* from toxic amounts of LPC.

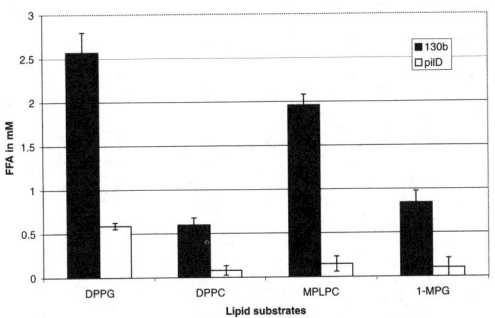

**FIGURE 3** Release of FFA from DPPG, DPPC, MPLPC, and 1-MPG by culture supernatants of *L. pneumophila* in comparison to a *pilD*-deficient mutant. Legionellae were grown in buffered yeast extract (BYE) broth. Lipolytic activities were determined by detection of FFA release after incubation of culture supernatant with DPPG, DPPC, MPLPC, and 1-MPG, respectively, for 15 h. Data are means ± standard deviation of four experiments and are shown as the difference between fatty acids released by bacterial supernatant and by negative control (BYE broth).

## ACKNOWLEDGMENTS

Antje Flieger was supported by grants from Boehringer-Ingelheim-Pharma-KG (Biberach, Germany), the Boehringer-Ingelheim-Foundation (Mainz, Germany), and the *fortuene* Fund (179-1 and 179-2, University Hospital of Tübingen, Germany). Shimei Gong was supported by the *fortuene* Fund (305-1 and 305-2, University Hospital of Tübingen, Germany).

## REFERENCES

1. **Aragon, V., S. Kurtz, A. Flieger, B. Neumeister, and N. P. Cianciotto.** 2000. Secreted enzymatic activities of wild-type and pilD-deficient *Legionella pneumophila*. *Infect. Immun.* **68:** 1855–1863.

2. **Aronson, J. F., and L. W. Johns.** 1977. Injury of lung alveolar cells by lysolecithin. *Exp. Mol. Pathol.* **27:**35–42.

3. **Camilli, A., L. G. Tilney, and D. A. Portnoy.** 1993. Dual roles of plcA in *Listeria monocytogenes* pathogenesis. *Mol. Microbiol.* **8:**143–157.

4. **Dennis, E. A.** 1997. The growing phospholipase A2 superfamily of signal transduction enzymes. *Trends Biochem. Sci.* **22:**1–2.

5. **Finnerty, W. R., R. A. Makula, and J. C. Feeley.** 1979. Cellular lipids of the Legionnaires' disease bacterium. *Ann. Intern. Med.* **90:**631–634.

6. **Flieger, A., S. Gong, M. Faigle, M. Deeg, P. Bartmann, and B. Neumeister.** 2000. Novel phospholipase A activity secreted by *Legionella* species. *J. Bacteriol.* **182:**1321–1327.

7. **Flieger, A., S. Gong, M. Faigle, H. A. Mayer, U. Kehrer, J. Mußotter, P. Bartmann, and B. Neumeister.** 2000. Phospholipase A secreted by *Legionella pneumophila* destroys alveolar surfactant phospholipids. *FEMS Microbiol. Lett.* **188:**129–133.

8. **Flieger, A., S. Gong, M. Faigle, S. Stevanovic, N. P. Cianciotto, and B. Neumeister.** 2001. Novel lysophospholipase A secreted by *Legionella pneumophila. J. Bacteriol.* **183:**2121–2124.

9. **Kume, N., M. I. Cybulsky, and M. A. Gimbrone, Jr.** 1992. Lysophosphatidylcholine, a component of atherogenic lipoproteins, induces mononuclear leukocyte adhesion molecules in cultured human and rabbit arterial endothelial cells. *J. Clin. Invest.* **90:**1138–1144.

10. **Lang, F., G. L. Busch, and H. Volkl.** 1998. The diversity of volume regulatory mechanisms. *Cell. Physiol. Biochem.* **8:**1–45.

11. **Liles, M. R., P. H. Edelstein, and N. P. Cianciotto.** 1999. The prepilin peptidase is required for protein secretion by and the virulence of the intracellular pathogen *Legionella pneumophila. Mol. Microbiol.* **31:**959–970.

12. **Neumeister, B., S. Schoniger, M. Faigle, M. Eichner, and K. Dietz.** 1997. Multiplication of different *Legionella* species in Mono Mac 6 cells and in *Acanthamoeba castellanii. Appl. Environ. Microbiol.* **63:**1219–1224.

13. **Rossier, O., and N. P. Cianciotto.** 2001. Type II protein secretion is a subset of the PilD-dependent processes that facilitate intracellular infection by *Legionella pneumophila. Infect. Immun.* **69:**2092–2098.

14. **Simons, J. W., F. Gotz, M. R. Egmond, and H. M. Verheij.** 1998. Biochemical properties of staphylococcal (phospho)lipases. *Chem. Phys. Lipids* **93:**27–37.

# IN VITRO SECRETION KINETICS
# OF *LEGIONELLA PNEUMOPHILA*
# COMPARED WITH THOSE OF
# NON-*L. PNEUMOPHILA* SPECIES

*Antje Flieger, Shimei Gong, Marion Faigle,*
*Hinnak Northoff, and Birgid Neumeister*

# 5

The genus *Legionella* consists of more than 40 species. *L. pneumophila* is the most frequently isolated species in patients suffering from Legionnaires' disease. However, unique virulence factor(s) that contribute to the epidemiological importance of *L. pneumophila* are not known. It has been shown recently that a mutation in the *pilD* gene of *L. pneumophila* influences protein secretion and leads to a decrease of bacterial virulence (1, 6, 9). *pilD*-dependent secreted enzyme activities include protease, acid phosphatase, and both phospholipase A (PLA) and lysophospholipase A (LPLA) activities (1, 6, 9). In this chapter, we characterize the secretion kinetics of putative virulence factors of *L. pneumophila* in comparison with those of non-*L. pneumophila* species during the phase of growth, when nutritional factors may become limited.

*Antje Flieger* Department of Microbiology-Immunology, Northwestern University Medical School, 320 E. Superior St., Searle 6-573, Chicago, IL 60611. *Shimei Gong* Department of Microbiology and Immunology, Chandler Medical Center, University of Kentucky, 800 Rose St., Lexington, KY 40536. *Marion Faigle, Hinnak Northoff, and Birgid Neumeister* Abteilung für Transfusionsmedizin, Universitätsklinikum Tübingen, Otfried-Müller-Str. 4/1, D-72076 Tübingen, Germany.

## ENZYME SECRETION PATTERN OF DIFFERENT LEGIONELLAE

To investigate the secretion pattern of different *Legionella* species (Table 1), culture supernatants were evaluated for acid phosphatase, protease, PLA, and LPLA activities. For acid phosphatase, the release of *p*-nitrophenol (*p*-NP) from *p*-nitrophenylphosphate was detected at pH 6. Protease activity was determined by the cleavage of azocaseine. PLA was estimated by the release of free fatty acids (FFA) from dipalmitoylphosphatidylcholine (DPPC). LPLA was detected by the release of FFA from monopalmitoyl lysophosphatidylcholine (MPLPC). The experiments revealed that the examined enzyme activities seem to be secreted throughout the whole *Legionella* genus, except *L. longbeachae* and *L. micdadei* lack the majority of the activities tested (Table 1). This was already noticed for PLA secretion in two different isolates of *L. micdadei* (4). However, in former experiments, PLA activity was found in culture supernatants of another isolate of *L. longbeachae* (4). Differences in PLA secretion of different isolates within one *Legionella* species (*L. steigerwaltii*) have already been described (4). *L. pneumophila* and *L. gormanii* secreted the highest amounts of protease (Table 1). *L. gormanii, L. dumoffii,* and *L. steigerwaltii* were most active in phosphatase

*Legionella*, Edited by Reinhard Marre et al.
© 2002 ASM Press, Washington, D.C.

**TABLE 1** *Legionella* strains used and maximal enzyme activities of their culture supernatants

| *Legionella* species[a] | Serogroup (subtype) | Source[b] | Abbreviation | Activity[c] | | | |
|---|---|---|---|---|---|---|---|
| | | | | PLA | LPLA | Protease | Acid phosphatase |
| *L. pneumophila* | 1 (Wadsworth) strain 130b | N. P. Cianciotto, Chicago, Ill. | Lp1-130b | + (18 h) | ++ (22 h) | ++ | + |
| *L. pneumophila* | 1 (Philadelphia-1) | CDC stock 5 | Lp1-CDC | + (22 h) | ++ (>22 h) | ++ | + |
| *L. pneumophila* | 1 (Pontiac-1) | G. Ruckdeschel, München, Germany | Lp1P-c | + (18 h) | ++ (22 h) | ++ | + |
| *L. dumoffii* | | CDC F1407 | Ld-CDC | +/− (>22 h) | + (22 h) | + | +++ |
| *L. gormanii* | | CDC F462 | Lg-CDC | +++ (22 h) | ++ (18 h) | ++ | +++ |
| *L. longbeachae* | 1 | ATCC 33462 | Ll-ATCC | +/− | − | − | − |
| *L. micdadei* | | CDC F976 | Lm-CDC | − | +/− | +/− | − |
| *L. steigerwaltii* | | CDC 464 | Ls-CDC | ++ (14 h) | + (10 h) | + | ++ |

[a] The *L. pneumophila* strains are human isolates; the other species originate from environmental sources.
[b] CDC, Centers for Disease Control and Prevention, Atlanta, Ga. Strains kindly provided by Barry Fields.
[c] Culture supernatants were investigated for maximal PLA, LPLA, protease, and acid phosphatase activities. −, not detectable; +++, high amounts. The time point for maximal enzyme activity during growth of bacteria is given in parentheses.

secretion (Table 1). *L. gormanii, L. steigerwaltii,* and *L. pneumophila* exhibited the highest PLA activity, and both *L. gormanii* and one of the tested *L. pneumophila* strains exhibited the most prominent LPLA activity (Table 1). In general, distinct *Legionella* species secreted different amounts of the tested enzyme activities, whereas different isolates of the species *L. pneumophila* resembled each other in their secreted hydrolytic activity. Interestingly, *L. pneumophila* is not the species that generally produces the highest amounts of the tested enzymatic activities (Table 1). However, when the order of secretion of PLA and LPLA is regarded in detail, it is obvious that PLA reaches the most prominent activity prior to LPLA only in *L. pneumophila*, whereas non-*L. pneumophila* species secreted maximal LPLA activity simultaneously or prior to PLA activity (Table 1). The ratio and the time of secretion of both activities (PLA generates lysophosphatidylcholine [LPC], whereas LPLA degrades LPC) may be important for the generation and enrichment of LPC, which has several functions that may contribute to pathogenesis such as induction of inflammation, impairment of lung function, cytotoxic and pore-forming activity, and signal transduction. Accumulation of LPC could therefore be an important mechanism in the development of Legionnaires' disease (2, 3, 5, 7, 8, 10, 12, 13, 14).

## GENERATION OF LYSOPHOSPHATIDYLCHOLINE (LPC)
To estimate the amount of LPC generated from culture supernatants of different *Legionella* species (Table 1), we incubated culture supernatants with DPPC and analyzed the lipids by thin-layer chromatography. Culture supernatants from the exponential growth phase of both *L. pneumophila* and *L. steigerwaltii* generated considerable amounts of LPC (Table 2). LPC was also produced by *L. gormanii* but not before bacteria entered the stationary phase. Due to their low PLA activity, *L. dumoffii* and *L. micdadei* did not enrich the LPC. The generation of LPC by *L. steigerwaltii* and *L. gor-*

**TABLE 2**  Generation of LPC after incubation of DPPC with culture supernatants of different *Legionella* species and strains from different times of growth in BYE broth[a]

| *Legionella* strain[b] | Generation of LPC at: | | | | | | |
|---|---|---|---|---|---|---|---|
| | 0 h | 8 h | 10 h | 14 h | 18 h | 22 h | 36 h |
| Lp1-130 b | − | − | + | ++ | ++ | ++ | + |
| Lp1-CDC | ND | ND | ND | ND | ND | ND | ND |
| Lp1P-c | − | − | +/− | + | + | + | + |
| Ld-CDC | − | +/− | − | − | − | +/− | − |
| Lg-CDC | − | − | − | − | − | ++ | − |
| Ll-ATCC | ND | ND | ND | ND | ND | ND | ND |
| Lm-CDC | − | − | − | − | − | − | − |
| Ls-CDC | − | − | + | +++ | ++ | + | − |

[a] −, not detectable; +++, high amounts of activity; ND, not determined.
[b] See Table 1 for definition of strain abbreviations.

*manii* can be explained by the very potent PLA activity compared with a more moderate LPLA activity. It has been shown recently that PLA secretion starts with the mid-exponential growth phase and reaches maximal extent with entry into the stationary growth phase (6). Therefore, it is conceivable that in contrast to *L. pneumophila, L. steigerwaltii* and *L. gormanii* might not be able to enrich dangerous amounts of LPC in vivo since they are not able to multiply within monocytic host cells (11). LPLA activity is high compared with PLA activity in *L. pneumophila* (Table 1). However, *L. pneumophila* may be able to generate LPC due to PLA secretion prior to LPLA. These data are in good correlation with former experiments where we have already shown that *L. pneumophila* generates LPC from lung surfactant (5).

## ACKNOWLEDGMENTS

Antje Flieger was supported by grants from Boehringer-Ingelheim-Pharma-KG (Biberach, Germany), the Boehringer-Ingelheim-Foundation (Mainz, Germany), and the *fortuene* Fund (179-1 and 179-2, University Hospital of Tübingen, Germany). Shimei Gong was supported by by *fortuene* Fund (305-1 and 305-2, University Hospital of Tübingen, Germany).

## REFERENCES

1. **Aragon, V., S. Kurtz, A. Flieger, B. Neumeister, and N. P. Cianciotto.** 2000. Secreted enzymatic activities of wild-type and *pilD*-deficient *Legionella pneumophila. Infect. Immun.* **68:** 1855–1863.
2. **Aronson, J. F., and L. W. Johns.** 1977. Injury of lung alveolar cells by lysolecithin. *Exp. Mol. Pathol.* **27:**35–42.
3. **Dennis, E. A.** 1997. The growing phospholipase A2 superfamily of signal transduction enzymes. *Trends Biochem. Sci.* **22:**1–2.
4. **Flieger, A., S. Gong, M. Faigle, M. Deeg, P. Bartmann, and B. Neumeister.** 2000. Novel phospholipase A activity secreted by *Legionella* species. *J. Bacteriol.* **182:**1321–1327.
5. **Flieger, A., S. Gong, M. Faigle, H. A. Mayer, U. Kehrer, J. Mußotter, P. Bartmann, and B. Neumeister.** 2000. Phospholipase A secreted by *Legionella pneumophila* destroys alveolar surfactant phospholipids. *FEMS Microbiol. Lett.* **188:**129–133.
6. **Flieger, A., S. Gong, M. Faigle, S. Stevanovic, N. P. Cianciotto, and B. Neumeister.** 2001. Novel lysophospholipase A secreted by *Legionella pneumophila. J. Bacteriol.* **183:**2121–2124.
7. **Holm, B. A., L. Keicher, M. Y. Liu, J. Sokolowski, and G. Enhorning.** 1991. Inhibition of pulmonary surfactant function by phospholipases. *J. Appl. Physiol.* **71:**317–321.
8. **Kume, N., M. I. Cybulsky, and M. A. Gimbrone, Jr.** 1992. Lysophosphatidylcholine, a component of atherogenic lipoproteins, induces mononuclear leukocyte adhesion molecules in cultured human and rabbit arterial endothelial cells. *J. Clin. Invest.* **90:**1138–1144.
9. **Liles, M. R., P. H. Edelstein, and N. P. Cianciotto.** 1999. The prepilin peptidase is required for protein secretion by and the virulence of the intracellular pathogen *Legionella pneumophila. Mol. Microbiol.* **31:**959–970.

10. **Lindahl, M., A. R. Hede, and C. Tagesson.** 1986. Lysophosphatidylcholine increases airway and capillary permeability in the isolated perfused rat lung. *Exp. Lung Res.* **11**:1–12.

11. **Neumeister, B., S. Schoniger, M. Faigle, M. Eichner, and K. Dietz.** 1997. Multiplication of different *Legionella* species in Mono Mac 6 cells and in *Acanthamoeba castellanii. Appl. Environ. Microbiol.* **63**:1219–1224.

12. **Niewoehner, D. E., K. Rice, A. A. Sinha, and D. Wangensteen.** 1987. Injurious effects of lysophosphatidylcholine on barrier properties of alveolar epithelium. *J. Appl. Physiol.* **63**:1979–1986.

13. **Prokazova, N. V., N. D. Zvezdina, and A. A. Korotaeva.** 1998. Effect of lysophosphatidylcholine on transmembrane signal transduction. *Biochem. Mosc.* **63**:31–37.

14. **Weltzien, H. U.** 1979. Cytolytic and membrane-perturbing properties of lysophosphatidylcholine. *Biochim. Biophys. Acta* **559**:259–287.

# IRON REQUIREMENTS OF AND ACQUISITION OF IRON BY *LEGIONELLA PNEUMOPHILA*

*Nicholas P. Cianciotto, Sherry Kurtz, Kevin Krcmarik, Sejal Mody, Uttara Prasad, Marianne Robey, Joseph Salerno, and V. K. Viswanathan*

# 6

*Legionella pneumophila* is remarkable for its ability to flourish within a wide variety of aquatic environments, as well as within mammalian, including human, hosts. As is reflected in this book, this capacity depends upon the actions of myriad bacterial factors. In our laboratory, we have examined a number of aspects of *Legionella* genetics, physiology, and pathogenicity. Several of these—pilus production, PilD-dependent infectivity, type II protein secretion, degradative exoenzymes, and resistance to cationic peptides—are the topics for other chapters in this book. Here, we discuss our current understanding of the relationship between *L. pneumophila* and the metal iron. After summarizing the work of a number of laboratories that demonstrated the importance of iron for *Legionella*, we will highlight our recent advances toward uncovering mechanisms of *L. pneumophila* iron acquisition.

Earlier studies indicated that iron is a key requirement for *L. pneumophila* extracellular replication, intracellular infection, and virulence. Indeed, buffered charcoal yeast extract, the standard medium for culturing legionellae, is notable for containing a large amount of added iron. Similarly, legionellae are most readily isolated from water systems that contain elevated iron levels. As determined on bacteriologic media, the ferric or ferrous iron requirement for *L. pneumophila* has been estimated to be 3 to 13 $\mu$M for minimal growth and $>20$ $\mu$M for optimal growth (11, 14, 19). However, on the basis of some of our recent findings, these values are likely overestimates (see below). In artificial media, the iron is generally in the form of ferric pyrophosphate, although ferric citrate, ferric chloride, ferric nitrate, and ferrous sulfate have also been used successfully. Furthermore, we have demonstrated that *L. pneumophila* can bind and utilize hemin as a sole source of iron (15). As with other bacteria, iron is required by *L. pneumophila* for its role as a cofactor in critical enzymes, including a superoxide dismutase and aconitase (14). However, a variety of studies indicate that iron acquisition is particularly relevant for *Legionella* pathogenesis. Three lines of evidence signal that the ability of *L. pneumophila* to replicate within mammalian cells depends upon iron: First, human monocytes and macrophages treated with iron chelators such as desferrioxamine, apotransferrin, or

*Nicholas P. Cianciotto, Sherry Kurtz, Kevin Krcmarik, Sejal Mody, Uttara Prasad, Marianne Robey, Joseph Salerno, and V. K. Viswanathan* Department of Microbiology-Immunology, Northwestern University Medical School, Chicago, IL 60611.

*Legionella*, Edited by Reinhard Marre et al.
© 2002 ASM Press, Washington, D.C.

apolactoferrin do not support *Legionella* replication (3). Second, the cytokine interferon-γ inhibits bacterial growth by reducing the amount of iron in the host cell (2). Third, macrophages from A/J mice become permissive for intracellular infection following the addition of iron (5).

Three additional observations further highlight the importance of iron acquisition for *L. pneumophila* virulence. First, the introduction of supplemental iron into experimental animals increases their susceptibility to *Legionella* infection. Second, *L. pneumophila* grown under iron-depleted conditions exhibits a reduced ability to cause disease (10). Third, an avirulent strain, derived by prolonged plate passage of the wild type, has an elevated iron requirement, although both parent and mutant accumulate equal amounts of the metal (11).

Although the importance of iron for *L. pneumophila* has always been clear, the mechanisms by which the bacterium acquires iron, especially intracellular iron, had remained largely obscured. *L. pneumophila* can degrade transferrin and use the released iron for growth (9). However, this form of iron acquisition is not likely to promote intracellular infection, since the microbial phagosome lacks transferrin, and the bacterium itself does not bind the host chelator (4, 11, 18). *L. pneumophila* can bind lactoferrin, but this interaction is actually bactericidal (1). A cytoplasmic and a periplasmic ferric reductase have been identified in *L. pneumophila* (9, 16). These enzymes undoubtedly facilitate iron assimilation after the initial uptake of the metal, but their roles in pathogenesis have not been delineated. Among all of the past considerations regarding *Legionella* iron acquisition, it is the issue of siderophores that has been the most controversial. In the early 1980s, it was reported that *L. pneumophila* does not produce siderophores (19). This conclusion was based upon the negative results that were obtained from a standard bioassay, as well as the Arnow and Csaky assays, the customary methods for detecting

catecholates and hydroxamates. The question of *Legionella* siderophores was revisited using the chrome azurol S (CAS) assay, a procedure that detects iron chelators independently of their structure (6). This study identified *L. pneumophila* supernatants with CAS reactivity, suggesting the existence of a noncatecholate, nonhydroxamate siderophore. However, our later work determined that the CAS reactivity was the assay medium's cysteine (13). When the CAS assay was repeated using supernatants from cultures generated with cysteine-free media, we also did not detect any siderophore activity. A later study, which employed chemostat cultures, also failed to identify any CAS, Arnow, or Csaky reactive substances in iron-starved *L. pneumophila* cultures (9). These data, along with the belief that *L. pneumophila* survives much of the time as an intracellular parasite, had promoted the notion that *Legionella* does not (need to) produce siderophores.

With this background of largely negative results, we initially applied a broad genetic approach toward identifying *Legionella* mechanisms of iron acquisition. As part of a first genetical approach, a genomic library of *L. pneumophila* serogroup 1 strain 130b (Wadsworth, ATCC BAA-74) was screened for a *Legionella* locus that conferred hemin binding upon *Escherichia coli*. A single gene, designated as *hbp* for *hemin binding promotion*, was identified by this method (15). The *hbp* gene was predicted to encode a secreted, 15.5-kDa protein, which did not bear significant homology with any known protein. To determine the importance of this gene in *L. pneumophila*, we used allelic exchange to construct an *hbp* deficient strain. The mutant displayed a 42% reduction in hemin binding, confirming that *hbp* potentiates hemin acquisition by *L. pneumophila*. The strain, however, was unaltered in its ability to grow within U937 macrophages or *Hartmannella* amoebae, indicating that *hbp* is not required for intracellular infection (15). These data suggest that heme acquisition is not required during *Legionella* intracellular infection. They do not, however, prove that heme acquisition is inoperative during *L. pneumophila* infection of the mammalian host.

As a second genetic approach, we mutagenized strain 130b with mini-Tn*10*, and then screened for mutants that were hypersensitive to the iron chelator EDDA and/or resistant to streptonigrin, an antibiotic whose effect requires high intracellular iron (17). Seventeen *L. pneumophila* strains that appeared defective for iron acquisition were obtained. Eleven of these mutants were both sensitive to EDDA and resistant to streptonigrin. Six were also defective for infection of human U937 cells. The mutants displayed prolonged lag phases and in some cases, replicated at a slower rate. Overall, the reduced recoveries of the mutants, relative to the wild type, ranged from 3- to 1,000-fold. The isolation of these mutants offered genetic proof that iron acquisition is critical for intracellular infection by *L. pneumophila* (17).

Strain NU216, an EDDA-hypersensitive mutant displaying a severe intracellular lag phase and a slow rate of replication, was studied further (20). Within U937 cells, NU216 and its allelic equivalent NU216R were approximately 100-fold more sensitive than the wild type to treatment with desferrioxamine, confirming that they are defective for intracellular iron acquisition. To determine whether NU216R was attenuated for virulence, we assessed its ability to cause disease in guinea pigs following intratracheal inoculation (20). NU216R-infected animals yielded 1,000-fold fewer bacteria from their lungs and spleen compared with wild-type-infected animals that had received a 50-fold lower dose. Moreover, NU216R-infected animals subsequently cleared the bacteria from these sites. Infection with the mutant did not elicit a high fever, weight loss, or ruffled fur. Sequence analysis revealed that the mutation in NU216R lies in the first gene of a two-gene operon (20). This gene (*iraA*) encodes a 272-amino acid protein that shows sequence similarity to methyltransferases. The second gene

(*iraB*) encodes a 501-amino acid protein that is highly similar to di/tripeptide transporters from both prokaryotes and eukaryotes. A new mutant containing a disruption in *iraB* showed reduced growth under iron-depleted extracellular conditions, but it did not have a defect in macrophages. These data suggest that *iraA* is critical for virulence of *L. pneumophila*, while *iraB* is involved in a novel method of iron acquisition that may utilize iron-loaded peptides (20).

The EDDA-hypersensitive mutant NU208 was also dramatically impaired for replication in U937 cells, and its infectivity defect was exacerbated by treatment of the macrophages with desferrioxamine. A reconstruction of the NU208 mutation confirmed that the iron acquisition and infectivity defects were due to the transposon insertion and not a spontaneous second-site mutation. Sequence analysis demonstrated that the transposon disruption lies within a gene that is highly similar to the cytochrome c maturation gene, *ccmC*. *ccmC* is generally recognized for its role in the heme export step of cytochrome biogenesis. Indeed, NU208 lacked cytochrome c. Importantly, three additional *L. pneumophila* mutants, which had been identified for their diminished cytopathicity toward U937 cells, contained mutations in *ccmC* as well as a second cytochrome c biogenesis gene, *ccmF*. All *ccm* mutants were defective for growth within *Hartmannella* and *Acanthamoeba* amoebae. Like the *ccmC* mutants, the *ccmF* mutant was impaired for growth in media lacking iron supplements but grew normally in iron-supplemented media. Together, these data indicate the *Legionella ccm* locus promotes both intracellular infection and iron acquisition by a potentially novel mechanism. Complete sequence analysis of the *ccm* locus from strain 130b identified *ccmA-H*. Interestingly, however, we also observed that a 1.7-kb insertion sequence element, containing two novel open reading frames (ORFs), was positioned between *ccmB* and *ccmC*. This element (ISLp*1*) was present in multiple copies in some strains of *L. pneumophila* but was absent from others. These latter findings represent the first evidence for a transposable element in *Legionella* and the first identification of an *L. pneumophila* strain-specific gene. Our observations represent the fourth example of a linkage between *ccm* genes and bacterial iron acquisition, complementing recent studies with *Paracoccus, Pseudomonas,* and *Rhizobium* species. The manner in which *ccm* promotes iron acquisition is unclear, although in the case of *Pseudomonas,* the *ccm* mutants had altered siderophore expression. The infectivity defects of our mutants indicate, for the first time, that *ccm* genes can be necessary for bacterial growth within an intracellular niche.

The final putative iron acquisition mutant to be considered here is NU225. Although this strain has a marked resistance to streptonigrin, it has proven to be nearly equivalent to the wild type in terms of intracellular infectivity. The miniTn*10* insertion in NU225 maps to an ORF that has only one known analog, the so-called *orfZ* of *Streptomyces hygroscopicus*. Interestingly, the *Streptomyces* gene lies at the end of a rapamycin biosynthetic gene cluster, but it has not yet been formally ascribed any function. Thus, it is tempting to speculate that the mutation in NU225 has abolished some form of nonribosomal peptide synthesis, a process that has been linked to siderophore production in bacteria such as *Mycobacterium* species.

As a third genetic approach toward examining *L. pneumophila* iron acquisition, strain 130b was randomly mutated with a miniTn*10'lacZ* transposon, and the resulting gene fusions were tested for iron regulation by assessing β-galactosidase production in the presence and absence of iron chelators (8). In other bacteria, iron- and Fur-regulated genes are important for infection and iron acquisition. We had previously demonstrated that *Legionella* produces Fur, a protein that can repress gene transcription in response to iron concentration (7). Mutant NU229 possessed a *lacZ* fusion that was stably iron-regulated (8). That fusion was also demonstrated to be Fur-

regulated, on the basis of the derepression that occurred when the gene construct was introduced into a manganese-resistant Fur⁻ derivative of strain 130b. Extracellular growth of NU229 in bacteriological media was similar to that of the wild type. To assess the role of the *frgA* gene in intracellular infection, we determined the relative ability of NU229 to grow within U937 cell monolayers (8). Quantitative infection assays demonstrated that NU229 was impaired ca. 80-fold in intracellular growth. Reconstruction of the mutant by allelic exchange proved that the defect was due to the inactivation of *frgA* and not a spontaneous second-site mutation. Subsequently, *trans*-complementation of the mutation demonstrated that the infectivity defect was directly due to the loss of FrgA. Nucleotide sequence analysis revealed that the 63-kDa FrgA is analogous to the aerobactin synthetases IucA and IucC of *E. coli*. This finding raised the intriguing possibility that *L. pneumophila* encodes a hydroxymate siderophore, which is particularly relevant for intracellular replication (8). Supporting this notion, we have recently found a second *Legionella* gene (*frgB*) that is homologous with the *iucA/iucC*. Since *frgA* appeared to be specific to the *L. pneumophila* species, we have designated the hypothetical *Legionella* siderophore as pneumobactin.

Given the results of our genetic analysis, we sought once again to gain biochemical evidence for *L. pneumophila* siderophores. In this case, we were able to demonstrate that supernatants from *L. pneumophila* cultures contain a nonproteinaceous, high-affinity, iron chelator (12). More specifically, when aerobically grown in a low-iron, chemically defined medium, *L. pneumophila* secreted a substance that was reactive in the CAS assay. Importantly, the siderophore-like activity was observed only when the cultures were inoculated to relatively high density with bacteria that had been grown to log or early stationary phase. Inocula derived from late stationary phase cultures, despite ultimately growing, failed to result in the elaboration of siderophore-like activity. The *Legionella* CAS reactivity was detected in the supernatants of strains 130b and Philadelphia 1, as well as those from representatives of other serogroups and other *Legionella* species (12). The CAS reactive substance was resistant to boiling and protease treatment and was associated with the <1-kDa fraction. As would also be expected for a siderophore, the addition of 0.5 or 2.0 $\mu$M iron to the cultures repressed the expression of the CAS reactive substance. Control experiments determined that the CAS reactivity was not due to cysteine, phosphate, or citrate that might have been in the medium and/or produced by *Legionella* secondary metabolism. The supernatants were negative in the Arnow, Csaky, and Rioux assays, indicating that the *Legionella* siderophore was not a classic catecholate or hydroxamate and hence, might be of novel structure (12). Since the CAS reactivity was produced by the *frgA* mutant NU229, it is not pneumobactin. Thus, we have tentatively designated the *L. pneumophila* siderophore as legiobactin. The discovery of legiobactin represents the first hard evidence against the long-held view of *L. pneumophila* as a bacterium that does not elaborate siderophores. It is likely that the novel influence of the bacterial inoculum on siderophore production is the main reason that we, and others, failed to detect legiobactin in the past. The discovery of legiobactin and its promotion of growth in media lacking iron also indicate that the *L. pneumophila* requirement for iron is not as great as had been intimated and may even be <1 $\mu$M (12).

We have recently identified, in the developing *L. pneumophila* Philadelphia-1 genome database as well as in our strain 130b, genes that are homologous with *pvc* and *pvd* genes of *Pseudomonas* and *Burkholderia*. The *pvc* and *pvd* genes are involved in the biosynthesis of the siderophores pyoverdin and ornibactin. Thus, *L. pneumophila* might be capable of producing a pyoverdin-like siderophore, in addition to elaborating legiobactin and pneumobactin. Alternately, it is possible that legiobactin is actually a pyoverdin-like siderophore. We have recently mutated one of the

*pvc*-like genes and found the resulting mutant is impaired for growth in low-iron media. Ongoing studies are assessing the CAS reactivity and infectivity of this and related mutants.

Two other genes evident in the data released from the *L. pneumophila* sequencing project that we have targeted for further investigation are *feoB* and *tonB*. In other systems, these genes, among other things, promote ferrous iron import. Using allelic exchange, we have constructed a *feoB* mutant and are currently assessing its behavior within and outside of host cells.

In summary, we believe that *L. pneumophila* possesses multiple pathways for iron acquisition (Fig. 1). The organism may produce as many as three siderophores; there is biochemical evidence for legiobactin, and genetic data for the existence of hydroxamate- and pyoverdin-like iron chelators. The membrane-associated Ccm complex is clearly required for optimal iron assimilation; however, additional work is needed to determine the molecular mechanisms involved. Based upon precedent, it is possible that a *ccm* gene product(s) influences *Legionella* siderophore production. Since the *ccm* mutants were not impaired for the observed CAS reactivity, that siderophore would appear not to be legiobactin. The *iraAB* locus is predicted to encode a peptide membrane transporter. As depicted here, we speculate that the IraAB system promotes iron acquisition by importing iron-loaded peptides. Alternatively, transported di/tripeptides might be involved in the expression of a peptidic siderophore. We have shown that *L. pneumophila* can bind and use hemin, in part through the action of the Hbp protein. This suggests that the *Legionella* parasite, like a number of other pathogenic bacteria, may utilize a variety of heme-containing proteins as iron sources. The existence of an *L. pneumophila feoB* gene suggests that the organism has the capacity to transport ferrous iron. Thus, it is possible that one of the organism's niches is relatively reduced, such that ferrous iron is prevalent. On the other hand, the FeoB

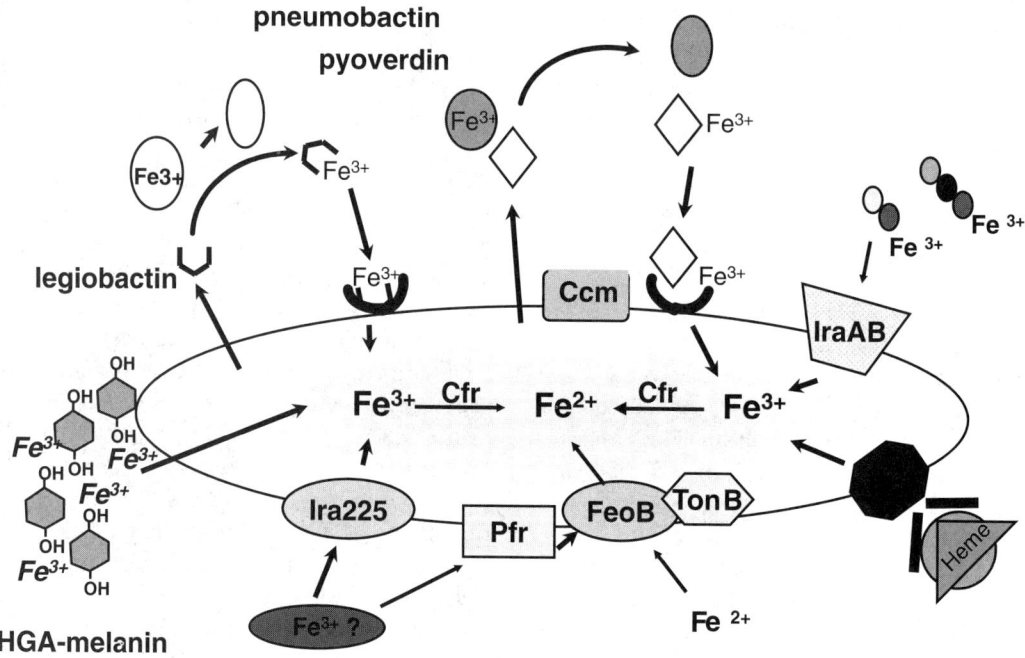

**FIGURE 1** Potential iron acquisition pathways of *Legionella pneumophila*. See text for details.

inner membrane permease may (also) exist to assimilate $Fe^{2+}$ that had been generated in the periplasm, by the reduction of acquired $Fe^{3+}$. The fact that *L. pneumophila* possesses a periplasmic ferric reductase (Pfr) is compatible with such a scenario. However, the existence of a *Legionella* cytoplasmic ferric reductase (Cfr) suggests that not all iron reductions occur in the periplasm. The preliminary characterization of NU225 and other mutants identified in our genetic screens suggests that yet additional iron uptake pathways (e.g., Ira225) are operative in *L. pneumophila*. Finally, we have observed that the formation of HGA-melanin, the pigment evident in *L. pneumophila* stationary phase supernatants, is iron-dependent. This observation, plus the finding that fractions enriched for melanin retain iron, suggests that the *Legionella* pigment acts as an extracellular sink for excess iron. The existence of multiple iron uptake systems in *L. pneumophila* is quite compatible with the fact that the bacterium resides within such a wide variety of environments. It is likely that many of them are relevant for *Legionella* intracellular infection and pathogenesis.

## REFERENCES

1. **Bortner, C. A., R. R. Arnold, and R. D. Miller.** 1989. Bactericidal effect of lactoferrin on *Legionella pneumophila*: effect of the physiological state of the organism. *Can. J. Microbiol.* **35:**1048–1051.
2. **Byrd, T. F., and M. A. Horwitz.** 1989. Interferon gamma-activated human monocytes downregulate transferrin receptors and inhibit the intracellular multiplication of *Legionella pneumophila* by limiting the availability of iron. *J. Clin. Invest.* **83:**1457–1465.
3. **Byrd, T. F., and M. A. Horwitz.** 1991. Lactoferrin inhibits or promotes *Legionella pneumophila* intracellular multiplication in nonactivated and interferon gamma-activated human monocytes depending upon its degree of iron saturation. Iron-lactoferrin and nonphysiologic iron chelates reverse monocyte activation against *Legionella pneumophila*. *J. Clin. Invest.* **88:**1103–1112.
4. **Clemens, D. L., and M. A. Horwitz.** 1995. Characterization of the *Mycobacterium tuberculosis* phagosome and evidence that phagosomal maturation is inhibited. *J. Exp. Med.* **181:**257–270.

5. **Gebran, S. J., C. Newton, Y. Yamamoto, R. Widen, T. W. Klein, and H. Friedman.** 1994. Macrophage permissiveness for *Legionella pneumophila* growth modulated by iron. *Infect. Immun.* **62:**564–568.

6. **Goldoni, P., P. Visca, M. C. Pastoris, P. Valenti, and N. Orsi.** 1991. Growth of *Legionella* spp. under conditions of iron restriction. *J. Med. Microbiol.* **34:**113–118.

7. **Hickey, E. K., and N. P. Cianciotto.** 1994. Cloning and sequencing of the *Legionella pneumophila fur* gene. *Gene* **143:**117–121.

8. **Hickey, E. K., and N. P. Cianciotto.** 1997. An iron- and fur-repressed *Legionella pneumophila* gene that promotes intracellular infection and encodes a protein with similarity to the *Escherichia coli* aerobactin synthetases. *Infect. Immun.* **65:**133–143.

9. **James, B. W., W. S. Mauchline, P. J. Dennis, and C. W. Keevil.** 1997. A study of iron acquisition mechanisms of *Legionella pneumophila* grown in chemostat culture. *Curr. Microbiol.* **34:**238–243.

10. **James, B. W., W. S. Mauchline, R. B. Fitzgeorge, P. J. Dennis, and C. W. Keevil.** 1995. Influence of iron-limited continuous culture on physiology and virulence of *Legionella pneumophila. Infect. Immun.* **63:**4224–4230.

11. **Johnson, W., L. Varner, and M. Poch.** 1991. Acquisition of iron by *Legionella pneumophila*: role of iron reductase. *Infect. Immun.* **59:**2376–2381.

12. **Liles, M. R., T. Aber Scheel, and N. P. Cianciotto.** 2000. Discovery of a nonclassical siderophore, legiobactin, produced by strains of *Legionella pneumophila. J. Bacteriol.* **182:**749–757.

13. **Liles, M. R., and N. P. Cianciotto.** 1996. Absence of siderophore-like activity in *Legionella pneumophila* supernatants. *Infect. Immun.* **64:**1873–1875.

14. **Mengaud, J. M., and M. A. Horwitz.** 1993. The major iron-containing protein of *Legionella pneumophila* is an aconitase homologous with the human iron-responsive element-binding protein. *J. Bacteriol.* **175:**5666–5676.

15. **O'Connell, W. A., E. K. Hickey, and N. P. Cianciotto.** 1996. A *Legionella pneumophila* gene that promotes hemin binding. *Infect. Immun.* **64:**842–848.

16. **Poch, M. T., and W. Johnson.** 1993. Ferric reductases of *Legionella pneumophila. Biometals* **6:**107–114.

17. **Pope, C. D., W. O'Connell, and N. P. Cianciotto.** 1996. *Legionella pneumophila* mutants that are defective for iron acquisition and assimilation and intracellular infection. *Infect. Immun.* **64:**629–636.

18. **Quinn, F. D., and E. D. Weisberg.** 1988. Killing of *Legionella pneumophila* by human serum and iron-binding agents. *Curr. Microbiol.* **17:**111–116.

19. **Reeves, M. W., L. Pine, J. B. Neilands, and A. Balows.** 1983. Absence of siderophore activity in *Legionella* species grown in iron-deficient media. *J. Bacteriol.* **154:**324–329.

20. **Viswanathan, V. K., P. H. Edelstein, C. D. Pope, and N. P. Cianciotto.** 2000. The *Legionella pneumophila iraAB* locus is required for iron assimilation, intracellular infection, and virulence. *Infect. Immun.* **68:**1069–1079.

# RESISTANCE OF *LEGIONELLA PNEUMOPHILA* TO CATIONIC ANTIMICROBIAL PEPTIDES

*Marianne Robey, William O'Connell, and Nicholas P. Cianciotto*

# 7

Cationic antimicrobial peptides (CAMP) form an important part of the innate immune response in many organisms ranging from humans to amoebae (5). These peptides are thought to elicit death by insertion into and lysis of bacterial membranes (5). As a facultative intracellular pathogen of both humans and amoebae, *Legionella pneumophila* must contend with the bactericidal action of CAMPs for successful proliferation within the host. The fact that CAMP resistance mechanisms exist in *L. pneumophila* is suggested by several lines of evidence. For example, *L. pneumophila* is inherently resistant to the CAMP, polymyxin B (PmB) (2). Furthermore, *L. pneumophila* mutants have been generated that are capable of survival despite delivery to the macrophage phagolysosome (6). Also, recent evidence suggests that phagolysosomal fusion does occur late in the intracellular infection cycle (9). While characterizing a gene involved in iron acquisition, *hbp*, we identified an open reading frame, the product of which exhibited homology (42% identity, 57% similarity, and

protein products of identical size) with the product of the *pagP* (*phoP-activated gene P*) gene in *Salmonella enterica* serovar Typhimurium, involved in CAMP resistance and PagP in *Escherichia coli* (1, 4, 7). Investigations were undertaken to investigate the role of the *pagP*-like gene in *L. pneumophila* in CAMP resistance and intracellular infections.

## GENERATION OF *L. PNEUMOPHILA* MUTANTS
Mutants were generated by introduction of a kanamycin cassette into the chromosomal copy of the *pagP*-like gene in *L. pneumophila* serogroup 1 strain 130b (Wadsworth, BAA-74) by allelic exchange using a *sacB*, chloramphenicol resistance plasmid (7). Mutant phenotypes of chloramphenicol and sucrose sensitivity and kanamycin resistance were verified by PCR and Southern hybridization (7). Two independent mutants, NU260 and NU261, were used in subsequent investigations, although for clarity only data from NU260 are presented here.

## CAMP RESISTANCE OF *L. PNEUMOPHILA* MUTANTS
To investigate the role of the *pagP*-like gene in CAMP resistance, the MICs of PmB, a bac-

_____

*Marianne Robey, William O'Connell, and Nicholas P. Cianciotto* Department of Microbiology-Immunology, Northwestern University Medical School, Chicago, IL 60611.

*Legionella*, Edited by Reinhard Marre et al.
© 2002 ASM Press, Washington, D.C.

terially derived CAMP, and C18G, a synthetic CAMP based on human platelet activating factor IV (Table 1), were assessed for the mutants generated (4). Following incubation at 37°C for 30 h, the lowest concentration of C18G or PmB resulting in no visible growth was deemed to be the MIC. The MICs of both PmB and C18G were decreased in NU260 compared with the wild type (Table 1). Taken together with the significant degree of sequence homology with PagP in *Salmonella*, these data indicate that the *L. pneumophila* counterpart of PagP plays a role in CAMP resistance. We therefore designate this gene *rcp*, for resistance to cationic antimicrobial peptides.

## INTRACELLULAR INFECTIONS WITH MACROPHAGES AND AMOEBAE

To assess the role of *rcp* in an intracellular environment, a phenotype not previously investigated for any *pagP*-like gene, U937 macrophages were infected with either 130b or NU260 and then the numbers of bacteria were monitored over time. Assessment of the intracellular growth kinetics of *L. pneumophila* in U937 macrophages was performed as previously reported (7). At 0 h, equivalent num-

bers of bacteria were recovered between 130b and NU260 (Fig. 1A). Thus, there was no obvious defect in the initial stages of infection, i.e., attachment and invasion. However, the mutant exhibited reduced recovery compared with the wild-type parent by 1 log at 18 h postinoculation (p.i.) (Fig. 1A). The difference in numbers of recovered bacteria diminished at later time points, until by 72 h, similar numbers of mutant and wild type were recovered (Fig. 1A and data not shown). No difference between the abilities of NU260 and 130b to survive in the medium used to culture the macrophages was noted (data not shown). Taken together, these data suggest that *rcp* promotes the ability of *L. pneumophila* to replicate and/or survive in macrophages.

Intracellular growth of both wild type and mutant was also tested in a coculture assay with *Hartmannella vermiformis*. This amoeba is known to support the growth of *L. pneumophila* and was isolated from a clinical case of legionellosis. Coculture assays were performed as previously described (7). Both 130b and NU260 were recovered in similar numbers until 24 h p.i. (Fig. 1B). However, by 72 h p.i., the mutant exhibited a nearly 1,000-fold reduction in numbers compared with the wild type (Fig. 1B). No difference in the abilities of the *rcp* mutant and 130b to survive in the assay media were noted (data not shown). *Trans*-complementation of NU260 to wild-type levels was achieved in an *H. vermiformis* coculture by introduction of the intact *rcp* gene encoded on a low copy number plasmid (data not shown). Similar to the case with macrophages, the growth defect of the mutant during coculture with *H. vermiformis* could be due to a decreased ability to replicate and/or survive intracellularly. Alternatively, it could also involve alterations in invasion. Growth of both the *rcp* mutant and the wild-type parent was shown to be highly similar in both buffered yeast extract (BYE) broth and a chemically defined medium (CDM), suggesting that differences observed between the numbers of recovered bacteria in amoebae and macro-

**TABLE 1**  CAMP susceptibility of *L. pneumophila* strains[a]

| CAMP | Growth condition | Strain | MIC ($\mu$g/ml) |
|------|------------------|--------|-----------------|
| PmB | BYE | 130b | 12.5 |
| | | NU260 | 6.2 |
| | CDM | 130b | 3.1 |
| | | NU260 | 3.1 |
| | 0.005 mM Mg$^{2+}$ CDM | 130b | 12.5 |
| | | NU260 | 6.2 |
| C18G | BYE | 130b | 16 |
| | | NU260 | 8 |
| | CDM | 130b | 16 |
| | | NU260 | 4–8 |
| | 0.005 mM Mg$^{2+}$ CDM | 130b | 64 |
| | | NU260 | 16 |

[a] The bacteria were grown in triplicate to mid-exponential phase in the indicated media and then, after dilution to $5 \times 10^4$ CFU/ml, were exposed to PmB or C18G. Similar MICs were obtained in a replicate experiment (data not shown) (3).

**A**

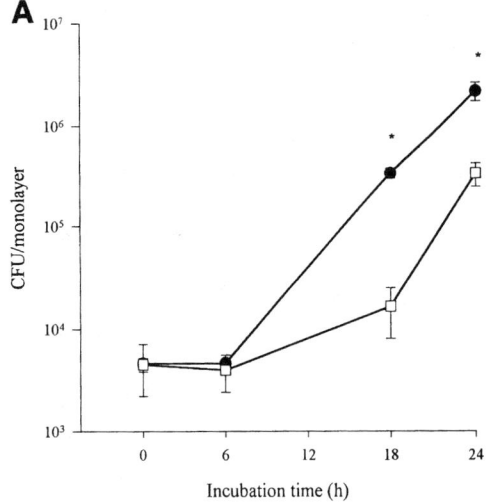

**B**

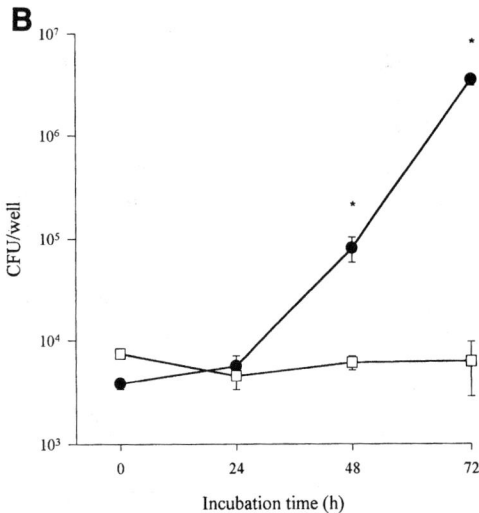

**FIGURE 1** Intracellular infection with *L. pneumophila* strains. (A) U937 cell monolayers (*n* = 3) were infected at a multiplicity of infection (MOI) of 1 with strain 130b (●) and NU260 (□). Asterisks indicate significant differences (*P* < 0.01; Student's *t* test) in numbers of recovered bacteria between 130b and NU260. (B) Monolayers of *H. vermiformis* amoebae (*n* = 3) were infected with wild-type 130b (●) and mutant NU260 (□) at an MOI of 0.01. Asterisks indicate significant differences (*P* < 0.05 at 48 h or 0.005 at 72 h; Student's *t* test). Comparable results were obtained in triplicate experiments, and the data presented here are from one representative experiment.

phages were not due to generalized growth defects (data not shown and Fig. 2A).

## MAGNESIUM-REGULATED PHENOTYPE OF *L. PNEUMOPHILA* STRAINS

In *Salmonella, pagP* is transcriptionally activated by the PhoPQ two-component regulator in response to low $Mg^{2+}$ conditions (4). Consequently, bacterial growth in low $Mg^{2+}$ minimal media increases the CAMP resistance generated by *pagP*. Thus, we hypothesized that the *L. pneumophila rcp* mutant might also have an $Mg^{2+}$-regulated CAMP-resistant phenotype. First, we investigated the growth of NU260 in CDM containing reduced amounts of $Mg^{2+}$. In 0.005 mM $Mg^{2+}$ CDM, NU260 entered into stationary phase earlier than 130b, although growth rate was unaffected (Fig. 2B). Thus, the *L. pneumophila rcp* gene appears to be involved in growth and/or survival in low-$Mg^{2+}$ media. The growth characteristics of the *rcp* mutant in low-$Mg^{2+}$ media were very similar to those observed in *Salmonella* strains with mutations in *phoP*, or the $Mg^{2+}$ transporters, *mgtA* and *mgtCB* (8). Given the reduced ability of the *L. pneumophila rcp* mutant to grow in low-$Mg^{2+}$ media, we tested its relative resistance to C18G and PmB after growth in CDM containing various amounts of $Mg^{2+}$. CAMP resistance to PmB or C18G was increased by growth in low-$Mg^{2+}$ CDM in both 130b and NU260 (Table 1). However, there was a greater increase in the wild type, suggesting that *rcp* is partly responsible for $Mg^{2+}$-dependent CAMP resistance and that other, as yet unidentified, CAMP resistance mechanisms appear to be operational in *L. pneumophila*.

## CONCLUDING REMARKS

These investigations mark the first identification of an *L. pneumophila* gene involved in CAMP resistance, the novel finding that *rcp* is required for growth and/or survival in low-$Mg^{2+}$ media, and the first demonstration of increased *Legionella* CAMP resistance due to

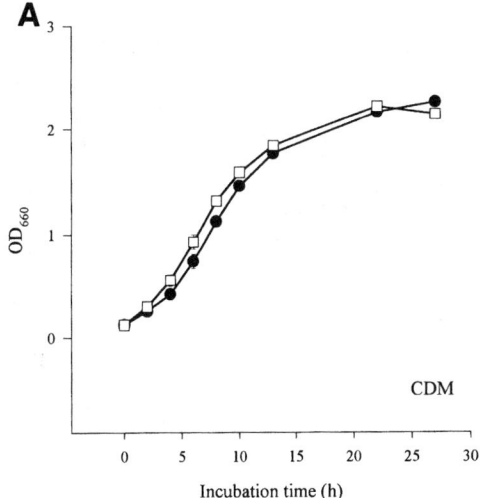

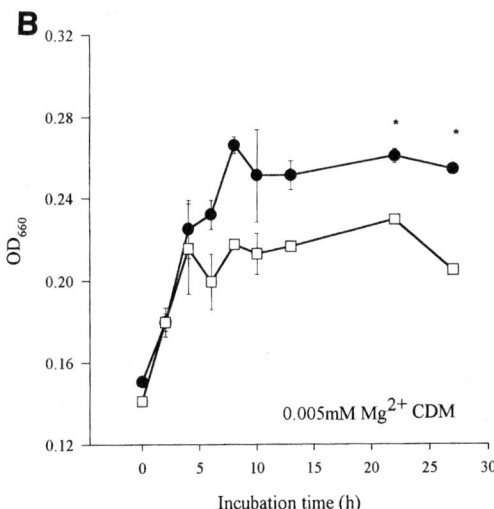

**FIGURE 2** Growth of *L. pneumophila* strains in low-Mg$^{2+}$ liquid medium. Wild-type strain 130b (●) and mutant NU260 (□) were compared for growth in CDM (A), and CDM with 0.005 mM Mg$^{2+}$ cations (B). Growth was assessed by measuring the optical density at 660 nm of triplicate cultures at various times of incubation. Asterisks indicate significant ($P < 0.05$; Student's *t* test) differences between the 130b and NU260 cultures. Standard deviations are shown, but the error bars are too small to be observed in panels A and B. This experiment was performed in triplicate with comparable results and representative data are presented here.

low-Mg$^{2+}$ conditions. Furthermore, this is the first indication of the requirement for CAMP resistance during intracellular growth and/or survival in both human macrophages and amoebae. However, is it conceivable that *rcp* has another, as yet uncharacterized role during intracellular infection. The regulation of *pagP* by PhoPQ in response to low Mg$^{2+}$ has prompted speculation that the *Salmonella*-containing phagosome is an Mg$^{2+}$-limiting environment. Whether the *L. pneumophila* intraphagosomal environment is similarly low in Mg$^{2+}$ remains to be seen. Mg$^{2+}$-regulated behavior of the *L. pneumophila rcp* mutant may be indicative of the presence of a PhoPQ homologue in legionellae. In *Salmonella* and *E. coli*, PagP functions as a palmitoyl transferase, able to modify the lipid A component of lipopolysaccharide by addition of palmitate (1, 4). The increased acylation is believed to promote resistance to CAMPs by decreasing membrane fluidity and preventing insertion of the peptide (4). Lipid A modifications that increase bacterial CAMP resistance are an emerging theme in gram-negative bacteria. Due to the high degree of sequence homology and the similar function of both PagP and Rcp, similar lipid A modifications could be promoted by the *L. pneumophila rcp* gene.

## REFERENCES

1. Bishop, R. E., H. S. Gibbons, T. Guina, M. S. Trent, S. I. Miller, and C. R. Raetz. 2000. Transfer of palmitate from phospholipids to lipid A in outer membranes of Gram-negative bacteria. *EMBO J.* **19:**5071–5080.
2. Edelstein, P. H., and S. M. Finegold. 1979. Use of a semiselective medium to culture *Legionella pneumophila* from contaminated lung specimens. *J. Clin. Microbiol.* **10:**141–143.
3. Giacometti, A., O. Cirioni, F. Barchiesi, M. S. Del Prete, M. Fortuna, F. Caselli, and G. Scalise. 2000. *In vitro* susceptibility tests for cationic peptides: comparison of broth microdilution methods for bacteria that grow aerobically. *Antimicrob. Agents Chemother.* **44:**1694–1696.
4. Guo, L., K. B. Lim, C. M. Poduje, M. Daniel, J. S. Gunn, M. Hackett, and S. I. Miller. 1998. Lipid A acylation and bacterial resistance

against vertebrate antimicrobial peptides. *Cell* **95:** 189–198.

5. **Hancock, R. E., and M. G. Scott.** 2000. The role of antimicrobial peptides in animal defenses. *Proc. Natl. Acad. Sci. USA* **97:**8856–8861.

6. **Horwitz, M. A.** 1987. Characterisation of avirulent mutant *Legionella pneumophila* that survive but do not multiply within human monocytes. *J. Exp. Med.* **166:**1310–1328.

7. **O'Connell, W. A., E. K. Hickey, and N. P. Cianciotto.** 1996. A *Legionella pneumophila* gene that promotes hemin binding. *Infect. Immun.* **64:** 842–848.

8. **Soncini, F. C., E. Garcia Vescovi, F. Solomon, and E. A. Groisman.** 1996. Molecular basis of the magnesium deprivation response in *Salmonella typhimurium*: identification of PhoP-regulated genes. *J. Bacteriol.* **178:**5092–5099.

9. **Sturgill-Koszycki, S., and M. S. Swanson.** 2000. *Legionella pneumophila* replication vacuoles mature into acidic, endocytic organelles. *J. Exp. Med.* **192:**1261–1272.

# FUNCTION AND EXPRESSION OF *LEGIONELLA PNEUMOPHILA* SURFACE FACTORS

*Klaus Heuner, Michael Steinert, Claudia Dietrich,*
*Gunter Fischer, Rolf Köhler, and Jörg Hacker*

# 8

Surface structures commonly play an important role in bacterial pathogenicity. In *Legionella pneumophila*, various factors contribute to pathogenicity and some of them are located on the bacterial surface or secreted into the medium. Adherence and the entry of the bacterium into the host cell is the crucial step in the infection cycle of *L. pneumophila*. The major outer membrane protein (MOMP), the heat shock protein (Hsp60), and the major infectivity potentiator protein (Mip) are localized on the surface of the bacteria. The flagellum and the pili are also thought to have a role in adherence and entry of *Legionella* into alveolar macrophages and protozoa.

The MOMP protein binds the complement component C3 and mediates the uptake of *L. pneumophila* via the macrophage CR1 and CR3 receptors (1). But phagocytosis of *L. pneumophila* also occurs by a complement-independent mechanism. Another surface-associated factor is the Hsp60 protein,

probably involved in the attachment and entry of *L. pneumophila* to HeLa epithelial cells (9). The type IV pili of *L. pneumophila* are composed of the structural protein PilE. The PilE protein also mediates adherence of *L. pneumophila* to human monocytes, epithelial cells, and *Acanthamoeba castellanii* (24).

The Mip protein is a virulence factor necessary for the establishment of infection and for optimal intracellular survival of *L. pneumophila* in alveolar macrophages. The 24-kDa protein exhibits peptidyl-prolyl *cis/trans* isomerase (PPIase) activity. An additional cytoplasmic PPIase of *L. pneumophila* has been described. The *lcy* gene encodes a cyclophilin with a molecular mass of 18 kDa. A sequence comparison revealed significant similarity to the cyclophilin of *Escherichia coli*. The enzymatic activity could be inhibited by cyclosporin A (23).

Motility of *L. pneumophila* is mediated by the flagellum of the bacterium. The flagellum positively affects the establishment of infection and supports the entry of *L. pneumophila* into human macrophages and protozoa. Flagellum expression is regulated by different environmental factors and is mediated by the alternative sigma-28 factor (FliA). This chapter will focus on the Mip protein and the function and expression of the flagellum of *L. pneumophila*.

*Klaus Heuner, Michael Steinert, Claudia Dietrich, Rolf Köhler, and Jörg Hacker* Institut für Molekulare Infektionsbiologie, Julius-Maximilians Universität Würzburg, Röntgenring 11, D-97070 Würzburg, Germany. *Gunter Fischer* Forschungsstelle "Enzymologie der Proteinfaltung" der Max-Planck-Gesellschaft, Weinbergweg 22, D-06120 Halle, Germany.

*Legionella*, Edited by Reinhard Marre et al.
© 2002 ASM Press, Washington, D.C.

## THE MAJOR INFECTIVITY POTENTIATOR PROTEIN (Mip)

Mip belongs to the group of FK506 binding proteins and exhibits PPIase activity that can be effectively inhibited by the immunosuppressants rapamycin and FK506. It is a surface protein and represents a virulence factor that is necessary for optimal intracellular survival of *L. pneumophila* in macrophages as well as in its protozoan host (5, 25). The *mip* gene is commonly found in all *Legionella* strains (4, 18, 19). Mip homolog proteins are also found in *Chlamydia trachomatis, Salmonella enterica* serovar Typhimurium, *Coxiella burnetii, Rickettsia* spp., *Ehrlichia* spp., and the eukaryotic parasite *Trypanosoma cruzii*. DNA sequence analysis of different *L. pneumophila* strains revealed minor amino acid substitutions that did not affect the isomerase property of the enzyme (15). Furthermore, sequence comparison of 35 *Legionella* species revealed 69 to 97% conserved nucleotides, and no apparent differences were determined that would predict a functional difference for Mip from virulent and nonvirulent species (18).

Using a Mip::Gfp fusion protein, it was shown that the *mip* gene is expressed constitutively during intracellular growth of *Legionella* (14). An earlier study showed that *mip* gene expression was lowest during lag phase, then increased and peaked at late log/early stationary phase during extracellular growth. In this study a *mip::lacZ* gene fusion was used to analyze *mip* expression (7).

The Mip protein forms a homodimer on the bacterial surface; each monomer consists of a proximal and a peripheral domain. The contact regions between the two monomers seem to be located at the N-terminal part of the protein (8, 15, 21, 22). A *mip* minus mutant strain can be complemented for intracellular replication by in *trans* expression of Mip variants, which are significantly reduced in PPIase activity (25). Complementation of the *mip* mutant strain with truncated Mip that is not able to form a dimeric structure, but exhibits full PPIase activity, revealed that dimerization but not the half-site isomerase activity

of Mip is necessary for full virulence in a monocellular (*A. castellanii*) system. However, in the guinea pig model of infection, isomerase activity of the dimeric enzyme seems to be necessary for establishing full virulence of *Legionella* (R. Köhler, J. Fanghänel, B. König, E. Lüneberg, G. Fischer, M. Frosch, M. Steinert, and J. Hacker, 5th Int. Conf. *Legionella*, abstr. P19, 2000).

## THE ROLE OF MOTILITY AND THE REGULATION OF FLAGELLUM EXPRESSION

*L. pneumophila* contains a single, monopolar flagellum (Fig. 1A). The flagellum is composed of one major subunit (FlaA), which exhibits a molecular mass of 48 kDa and is encoded by the *flaA* gene (10). *L. pneumophila* is motile, yet swarming onto the surface of low concentrated agar plates has not been reported. Motility might be an important factor to find a new host for another cycle of intracellular replication and for colonization of new habitats. In addition, there is some evidence that the flagellum might also be a virulence-associated factor. Flagellated bacteria have been found in lung alveolar spaces of patients with legionellosis. It was shown that expression of the virulent phenotype and motility is regulated coordinately (2, 3, 17, 20). However, other reports do not suppport a direct link between virulence and motility.

To elucidate the role of the flagellum during the infection process, we generated a specific FlaA-negative strain of *L. pneumophila* Corby (KH3). The mutant strain is nonmotile and does not exhibit flagellar structures (Fig. 1B). A gentamicin infection assay revealed a clear difference in the number of intracellular bacteria at the onset of multiplication. Two hours after coincubation ($t = 0$) with *A. castellanii* or HL-60 cells, 10 to 50 times fewer organisms of strain KH3 than the wild type were found inside the host cells, while the complemented strain CD10 exhibited the wild-type phenotype in both host cell systems (Fig. 2). The rate of intracellular multiplication was not affected and the *flaA*-negative

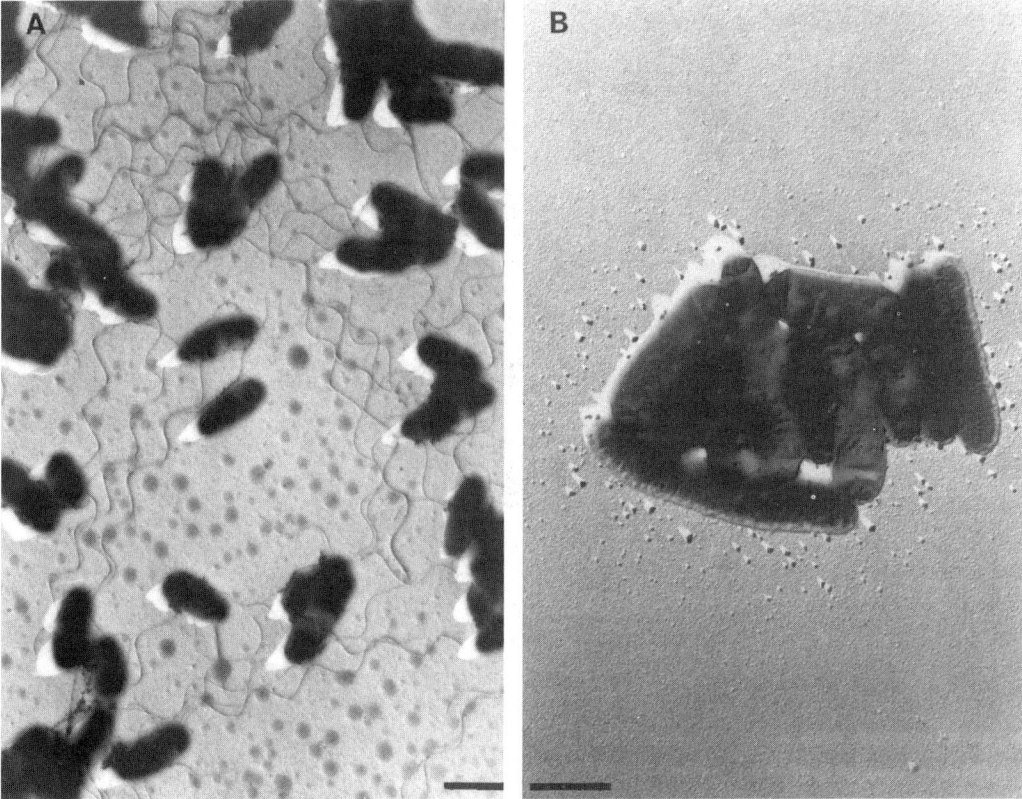

**FIGURE 1**  Electron micrographs showing the flagellated wild-type strain *L. pneumophila* Corby (A) and the nonflagellated mutant strain KH3 (B). Bacteria were grown to stationary phase at 30°C, suspended in water, and applied to Formvar coated copper grids. Samples were shadowed with platinum-palladium and examined with a Zeiss 10A transmission electron microscope. Bars, 0.5 μm.

mutant strain showed even a slightly higher rate of multiplication than that of the wild-type strain after 24 h (Fig. 2). In summary, we could demonstrate that the flagellum positively affects the establishment of infection by facilitating the encounter of the host cell, as well as by enhancing the invasion capacity, while adhesion and intracellular replication of *L. pneumophila* were unaffected (6).

L. pneumophila is found in very different habitats and it is able to replicate intracellularly in many host cells. Therefore, *Legionella* has to modulate gene expression to be able to survive in these different environments. We recently demonstrated that regulation of *flaA* expression is modulated by different environmental factors, such as temperature, growth phase, osmolarity, viscosity, and the nutrient stage (Fig. 3) (10, 12). *Legionella* replicating intracellularly are nonflagellated but at the end of the infection they become motile (3, 20). We recently showed that the *flaA* gene is transcribed as a monocistronic unit and contains a typical sigma-28 consensus sequence, which is recognized by the alternative sigma factor FliA (10, 11). The *fliA* gene was cloned by complementation of an *E. coli fliA* mutant strain. FliA of *L. pneumophila* is able to restore the flagellation and motility defect of the *E. coli* mutant strain and was shown to direct transcription initiation from the *flaA*-specific promoter (11). Most of the *Legionella* strains are

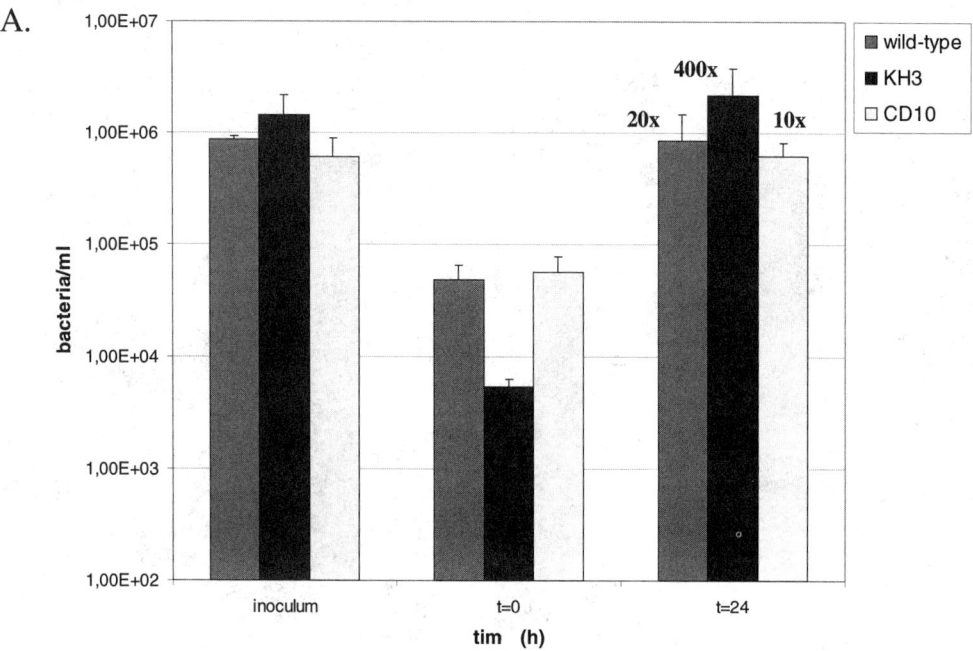

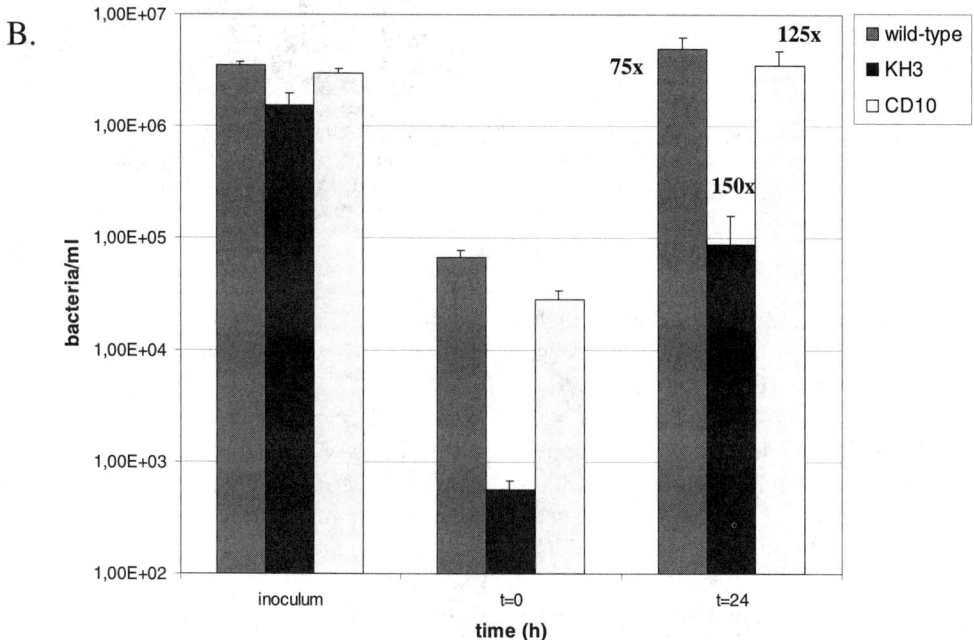

**FIGURE 2** Gentamicin assay of *L. pneumophila* Corby wild-type, the *flaA* mutant strain (KH3), and the complemented mutant strain (CD10) with *A. castellanii* (A) and HL-60 cells (B). Host cells were incubated with legionellae at a multiplicity of infection of 10 for 2 h. Extracellular bacteria were killed by incubation with gentamicin (80 μg/ml) for 1 h, and the CFUs were determined by plating on ABCYE agar plates (*t* = 0). The rate of intracellular multiplication (*t* = 0 to *t* = 24) is given above or beneath the error bars. Error bars indicate the standard deviation obtained from three independent experiments.

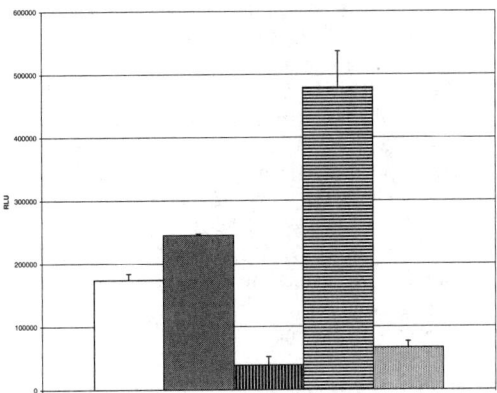

**FIGURE 3** Effects of different environmental factors on the flagellin expression of *L. pneumophila* Corby (pKH23, p*flaA-luxAB* fusion). *L. pneumophila* was grown in YEB medium at 37°C supplemented with 1% glucose, 30 mM serine, 200 mM sucrose (osmolarity), or 6% polyvinylpyrrolidone (PVP) (viscosity). Cells were harvested at the late exponential growth phase and luciferase activity was measured and is given in relative light units (RLU). Error bars indicate the standard deviation obtained from three independent experiments. □, control; ■, 1% glucose; ▦, 30 mM serine; ▤, 200 mM sucrose; ▦, 6% PVP.

flagellated and these strains also contain a *flaA* homologous gene (10, 16).

As mentioned above, the expression of the virulent phenotype of *L. pneumophila* seems to be linked genetically to flagellum expression. Therefore the search for genes regulating *flaA* expression appears to be a good tool for cloning other factors regulating virulence. We screened an expression library of *L. pneumophila* Corby for its ability to reduce expression from a Lp-*flaA* promoter in *E. coli* YK410. Using this approach, we identified a gene locus encoding a DNA binding protein (FlaR), which is a member of the LysR family of transcriptional regulators. Gel retardation experiments revealed that FlaR is able to bind to its own promoter and to a lesser extent to the promoter of the *flaA* gene. Southern blot analysis revealed homologous genes in various *L. pneumophila* strains, but *flaR* seems to be an *L. pneumophila*-specific locus, since no non-*L. pneumophila* strain tested so far showed a homologous gene (13).

## CONCLUSION

The *mip* gene was shown to be a gene commonly found in the genus *Legionella* and it was shown that Mip is a virulence factor of *L. pneumophila* supporting the intracellular survival of *L. pneumophila* in human macrophages. In contrast, the *flaR* gene is an example of an *L. pneumophila*-specific gene. Many virulence genes have been cloned so far, but less is known about their regulation. Analysis of genes influencing *flaA* expression may be a useful tool for cloning factors involved in the regulation of virulence of *L. pneumophila*. The screening and analysis of such factors will contribute to a better understanding of mechanisms regulating the virulence of *L. pneumophila*.

## REFERENCES

1. **Bellinger-Kawahara, C., and M. A. Horwitz.** 1990. Complement component C3 fixes selectively to the major outer membrane protein (MOMP) of *Legionella pneumophila* and mediates phagocytosis of liposome-MOMP complexes by human monocytes. *J. Exp. Med.* **172:**1201–1210.

2. **Bosshardt, S. C., R. F. Benson, and B. S. Fields.** 1997. Flagella are a positive predictor for virulence in *Legionella*. *Microb. Pathog.* **23:**107–112.

3. **Byrne, B., and M. S. Swanson.** 1998. Expression of *Legionella pneumophila* virulence traits in response to growth conditions. *Infect. Immun.* **66:**3029–3034.

4. **Cianciotto, N. P., J. M. Bangsborg, B. I. Eisenstein, and N. C. Engleberg.** 1990. Identification of *mip*-like genes in the genus *Legionella*. *Infect. Immun.* **58:**2912–2918.

5. **Cianciotto, N. P., and B. S. Fields.** 1992. *Legionella pneumophila mip* gene potentiates intracellular infection of protozoa and human macrophages. *Proc. Natl. Acad. Sci. USA* **89:** 5188–5191.

6. **Dietrich, C., K. Heuner, B. C. Brand, J. Hacker, and M. Steinert.** 2001. Flagellum of *Legionella pneumophila* positively affects the early phase of infection of eukaryotic host cells. *Infect. Immun.* **69:**2116–2122.

7. **Dumais-Pope, C., W. O'Connell, and N. P. Cianciotto.** 1993. Distribution and regulation of the *Legionella mip* gene, p. 70–72. *In* J. M. Barbaree, R. F. Breiman, and A. P. Dufour (ed.), *Legionella: Current Status and Emerging Perspectives.* ASM Press, Washington, D.C.

8. **Fischer, G., H. Bang, B. Ludwig, K. Mann, and J. Hacker.** 1992. Mip protein of *Legionella pneumophila* exhibits peptidyl-prolyl-cis/trans isomerase (PPlase) activity. *Mol. Microbiol.* **6:** 1375–1383.

9. **Garduno, R. A., E. Garduno, and P. S. Hoffman.** 1998. Surface-associated hsp60 chaperonin of *Legionella pneumophila* mediates invasion in a HeLa cell model. *Infect. Immun.* **66:**4602–4610.

10. **Heuner, K., L. Bender-Beck, B. C. Brand, P. C. Lück, K.-H. Mann, R. Marre, M. Ott, and J. Hacker.** 1995. Cloning and genetic characterization of the flagellum subunit gene (*flaA*) of *Legionella pneumophila* serogroup 1. *Infect. Immun.* **63:**2499–2507.

11. **Heuner, K., J. Hacker, and B. C. Brand.** 1997. The alternative sigma factor $\sigma^{28}$ of *Legionella pneumophila* restores flagellation and motility to an *Escherichia coli fliA* mutant. *J. Bacteriol.* **179:**17–23.

12. **Heuner, K., B. C. Brand, and J. Hacker.** 1999. The expression of the flagellum of *Legionella pneumophila* is modulated by different environmental factors. *FEMS Microb. Lett.* **175:**69–77.

13. **Heuner, K., C. Dietrich, M. Steinert, U. B. Göbel, and J. Hacker.** 2000. Cloning and characterization of a *Legionella pneumophila* specific gene encoding a member of the LysR family of transcriptional regulators. *Mol. Gen. Genet.* **264:** 204–211.

14. **Köhler, R., A. Bubert, W. Goebel, M. Steinert, J. Hacker, and B. Bubert.** 2000. Expression and use of the green fluorescent protein as a reporter system in *Legionella pneumophila. Mol. Gen. Genet.* **262:**1060–1069.

15. **Ludwig, B., J. Rahfeld, B. Schmidt, K. Mann, E. Wintermeyer, G. Fischer, and J. Hacker.** 1994. Characterization of Mip proteins of *Legionella pneumophila. FEMS Microbiol. Lett.* **118:**23–30.

16. **Ott, M., P. Messner, J. Heesemann, R. Marre, and J. Hacker.** 1991. Temperature-dependent expression of flagella in *Legionella. J. Gen. Microbiol.* **137:**1955–1961.

17. **Pruckler, J. M., R. F. Benson, M. Moyenuddin, W. T. Martin, and B. S. Fields.** 1995. Association of flagellum expression and intracellular growth of *Legionella pneumophila. Infect. Immun.* **63:**4928–4932.

18. **Ratcliff, R. M., S. C. Donnellan, J. A. Lanser, P. A. Manning, and M. W. Heuzenroeder.** 1997. Interspecies sequence differences in the Mip protein from the genus *Legionella*: implications for function and evolutionary relatedness. *Mol. Microbiol.* **25:**1149–1158.

19. **Ratcliff, R. M., J. A. Lanser, P. A. Manning, and M. W. Heuzenroeder.** 1998. Sequence-based classification scheme for the genus *Legionella* targeting the mip gene. *J. Clin. Microbiol.* **36:**1560–1567.

20. **Rowbotham, T. J.** 1986. Current views on the relationships between amoebae, legionellae and man. *Isr. J. Med. Sci.* **22:**678–689.

21. **Schmidt, B., J. Rahfeld, A. Schierhorn, B. Ludwig, J. Hacker, and G. Fischer.** 1994. A homodimer represents an active species of the peptidyl-prolyl cis/trans isomerase FKBP25mem from *Legionella pneumophila. FEBS Lett.* **352:**185–190.

22. **Schmidt, B., S. Konig, D. Svergun, V. Volkov, G. Fischer, and M. H. Koch.** 1995. Small-angle X-ray solution scattering study on the dimerization of the FKBP25mem from *Legionella pneumophila. FEBS Lett.* **372:**169–172.

23. **Schmidt, B., T. Tradler, J. U. Rahfeld, B. Ludwig, B. Jain, K. Mann, K. P. Rucknagel, B. Janowski, A. Schierhorn, G. Kullertz, J. Hacker, and G. Fischer.** 1996. A cyclophilin-like peptidyl-prolyl cis/trans isomerase from *Legionella pneumophila*—characterization, molecular cloning and overexpression. *Mol. Microbiol.* **21:**1147–1160.

24. **Stone, B. J., and Y. Abu Kwaik.** 1998. Expression of multiple pili by *Legionella pneumophila*: identification and characterization of a type IV pilin gene and its role in adherence to mammalian and protozoan cells. *Infect. Immun.* **66:**1768–1775.

25. **Wintermeyer, E., B. Ludwig, M. Steinert, B. Schmidt, G. Fischer, and J. Hacker.** 1995. Influence of site specifically altered Mip proteins on intracellular survival of *Legionella pneumophila* in eukaryotic cells. *Infect. Immun.* **63:**4576–4583.

# LOCALIZATION OF *LEGIONELLA PNEUMOPHILA* Mip PROTEIN INSIDE PHAGOSOMES OF *ACANTHAMOEBA CASTELLANII*

*Jürgen H. Helbig, P. Christian Lück,*
*Enno Jacobs, and Martin Witt*

# 9

More than 10 years ago, genetic analysis successfully characterized for the first time a virulence-associated gene in *Legionella pneumophila*. Following the phenotypic findings, the gene was named *m*acrophage *i*nfectivity *p*otentiator (*mip*) (3, 6). The Mip protein has been shown to contribute to the infection of both protozoa and human macrophages (4). The 24-kDa Mip protein belongs to the FK506 binding protein (FKBP) family of peptidyl-prolyl *cis/trans* isomerases (PPIase) catalyzing the slow *cis/trans* isomerization of prolyl peptide bonds in oligopeptides and proteins (7, 9). However, no experimental evidence demonstrated the necessity of *L. pneumophila* PPIase activity being involved in the pathomechanism of this intracellular bacterium. To get morphological evidence for the virulence association of the Mip protein, we applied the immunogold technique to localize this protein on legionellae before and after invasion of *Acanthamoeba castellanii*, one of the protozoan species that serve as a natural host in the environment.

*A. castellanii* was infected with *L. pneumophila* serogroup 1 strain Corby as described elsewhere (12). This virulent strain is able to multiply 100- to 1,000-fold in *A. castellanii* within 2 days (11). After an incubation time of 4 h at room temperature, protozoa cells were prepared for immunogold electron microscopy. Briefly, cells were fixed by paraformaldehyde, subsequently incubated with sucrose, cryosubstituted with methanol, embedded in Lowicryl HM20 (Plano, Marburg, Germany), and polymerized with UV irradiation. Ultrathin sections were mounted on pioloform-coated slot nickel grids (Plano), preincubated with 10% normal goat serum, and incubated with the Mip-specific monoclonal antibody (MAb) 22/1 (10). After incubation with 10-nm gold conjugated anti-mouse immunoglobulin G (IgG)/IgM (Biocell, Cardiff, United Kingdom), ultrathin sections were contrasted with uranyl acetate and lead citrate, respectively. The MAb 22/1 was established to detect a genus-wide conserved epitope of *Legionella* Mip protein without cross-reactivity to other prokaryotic and eukaryotic cells (10). In addition to localization of Mip protein inside replicative phagosomes of amoeba, agar-grown legionellae were also immunogold-labeled according to the same procedure.

*Jürgen H. Helbig, P. Christian Lück, and Enno Jacobs* Institute of Medical Microbiology and Hygiene, Technical University Dresden, D-1307 Dresden, Germany. *Martin Witt* Institute of Anatomy, Technical University Dresden, D-1307 Dresden, Germany.

*Legionella*, Edited by Reinhard Marre et al.
© 2002 ASM Press, Washington, D.C.

Mip protein of in vitro cultured legionellae is regularly distributed in the bacterial cell wall/cytomembrane complex (Fig. 1). Cytoplasmic localization of the *Legionella* Mip was not detected. Four hours after uptake of agar-grown legionellae by *A. castellanii* cells, Mip protein was localized inside phagosomes of the host cells. Figure 2A shows a *Legionella* cell with immunogold-labeled Mip protein on the bacterial surface. It was surprising to find many gold particles separated from the *Legionella* membranes, in contrast to the number of labeled Mip structures associated with the bacterial outer membrane (Fig. 2A and B). Control staining of noninfected *Acanthamoeba* cells with MAb 22/1 always led to unlabeled compartments (data not shown). These findings make clear that legionellae shed Mip protein inside the phagosome of protozoa. A separation of this protein from fixed bacteria due to the preparation for electron microscopy could be excluded because a directed ultrastructural arrangement on multilamellar structures inside the phagosomes was found (Fig. 2). Bergk et al. (2) reported recently that *Acanthamoeba* produces respirable vesicles contain-

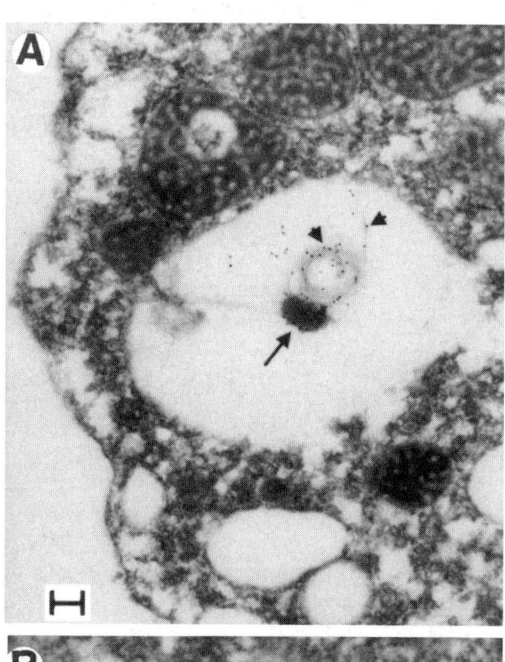

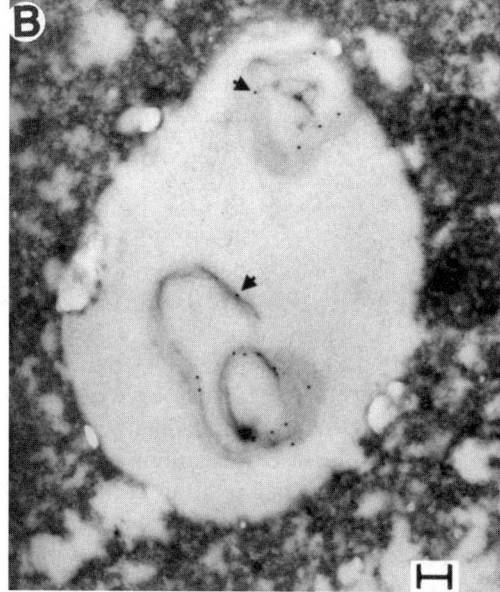

FIGURE 2  *A. castellanii* 4 h after infection with *L. pneumophila*. Ultrathin sections of Lowicryl HM20-embedded cells were labeled with Mip-specific monoclonal antibody MAb 22/1. The arrow points to a *Legionella* cell inside a phagosome (A); arrowheads point to released Mip deposited on membranes with myelin forms (A, B). Bar, 0.5 μm.

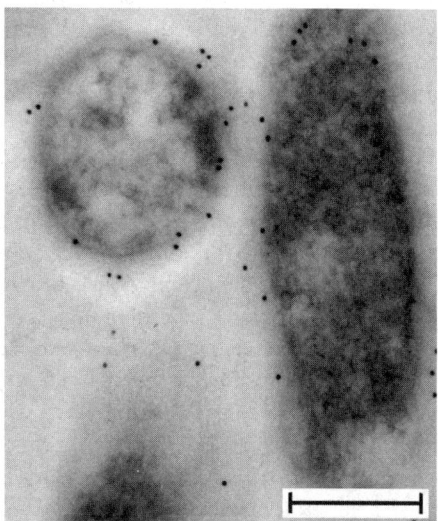

FIGURE 1  Immunogold labeling of agar-grown *L. pneumophila*. Ultrathin sections of Lowicryl HM20-embedded cells were labeled with Mip-specific monoclonal antibody MAb 22/1. Bar, 0.5 μm.

ing live *L. pneumophila* cells. Bacteria in these vesicles appeared to be wrapped in membranes with myelin forms. These multilamellar structures are visible in the phagosomes by using transmission electron microscopy (2). Our study indicated the localization of labeled Mip protein on such multilamellar host cell membranes. Therefore, it can be assumed that the isomerase activity of Mip is also involved in creation of these structures.

In the last years, many studies used transmission electron microscopy for demonstrating the sequence of events of the intracellular infection of amoeba with legionellae (1, 5, 8), as well as the immunogold technique for labeling of host cell proteins such as BiP, which is involved in a chaperoning function of proteins across the membrane of the endoplasmatic reticulum (1). Immunogold labeling of virulence-associated *Legionella* components inside the replicative phagosomes was not performed in these studies. We have found the presence of shedded Mip protein in the early phase of intracellular multiplication of legionellae. Since no information existed on the natural receptor/substrate of the Mip protein PPIase until now, it can only be speculated that isomerase activity is involved in the protein folding process during the infectivity process. Shedded Mip protein molecules, which are integrated in multilamellar membranes inside the phagosome, are more effective than only bacterial membrane-bound enzyme molecules. Our study used only *A. castellanii* as host cells. Nevertheless, shedding of Mip protein inside replicative phagosomes of human macrophages can also be assumed because *L. pneumophila* uses similar mechanisms to parasitize protozoa as well as mammalian host cells (8). Whether mammalian phagosomes are also able to develop multilamellar membranes with integrated Mip protein must be elucidated in further studies.

## ACKNOWLEDGMENTS

We acknowledge Martina Rossmann and Sigrid Gäbler for excellent technical assistance and Volker Bellmann for preparing the photographs.

## REFERENCES

1. **Abu Kwaik, Y.** 1996. The phagosome containing *Legionella pneumophila* within the protozoan *Hartmanella vermiformis* is surrounded by the rough endoplasmic reticulum. *Appl. Environ. Microbiol.* **62:**2022–2028.
2. **Bergk, S. G., R. S. Ting, G. W. Turner, and R. J. Ashburn.** 1998. Production of respirable vesicles containing live *Legionella pneumophila* cells by two *Acanthamoeba* spp. *Appl. Environ. Microbiol.* **64:**279–286.
3. **Cianciotto, N. P., B. I. Eisenstein, C. H. Mody, G. B. Toews, and N. C. Engleberg.** 1989. A *Legionella pneumophila* gene encoding a species-specific surface protein potentiates initiation of intracellular infection. *Infect. Immun.* **57:** 1255–1262.
4. **Cianciotto, N. P., and B. S. Fields.** 1992. *Legionella pneumophila mip* gene potentiates intracellular infection of protozoa and human macrophages. *Proc. Natl. Acad. Sci. USA* **89:** 5188–5191.
5. **Cerillo, J. D., S. Falkow, and L. Tompkins.** 1994. Growth of *Legionella pneumophila* in *Acanthamoeba castellanii* enhances invasion. *Infect. Immun.* **62:**3254–3261.
6. **Engleberg, N. C., C. Carter, D. R. Weber, N. P. Cianciotto, and B.I. Eisenstein.** 1989. DNA sequence of *mip*, a *Legionella pneumophila* gene associated with macrophage infectivity. *Infect. Immun.* **57:**1263–1270.
7. **Fischer, G., H. Bang, B. Ludwig, K. Mann, and J. Hacker.** 1992. Mip protein of *Legionella pneumophila* exhibits peptidyl-prolyl-*cis*/*trans* isomerase (PPIase) activity. *Mol. Microbiol.* **6:** 1375–1383.
8. **Gao, L.-Y., O. S. Harb, and Y. Abu Kwaik.** 1997. Utilization of similar mechanisms by *Legionella pneumophila* to parasitize two evolutionarily distant host cells, mammalian macrophages and protozoa. *Infect. Immun.* **65:**4738–4746.
9. **Hacker, J., and G. Fischer.** 1993. Immunophilins: structure–function relationship and possible role in pathogenicity. *Mol. Microbiol.* **11:** 445–456.
10. **Helbig, J. H., B. Ludwig, P. C. Lück, A. Groh, W. Witzleb, and J. Hacker.** 1995. Monoclonal antibodies to *Legionella* Mip proteins recognize genus- and species-specific epitopes. *Clin. Diagn. Lab. Immunol.* **2:**160–165.
11. **Steinert, M., M. Ott, P. C. Lück, E. Tannich, and J. Hacker.** 1994. Studies on the uptake and intracellular replication of *Legionella pneumophila* in protozoa and in macrophage-like cells. *FEMS Microbiol. Ecol.* **15:**299–308.
12. **Wintermeyer, E., B. Ludwig, M. Steinert, B. Schmidt, G. Fischer, and J. Hacker.** 1995. Influence of site specifically altered Mip proteins on intracellular survival of *Legionella pneumophila* in eukaryotic cells. *Infect. Immun.* **63:**4576–4583.

# CHANGES IN THE *lag-1* LOCUS OF *LEGIONELLA PNEUMOPHILA* SEROGROUP 1 STRAINS RESULT IN DIFFERENT LIPOPOLYSACCHARIDES RECOGNIZED BY MONOCLONAL ANTIBODIES BUT DO NOT INFLUENCE VIRULENCE

*P. Christian Lück, Markus Schuppler, and Jürgen H. Helbig*

## 10

It is well established that *Legionella pneumophila* is an important cause of nosocomial and community-acquired pneumonia (1). *L. pneumophila* serogroup 1, the most prevalent serogroup, can be divided into several subtypes by using monoclonal antibodies (MAb) (3, 5).

Lipopolysaccharide (LPS) produced by *L. pneumophila* is a major immunogenic cell surface determinant that confers serogroup/MAb subgroup specificity (5, 9, 14). *Legionella* LPS can activate both the classical and the alternative complement pathways (14), but it is 1,000-fold less active than *Salmonella* LPS in inducing cytokine secretion in macrophage-like cells (12). Lüneberg et al. (9) showed recently that changes in the LPS MAb binding patterns are associated with changes in the virulence properties of *L. pneumophila*. Despite these findings, the role of the LPS in the pathogenesis of Legionnaires' disease remains obscure.

Several studies showed that a majority of clinical isolates, especially strains associated with outbreaks, carried an LPS epitope that

reacts with MAb 2 of the international standard panel (2, 5) and our MAb 3/1 (3, 4, 7). The epitope recognized by these antibodies has been referred to as the "virulence-associated" antigen. We determined that MAb 3/1 recognizes an epitope associated with the 8-*O*-acetyl group on the legionaminic acid that was identified as the basic component of *L. pneumophila* serogroup 1 LPS (4, 14). Recently, a gene designated *lag-1* was identified that encodes an *O*-acetyl-transferase that is responsible for the O acetylation of the legionaminic acid and the binding of MAb 3/1 to serogroup 1 LPS (13).

We used genetic fingerprinting to investigate several *L. pneumophila* serogroup 1 strains originated from the same source that differed in their reactivity with MAb 3/1 but were indistinguishable or very similar (6). In detail, we analyzed the genetic background responsible for this phenomenon. Furthermore, we investigated whether the loss of the reactivity with MAb 3/1 resulted in differences in the multiplication in *Acanthamoeba castellanii* and macrophage cells.

The strains investigated in this chapter are listed in Table 1. Typing by using MAbs was carried out as described (3, 7). The *lag-1* gene was amplified from chromosomal DNA and sequenced using an ABI 377 sequencer (Ap-

*P. Christian Lück, Markus Schuppler, and Jürgen H. Helbig* Institut für Medizinische Mikrobiologie und Hygiene, TU Dresden, Fiedlerstrasse 42, D-01307 Dresden, Germany.

**TABLE 1** Characterization of the *lag-1* locus in *L. pneumophila* serogroup 1 strains originated from the same source

| Strain | Origin | Monoclonal subtype[a] | Reactivity with MAb 3/1 | Changes in the *lag-1* locus | Intracellular multiplication rate in *Acanthamoeba*[c] |
|---|---|---|---|---|---|
| Corby | Patient | Knoxville | + | Complete gene | 2.43 |
| Corby TF3/1 | Spontaneous mutant | Denver | 0 | Mutation 169 C → T, Ser → Leu | 2.38 |
| Philadelphia-1 (AM511) | Patient | Philadelphia | + | Complete gene | yes (11) |
| CS 322 | Spontaneous mutant | Olda | 0 | Deletion of the complete gene | yes (11) |
| Wien 42 | Water[b] | Philadelphia | + | Complete gene | 1.93 |
| Wien 47-14 | Water | Olda | 0 | Deletion of the complete gene | 2.24 |
| DK 666 | Water[b] | Benidorm | + | Complete gene | 2.90 |
| DK 683 | Water | Bellingham | 0 | Insertion in the *lag* gene (introduction of a stop codon at nucleotide 962 resulting in a truncated ORF) | 1.84 |
| London 11 | Water | Philadelphia | + | Complete gene | nt[d] |
| London 15 | Water | Olda | 0 | Deletion of the complete gene | nt |
| London 12 | Water | Benidorm | + | Complete gene | nt |
| London 17 | Water | Oxford | 0 | Deletion of the complete gene | nt |

[a] According to Joly et al. (7).
[b] Identical strains were isolated from patient.
[c] Multiplication rate is expressed as log-value (CFU at 24 h after infection/CFU at time zero).
[d] nt, not tested.

plied Biosystems, Weiterstadt, Germany). DNA sequences were aligned using the software package Lasergene (DNA-Star Inc.). Pulsed-field gel electrophoresis and Southern blotting were carried out using a CHEF II apparatus (BioRad, Munich, Germany) (6), and nonradioactive detection was conducted with the ECL-kit (Pharmacia-Amersham, Braunschweig, Germany). The intracellular uptake and multiplication in *A. castellanii* and U937 macrophage-like cells was performed as described previously (8). DNA sequence analysis of the *lag-1* locus from *L. pneumophila* serogroup 1 strains revealed that all MAb 3/1-positive strains harbored *lag-1* genes of identical size (1074 bp). The alignment of the *lag-1* sequences showed that strains belonging to the MAb type Philadelphia clustered in one DNA group and strains of the MAb types Knoxville and Benidorm clustered in a second DNA group. Both the DNA and the amino acid sequences of the coding region of the *lag-1* gene revealed only 90% homology between Philadelphia-like and Knoxville/Benidorm-like strains. Within each of these DNA groups, the strains have very similar *lag-1* genes with an identity of more than 99.5%. In all MAb 3/1-positive strains, downstream of the *lag-1* gene, in an opposite orientation, we identified an open reading frame (ORF) that showed high similarity to ORF 2 of the *L. pneumophila* LPS biosynthesis cluster described by Lüneberg et al. (10). Strains not reacting with MAb 3/1 either lost the complete gene or contained a mutation or insertions within the *lag-1* gene, resulting in altered Lag proteins (Table 1). In all strains that lost the *lag-1* gene, ORF 2 of the LPS biosynthesis cluster was found to be adjacent to ORF 3 (10). In strains Corby and Philadelphia (13), the changes in the *lag-1* gene occurred under in vitro conditions. But pairs of MAb 3/1-positive and -negative strains could also be isolated from the same water supplies. Thus, such genetic variations might occur in the environment, too. In summary, our results suggests that the *lag-1* gene may be an unstable genetic element.

We used *A. castellanii*, U937 cells, and primary alveolar macrophages from guinea pigs to determine whether changes in LPS structure result in differences in uptake and intracellular multiplication of the strains Corby, Corby TF 3/1, Wien 42, and Wien 47-14. There were no discernable differences between wild-type strains and the mutants in uptake or intracellular multiplication in each of these host cell systems. These results are in agreement with the observation of Mintz et al., who also found no reduction of virulence characteristics of their *lag-1* mutant (11).

These results suggest that the MAb 3/1 epitope may contribute to the virulence properties of *L. pneumophila* in a subtle manner. Zähringer et al. (14) determined that 8-*O* acetylation of *Legionella* LPS increased the hydrophobicity of legionellae which, in turn, may account for the ability of the organisms to form stable aerosols. Aerolization of contaminated water has been determined to be the major source of transmission during outbreaks of community-acquired Legionnaires' disease. In support of this idea, we found that the majority of clinical isolates from community-acquired cases bound MAb 3/1, whereas only 35% of nosocomial isolates bound this antibody (chapter 52). The data from the present study support this view since in two cases, both MAb 3/1-positive and MAb 3/1-negative strains were isolated from the same environmental source, but only the MAb 3/1-positive strains caused community-acquired pneumonia in two patients. Thus, the MAb 3/1 epitope might be important for infectiousness, but once the legionellae come in close contact to host cells, the ability to infect cells and to multiply within cells does not depend on the presence of the MAb 3/1 epitope. Another explanation for this phenomenon might be that the complex unspecific and specific defense mechanisms in immunocompetent patients enables the elimination of MAb 3/1-negative strains more efficiently.

## ACKNOWLEDGMENTS

We thank Tim G. Harrison, London, United Kingdom; Clifford S. Mintz, Miami, Fla.; Soren A.

Uldum, Copenhagen, Denmark; and Günther Wewalka, Vienna, Austria, for providing *Legionella* strains. We gratefully acknowledge the technical assistance of Jutta Paasche, Sylvia Petsche, Kerstin Seeliger, Susanne Thomas, and Sigrid Gäbler.

This study was supported by the Deutsche Forschungsgemeinschaft (Lu 485/1-2).

## REFERENCES

1. **Breiman, R. F., and J. C. Butler.** 1998. Legionnaires' disease: clinical, epidemiological, and public health perspectives. *Semin. Respir. Infect.* **13:**84–89.
2. **Dournon, E., W. F. Bibb, P. Rajagopalan, N. Desplaces, and R. M. McKinney.** 1988. Monoclonal antibody reactivity as a virulence marker for *Legionella pneumophila* serogroup 1 strains. *J. Infect. Dis.* **157:**496–501.
3. **Helbig, J. H., J. B. Kurtz, M. Castellani Pastoris, C. Pelaz, and P. C. Lück.** 1997. Antigenic lipopolysaccharide components of *Legionella pneumophila* recognized by monoclonal antibodies: possibilities and limitations for division of the species and serogroups. *J. Clin. Microbiol.* **35:** 2841–2845.
4. **Helbig, J. H., P. C. Lück, Y. A. Knirel, W. Witzleb, and U. Zähringer.** 1995. Molecular characterization of a virulence-associated epitope on the lipopolysaccharide of *Legionella pneumophila* serogroup 1. *Epidemiol. Infect.* **115:**71–78.
5. **Joly, J. R., R. M. McKinney, J. H. Tobin, W. F. Bibb, I. D. Watkins, and D. Ramsay.** 1986. Development of a standardized subgrouping scheme for *Legionella pneumophila* serogroup 1 using monoclonal antibodies. *J. Clin. Microbiol.* **23:**768–771.
6. **Lück, P. C., R. J. Birtles, and J. H. Helbig.** 1995. Correlation of MAb subgroups with genotype in closely related *Legionella pneumophila* serogroup 1 strains from a cooling tower. *J. Med. Microbiol.* **43:**50–54.
7. **Lück, P. C., J. H. Helbig, W. Ehret, R. Marre, and W. Witzleb.** 1992. Subtyping of *Legionella pneumophila* serogroup 1 strains isolated in Germany using monoclonal antibodies. *Zentralbl. Bakteriol.* **277:**179–187.
8. **Lück, P. C., J. W. Schmitt, A. Hengerer, and J. H. Helbig.** 1998. Subinhibitory concentrations of antimicrobial agents reduce the uptake of *Legionella pneumophila* into *Acanthamoeba castellanii* and U937 cells by altering the expression of virulence-associated antigens. *Antimicrob. Agents Chemother.* **42:**2870–2876.
9. **Lüneberg, E., U. Zähringer, Y. A. Knirel, D. Steinman, M. Hartmann, I. Steinmetz, M. Rohde, J. Köhl, and M. Frosch.** 1998. Phase-variable expression of lipopolysaccharide contributes to the virulence of *Legionella pneumophila*. *J. Exp. Med.* **188:**49–60.
10. **Lüneberg, E., N. Zetzmann, D. Alber, Y. A. Knirel, O. Kooistra, U. Zähringer, and M. Frosch.** 2000. Cloning and functional characterization of a 30 kb gene locus required for lipopolysaccharide biosynthesis in *Legionella pneumophila*. *Int. J. Med. Microbiol.* **290:**37–49.
11. **Mintz, C. S., and C. H. Zou.** 1992. Isolation and characterization of a lipopolysaccharide mutant of *Legionella pneumophila*. *FEMS Microbiol. Lett.* **93:**249–254.
12. **Neumeister, B., M. Faigle, M. Sommer, U. Zähringer, F. Stelter, R. Menzel, C. Schütt, and H. Northoff.** 1998. Low endotoxic potential of *Legionella pneumophila* lipopolysaccharide due to failure of interaction with the monocyte lipopolysaccharide receptor CD14. *Infect. Immun.* **66:**4151–4157.
13. **Zou, C. H., Y. A. Knirel, J. H. Helbig, U. Zahringer, and C. S. Mintz.** 1999. Molecular cloning and characterization of a locus responsible for O-acetylation of the O-polysaccharide of *Legionella pneumophila* serogroup 1 lipopolysaccharide. *J. Bacteriol.* **181:**4137–4141.
14. **Zähringer, U., Y. A. Knirel, B. Lindner, J. H. Helbig, A. Sonesson, R. Marre, and E. T. Rietschel.** 1995. The lipopolysaccharide of *Legionella pneumophila* serogroup 1 (strain Philadelphia-1): chemical structure and biological significance, p. 113–139. *In Bacterial Endotoxins: Lipopolysaccharides from Gene to Therapy.* Wiley-Liss, Inc., New York, N.Y.

# PHASE VARIATION OF LIPOPOLYSACCHARIDE AND OTHER VIRULENCE DETERMINANTS IN *LEGIONELLA PNEUMOPHILA*

*Edeltraud Lüneberg*

## 11

*Legionella pneumophila* is an intracellular parasite of free-living amoeba species. In natural or man-made freshwater systems, *L. pneumophila* is frequently found in tight association with biofilms. To date, there is no experimental evidence for replication of *Legionella* outside a host cell in its natural habitat. In the human host, *L. pneumophila* is an intracellular pathogen of alveolar macrophages and blood monocytes. Withstanding those different environmental conditions by *L. pneumophila* requires elaborate adaptive response mechanisms.

## PHASE VARIATION IN *L. PNEUMOPHILA*

We have recently described the phase-variable expression of a lipopolysaccharide (LPS) epitope in *L. pneumophila* serogroup 1 strains (3). LPS phase variation is detected with monoclonal antibody (MAb) 2625, which binds the wild-type, but not the phase variant (mutant), strain. The colonies of the mutant can also be distinguished microscopically from the wild-type colonies. Associated with LPS phase variation, we observed the loss of virulence and

serum resistance in the mutant strain. The wild-type strain RC1 replicates in the human macrophage-like cell line HL60 and in the amoeba *Acanthamoeba castellanii* and causes severe pneumonia in the guinea pig animal model. In contrast, the phase variant strain 811 is unable to replicate in HL60 cells (Fig. 1) and in amoebae, and only low numbers of bacteria are recovered from the lungs of infected guinea pigs. Phase variation is promoted under in vivo conditions in the guinea pig animal model as well as upon incubation in heat-inactivated serum, which is suggestive for environmental conditions as a trigger or enhancer of phase variation (3).

Furthermore, electron microscopy studies revealed that the mutant does not express pili and flagella. In addition, the mutant exhibits a less negative net cell surface charge as determined by whole cell electrophoretic mobility assay. The phenotypic alterations affected by phase variation are summarized in Table 1. It is noteworthy that revertands from mutant 811 accomplish full virulence (Fig. 1) and also retain all other phenotypic characteristics of the wild type.

The LPS structure of *L. pneumophila* serogroup 1 has been extensively studied (1, 6). Thorough investigation of the LPS structure by nuclear magnetic resonance (NMR) spec-

*Edeltraud Lüneberg*   Institute of Hygiene and Microbiology, University of Wuerzburg, D-97080 Wuerzburg, Germany.

*Legionella*, Edited by Reinhard Marre et al.

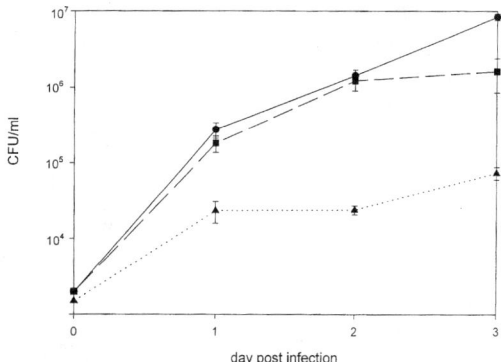

**FIGURE 1** Infection of HL60 cells with *L. pneumophila*. After 2 h of coincubation of host cells and bacteria, extracellularly remaining bacteria were killed by gentamicin. The CFU determined at day 0 therefore represent intracellular bacteria. Symbols: circles, wild-type RC1; triangles, mutant 811; squares, 811-rev. CFU are shown as mean of duplicates. Reprinted from the *Journal of Experimental Medicine* (3) with permission of the publisher.

troscopy of wild-type RC1 and phase-variant 811 revealed a hitherto unknown modification of bacterial polysaccharides in the wild-type strain. N-linked methyl groups as substituents of the 5-acetimidoylamino group of a single legionaminic acid residue could be identified as the epitope or as part of the epitope of MAb 2625 (2).

In a previous study we described cloning and sequencing of a cluster of 25 genes required for LPS biosynthesis in *L. pneumophila* (4). The genes were cloned from the avirulent OLDA strain 5097 (ATCC 43109). The spontaneous, stable LPS mutant 137 (derived from 5097), which did not bind MAb 2625, could

**TABLE 1** Phenotypic characteristics affected by phase variation in *L. pneumophila*

| |
|---|
| Virulence |
| Serum resistance |
| Binding of MAb 2625 |
| N-methyl substitution of legionaminic acid |
| Lipid A structure |
| Piliation |
| Flagellation |
| Net surface charge |

be complemented with open reading frame (ORF) 8 of the gene cluster. ORF 8 exhibited homologies to bacterial methyl transferases. When ORF 8 was deleted in the virulent strain RC1, the resulting mutant 5215 indeed did not bind MAb 2625 and did not carry the N-methyl substituents in its legionaminic acid (2). However, mutant 5215 was as virulent as the parent wild type. These data confirmed our hypothesis that the LPS epitope bound by MAb 2625 does not directly influence the virulence of *L. pneumophila*.

Further differences in the LPS structure of wild-type RC1 and mutant 811 could be observed in the composition of the lipid A moiety. The profile of the primarily long-chain 3-hydroxylated fatty acids was shifted to shorter chains by about two carbons on average in phase-variant 811 compared with wild-type RC1 (chapter 14). These alterations may influence the architecture of the outer membrane of mutant 811, which again could have an impact on susceptibility of the bacteria to serum complement attack.

Virulent *L. pneumophila* strains including RC1 are relatively resistant to lysis by serum complement factors, whereas from the phase-variant strain 811, no viable bacteria could be recovered after 15 min of incubation in 40% normal human serum at 37°C (3). Further investigation of the drastic effect of phase variation on serum resistance revealed that C3b bound to *L. pneumophila* cells is rapidly inactivated, since iC3b is by far the predominant molecule deposited on the bacterial cell surface. Rapid C3b degradation, a mechanism to circumvent further complement activation, seems to be a general property of *L. pneumophila* since it could be observed in all of the numerous investigated strains. In mutant 811, rapid C3b inactivation occurs to an even higher extent than in wild-type RC1. However, in both strains a minor portion of C3b bound to the bacterial cell is not inactivated and proceeds in the activation process to initiate assembly of the membrane attack complex (MAC), as was determined by C5a release. MAC deposition occurs in both strains, wild-type RC1 and mutant 811, but again to a higher extent in mutant 811 (chapter 12). The reason that mutant 811 is efficiently lysed by serum complement and wild-type RC1 is not remains to be defined. Genetically defined mutants with variations in lipid A structure may be a valuable tool to further address this question.

## MOLECULAR MECHANISM OF PHASE VARIATION IN *L. PNEUMOPHILA*

Diversity of surface carbohydrates achieved by means of reversible switching of sugar epitopes has been described for numerous pathogenic bacteria. Changes in the number of tetrametic nucleotides or in the length of polynucleotide stretches by slipped-strand mispairing are responsible for alterations in expression of LPS biosynthesis genes, for example in *Haemophilus influenzae* and in pathogenic *Neisseria*. However, none of the 25 genes involved in LPS biosynthesis of *L. pneumophila* exhibited structural features indicative for a molecular switch mechanism. In contrast, we identified the molecular mechanism responsible for LPS phase variation and loss of virulence in *L. pneumophila* as being attributed to chromosomal insertion and excision of an unstable 30-kb genetic element of presumably phase origin (5). In the virulent wild-type strain RC1, the 30-kb element is located in the chromosome, whereas excision from the chromosome and replication as a high-copy plasmid resulted in the mutant phenotype. Correlation of the presence of the 30-kb element and the occurrence of phase variation was confirmed by investigation of a number of strains other than RC1. Sequence analysis of the 30-kb plasmid revealed 30 putative ORFs. A schematic drawing of the 30-kb plasmid p811 is shown in Fig. 2. Some of the genes exhibited homologies to viral or bacteriophage genes and we therefore presume that the 30-kb element may be of phage origin, even though phage release could not be induced by mitomycin C. The most striking sequence homologies were observed for ORFs B, C, and G, which shared similarities with RecE, RecT, and RusA, re-

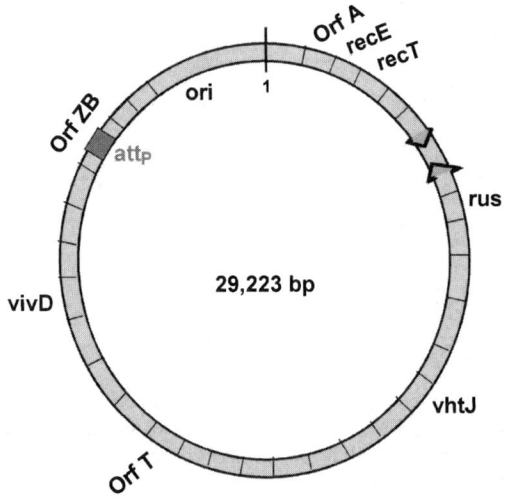

**FIGURE 2** Schematic drawing of the 30-kb plasmid isolated from mutant 811. ORF A is indicated and the other ORFs are positioned clockwise. One putative transcriptional unit starts from ORF A and terminates at ORF E as indicated by an arrowhead. The second predicted transcriptional unit covers ORF ZD to ORF F, the direction of transcription being opposite to ORF A to E. The attachment site located in ORF ZB is indicated (att$_p$). Sequence homologies of some of the ORFs are depicted on the outer side. Reprinted from *Molecular Microbiology* (5) with permission of the publisher.

spectively. These proteins are involved in DNA recombination events. Analysis of *recA* deletion mutants of different *L. pneumophila* strains harboring the 30-kb sequence showed that excision of the 30-kb element from the chromosome occurred in a RecA-independent way (5).

None of the genes encoded on plasmid p811 showed any relatedness to LPS biosynthesis genes, and hence no possible event leading to LPS phase variation could be deduced from the 30-kb sequence. The chromosomal insertion site of the 30-kb element was mapped and sequenced. An 18-bp attachment site was found both on plasmid p811 and on the chromosome. By integration of p811 into the chromosome, ORF ZB on plasmid p811 is interrupted. The chromosomal attachment site is located in an intergenic region and does not interrupt a coding sequence. The genes adjacent to the chromosomal insertion site did not show homologies to known proteins when database searches were performed (5).

By comparative proteome analysis of wild-type RC1 and mutant 811, we identified 28 differentially synthesized proteins. Among those found in the mutant strain but not in the wild-type bacteria were the two proteins encoded by ORF S and ORF T on the 30-kb plasmid. These findings allow the conclusion that genes located on the 30-kb element are expressed during the episomal high-copy plasmid stage.

The mechanism that leads to loss of virulence in the mutant phenotype is presently unknown. From the number of phenotypic alterations observed in the mutant strain upon phase variation (Table 1), the involvement of a regulatory factor can be assumed. It is conceivable that genes encoded on the 30-kb element are abundantly expressed during the episomal stage of the 30-kb element and that those gene products interfere with a regulatory protein in a way that inhibits the normal function of the regulator. However, at this point of our investigation it is not clear what kind of regulator could be affected. It is also conceivable that a site on the 30-kb element is titrating a transcription factor and thereby leads to alterations in gene expression. Over-expression of the genes encoded on p811 and high-copy introduction of the noncoding regions of p811 should identify the site(s) responsible for phase variation in future studies.

The selective advantage of phase variation by means of chromosomal integration and excision of a 30-kb unstable genetic element for survival and virulence of *L. pneumophila* remains to be investigated. Excision of the 30-kb sequence from the chromosome is enhanced under in vivo conditions in the guinea pig animal model and upon serum incubation, a fact that suggests that host factors are involved in this process. On the other hand, the episomal status causes loss of virulence and serum resistance, an obvious disadvantage for infection of a host organism. But

in its natural aquatic environment, *L. pneumophila* may benefit from phase variation by gaining additional adaptive properties. The colony material of the mutant strains is very sticky and appears slimy when suspended in aqueous solutions, which may facilitate adherence to and survival in biofilms outside a host cell and may protect the cells from dehydration as well. However, these hypotheses remain to be investigated and the unstable 30-kb element of *L. pneumophila* may be one mechanism among others to facilitate adaptation of the bacteria. Moreover, phages represent elements that promote genome plasticity by horizontal DNA exchange and we presume that further *L. pneumophila* bacteriophages will be described in the future.

## REFERENCES

1. **Knirel, Y. A., H. Moll, and U. Zähringer.** 1996. Structural study of a highly O-acetylated core of *Legionella pneumophila* serogroup 1 lipopolysaccharide. *Carbohydr. Res.* **293:**223–234.
2. **Kooistra, O., E. Lüneberg, Y. A. Knirel, M. Frosch, and U. Zähringer.** N-methylation in poly-legionaminic acid is associated with the phase-variable epitope of *Legionella pneumophila* serogroup 1 lipopolysaccharide. Submitted.
3. **Lüneberg, E., U. Zähringer, Y. A. Knirel, D. Steinmann, M. Hartmann, I. Steinmetz, M. Rohde, J. Köhl, and M. Frosch.** 1998. Phase-variable expression of lipopolysaccharide contributes to the virulence of *Legionella pneumophila*. *J. Exp. Med.* **188:**49–60.
4. **Lüneberg, E., N. Zetzmann, D. Alber, Y. A. Knirel, O. Kooistra, U. Zähringer, and M. Frosch.** 2000. Cloning and functional characterization of a 30 kb gene locus required for lipopolysaccharide biosynthesis in *Legionella pneumophila*. *Intern. J. Med. Microbiol.* **290:**37–49.
5. **Lüneberg, E., B. Mayer, N. Daryab, O. Kooistra, U. Zähringer, M. Rohde, J. Swanson, and M. Frosch.** 2001. Chromosomal insertion and excision of a 30 kb instable genetic element is responsible for phase variation of lipopolysaccharide and other virulence determinants in *Legionella pneumophila*. *Mol. Microbiol.* **39:**1259–1271.
6. **Zähringer, U., Y. A. Knirel, B. Lindner, J. H. Helbig, A. Sonesson, R. Marre, and E. T. Rietschel.** 1995. The lipopolysaccharide of *Legionella pneumophila* serogroup 1 (strain Philadelphia 1): chemical structure and biological significance. *Prog. Clin. Biol. Res.* **392:**113–139.

# MECHANISM OF SERUM RESISTANCE IN *LEGIONELLA PNEUMOPHILA*: COMPARISON OF WILD-TYPE AND MUTANT STRAINS AFTER PHASE VARIATION OF BACTERIAL SURFACE STRUCTURES

*Felix Gundling, Matthias Frosch, and Edeltraud Lüneberg*

# 12

For pathogenic bacteria, evasion from lysis by serum complement factors in the human host is essential for survival and virulence. Therefore, many pathogens have developed effective strategies to overcome eradication by complement. Such strategies include removal or destruction of complement factors, inhibition of complement activation, or imitation of complement protein by molecular mimicry (9).

*Legionella pneumophila* activates complement via both pathways, the classical and the alternative. The predominant activation was shown to occur through the classical pathway (6, 7). Classical pathway activation by *L. pneumophila* lipopolysaccharide (LPS) required natural immunoglobulin M (IgM) antibodies (6), whereas the major outer membrane protein (MOMP) bound C1q independent of the presence of antibodies (7). Uptake of *L. pneumophila* as an intracellular pathogen of human monocytes and macrophages into its host cells is facilitated by phagocytosis after binding to complement receptors CR1 and CR3. Complement factors C3b and iC3b bind to the *Le-gionella* MOMP (1). Virulent *L. pneumophila* strains, however, are resistant to complement-mediated lysis. Activation of complement is therefore advantageous, since it promotes uptake of legionellae into the host cells. Lysis by complement factors, on the other hand, is efficiently prevented in *L. pneumophila* by hitherto unknown mechanisms.

We have recently described the phase-variable expression of an LPS epitope in *L. pneumophila* serogroup 1 strains (4). LPS phase variation in associated with serum sensitivity and loss of virulence. We identified a 30-kb unstable genetic element as the molecular mechanism for phase variation, which is integrated into the chromosome in the virulent wild-type RC1. Excision of the 30-kb element from the chromosome and replication as a high-copy plasmid results in the avirulent mutant phenotype 811 (5). Wild-type RC1 and the phase-variant mutant 811 exhibited significant differences with regard to resistance to serum complement factors. Strain RC1 was relatively serum resistant, whereas when mutant 811 was incubated with 40% normal human serum at 37°C, no viable bacteria were recovered after 15 min (4). Therefore, the two strains provide a valuable tool for comparative investigation of serum resistance in *L. pneumophila*.

*Felix Gundling, Matthias Frosch, and Edeltraud Lüneberg* Institute of Hygiene and Microbiology, University of Wuerzburg, D-97080 Wuerzburg, Germany.

*Legionella*, Edited by Reinhard Marre et al.
© 2002 ASM Press, Washington, D.C.

## C3 DEPOSITION ON THE
## *L. PNEUMOPHILA* CELL SURFACE

Complement factor C3 is the central molecule of complement activation since it is the converging point of the classical and the alternative pathway. Conversion of C3 to C3b enables covalent binding of C3b to many bacterial surfaces. If particle-bound C3b is not inactivated, it contributes to amplification of the activation process and initation of membrane attack complex (MAC) assembly. Insertion of MAC into the target cell creates a pore and osmotic lysis leads to cell death (3).

First, we were interested to know whether a difference in C3 deposition between wild-type RC1 and mutant 811 could be observed. Bacteria were incubated in 40% normal human serum, which was a pool from 10 healthy donors. *Legionella*-specific antibodies were not detected by standard diagnostic methods (immunofluorescence test) in the sera. After time intervals of 3, 15, and 30 min, reactions were terminated by the addition of EGTA and incubation on ice water. Bacteria were then harvested by centrifugation and after three washing steps, bacterial proteins and serum proteins bound to the bacteria were separated by sodium dodecyl sulfate-polyacrylamide gel electrophoresis (SDS-PAGE). Proteins were subsequently blotted to nitrocellulose membranes, and for detection of C3 bound to the bacterial surface, filter membranes were incubated with monoclonal antibody (MAb) 755, which binds to the $\alpha$-chain of the human C3 molecule. The epitope bound by MAb 755 is located on the 45-kDa iC3b fragment (8).

These experiments revealed that iC3b is by far the most abundant molecule deposited on the *L. pneumophila* surface (Fig. 1). In contrast, C3b deposition is only visible as a very faint band or is even beyond the detection limit of the assay (Fig. 1). These data show that C3b, once bound to *L. pneumophila*, is rapidly degraded. This seems to be a general feature of *L. pneumophila* strains, since numerous strains other than RC1 were investigated with the same result. Immediate breakdown of bound ‚C3b could be one mechanism contributing to

serum resistance in *L. pneumophila*. However, the serum-sensitive mutant strain 811 exhibited an even higher degree of C3b degradation than the parent wild-type RC1 (Fig. 1). Therefore, additional mechanisms must exist in *L. pneumophila* that confer resistance to lysis by serum complement factors.

The predominant complement activation occurred via the classical pathway since only minor activation was observed when the classical pathway was inhibited by addition of EGTA to the reaction mixtures and alternative pathway activation was enabled by addition of $MgCl_2$ (Fig. 1). These findings are in accordance with previous studies on *L. pneumophila* complement activation (6, 7).

## COMPLEMENT ACTIVATION BY
## WILD-TYPE RC1 AND MUTANT 811

Because of the higher extent of C3b degradation observed in mutant 811 in comparison to wild-type RC1, we asked whether this could result from a stronger complement activation by mutant 811. To compare complement activation between the two strains, C3a release was determined. Essentially the same assay conditions as described for investigation of C3 deposition were used, and C3a release was quantified in the supernatant after pelleting of the bacteria. C3a quantification was performed with the aid of a MAb, which is specific to a neoepitope on C3a but does not bind C3 (2). As is shown in Fig. 2A, the amount of C3a release, and therefore C3 activation, is twice as high from mutant 811 as those from wild-type RC1. These differences in C3 activation can at least in part explain the increased iC3b deposition on mutant 811 compared with wild-type RC1.

To determine further complement activation due to the minor portion of not inactivated C3b bound to the *L. pneumophila* surface, C5a release was quantified from the same assay conditions as described before. Again a MAb that binds C5a but not C5 was used (2). C5a release showed the same quantitative relation between 811 and RC1 as was observed for C3a release (Fig. 2B). In contrast,

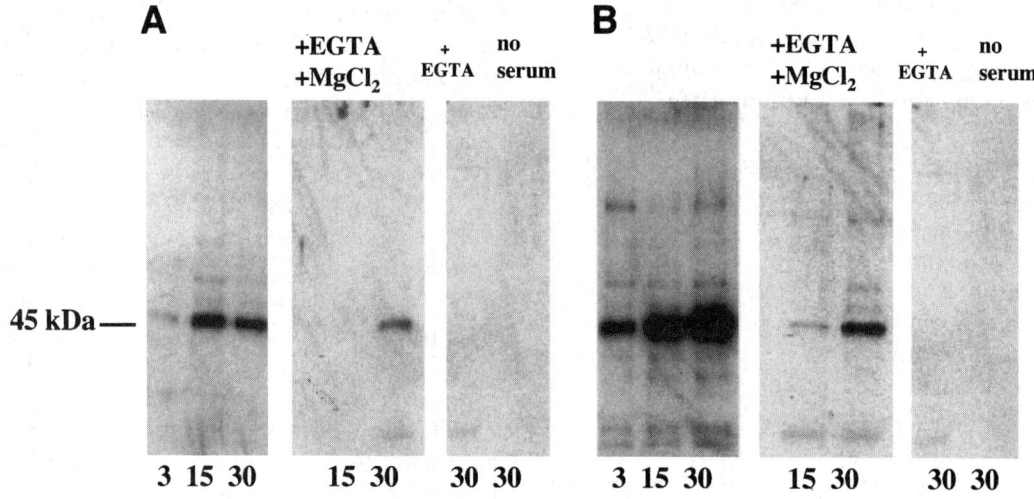

**FIGURE 1** C3 deposition on the cell surface of *L. pneumophila* wild-type strain RC1 (A) and mutant 811 (B) from 40% normal human serum. The predominant 45-kDa band represents the iC3b molecule as immunostained with MAb 755. Reaction mixtures with serum replaced by buffer and with EGTA added to inhibit complement activation were included as controls. Application of identical amounts of protein to each lane was confirmed by silver-stained SDS gels run in parallel.

MAC deposition occurred with comparable amounts on wild-type RC1 and mutant 811 (data not shown). Therefore, for the resistance of wild-type RC1 to complement lysis, hitherto unknown mechanisms must exist. In addition, electron microscopy studies revealed bleb formation in mutant 811 (not shown), which is indicative for membrane destruction.

### CONCLUSION

In summary, stronger complement activation occurs from mutant 811 compared with wild-

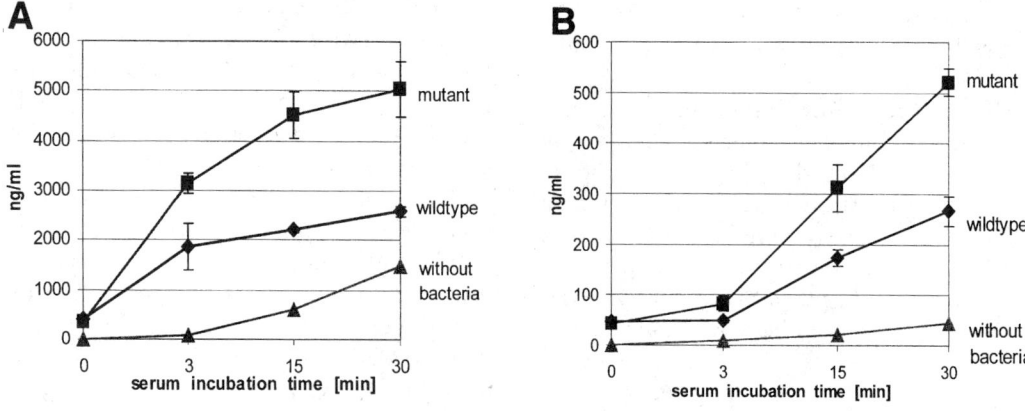

**FIGURE 2** Quantification of C3a release (A) and C5a release (B) from 40% normal human serum after incubation with *L. pneumophila* strains wild-type RC1 and mutant 811. For determination of C3a and C5a amounts, the ABICAP Immunoassay (Abion, Jülich, Germany) was used.

type RC1. Rapid C3b degradation appears to be a common property of *L. pneumophila*. In both strains, RC1 and 811, the most abundant portion of C3b is inactivated and iC3b is the predominant molecule deposited on the *L. pneumophila* surface. However, the amount of MAC bound to the bacteria differs only slightly when wild-type RC1 and mutant 811 are compared. Since RC1 is almost resistant to serum complement attack and 811 is not, additional mechanisms must prevent lysis of RC1. Proper insertion of MAC into the bacterial membrane is an essential prerequisite for lysis of the cell. The differences in lipid A composition observed between RC1 and 811 (chapter 14) could be responsible for the distinct fates of the two strains. However, only the generation and investigation of genetically defined *L. pneumophila* mutants will clarify the role of lipid A architecture in resistance to complement attack.

## REFERENCES

1. **Bellinger Kawahara, C., and M. A. Horwitz.** 1990. Complement component C3 fixes selectively to the major outer membrane protein (MOMP) of *Legionella pneumophila* and mediates phagocytosis of liposome-MOMP complexes by human monocytes. *J. Exp. Med.* **172:**1201–1210.
2. **Hartmann, H., B. Lübbers, M. Casaretto, W. Bautsch, A. Klos, and J. Köhl.** 1993. Rapid quantification of C3a and C5a using a combination of chromatographic and immunoassay procedures. *J. Immunol. Methods* **166:**35–44.
3. **Horstmann, R. D.** 1992. Target recognition failure by the nonspecific defense system: surface constituents of pathogens interfere with the alternative pathway of complement activation. *Infect. Immun.* **60:**721–727.
4. **Lüneberg, E., U. Zähringer, Y. A. Knirel, D. Steinmann, M. Hartmann, I. Steinmetz, M. Rohde, J. Köhl, and M. Frosch.** 1998. Phase-variable expression of lipopolysaccharide contributes to the virulence of *Legionella pneumophila*. *J. Exp. Med.* **188:**49–60.
5. **Lüneberg, E., B. Mayer, N. Daryab, O. Kooistra, U. Zähringer, M. Rohde, J. Swanson, and M. Frosch.** 2001. Chromosomal insertion and excision of a 30 kb instable genetic element is responsible for phase variation of lipopolysaccharide and other virulence determinants in *Legionella pneumophila*. *Mol. Microbiol.* **39:**1259–1271.
6. **Mintz, C. S., D. R. Schultz, P. I. Arnold, and W. Johnson.** 1992. *Legionella pneumophila* lipopolysaccharide activates the classical complement pathway. *Infect. Immun.* **60:**2769–2776.
7. **Mintz, C. S., P. I. Arnold, W. Johnson, and D. R. Schultz.** 1995. Antibody-independent binding of complement component C1q by *Legionella pneumophila*. *Infect. Immun.* **63:**4939–4943.
8. **Vogel, U., A. Weinberger, R. Frank, A. Müller, J. Köhl, J. P. Atkinson, and M. Frosch.** 1997. Complement factor C3 deposition and serum resistance in isogenic capsule and lipo-oligosaccharide sialic acid mutants of serogroup B *Neisseria meningitidis*. *Infect. Immun.* **65:**4022–4029.
9. **Würzner, R.** 1999. Evasion of pathogens by avoiding recognition or eradication by complement, in part via molecular mimicry. *Mol. Immunol.* **36:**249–260.

# CHARACTERIZATION OF THE
# *LEGIONELLA PNEUMOPHILA* DnaJ-LIKE
# PROTEIN DjlA: VIRULENCE
# ATTENUATION OF *djlA* MUTANTS

Werner Brabetz, Helmut Brade,
Matthias Frosch, and Edeltraud Lüneberg

# 13

We have recently described cloning and characterization of the Kdo-transferase-encoding gene *waaA* (*kdtA*) of *Legionella pneumophila* serogroup 1, subgroup Philadelphia (2). Located 155 bp upstream from the *waaA* gene, an 888-bp open reading frame (ORF), which could encode a 296-amino acid protein with a calculated molecular weight of 34.1 kDa, was found. The deduced amino acid sequence revealed homologies to DjlA proteins from other gram-negative bacteria, e.g., 39% identity to DjlA of *Coxiella burnetii* (9), 33% identity to DjlA of *Haemophilus influenzae* (5), and 32% identity to DjlA of *Escherichia coli* (1, 8), respectively. A physical map of the cloning plasmid pLPO28 is depicted in Fig. 1A.

The bacterial DnaJ-like protein DjlA is composed of two functional domains, an N-terminal transmembrane domain of type III topology and a J domain at the C terminus. The J domain mediates binding to DnaK and is in DnaJ chaperone proteins (Hsp40) located at the N terminus. DjlA is considered to be a chaperone/cochaperone involved in assembly and activity of membrane proteins, including two-component signal-transduction systems, e.g., RcsC/RcsB. Colanic acid capsule production in *E. coli* K-12 is regulated via RcsC/RcsB-mediated activation of the *cps* operon. Overexpression of *djlA* in *E. coli* triggers colanic acid polysaccharide capsule synthesis. Colanic acid capsule production is not normally observed in *E. coli* at 37°C, but can be induced by osmotic shock or low temperature and is therefore considered an adaptive response to environmental conditions (3, 4, 6, 7, 9). Since our groups have been interested in bacterial surface polysaccharides for many years, we further investigated the *L. pneumophila* DjlA protein.

## OVEREXPRESSION OF THE
## *L. PNEUMOPHILA djlA* GENE
To overexpress the *L. pneumophila djlA* gene in *L. pneumophila* and in *E. coli*, the gene was subcloned and placed under the control of its own promoter and under the control of the $P_{trc}$ promoter, respectively. The plasmid constructs (Fig. 1B and C) were used to transform *L. pneumophila* and *E. coli* strains. Overexpression of the *L. pneumophila djlA* gene in *E. coli* K-12 resulted in a mucoid phenotype due to colanic acid capsule production. However,

*Werner Brabetz and Helmut Brade*   Department of Immune Chemistry and Biochemical Microbiology, Research Center Borstel, D-23845 Borstel, Germany.   *Matthias Frosch and Edeltraud Lüneberg*   Institute of Hygiene and Microbiology, University of Wuerzburg, D-97080 Wuerzburg, Germany.

*Legionella*, Edited by Reinhard Marre et al.
© 2002 ASM Press, Washington, D.C.

**A)**

pLPO28
6.3 kb

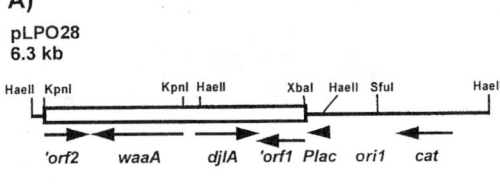

**B)**

pSU2718
2.3 kb

pJKB74
4.0 kb

pJKB75
4.0 kb

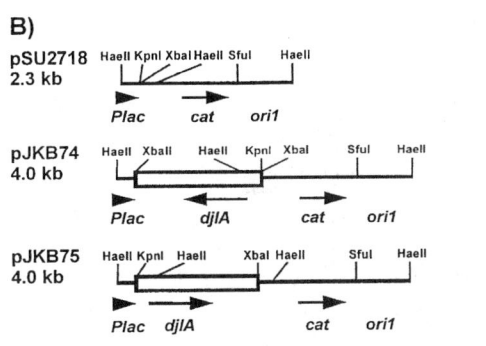

**C)**

pJKB70
4.1 kb

pJKB71
5.0 kb

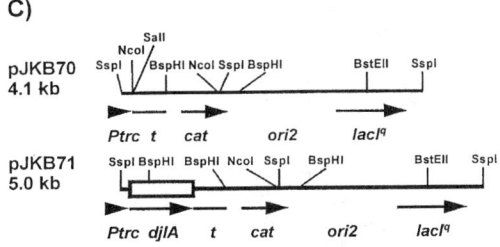

FIGURE 1 (A) Physical map of plasmid pLPO28, which harbors the *L. pneumophila djlA* gene from strain Philadelphia (ATCC 33152). (B) Plasmid constructs for overexpression of the *L. pneumophila djlA* gene with its own promoter. (C) Plasmids constructed for *djlA* overexpression under p$_{trc}$ control.

overexpression of the *L. pneumophila djlA* gene under p$_{trc}$ control was lethal to *E. coli* at 37°C (Table 1). Induction of the p$_{trc}$ promoter by IPTG (isopropyl-β-D-thiogalactopyranoside) caused lethality also at 30°C in *E. coli*. These results are in accordance with previous studies on the *C. burnetii* (9) and *E. coli* (7) *djlA* gene, respectively, and suggest that *djlA* is normally tightly regulated.

In contrast, in *L. pneumophila*, p$_{trc}$-mediated *djlA* overexpression was lethal to the bacteria at any of the investigated temperatures, whereas *L. pneumophila* was able to tolerate moderate *djlA* overexpression under the con-

trol of the *L. pneumophila djlA* promoter (Table 1).

## DELETION OF THE *djlA* GENE IN *L. PNEUMOPHILA*

To further characterize the functional importance of the *djlA* gene product in *L. pneumophila*, we constructed *djlA* deletion mutants. From sequence analysis of pLPO28 the *djlA* gene did not appear to be organized in an operon, but rather represented a monocistronically transcribed gene (Fig. 1A). The *djlA* gene was interrupted by deletion of an internal 600-bp *Bsm*I fragment and insertion of a kanamycin resistance cassette. The construct was ligated into plasmid pLAW344, which allows counter-selection for homologous recombination due to the presence of the *sacB* gene. The resulting plasmid pMH32 was used to transform the *L. pneumophila* serogroup 1 strains OLDA RC1, OLDA R458, Philadelphia AM511, and Corby, respectively. Homologous recombination by double cross-over was confirmed by Southern blot analysis and PCR in the mutant strains. The *djlA* mutants of all four strains did not exhibit alterations in growth rate in buffered yeast extract (BYE) broth when compared with the appropriate wild type, suggesting that *djlA* is not an essential gene in *L. pneumophila*. In *E. coli*, *djlA* also proved not to be essential for viability of the bacteria (4, 7, 9). Cell morphology was investigated by Gram stain and immunofluorescence testing and was found to be unaffected in the *L. pneumophila djlA* mutants. Also, we did not observe any alterations in the LPS phenotype, as determined with the monoclonal antibody typing panel. Incubation with a pool of 40% normal human serum revealed that the *djlA* mutants were as serum-resistant as the parent wild-type strains.

## VIRULENCE ATTENUATION OF *djlA* MUTANTS

The *djlA* mutant strains RC1 *djlA*⁻, R458 *djlA*⁻, AM511 *djlA*⁻ and Corby *djlA*⁻, respectively, were assessed for virulence in the HL-60 infection assay. The human

**TABLE 1**  Overexpression of the *L. pneumophila djlA* gene in *E. coli* and in *L. pneumophila*

| Strain | Plasmid | Description | Growth at following temperature[c] | | |
|---|---|---|---|---|---|
| | | | 25°C | 30°C | 37°C |
| *L. pneumophila*[a] | pSU2718 | Control plasmid | + | + | + |
| *L. pneumophila*[a] | pJKB74 | *djlA* promoter | + | + | + |
| *L. pneumophila*[a] | pJKB75 | *djlA* promoter | + | + | + |
| *E. coli*[b] | pSU2718 | Control plasmid | ND | ND | + |
| *E. coli*[b] | pJKB74 | *djlA* promoter | +/m | +/m | +/m |
| *E. coli*[b] | pJKB75 | *djlA* promoter | +/m | +/m | +/m |
| *L. pneumophila*[a] | pJKB70 | Control plasmid | + | + | + |
| *L. pneumophila*[a] | pJKB71 | $p_{trc}$ promoter | − | − | − |
| *E. coli*[b] | pJKB70 | Control plasmid | + | + | + |
| *E. coli*[b] | pJKB71 | $p_{trc}$ promoter | +/m | +/m | − |

[a] *L. pneumophila* strains Philadelphia (ATCC 33152) and RC1 (subgroup OLDA) were transformed with identical results in both strains.
[b] Transformation of *E. coli* strains DH5α and XL1Blue revealed identical results.
[c] +, viable transformants isolated; −, no viable bacteria following transformation; m, mucoid phenotype.

macrophage-like cell line was infected with the bacteria, and plating at 24, 48, and 72 h postinfection was performed to determine the number of viable bacteria. Whereas the wild-type strains replicated by 2 to 3 logs within 3 days postinfection, the number of mutant bacteria increased by only 1 log. The obtained CFU counts for strains R458 and Corby and the corresponding mutants are depicted in Fig. 2. Thus, deletion of the *djlA* gene resulted in reduced virulence in all investigated *L. pneumophila* strains.

To our knowledge, this is the first report of an influence on virulence by the *djlA* gene

product in pathogenic bacteria. However, we do not know by which mechanism virulence attenuation is achieved in the *L. pneumophila djlA* mutants.

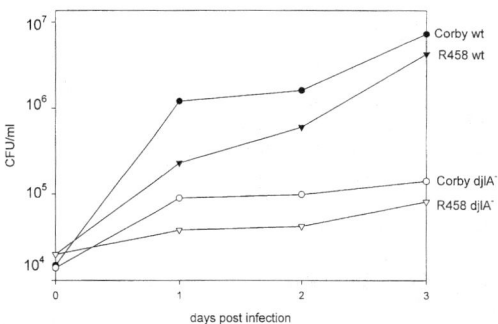

**FIGURE 2**  Infection of HL-60 cells with *L. pneumophila* wild-type and *djlA* mutant strains. Bacterial CFU were determined at 24, 48, and 72 h postinfection and are shown as means of duplicate values. Experiments were repeated three times.

**REFERENCES**

1. **Blattner, F. R., G. Plunkett III, C. A. Bloch, N. T. Perna, V. Burland, M. Riley, J. Collado-Vides, J. D. Glassner, C. K. Rode, G. F. Mayhew, J. Gregor, N. W. Davis, H. A. Kirkpatrick, M. A. Goeden, D. J. Rose, B. Mau, and Y. Shao.** 1997. The complete genome sequence of *Escherichia coli* K-12. *Science* **277:**1453–1474.

2. **Brabetz, W., C. E. Schirmer, and H. Brade.** 2000. 3-Deoxy-D-*manno*-oct-2-ulosonic acid (Kdo) transferase of *Legionella pneumophila* transfers two Kdo residues to a structurally different lipid A precursor of *Escherichia coli. J. Bacteriol.* **182:**4654–4657.

3. **Clarke, D. J., I. B. Holland, and A. Jacq.** 1997. Point mutations in the transmembrane domain of DjlA, a membrane-linked DnaJ-like protein, abolish its function in promoting colanic acid production via the Rcs signal transduction pathway. *Mol. Microbiol.* **25:**933–944.

4. **Clarke, D. J., A. Jacq, and I. B. Holland.** 1996. A novel DnaJ-like protein in *Escherichia coli* inserts into the cytoplasmic membrane with a type III topology. *Mol. Microbiol.* **20:**1273–1286.

5. **Fleischmann, R. D., M. D. Adams, O. White, R. A. Clayton, E. F. Kirkness, A. R. Kerlavage, C. J. Bult, J.-F. Tomb, B. A. Dougherty, J. M. Merrick, K. McKenney, G. Sutton, W. Fitzhugh, C. A. Fields, J. D. Gocayne, J. D. Scott, R. Shirley, L.-E. Liu,**

A. Glodek, J. M. Kelley, J. F. Weidman, C. A. Phillips, T. Spriggs, E. Hedblom, M. D. Cotton, T. R. Utterback, M. C. Hanna, D. T. Nguyen, D. M. Saudek, R. C. Brandon, L. D. Fine, J. L. Fritchman, J. L. Fuhmann, N. S. M. Geoghagen, C. L. Gnehm, L. A. McDonald, K. V. Small, C. M. Fraser, H. O. Smith, and J. C. Venter. 1995. Whole-genome random sequencing and assembly of *Haemophilus influenzae* Rd. *Science* **269:**496–512.

6. **Genevaux, P., A. Wawrzynow, M. Zylicz, C. Georgopoulos, and W. L. Kelley.** 2001. DjlA is a third DnaK co-chaperone of *Escherichia coli* and DjlA-mediated induction of colanic acid capsule requires DjlA-DnaK interaction. *J. Biol. Chem.* **276:**7906–7912.

7. **Kelley, W. J., and C. Georgopoulos.** 1997. Positive control of the two-component RcsC/B signal transduction network by DjlA: a member of the DnaJ family of molecular chaperones in *Escherichia coli. Mol. Microbiol.* **25:**913–931.

8. **Yura, T., H. Mori, H. Nagai, T. Nagata, A. Ishihama, N. Fujita, K. Isono, K. Mizobuchi, and A. Nakata.** 1992. Systematic sequencing of the *Escherichia coli* genome: analysis of the 0-2.4 min region. *Nucleic Acids Res.* **20:**3305–3308.

9. **Zuber, M., T. A. Hoover, and D. L. Court.** 1995. Analysis of a *Coxiella burnetii* gene product that activates capsule synthesis in *Escherichia coli:* requirement for the heat shock chaperone DnaK and the two-component regulator RcsC. *J. Bacteriol.* **177:**4238–4244.

# PHASE VARIATION IN *LEGIONELLA PNEUMOPHILA* SEROGROUP 1, SUBGROUP OLDA, STRAIN RC1 INFLUENCES LIPID A STRUCTURE

*Oliver Kooistra, Yuriy A. Knirel, Edeltraud Lüneberg, Matthias Frosch, and Ulrich Zähringer*

## 14

## PHASE VARIATION IN *LEGIONELLA PNEUMOPHILA*

A change in the lipopolysaccharide (LPS) upon phase variation in *L. pneumophila* serogroup 1, subgroup OLDA, wild-type strain RC1 was detected with the aid of LPS-specific monoclonal antibody MAb 2625 (5). A spontaneous mutant strain, termed 811, was isolated and found to be negative for MAb 2625 binding, avirulent in animal model, and serum sensitive. In contrast to the parental virulent wild-type strain RC1, phase-variant strain 811 (i) exhibits a significantly reduced ability to replicate in guinea pigs, (ii) is unable to replicate intracellularly in the macrophage-like cell line HL-60, and (iii) is lysed by serum complement components (5). Preliminary data obtained with the whole LPS in a tumor necrosis factor-$\alpha$ induction assay suggested that LPS of phase-variant 811 has an attenuated inducing potential on mononuclear cells compared with that of wild-type RC1.

Chromosomal insertion and excision of a 30-kb instable genetic element of possibly phage origin was identified as the molecular mechanism for phase variation. In the wild-type strain, the 30-kb element is located on the chromosome, whereas excision from the chromosome and replication as a high-copy plasmid result in the phase-variant phenotype, which is characterized by an alteration in an LPS epitope and the loss of virulence (4).

## *LEGIONELLA PNEUMOPHILA* LPS STRUCTURE

The chemical structure of *L. pneumophila* serogroup 1 strain Philadelphia 1 LPS has been extensively studied (11). The O-antigen of the LPS is a homopolymer of the 5-*N*-acetimidoyl-7-*N*-acetyl derivative of 5,7-diamino-3,5,7,9-tetradeoxy-D-*glycero*-D-*galacto*-non-2-ulosonic acid, termed legionaminic acid (1, 10). Similarities in the biosynthesis pathway of legionaminic acid and neuraminic acid (5-amino-3,5-dideoxy-D-*glycero*-D-*galacto*-non-2-ulosonic acid) have been described (6). In serogroup 1 strains of the Pontiac group containing the O-acetyl transferase-encoding gene *lag-1* (12), e.g., strain Philadelphia 1, legionaminic acid is quantitatively 8-O-acetylated (1). In all serogroup 1 strains, including those of subgroup OLDA,

*Oliver Kooistra and Ulrich Zähringer* Division of Immunochemistry, Research Center Borstel, Center for Medicine and Biosciences, D-23845 Borstel, Germany. *Edeltraud Lüneberg and Matthias Frosch* Institute for Hygiene und Microbiology, University of Würzburg, D-97080 Würzburg, Germany. *Yuriy A. Knirel* N. D. Zelinsky Institute of Organic Chemistry, Russian Academy of Sciences, 117913 Moscow, Russia.

*Legionella*, Edited by Reinhard Marre et al.
© 2002 ASM Press, Washington, D.C.

the first three legionaminic acid residues next to the core in the short-O-antigen LPS (<10 legionaminic acid residues) are 8-O-acetylated in a *lag-1*-independent manner (3).

The core of the LPS is a nonasaccharide that lacks heptose and phosphate, contains abundant 6-deoxy sugars, and is highly O- and N-acetylated (2, 3, 8). The lipid A of *L. pneumophila* strain Philadelphia 1 consists of a 1,4'-bisphosphorylated backbone of a β-(1 → 6)-linked disaccharide of 2,3-diamino-2,3-dideoxyglucose, β-Glc*p*N3N-(1 → 6)-Glc*p*N3N (11), substituted with unusual long-chain, branched, and dihydroxylated fatty acids (7), the features that may account for its low endotoxic potential (9).

## THE INFLUENCE OF PHASE VARIATION ON THE POLYSACCHARIDE STRUCTURE OF LPS

The MAb 2625 epitope is present in wild-type RC1 cells and is lost in the spontaneous mutant 811 upon phase variation. Nuclear magnetic resonance (NMR) spectroscopic studies revealed a hitherto unknown modification of bacterial polysaccharides in wild-type RC1, namely N-methylation of the 5-acetimidoylamino group of a single legionaminic acid residue located in the O-antigen proximal to the core. Two major N-methylated substituents, the (N,N-dimethylacetimidoyl)amino and acetimidoyl(N-methyl)amino groups, could be allocated to the long-O-antigen (>30 legionaminic acid residues) and middle-O-antigen (~15 legionaminic acid residues) LPS species, respectively. N-Methylation of legionaminic acid that was suppressed in phase-variant 811 correlated with the presence of the MAb 2625 epitope (O. Kooistra, E. Lüneberg, Y. A. Knirel, M. Frosch, and U. Zähringer, submitted for publication). A gene locus required for LPS biosynthesis was characterized (6), and genes responsible for biosynthesis of the MAb 2625 epitope were identified and deleted. The resultant isogenic mutant did not bind MAb 2625, but was as virulent as the parental wild-

type strain and, therefore, N-methylation is not required for virulence (Kooistra et al., submitted).

Comprehensive analysis using NMR spectroscopy and matrix-assisted laser desorption ionization–time of flight mass spectrometry (MALDI-TOF MS) of the core oligosaccharide of wild-type RC1 and phase-variant 811 revealed no structural differences from each other and from the strain Philadelphia 1 core oligosaccharide studied earlier (2, 3, 8).

## THE INFLUENCE OF PHASE VARIATION ON THE LIPID A STRUCTURE

Lipid A was prepared by mild acid hydrolysis (0.1 M NaOAc-HOAc buffer, pH 4.4, 100°C, 4 h) of LPS each of wild-type RC1 and phase-variant 811 followed by centrifugation and lyophilization of the pellet. The crude preparation was purified by high-pressure liquid chromatography (HPLC); fractions containing lipid A were detected by thin-layer chromatography (TLC), appropriately pooled, extracted with chloroform, and dried.

The lipid A backbone of each strain was analyzed after mild hydrazinolysis (37°C, 30 min) and strong alkaline hydrolysis (4 M KOH, 120°C, 16 h) of lipid A followed by gel-permeation chromatography of the water-soluble portion. Two-dimensional NMR spectroscopic studies, including $^1$H, $^1$H COSY, TOCSY, H-detected $^1$H, $^{13}$C HMQC, and H-detected $^1$H, $^{31}$P HMQC, revealed that both strains shared the same 1,4'-bisphosphorylated β-D-Glc*p*N3N-(1 → 6)-α-D-Glc*p*N3N disaccharide backbone as found earlier in strain Philadelphia 1 (11). The D configuration of GlcN3N was confirmed by gas-liquid chromatography (GLC) analysis of the acetylated (R)-2-butyl glycosides compared with the derivatives obtained from the authentic compound.

Fatty acids of lipid A from each strain were analyzed by GLC and combined GLC/MS as the methyl esters prepared by methanolysis (2 M HCl/MeOH, 24 h, 120°C) followed by trimethylsilylation with N,O-bis-

(trimethylsilyl)-trifluoroacetamide, as described (7). Analysis revealed the presence in both strains of comparable amounts of the secondary nonhydroxylated fatty acids and the characteristic very-long-chain fatty acids [27:0(1,27-dioic) and 28:0(27-oxo)] (Table 1), which are typically linked to the primary mono- and di-hydroxylated fatty acids (11). The content of the primary short-chain branched (*iso* and *anteiso*) and normal 3-hydroxylated and 2,3-dihydroxylated tetradecanoic acid [14:0(3-OH) and 14:0(2,3-di-OH)] that are amide-bound at positions 3 and 3′ of the GlcN3N-

disaccharide (11), was similar in both strains as well (Table 1). However, the profile of the primary long-chain 3-hydroxylated fatty acids that are amide-bound at positions 2 and 2′ of the GlcN3N-disaccharide (11) was shifted to shorter chains, on average by about two carbons in phase-variant 811 compared with wild-type RC1 (Table 1). In wild-type RC1, the major fatty acid was identified as *n*20:0(3-OH) and was accompanied by lower amounts of *n*18:0(3-OH), *n*19:0(3-OH), *n*21:0(3-OH), and *n*22:0(3-OH). In phase-variant 811, mainly *n*16:0(3-OH) and *n*18:0(3-OH) were present, together with rel-

**TABLE 1**  Fatty acid composition of lipid A from wild-type RC1 and phase-variant 811[a]

| Fatty acid[b] | nmol of fatty acid/mg of lipid A[c] | |
|---|---|---|
| | Wild-type RC1 | Phase-variant 811 |
| *i*14:0 | 6.60 | 5.65 |
| *i*15:0 | 8.20 | 9.40 |
| *a*15:0 | 14.65 | 12.17 |
| *i*16:0 | 89.21 | 101.23 |
| *n*16:0 | 35.43 | 24.97 |
| *i*17:0 | 5.13 | 5.33 |
| *a*17:0 | 34.16 | 37.72 |
| *i*18:0 | 11.27 | 5.94 |
| *i*14:0(2,3-di-OH) | 82.18 | 89.01 |
| *n*14:0(2,3-di-OH) | 13.70 | 9.30 |
| *i*14:0(3-OH) | 132.00 | 148.89 |
| *n*14:0(3-OH) | 17.99 | 16.28 |
| *a*15:0(3-OH) | 3.76 | 6.29 |
| *i*16.0(3-OH) | 0.81 | 10.66 |
| *n*16:0(3-OH) | 3.80 | 33.33 |
| *n*17:0(3-OH) | 3.95 | 21.36 |
| *i*18:0(3-OH) | 4.73 | 20.38 |
| *n*18:0(3-OH) | 34.49 | 54.65 |
| *a*19:0(3-OH) | 6.30 | 8.73 |
| *n*19:0(3-OH) | 14.80 | 18.47 |
| *i*20:0(3-OH) | 10.94 | 5.24 |
| *n*20:0(3-OH) | 90.83 | 10.95 |
| *n*21:0(3-OH) | 21.28 | 1.79 |
| *i*22:0(3-OH) | 11.10 | 0.03 |
| *n*22:0(3-OH) | 11.75 | 0.03 |
| 27:0(1,27-dioic) | 17.87 | 37.87 |
| 28:0(27-oxo) | 25.95 | 44.69 |

[a] The content of the fatty acids was calculated using response factors and was related to *n*13:0(3-OH), *n*17:0, and *n*28:0, which served as internal standards.

[b] Fatty acids are denoted by the total number of carbons with prefixes *a* for *anteiso*-branching, *i* for *iso*-branching, *n* for normal chain, and OH for hydroxyl substitution with the position indicated.

[c] Fatty acids present in both strains in a content less than 5 nmol mg$^{-1}$ are not shown.

atively high amounts of n17:0(3-OH), i18:0(3-OH), and n19:0(3-OH), but almost no 3-hydroxylated fatty acids with a longer chain than 20 carbons.

These results were confirmed by negative ion mode MALDI-TOF MS of purified lipid A. To simplify the interpretation of the complex mass spectra, the heterogeneity caused by the acyloxyacyl residues was eliminated by de-O-acylation with anhydrous hydrazine (37°C, 30 min). The MALDI-TOF mass spectra of the resultant tetraacyl lipid A clearly showed the profile of the amide-linked fatty acids (Fig. 1). In wild-type RC1, the major tetraacyl lipid A species contained one residue each of 14:0(3-OH) and 14:0(2,3-di-OH) and two

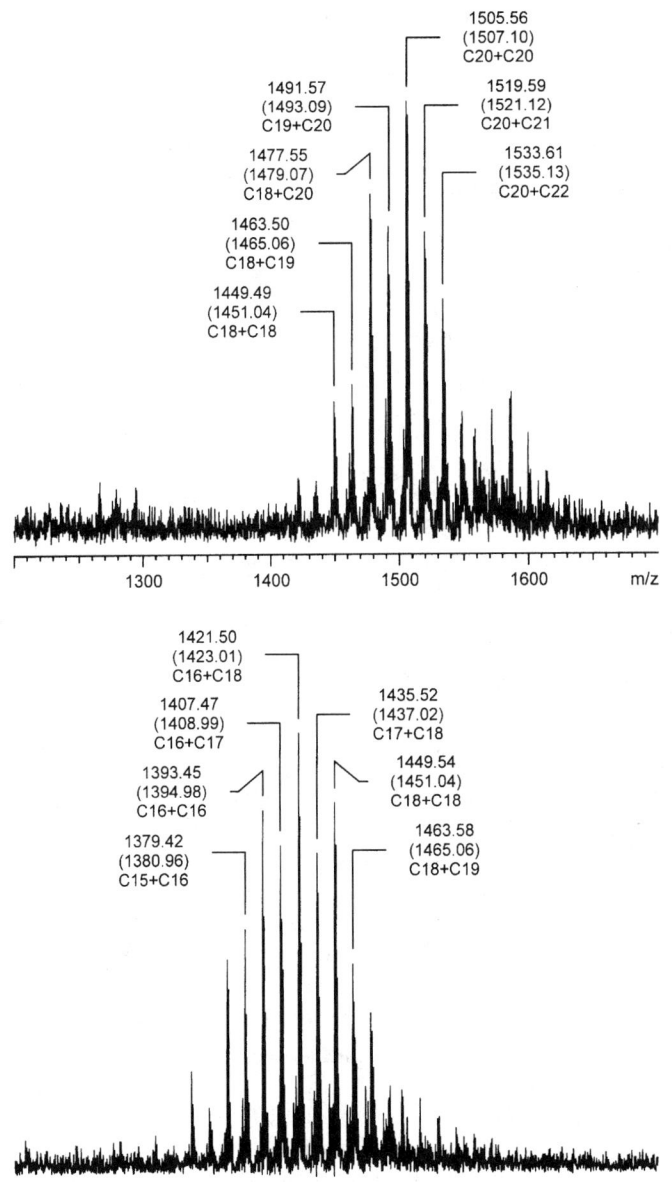

**FIGURE 1** Parts of negative ion mode MALDI-TOF mass spectra of tetraacyl lipid A from *L. pneumophila* serogroup 1, subgroup OLDA, wild-type RC1 (top panel) and phase-variant 811 (bottom panel). Tetraacyl monophosphoryl lipid A was prepared by de-O-acylation with hydrazine; one of the phosphate groups (most likely at position 1) was split, probably due to overheating during work-up of the reaction mixture with acetone. The $m/z$ value for [M-H]$^-$ ions, the calculated chemical molecular mass (in parentheses), and the deduced chain length (the total number of carbons) of the 3-hydroxylated fatty acids at positions 2 and 2′ are given for each major ion peak of tetraacyl lipid A with one residue each of 14:0(3-OH) and 14:0(2,3-di-OH) at positions 3 and 3′. The mass spectra were acquired in reflector configuration with 2,5-dihydroxybenzoic acid as matrix.

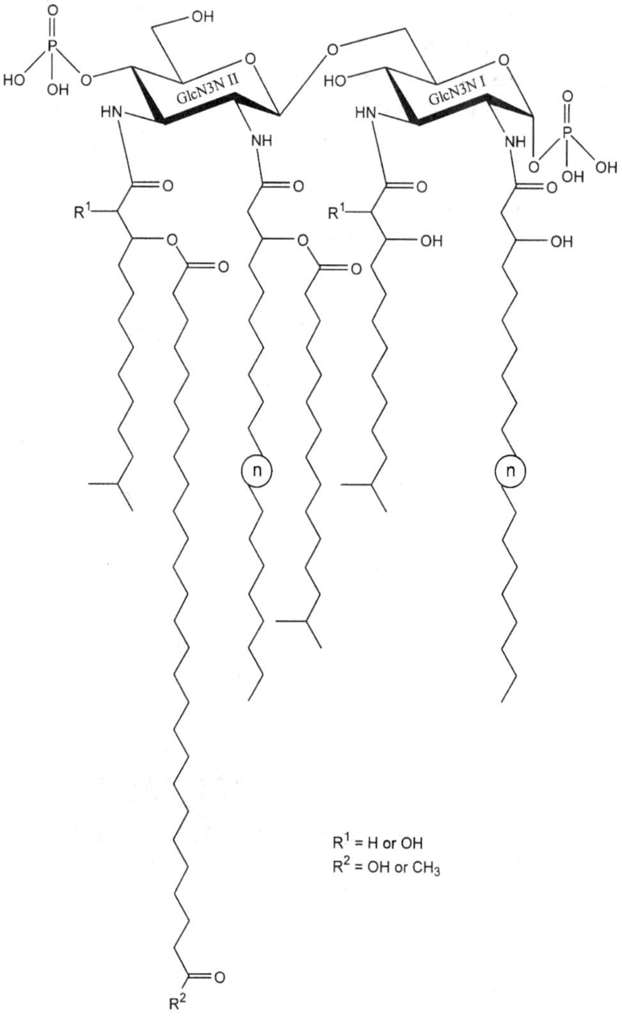

**FIGURE 2** Proposed structure of the major lipid A from *L. pneumophila* serogroup 1, subgroup OLDA, wild-type RC1, and phase-variant 811. The position of the fatty acids is shown according to published data (11). The chain length of the 3-hydroxylated fatty acids at positions 2 and 2′ is indicated as the total number of carbons $n = 20$ at both GlcN3N residues in wild-type RC1. In the avirulent phase variant 811, the chain length of the 3-hydroxylated fatty acids at positions 2 and 2′ is $n = 16$ at one and $n = 18$ at the other GlcN3N residue.

residues of 20:0(3-OH) (Fig. 2). In phase-variant 811, the major species contained one residue each of 14:0(3-OH), 14:0(2,3-di-OH), 16:0(3-OH), and 18:0(3-OH) (Fig. 2). Analysis of in-source laser-induced fragment ions for the monomers from the tetraacyl lipid A of phase-variant 811 showed the even distribution of the 3-hydroxylated fatty acids among the two GlcN3N residues in the lipid A backbone.

## CONCLUSIONS

The data obtained demonstrated that various phenotypic alterations may occur upon phase variation in *L. pneumophila* serogroup 1, and the loss of the MAb 2625 epitope is only one of them. LPS biosynthesis pathways involved in assembly of lipid A were also affected by phase variation, which resulted in a specifically altered lipid A structure with a modified profile of fatty acids of a particular type. The core oligosaccharide, the lipid A backbone, and the lipid A phosphorylation pattern remained unaffected.

These data suggested that phase variation in *L. pneumophila* is regulated by a complex interplay of different genes. Phase variation may affect a regulatory factor, which influences

LPS biosynthesis, virulence, and serum resistance. Further studies are necessary to elucidate such a factor(s) and its role in the bacterial cell.

## ACKNOWLEDGMENTS

We thank B. Lindner and H. Lüthje for performing MALDI-TOF MS, H.-P. Cordes for running NMR spectra, H. Moll for expert help with GLC/MS, and K. Jakob for skillful technical assistance.

## REFERENCES

1. **Knirel, Y. A., E. T. Rietschel, R. Marre, and U. Zähringer.** 1994. The structure of the O-specific chain of *Legionella pneumophila* serogroup 1 lipopolysaccharide. *Eur. J. Biochem.* **221:**239–245.
2. **Knirel, Y. A., H. Moll, and U. Zähringer.** 1996. Structural study of a highly O-acetylated core of *Legionella pneumophila* serogroup 1 lipopolysaccharide. *Carbohydr. Res.* **293:**223–234.
3. **Kooistra, O., E. Lüneberg, B. Lindner, Y. A. Knirel, M. Frosch, and U. Zähringer.** 2001. Complex O-acetylation in *Legionella pneumophila* serogroup 1 lipopolysaccharide. Evidence for two genes involved in 8-O-acetylation of legionaminic acid. *Biochemistry* **40:**7630–7640.
4. **Lüneberg, E., B. Mayer, N. Daryab, O. Kooistra, U. Zähringer, M. Rohde, J. Swanson, and M. Frosch.** 2001. Chromosomal insertion and excision of 30 kb instable genetic element is responsible for phase variation of lipopolysaccharide and other virulence determinants in *Legionella pneumophila. Mol. Microbiol.* **39:**1259–1271.
5. **Lüneberg, E., U. Zähringer, Y. A. Knirel, D. Steinmann, M. Hartmann, I. Steinmetz, M. Rohde, J. Kohl, and M. Frosch.** 1998. Phase-variable expression of lipopolysaccharide contributes to the virulence of *Legionella pneumophila. J. Exp. Med.* **188:**49–60.
6. **Lüneberg, E., N. Zetzmann, D. Alber, Y. A. Knirel, O. Kooistra, U. Zähringer, and M. Frosch.** 2000. Cloning and functional characterization of a 30 kb gene locus required for lipopolysaccharide biosynthesis in *Legionella pneumophila. Int. J. Med. Microbiol.* **290:**37–49.
7. **Moll, H., A. Sonesson, E. Jantzen, R. Marre, and U. Zähringer.** 1992. Identification of 27-oxo-octacosanoic acid and heptacosane-1,27-dioic acid in *Legionella pneumophila. FEMS Microbiol. Lett.* **92:**1–6.
8. **Moll, H., Y. A. Knirel, J. H. Helbig, and U. Zähringer.** 1997. Identification of an α-D-Man *p*-(1 → 8)-Kdo disaccharide in the inner core region and the structure of the complete core region of the *Legionella pneumophila* serogroup 1 lipopolysaccharide. *Carbohydr. Res.* **304:** 91–95.
9. **Neumeister, B., M. Faigle, M. Sommer, U. Zähringer, F. Stelter, R. Menzel, C. Schütt, and H. Northoff.** 1998. Low endotoxic potential of *Legionella pneumophila* lipopolysaccharide due to failure of interaction with the monocyte lipopolysaccharide receptor CD14. *Infect. Immun.* **66:** 4151–4157.
10. **Tsvetkov, Y. E., A. S. Shashkov, Y. A. Knirel, and U. Zähringer.** 2001. Synthesis and identification in bacterial lipopolysaccharides of 5,7-diacetamido-3,5,7,9-tetradeoxy-D-*glycero*-D-*galacto*- and -D-*glycero*-D-*talo*-non-2-ulosonic acids. *Carbohydr. Res.* **331:**233–237.
11. **Zähringer, U., Y. A. Knirel, B. Lindner, J. H. Helbig, A. Sonesson, R. Marre, and E. T. Rietschel.** 1995. The lipopolysaccharide of *Legionella pneumophila* serogroup 1 (strain Philadelphia 1): chemical structure and biological significance. *Prog. Clin. Biol. Res.* **392:**113–139.
12. **Zou, C. H., Y. A. Knirel, J. H. Helbig, U. Zähringer, and C. S. Mintz.** 1999. Molecular cloning and characterization of a locus responsible for O-acetylation of the O-polysaccharide of *Legionella pneumophila* serogroup 1 lipopolysaccharide. *J. Bacteriol.* **181:**4137–4141.

# THE *LEGIONELLA PNEUMOPHILA* LIFE CYCLE: CONNECTIONS BETWEEN GROWTH PHASE, VIRULENCE EXPRESSION, AND REPLICATION VACUOLE BIOGENESIS

*Michele S. Swanson and Michael A. Bachman*

# 15

Seminal studies by Horwitz and colleagues established that a principal tactic of pathogenic *Legionella pneumophila* is to disarm macrophages by establishing a phagosome that does not acidify or merge with degradative lysosomes (10, 11). Consequently, this gram-negative bacterium can replicate within the belly of the mononuclear beast (12). Recent research in our laboratory has revealed another remarkable talent of *L. pneumophila*: the capacity to survive and apparently replicate within phagolysosomes (17). We will incorporate these two seemingly paradoxical observations within a model for the *L. pneumophila* life cycle in which expression of virulence traits is determined by growth conditions. After describing the model, we will review its experimental basis, then discuss a number of intriguing questions it raises.

## A MIGRATORY LIFESTYLE

Although best known as a causative agent of pneumonia, *L. pneumophila* truly thrives in nature as a parasite of freshwater amoebae. Indeed, since the 1980s, approximately 1,000 cases of legionellosis have been reported annually to the Centers for Disease Control and Prevention (4), yet not a single instance of person-to-person transmission of the bacterium has been documented. Therefore, the selective pressure to reproduce in the aquatic niche must be a dominant evolutionary force. To persist in the environment, *L. pneumophila* that is confronted with feeding amoebae must avoid digestion and instead establish a protected site for intracellular replication. After exhausting the resources of its host, the bacterial progeny must vacate the premises to search out a more fertile locale. The bacteria may take up residence with a consortium of microbes within a biofilm community (see chapters 17, 30, and 31). When *L. pneumophila* encounters grazing amoebae, its prowess as a parasite becomes paramount.

If humans inhale water contaminated with *L. pneumophila*, the microbe can also replicate within alveolar macrophages. A robust cell-mediated immune response can vanquish the invader; if immunity is compromised, a deadly pneumonia can develop. Although *L. pneumophila* can replicate within human phagocytes, it cannot escape by the respiratory route. Thus, the encounter is disadvantageous to both the displaced bacterium and its accidental human host.

*Michele S. Swanson and Michael A. Bachman*   Department of Microbiology and Immunology, University of Michigan Medical School, Ann Arbor, MI 48109-0620.

*Legionella*, Edited by Reinhard Marre et al.
© 2002 ASM Press, Washington, D.C.

## A MODEL THAT CONNECTS GROWTH CONDITIONS, VIRULENCE EXPRESSION, AND REPLICATION VACUOLE BIOGENESIS

On the basis of research conducted in our laboratory and elsewhere, we propose the following model for the *L. pneumophila* life cycle (Fig. 1 and 2). When ingested by amoebae or macrophages, *L. pneumophila* immediately modifies its phagosome. Factors exported via the Dot/Icm secretion system separate the vacuole from the endosomal pathway, while a different mechanism blocks fusion with the lysosomal compartment. During the next several hours, the isolated phagosome is engulfed within folds of endoplasmic reticulum. This

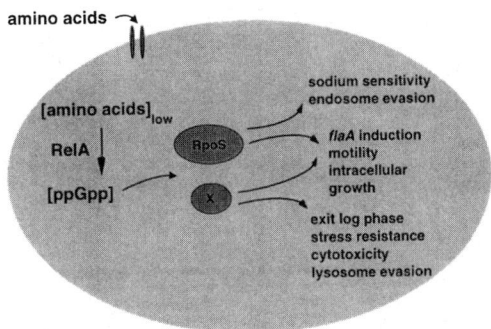

**FIGURE 2** A stringent response model for *L. pneumophila* virulence expression as a response to nutrient deprivation. When their amino acid supply is limited, bacteria accumulate uncharged tRNAs, which activate the ribosome-associated enzyme RelA. RelA converts GTP to the alarmone (p)ppGpp, a second messenger that positively activates the stationary phase sigma factor RpoS and an RpoS-independent regulatory factor (X). As a result, the bacteria exit the exponential growth phase and express a panel of traits that may promote bacterial survival and transmission in the environment. See the text for details.

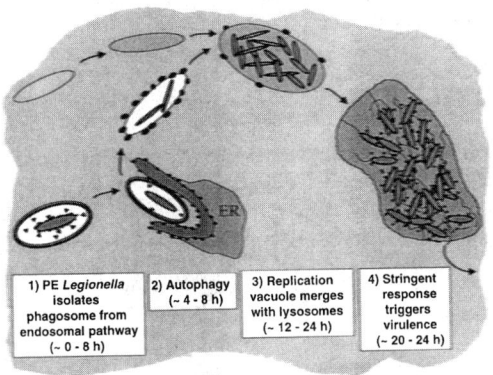

**FIGURE 1** A model for the *L. pneumophila* life cycle in which growth phase determines virulence expression and replication vacuole biogenesis. In the PE phase, *L. pneumophila* produces Dot-dependent (triangles) and –independent (coating) factors that immediately isolate its phagosome from the endosomal pathway (depicted as shaded vacuoles). During the next ~8 h, the bacterium remains in lag phase, induces acid resistance, and down-regulates expression of virulence factors, including those that block fusion with the endosomal pathway. Next, autophagy, an endoplasmic reticulum (ER)-dependent process, delivers the *L. pneumophila* phagosome to the lysosomal compartment, where replication continues. When nutrients become limiting, a stringent response-like mechanism induces virulence traits, including cytotoxicity, flagella, and factors that block phagosome maturation. Consequently, the bacterial progeny escape the spent host and seek a new replication site, where the cycle repeats. See text for details; times are approximate.

process resembles autophagy, a ubiquitous eukaryotic pathway in which organelles and other cytoplasmic constituents are sequestered by vacuoles derived from the endoplasmic reticulum for subsequent delivery to the lysosomes for digestion. Within its protected niche, *L. pneumophila* converts to a replicative form that tolerates acid and down-regulates expression of several virulence factors, including those that block phagosome maturation. Consequently, by 12 to 15 h after infection, the autophagy machinery can deliver the pathogen vacuole to a lysosome, a harsh but nutrient-rich compartment where bacterial replication continues.

By 20 or more hours after infection, the local amino acid supply dwindles, causing uncharged tRNAs to accumulate within the progeny bacteria (Fig. 2). As a result, the ribosome-associated enzyme RelA converts GTP to the alarmone (p)ppGpp. This second messenger positively activates RpoS, a stationary phase sigma factor that induces a number of traits that promote bacterial transmission to another phagocyte. In parallel, an RpoS-independent pathway(s) responds to (p)ppGpp by inducing additional virulence traits and resistance to certain environmental stresses. Thus, by a stringent response-like signaling mechanism, *L. pneumophila* responds to nutrient limitation by expressing a cytotoxin to escape from the spent host, increasing osmotic resistance to tolerate freshwater, and inducing motility to disperse and to contact a new host cell. Likewise, *L. pneumophila* regains the capacity to evade phagosome-lysosome fusion and to establish a protected niche within the next phagocyte, where the cycle repeats.

## *L. PNEUMOPHILA* BROTH CULTURES SWITCH PHENOTYPES IN RESPONSE TO GROWTH PHASE

A striking observation made by Brenda Byrne motivated our investigation of *L. pneumophila* virulence regulation. When broth cultures of *L. pneumophila* exit the exponential growth (E) phase, the bacteria become osmotically resistant, sodium sensitive, cytotoxic, motile, infectious, and competent to evade macrophage lysosomes (2). Expression of this "virulent" phenotype appears to be a response to starvation: replicating cells that are incubated in spent medium convert to the virulent form, whereas supplementation of these culture supernatants with amino acids prevents this phenotypic switch (2). Thus, *L. pneumophila* responds to nutrient limitation by coordinately expressing a panel of virulence traits.

## ONLY POST-EXPONENTIAL-PHASE *L. PNEUMOPHILA* EVADES THE ENDOCYTIC NETWORK

Analysis of phagosome maturation revealed one of the most striking differences between replicating and stationary-phase broth cultures of *L. pneumophila* (14) (Fig. 3). By applying a series of fluorescence microscopy assays, Amrita Joshi demonstrated that the majority of macrophage phagosomes containing postexponential (PE)-phase *L. pneumophila* remain separate from the endosomal pathway. In particular, vacuoles aged 2.5 min to 4 h lack the

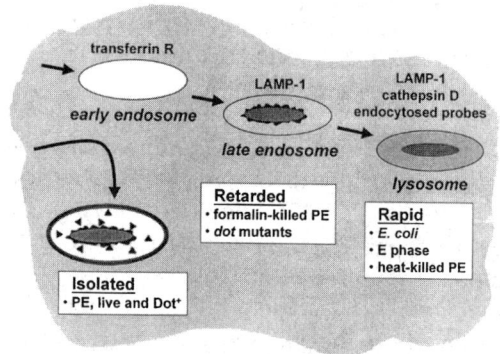

**FIGURE 3** Summary of the fate of virulent and avirulent *L. pneumophila* within macrophages. In the postexponential (PE) phase, *L. pneumophila* expresses Dot/Icm-dependent factors (triangles) to isolate the phagosome from the endosomal pathway. PE-phase bacteria must also produce a Dot/Icm-independent factor (coating) to block fusion with the terminal lysosomes, since *L. pneumophila* that lacks Dot/Icm function or has been killed by formalin colocalizes with the late endosomal protein LAMP-1 but not with other markers of the lysosomes. In contrast, exponential (E)-phase *L. pneumophila* traffic to lysosomes with the rapid kinetics observed for *E. coli* and heat-killed PE *L. pneumophila*. Early endosomes contain transferrin receptor (R), late endosomes contain LAMP-1, and lysosomes contain LAMP-1, cathepsin D, and accumulate endocytosed probes.

early endosomal protein transferrin receptor, the late endosomal and lysosomal glycoprotein LAMP-1, and the lysosomal protease cathepsin D. Moreover, phagosomes harboring PE *L. pneumophila* are inaccessible to each of four soluble or lipid fluorescent probes used to label the endocytic pathway either before or after infection. In contrast, ingested E-phase *L. pneumophila* fare no better than *Escherichia coli* or polystyrene beads: more than 70% reside within phagolysosomes, as judged by colocalization with LAMP-1, cathepsin D, and fluorescent endosomal probes.

Although entrance into the PE phase was a prerequisite for blocking phagosome maturation, neither bacterial viability nor a functional Dot/Icm transport complex was required to evade the terminal lysosomes (14) (Fig. 3). Whereas phagosomes containing formalin-killed PE-phase *L. pneumophila* rapidly accumulate the late endosomal protein LAMP-1, less than 20% acquire lysosomal cathepsin D or fluorescent endosomal probes. Likewise, live PE-phase *dotA* or *dotB* mutant bacteria reside in vacuoles that contain LAMP-1 but lack each of several lysosomal markers. Therefore, in response to starvation, *L. pneumophila* converts to a phagocyte-resistant form by producing two separable factors, or activities. A Dot-dependent factor isolates the phagosome from a LAMP-1-containing compartment, and a formalin-resistant, Dot-independent activity inhibits vacuolar accumulation of endocytosed material and delivery to the degradative lysosomes. By activating these dual mechanisms, progeny that are released into the freshwater and ingested by another amoebae can reestablish a protective intracellular niche.

## A STRINGENT RESPONSE-LIKE MECHANISM REGULATES *L. PNEUMOPHILA* VIRULENCE

Having observed the dramatic phenotypic switch displayed by nutrient-deprived *L. pneumophila*, we sought to understand its underlying mechanism. *E. coli* detects amino acid limitation in the form of the cognate uncharged tRNAs, which activate the ribosome-associated protein RelA. In response, RelA converts GTP to (p)ppGpp, a modified guanosine molecule that acts as a starvation signal for the cell and mediates a physiologic change known as the stringent response (3). In this rapid adaptation, synthesis of stable RNA and proteins are inhibited, growth rate immediately declines, and traits that promote survival in a nutrient-poor environment are induced.

Brian Hammer established that *L. pneumophila* utilize a stringent response-like signal transduction pathway to induce the virulent phenotype in response to starvation (8). In the PE phase or when subjected to amino-acid depletion, *L. pneumophila* accumulates the alarmone (p)ppGpp and converts to a virulent state, as judged by motility, cytotoxicity, and sodium sensitivity. (p)ppGpp appears to initi-ate this response, since *L. pneumophila* induced to express the *E. coli* RelA (p)ppGpp synthetase independently of nutrient depletion accumulate (p)ppGpp, exit the E phase, and express a similar pattern of traits correlated with virulence. Accordingly, when nutrients are limiting, (p)ppGpp acts as a second messenger to trigger expression of multiple traits likely to promote transmission of *L. pneumophila* to a more favorable site for replication.

## RpoS COORDINATES EXPRESSION OF CERTAIN VIRULENCE TRAITS WITH THE PE PHASE

Postulating that the transition from a replicative to a virulent phenotype reflects a new pattern of gene expression, we next investigated the role of a candidate transcription factor. In *E. coli*, (p)ppGpp positively activates expression of RpoS, the sigma factor that regulates the stationary-phase phenotype. Therefore, we examined whether *L. pneumophila* utilizes RpoS to coordinate virulence with the PE phase by constructing and analyzing isogenic wild-type and *rpoS* null mutant strains (1a). PE-phase *L. pneumophila* became cytotoxic by an RpoS-independent pathway, but its sodium sensitivity and maximal flagellin expression required RpoS. Likewise, induction of sodium sensitivity in response to experimentally induced (p)ppGpp synthesis was also RpoS-dependent. To replicate efficiently in macrophages, *L. pneumophila* required both RpoS-dependent and -independent pathways.

The intracellular growth defect of *rpoS* mutants is attributable to a failure to isolate their phagosomes from the endosomal pathway (1a). Like those containing the *dotA* type IV secretory mutant, phagosomes harboring either *rpoS* or *dotA rpoS* mutants rapidly acquire the late endosomal protein LAMP-1, but not the lysosomal marker Texas Red-ovalbumin. Thus, in the PE phase, RpoS may activate expression of Dot/Icm substrates to isolate *L. pneumophila* from the endocytic network. In parallel, other PE-phase transcription factors must act to block fusion with lysosomes and to induce cytotoxicity and stress resistance.

## INTRACELLULAR *L. PNEUMOPHILA* ALSO SWITCHES BETWEEN A REPLICATIVE AND A VIRULENT FORM

In phagocyte cultures, *L. pneumophila* recapitulates the phenotypic switch observed in broth. As is characteristic of E-phase cultures (2), bacteria replicating in macrophages are sodium resistant and noncytotoxic, and the cells do not produce flagella or transcribe *flaA* (1, 2, 8). Concomitant with macrophage lysis, *L. pneumophila* becomes sodium sensitive and cytotoxic, induces *flaA* expression, and assembles flagella.

The requirement for Dot/Icm type IV secretion by *L. pneumophila* cultured with macrophages may also be growth stage dependent. In the PE phase, the Dot/Icm complex appears to act during phagocytosis to isolate the *L. pneumophila* vacuole from the endosomal pathway (14, 15). Numerous mutants of the *dot/icm* family are mistargeted to the endosomal pathway within the earliest period examined, in some cases as early as 5 to 30 min after infection (19). However, once a protected vacuole is established, *L. pneumophila* may no longer require the Dot/Icm machinery to maintain its replication niche. For example, by using an inducible promoter to control *dotA* transcription, Roy and colleagues found that when *L. pneumophila* expresses DotA prior to contact with macrophages, but not after, the cells still replicate during the primary infection cycle (15). Furthermore, when provided with a wild-type partner to construct its privileged vacuole, *dotA* mutants can replicate (5). Thus, biogenesis of the *L. pneumophila* replication vacuole can be regarded as a two-stage process; isolation of the nascent phagosome from the endosomal pathway requires the Dot/Icm apparatus, but once replication begins, the complex is dispensable.

## *L. PNEUMOPHILA* VACUOLES MATURE INTO PHAGOLYSOSOMES IN MACROPHAGES

The stringent response model of *L. pneumophila* virulence regulation generated a surprising prediction: when conditions are favorable for growth, bacteria down-regulate expression of virulence traits. If so, how is replicating *L. pneumophila* protected from the degradative lysosomes? To determine the fate of *L. pneumophila* multiplying in macrophages, the interactions between the endosomal network and pathogen vacuoles throughout the primary infection period were examined.

From a series of cell biological studies, Sheila Sturgill-Koszycki obtained striking confirmation of the predictions generated by our in vitro studies. When replicating in macrophages, *L. pneumophila* loses the capacity to block phagosome maturation (17). Consistent with numerous studies published previously, after ingestion by macrophages, PE-phase *L. pneumophila* inhibits acidification and maturation of its phagosome. During a 6- to 10-h lag period, the vacuole associates with the endoplasmic reticulum (18); next, the bacteria replicate exponentially for 10 to 14 h until macrophage lysis releases dozens of progeny. It is during the E phase that a significant proportion of the *L. pneumophila* vacuoles acquire several lysosomal characteristics. By 16 to 18 h, 70% contain LAMP-1, 40% contain cathepsin D, and 50% acquire fluid-phase endosomal tracers that are added to the cultures either before or after infection. Moreover, those phagosomes that have merged with the endosomal pathway have an acidic pH, averaging 5.6.

Results obtained by four independent experimental approaches strengthen the hypothesis that *L. pneumophila* survives and replicates within lysosomal compartments (17). First, virtually every vacuole that harbors more than five bacteria also contains LAMP-1. Second, bacteria within endosomal vacuoles are viable, as judged by their capacity to respond to a metabolic inducer by expressing a *gfp* reporter gene. Third, replicating bacteria obtained from macrophages, but not broth, are acid resistant. Finally, inhibition of vacuole acidification and maturation by bafilomycin A1 or other agents actually inhibits bacterial replication.

Together, these observations indicate that during its lag period within isolated phagosomes, *L. pneumophila* senses and responds to intracellular signals by inducing acid resistance and down-regulating expression of factors that promote transmission. Consequently, after the pathogen phagosome is engulfed by autophagy, the vacuole matures, gradually acquiring lysosomal features. In exchange for braving these harsh conditions, presumably the bacteria gain, via endosomal traffic, a rich supply of nutrients to fuel their replication. Eventually, depletion or disruption of their amino acid supply triggers the stringent response pathway; consequently, *L. pneumophila* produces virulence factors that promote escape and transmission to more fertile territory.

## *COXIELLA* AND *LEISHMANIA* EMPLOY A SIMILAR STRATEGY TO REPLICATE IN MACROPHAGES

Similar to *L. pneumophila, Leishmania* and *Coxiella* species also switch between infectious and replicative forms that alternately block, then exploit, phagolysosome formation to replicate in macrophages. For example, when infectious promastigotes of the protozoa *Leishmania* are ingested by macrophages, phagosome maturation is blocked by lipophosphoglycan, a molecule abundant on the surface of non-replicating parasites. As promastigotes develop into the replicative amastigote form, lipophosphoglycan expression is down-regulated, the vacuole merges with the endosomal pathway, and the parasite replicates within an acidic phagolysosome (for a review, see reference 6).

The etiological agent of Q Fever, *Coxiella burnetti*, is an obligate intracellular pathogen closely related to *L. pneumophila*. Indeed, *C. burnetti* encodes homologues of *icmT, icmS,* and *icmK*, three genes *L. pneumophila* requires to grow intracellularly (16). Its stationary-phase form is an infectious small cell variant capable of delaying phagosome maturation (13), whereas its large cell variant form replicates within acidic phagolysosomes of macrophages (for a review, see reference 9). *C. burnetti* requires an acidic pH to trigger development of the dormant variant into the metabolically active form (7). In contrast, *L. pneumophila* differentiation from the PE-phase

virulent form to the replicative form appears to be pH-independent, since experimental neutralization of the endosomal pH arrested replication after it had initiated (17). Because *L. pneumophila* is amenable to genetic manipulation, it may serve as an experimental tool to investigate how this class of pathogens replicates in macrophages by first evading, then capitalizing on, the normally deadly lysosomal environment.

## UNFINISHED BUSINESS

Although we have tested several predictions of the stringent response model of virulence regulation, many questions remain. In this final section, we will discuss aspects of our current model that warrant more detailed investigation and experiments to extend our knowledge of *L. pneumophila* pathogenesis.

As yet, we lack direct evidence that *L. pneumophila* replicates in lysosomal compartments. For example, although a significant proportion of mature *L. pneumophila* vacuoles accumulate detectable quantities of lysosomal markers, not all of the vacuoles do so (17). However, two technical complications limit our ability to detect the population of vacuoles that contain endocytic markers. First, since vacuoles can be scored as positive only after accumulating detectable quantities of marker, the earliest point during infection when bacterial vacuoles interact with the endosomal pathway cannot be defined by our methods. Second, it is evident by phase microscopy of live infected cultures that macrophages containing large replication vacuoles round and detach from the coverslip. This population of cells is washed away during the immunofluorescence staining procedure; therefore, mature replication vacuoles are predicted to be under-represented in our microscopy data sets. To address directly whether *L. pneumophila* replicates in lysosomes, we can apply different microscopy techniques to record in live cells the interactions between replicating bacteria and the endosomal pathway.

Our cell biological studies documented that during the bacterial replication period, *L. pneumophila* vacuoles acquire a variety of lysosomal markers, including the protease cathepsin D. However, detection of an enzyme by immunofluorescence microscopy does not address whether it is biologically active. Investigation of whether *L. pneumophila* can tolerate, or perhaps exploit, the proteases of macrophage lysosomes to obtain amino acids needed for replication will require more sophisticated probes of macrophage biology.

In broth, *L. pneumophila* grows optimally at a neutral pH. Yet, mature vacuoles average pH 5.6, and bacteria replicating intracellularly are acid resistant (17). Presumably, during the several hours that its phagosome is isolated from the endocytic pathway, *L. pneumophila* senses some intracellular signal and responds by inducing pathways that confer acid resistance. As has been observed for other gram-negative bacilli, an early moderate decline in the vacuolar pH could trigger *L. pneumophila* acid resistance. Alternatively, factors present in macrophages may promote acid resistance by a more direct mechanism; for example, *L. pneumophila* may metabolize particular amino acids to generate protective basic compounds. Identification of both the eukaryotic and the bacterial factors that promote acid tolerance of intracellular *L. pneumophila* would advance significantly our understanding of pathogens that thrive in lysosomes.

The stringent response model depicts amino acid limitation as the signal that induces virulence, RelA as the sensor of that signal, (p)ppGpp as the second messenger in the signal transduction pathway, and RpoS as a transcription factor that coordinates virulence gene expression (1a, 2, 8) (Fig. 2). However, with the notable exception of our analysis of the fate of *rpoS* mutants in macrophages, the model relies heavily on data obtained from studies of broth cultures. Because the bona fide effectors of *L. pneumophila* virulence are not known, our regulation experiments depended on phenotypic assays of virulence. Only expression of flagellin, encoded by *flaA* and induced in the PE phase, can be monitored directly. A rigorous test of the hypothesis that a stringent response-like pathway triggers virulence of intracellular *L. pneumophila* requires that additional virulence reporters, and their cognate inducers, be identified and analyzed in phagocyte infection models.

The validity of the stringent response model of *L. pneumophila* virulence regulation should also be tested in experimental models that more closely mimic its natural aquatic reservoir or its pathogenesis in the human lung. For example, although cultures of macrophages or amoebae are valuable models to study bacterial replication, neither are adequate to measure whether cytotoxicity, or motility, promotes transmission of *L. pneumophila*. A/J mice provide a tractable model of legionellosis in the immunocompetent host, in which a 48-h period of bacterial replication is offset by a cell-mediated immune response that eventually clears the infection. Alternatively, guinea pigs can serve as experimental surrogates for a highly susceptible human host. In the environment, *L. pneumophila* likely persists in microbial biofilms as a transient resident of grazing amoebae. To dissect the environmental and bacterial factors that determine the fate of *L. pneumophila* in its natural reservoir, continuous-flow, multispecies biofilm models will be valuable experimental tools. By these approaches, the contribution of individual components of the stringent response model can be evaluated. Moreover, development of more physiological assays of *L. pneumophila* transmission will likely suggest new experimental approaches to identify the bacterial effectors dedicated to this stage of the life cycle.

By analogy to a number of other gram-negative pathogens, it is likely that multiple-signal transduction pathways operate in parallel to enable *L. pneumophila* to sense a variety of environmental signals and respond by an appropriate adaptation of its physiology or pattern of gene expression. As additional regulators of *L. pneumophila* virulence are identified, it will be interesting to learn whether they also exhibit temporal activity. In any case, the current growth-phase-dependent virulence paradigm can serve as a theoretical guide for future experimental approaches. The rational design of prevention and treatment protocols would be accelerated by the identification of the components of the virulence regulon, which together equip *L. pneumophila* to survive and replicate within bactericidal phagocytes of freshwater and of the human lung.

## ACKNOWLEDGMENTS

We thank members of our laboratory for their contributions to the ideas and experiments described here.

Our research is supported by grants from the NIH (AI 40694-01 and AI 44212-01). M. Bachman is supported by the University of Michigan Medical Scientist Training Program and the Presidential Initiatives Fund for Graduate Training in Microbial Pathogenesis.

## REFERENCES

1. **Alli, O. A. T., L.-Y. Gao, L. L. Pedersen, S. Zink, M. Radulic, M. Doric, and Y. Abu Kwaik.** 2000. Temporal pore formation-mediated egress from macrophages and alveolar epithelial cells by *Legionella pneumophila*. *Infect. Immun.* **68:**6431–6440.

1a. **Bachman, M. A., and M. S. Swanson.** 2001. RpoS co-operates with other factors to induce *Legionella pneumophila* virulence in the stationary phase. *Mol. Microbiol.* **40:**1201–1214.

2. **Byrne, B., and M. S. Swanson.** 1998. Expression of *Legionella pneumophila* virulence traits in response to growth conditions. *Infect. Immun.* **66:**3029–3034.

3. **Cashel, M., D. R. Gentry, V. J. Hernandez, and D. Vinella.** 1996. The stringent response, p. 1458–1496. *In* F. C. Neidhardt (ed.), *Escherichia coli and Salmonella: Cellular and Molecular Biology.* ASM Press, Washington, D.C.

4. **Centers for Disease Control and Prevention.** 1996. Summary of notifiable diseases, United States, 1996. *Morb. Mortal. Wkly. Rep.* **45:**40.

5. **Coers, J., C. Monahan, and C. R. Roy.** 1999. Modulation of phagosome biogenesis by *Legionella pneumophila* creates an organelle permissive for intracellular growth. *Nature Cell Biol.* **1:**451–453.

6. **Duclos, S., and M. Desjardins.** 2000. Subversion of a young phagosome: the survival strategies of intracellular pathogens. *Cell. Microbiol.* **2:**365–378.

7. **Hackstadt, T., and J. C. Williams.** 1981. Biochemical stratagem for obligate parasitism of eukaryotic cells by *Coxiella burnetti*. *Proc. Natl. Acad. Sci. USA* **78:**3240–3244.

8. **Hammer, B. K., and M. S. Swanson.** 1999. Co-ordination of *Legionella pneumophila* virulence with entry into stationary phase by ppGpp. *Mol. Microbiol.* **33:**721–731.

9. **Heinzen, R. A., T. Hackstadt, and J. E. Samuel.** 1999. Developmental biology of *Coxiella burnetii*. *Trends Microbiol.* **7:**149–154.

10. **Horwitz, M. A.** 1983. The Legionnaires' disease bacterium (*Legionella pneumophila*) inhibits phagosome lysosome fusion in human monocytes. *J. Exp. Med.* **158:**2108–2126.

11. **Horwitz, M. A., and F. R. Maxfield.** 1984. *Legionella pneumophila* inhibits acidification of its phagosome in human monocytes. *J. Cell. Biol.* **99:**1936–1943.

12. **Horwitz, M. A., and S. C. Silverstein.** 1980. Legionnaires' disease bacterium (*Legionella pneumophila*) multiplies intracellularly in human monocytes. *J. Clin. Invest.* **66:**441–450.

13. **Howe, D., and L. P. Mallavia.** 2000. *Coxiella burnetii* exhibits morphological change and delays phagolysosomal fusion after internalization by J774A.1 cells. *Infect. Immun.* **68:**3815–3821.

14. **Joshi, A. D., S. Sturgill-Koszycki, and M. S. Swanson.** 2001. Evidence that Dot-dependent and -independent factors isolate the *Legionella pneumophila* phagosome from the endocytic network in mouse macrophages. *Cell. Microbiol.* **3:**99–114.

15. **Roy, C. R., K. H. Berger, and R. R. Isberg.** 1998. *Legionella pneumophila* DotA protein is required for early phagosome trafficking decisions that occur within minutes of bacterial uptake. *Mol. Microbiol.* **28:**663–674.

16. **Segal, G., and H. A. Shuman.** 1999. Possible origin of the *Legionella pneumophila* virulence genes and their relation to *Coxiella burnetii*. *Mol. Microbiol.* **33:**669–670.

17. **Sturgill-Koszycki, S., and M. S. Swanson.** 2000. *Legionella pneumophila* replication vacuoles mature into acidic, endocytic organelles. *J. Exp. Med.* **192:**1261–1272.

18. **Swanson, M. S., and R. R. Isberg.** 1995. Association of *Legionella pneumophila* with the macrophage endoplasmic reticulum. *Infect. Immun.* **63:**3609–3620.

19. **Vogel, J. P., and R. R. Isberg.** 1999. Cell biology of *Legionella pneumophila*. *Curr. Opin. in Microbiol.* **2:**30–34.

# MORPHOLOGICAL AND PHYSIOLOGICAL EVIDENCE FOR A DEVELOPMENTAL CYCLE IN *LEGIONELLA PNEUMOPHILA*

*Rafael A. Garduño, Elizabeth Garduño, Margot Hiltz, David Allan, and Paul S. Hoffman*

# 16

*Legionella pneumophila*, an aquatic pathogen of freshwater protozoa and the cause of Legionnaires' disease in humans, must survive in water when between hosts. In the laboratory, it has been confirmed that this bacterium survives for months in tap water (12, 13) or even distilled water (7). When grown in HeLa cells, *L. pneumophila* clearly has two morphologically distinct intracellular forms (5). One of the forms, which arises late in infection and accumulates in infected HeLa cell cultures, can be purified using continuous density gradients of Percoll (5). Electron microscopy of these purified forms revealed the presence of a unique cell envelope characterized by a thick, electron-dense layer associated with the inner face of the outer membrane and/or the presence of multiple layers of cytoplasmic membrane (5). We have named these forms "mature bacteria" (4) or MIFs for "mature intracellular forms." By using the bacteriological Giménez stain, it was observed that MIFs are stained bright red (Giménez positive [Gim+])

(5), in contrast to *L. pneumophila* grown in vitro, which are stained green, bluish red, or grey (Giménez negative [Gim-]). These results agree with previous reports by other investigators on the existence of two morphological forms in *L. pneumophila* (10, 11) and *Legionella micdadei* (6), which also showed distinct staining phenotypes with carbol fuchsin.

Importantly, it has been reported that intracellular growth in amoebae enhances *L. pneumophila* infectivity and is accompanied by changes in morphology and Giménez staining with respect to agar-grown legionellae (1, 2, 11). We have also reported that MIFs are more infectious to HeLa cells than legionellae grown in agar or broth media (4, 5). These observations collectively suggest the possibility that this bacterium differentiates into an environmentally resilient and infectious form before leaving a dying infected host. We present here the cyclical nature of some morphological and physiological changes that take place in infected HeLa cells and during growth in vitro.

## CYCLIC MORPHOLOGICAL CHANGES OF *L. PNEUMOPHILA* IN INFECTED HeLa CELLS

Coverslip cultures of HeLa cells were infected with purified MIFs, and changes in Giménez

*Rafael A. Garduño and Paul S. Hoffman* Department of Medicine, Dalhousie University, Halifax, Nova Scotia B3H-4H7, Canada. *Elizabeth Garduño, Margot Hiltz, and David Allan* Department of Microbiology-Immunology, Dalhousie University, Halifax, Nova Scotia B3H-4H7, Canada.

staining were followed for up to 3 days. The bacterial strains used throughout these studies were Lp1-SVir and 2064, two virulent strains previously reported and characterized (4, 5). Giménez staining was performed exactly as reported by McDade (8). At and after 16 to 24 h of infection, foci of numerous bright green bacteria were observed, as well as long rods stained with a blue-red shade. Clearly, the foci of green bacteria and the long rods emerged from the bright red MIFs initially used to infect the HeLa cells. New MIFs accumulated in large numbers by day 3 after infection, but an accumulation of green forms or long blue-red rods was never observed.

Cultures with 100% green forms (after Giménez staining) were identified upon growth of *L. pneumophila* on buffered charcoal-yeast extract (BCYE) plates. Electron microscopy indicated that in contrast to MIFs, these green bacteria had a typical gram-negative envelope morphology, an electron-dense cytoplasm, and numerous ribosomes. When HeLa cells were infected with these 100% green forms, we also observed cell-associated foci of both green bacteria and long blue-red rods. Subsequently, a massive accumulation of MIFs, but no accumulation of the other forms, was observed. Evidently, MIFs arose from the green forms with a typical gram-negative ultrastructure, initially used to infect the HeLa cells. Rowbotham reported earlier that infection of amoebae resulted in the formation of small, highly motile, and infectious legionellae (11) that we believe are equivalent to the HeLa-derived MIFs reported here. Furthermore, infection of new hosts with these highly infectious forms gave rise to multiplicative, nonmotile forms showing the typical gram-negative ultrastructure (11). Collectively, our results (as those of Rowbotham) indicate a clear alternation between different forms associated with a distinct Giménez phenotype, and suggest that the foci of green bacteria observed in infected HeLa cells represent replicative bacteria (5).

## MORPHOLOGICAL CYCLIC CHANGES IN VITRO

Purified MIFs were placed in buffered yeast extract (BYE) and their growth was followed through viable cell counts. Giménez staining and electron microscopy (EM) were also performed at different times. Bacterial replication was invariably associated with the appearance of green forms (detected by Giménez staining) and EM indicated that these green forms either had a typical gram-negative ultrastructure or a very electron-dense cytoplasm and membranes with periplasmic vesicles and/or membrane coils (Fig. 1). Bacteria showing the ultrastructural features typical of MIFs were never observed undergoing cell division and their proportion noticeably decreased with time, once replication had started in the BYE cultures. We concluded that the green forms

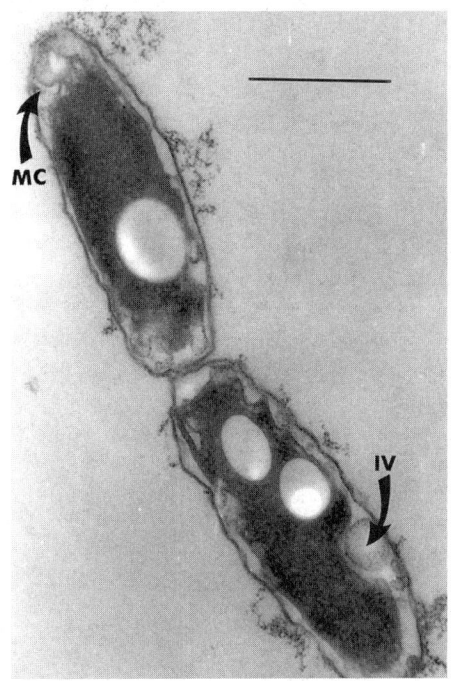

**FIGURE 1** Electron micrograph showing the typical ultrastructural features of the intermediate forms that arise after MIFs of the Lp1-SVir are inoculated into BYE broth. IV, intraperiplasmic vesicles; MC, membrane coils. Bar represents 0.5 μm.

arising in the BYE cultures were replicating bacteria that developed from the MIFs originally used as inoculum.

Changes in Giménez staining during the normal growth of *L. pneumophila* on BCYE plates or in BYE broth were then followed. Punctiform colonies had approximately 50% Gim(+) (red) bacteria, but 1-mm, 2-day-old colonies often had a predominant expression of the Gim(−) (green) phenotype. Larger, 2- to 3-day-old colonies, typically displayed a mixed population of Gim(+) and Gim(−) bacteria in different proportions, and >3-day-old colonies were always predominantly formed by red bacteria. Although no clear correlation could be established between growth phase in BYE and Giménez phenotype, high proportions of Gim(−) (green) legionellae were only observed immediately before or during early exponential growth, and postexponential cultures predominantly displayed the Gim(+) phenotype. For every growth cycle on BCYE agar or BYE broth, the changes described were repeated, clearly indicating that the red Gim(+) forms give rise to Gim(−) bacteria and vice versa.

## STATIONARY-PHASE BACTERIA VERSUS MIFs

While one might assume that stationary-phase bacteria in vitro are equivalent to MIFs (the in vivo stationary phase), microscopical evidence (general morphology and Giménez staining) clearly shows that they are different. For instance, at the EM ultrastructural level, stationary-phase legionellae had multiple invaginations of the inner membrane, but did not show all the features characteristic of the MIF ultrastructure. At the physiological level, MIFs and stationary-phase forms were similarly thermotolerant (~60 to 80% survival after a challenge of 57°C for 20 min) and survived well in distilled-deionized water (100% survival after a 2-week incubation in distilled deionized water [ddH₂O] at 37°C). However, they differed in their infectivity toward HeLa cells (4) and L929 murine fibroblasts (not shown). These features were lost

upon culturing and entering into an exponential replicative phase, where both stationary-phase bacteria and MIFs gave rise to a virtually identical phenotype.

Furthermore, MIFs and stationary-phase forms also differed on the expression of an ~20-kDa protein that was poorly expressed by exponential-phase-replicating *L. pneumophila*. As shown in Fig. 2A, MIFs synthesized this protein more actively than stationary-phase forms (as determined by sodium dodecyl sulfate-polyacrylamide gel electrophoresis [SDS-PAGE] and autoradiography after a 1-h pulse with 10 $\mu$Ci of $^{35}$S methionine) and

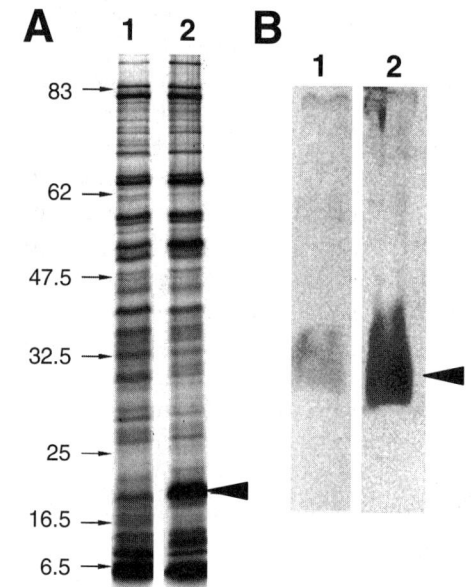

**FIGURE 2** An ~20-kDa protein is prominent in MIFs obtained from HeLa cells infected with Lp1-Vir. Autoradiogram (A) and immunoblot (B) from an SDS-PAGE gel run with whole cell lysates from stationary-phase bacteria grown in vitro (1) or MIFs (2). For autoradiography, bacteria were placed in distilled water for 4 h and then pulsed with radiolabelled methionine for 1 h. The blot was immunostained with a hyperimmune rabbit serum against the purified 20-kDa protein and a second antibody conjugated with alkaline phosphatase and then developed with NBT-BCIP. Numbers on the left of panel A indicate the position of molecular weight standards (×1,000) and the arrowheads on the right of the two panels point at the protein band of interest.

showed increased levels of the protein by immunoblotting (Fig. 2B). N-terminal amino acid sequence of this protein was commercially contracted to be done at the micro sequencing lab of the University of British Columbia (Vancouver), and turned out to be identical to the first 10 amino acids of a protein previously identified by Miyamoto et al. (9). Interestingly, this protein was entered into the database by Miyamoto et al. as Mip. However, the published N-terminal amino acid sequence of the *L. pneumophila* Mip, previously reported by Engleberg et al. (3), shows no homology at all with Miyamoto's or our 20-kDa protein, implying that the sequence deposited by Miyamoto et al. is distinct from Mip. We propose naming this gene *magA* for MIF-associated gene. The function of this protein in development remains to be determined.

In summary, *L. pneumophila* undergoes cyclical morphological and physiological changes that suggest the existence of a developmental program. The genes responsible for differentiation and the significance of a developmental cycle in the biology of Legionnaires' disease await to be explored.

## REFERENCES

1. **Cirillo, J. D., S. L. G. Cirillo, L. Yan, L. E. Bermudez, S. Falkow, and L. S. Tompkins.** 1999. Intracellular growth in *Acanthamoeba castellani* affects monocyte entry mechanisms and enhances virulence of *Legionella pneumophila. Infect. Immun.* **67:**4427–4434.

2. **Cirillo, J. D., S. Falkow, and L. S. Tompkins.** 1994. Growth of *Legionella pneumophila* in *Acanthamoeba castellani* enhances invasion. *Infect. Immun.* **62:**3254–3261.

3. **Engleberg, N. C., C. Carter, D. R. Weber, N. P. Cianciotto, and B. I. Eisenstein.** 1989.

4. **Garduño, R. A., E. Garduño, and P. S. Hoffman.** 1998. Surface-associated Hsp60 chaperonin of *Legionella pneumophila* mediates invasion in a HeLa cell model. *Infect. Immun.* **66:**4602–4610.

5. **Garduño, R. A., F. D. Quinn, and P. S. Hoffman.** 1998. HeLa cells as a model to study the invasiveness and biology of *Legionella pneumophila. Can. J. Microbiol.* **44:**430–440.

6. **Gress, F. M., R. L. Myerowitz, A. W. Pascule, C. R. Rinaldo Jr., and J. N. Dowling.** 1980. The ultrastructural morphologic features of Pittsburgh pneumonia agent. *Am. J. Pathol.* **101:**63–78.

7. **Lee, J. V., and A. A. West.** 1991. Survival and growth of *Legionella* species in the environment. *J. Appl. Bacteriol.* (Symp. Suppl.) **70:**121S–129S.

8. **McDade, J. E.** 1979. Primary isolation using guinea pigs and embryonated eggs, p. 70–76. *In* G. L. Jones and G. A. Hébert (ed.), *"Legionnaires'": the Disease, the Bacterium and Methodology.* U.S. Department of Health Education and Welfare, Public Health Service, Center for Disease Control, Bureau of Laboratories, Atlanta, Ga.

9. **Miyamoto, H., S. Yoshida, H. Taniguchi, M. H. Qin, H. Fujio, and Y. Mizuguchi.** 1993. Protein profiles of *Legionella pneumophila* Philadelphia-1 grown in macrophages and characterization of a gene encoding a novel 24 kDa *Legionella* protein. *Microb. Pathog.* **15:**469–484.

10. **Oldham, L. J., and F. G. Rodgers.** 1985. Adhesion, penetration and intracellular replication of *Legionella pneumophila*: an in vitro model of pathogenesis. *J. Gen. Microbiol.* **131:**697–706.

11. **Rowbotham, T. J.** 1986. Current views on the relationships between amoebae, legionellae and man. *Isr. J. Med. Sci.* **22:**678–689.

12. **Schofield, G. M.** 1985. A note on the survival of *Legionella pneumophila* in stagnant tap water. *J. Appl. Bacteriol.* **59:**333–335.

13. **Skaliy, D., and H. V. McEachern.** 1979. Survival of the Legionnaires' disease bacterium in water. *Ann. Intern. Med.* **90:**662–663.

DNA sequence of *mip*, a *Legionella pneumophila* gene associated with macrophage infectivity. *Infect. Immun.* **57:**1263–1270.

# *LEGIONELLA PNEUMOPHILA* PROLIFERATION IS NOT DEPENDENT ON INTRACELLULAR REPLICATION

*Susanne Surman, Glyn Morton, Bill Keevil, and Roy Fitzgeorge*

# 17

The complexities of the relationship between *Legionella pneumophila* and other microorganisms for the growth and survival of legionellae in the environment is still not fully understood, though it is generally believed that amoebae play an important role in the natural environment. Although strains of varying virulence are isolated from environmental sources, it is still generally accepted that intracellular replication is important for the ability of *L. pneumophila* to proliferate in the natural environment.

A continuous culture model water system was set up in the laboratory on the basis of that previously described (4). To model as closely as possible a naturally occurring water population, the initial inoculum was taken from the local mains water supply. To reduce the risk of bacterial selection by growth media and possible phenotypic alterations due to passage on laboratory media, the inoculum was obtained by filtering mains water and introduced directly into the system without any prior culture or other selection process.

The use of continuous culture allows the control of parameters including pH, nutrient concentration, temperature, and oxygen concentration. To maintain as natural a system as possible, pH and nutrient concentration were monitored but not controlled. By the definition of a "natural" system as described by Brock (1), it could be argued that because of this lack of complete control, this model was itself a "natural" system.

The model water system allowed the development of reproducible biofilms. A diverse but fairly constant consortium of aquatic microorganisms including fungi, bacteria, and protozoa could be maintained in this system. The relative numbers of planktonic to biofilm bacteria and the bacterial species isolated from this system were similar to those isolated in other studies, even where the system inoculum was from geographically distant sources (C. W. Mackerness, J. S. Colbourne, and C. W. Keevil, Proc. U.K. Symp. Health-Related Microbiology, abstr. 131, 1991; reference 11). This similarity in bacterial flora suggests that these species are ubiquitous within water systems; predominant organisms were *Pseudomonas*, *Flavobacterium*, *Methylobacterium*, *Acinetobacter*, and *Alcaligenes* spp.

*Susanne Surman* London Food Water & Environmental Microbiology Laboratory, Central Public Health Laboratory, 61 Colindale Ave., London NW9 5HT, United Kingdom.    *Glyn Morton* Department of Applied Biology, University of Central Lancashire, Preston PR1 2HE, United Kingdom.    *Bill Keevil and Roy Fitzgeorge* Centre for Applied Microbiology and Research, Porton Down, Salisbury SP4 0JG, United Kingdom.

*Legionella*, Edited by Reinhard Marre et al.
© 2002 ASM Press, Washington, D.C.

By microscopic examination of these bio-films and by the formation of plaques on the R2A plates used for enumeration, it was determined that this system contained many protozoa. The plaques were more readily observed in the undiluted planktonic and sessile phases. The predominant protozoa in the system were tentatively identified as *Hartmannella vermiformis* and *Acanthamoeba* spp., which are naturally occurring inhabitants of water systems, and their continued presence suggests that the environmental parameters of this system remained acceptable.

To investigate if legionellae could have the potential to replicate without multiplication within a protozoal host, an avirulent strain of *Legionella pneumophila* serogroup 1 Pontiac (Corby Strain) (CAC) was added to the system. This strain had previously been shown to be unable to infect and multiply within cultured alveolar macrophages and was not able to infect or cause death in guinea pigs that had been exposed to it (3, 10), and it did not infect protozoal hosts for legionellae (8). CAC achieved steady state when inoculated into the existing consortium of microorganisms but not when inoculated into the continuous culture model system as a pure culture.

Further investigations to eliminate any potential protozoan hosts by addition of cycloheximide to the model system were also carried out. Cycloheximide inhibits all three stages of protein synthesis in eukaryotic cells (initiation, elongation, and termination [5]) and has been used previously in ecological studies to inhibit protozoal bacteriovores without any detectable detrimental effect on the aerobic heterotrophic population (9).

A bioassay using growth inhibition of *Saccharomyces cerevisiae* was developed as a means of assessing the concentration of cycloheximide in the model system, and the system was maintained at a concentration of approximately 100 $\mu$M, which caused inhibition of the protozoal population, as determined by plaque inhibition and lack of observed motile trophozoites. This assay compared zones of in-

hibition with standard concentrations of cycloheximide.

The counts of the heterotrophic bacterial population and legionella increased in both the planktonic and sessile phases of the system following cycloheximide addition. Figure 1 shows the increase in *L. pneumophila* counts from 2.48 $\log_{10}$ CFU ml$^{-1}$ before cycloheximide addition to 4.92 $\log_{10}$ CFU ml$^{-1}$ in the planktonic phase after cycloheximide addition. Figure 2 shows an increase in legionella in the biofilm from 3.52 $\log_{10}$ CFU cm$^{-2}$ to 5.35 $\log_{10}$ CFU cm$^{-2}$.

Viability of the protozoal population was assessed by the formation of plaques on *Klebsiella aerogenes* lawn plates and by microscopic examination for the presence of motile amoebal trophozoites. Ten-milliliter samples of the

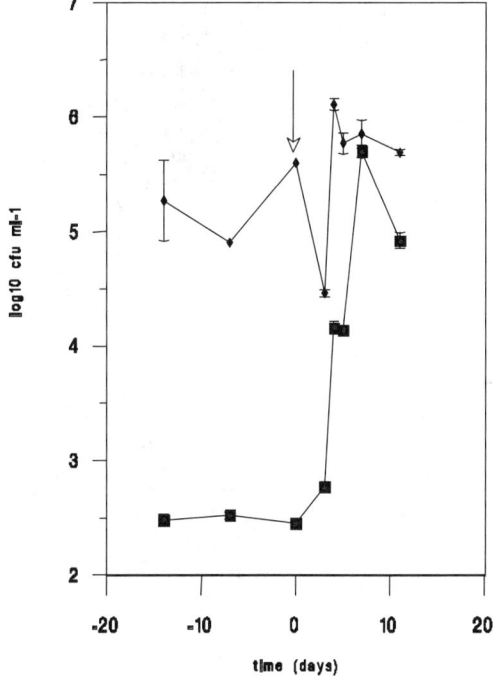

**FIGURE 1** The effect of cycloheximide on the planktonic bacterial population of the chemostat. Total counts of the heterotrophic population (♦) and the *L. pneumophila* population (■) in the planktonic phase of the continuous culture model system, before and following addition of cycloheximide (arrow), are shown (*n* = 3).

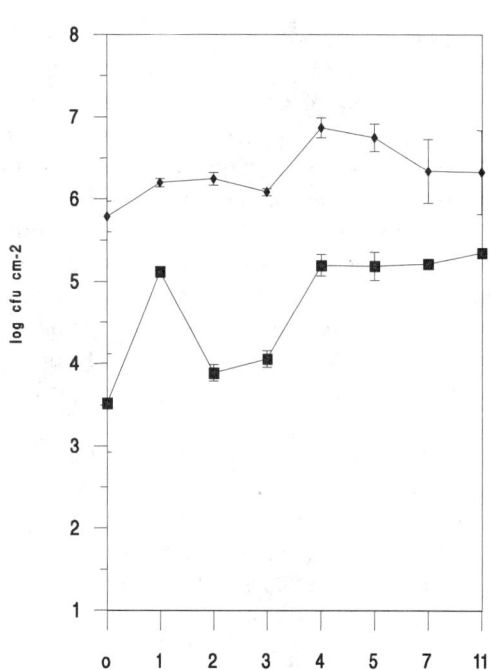

**FIGURE 2** The effect of cycloheximide on the biofilm bacterial population of the chemostat. Total biofilm counts (♦) and numbers of *L. pneumophila* (■) in the biofilm following cycloheximide addition are shown (*n* = 3).

planktonic phase were removed from the chemostat, centrifuged at 1,000 × *g* for 10 min, and the deposit inoculated onto the center of two replicate *K. aerogenes* lawn plates. For assessment of the viability of protozoa in the biofilm, two glass tiles were aseptically removed from the chemostat and each placed on the center of a *K. aerogenes* lawn. A control plate was inoculated from an amoebal suspension prepared with an axenic strain of *Acanthamoeba polyphaga*. The plates were then sealed in plastic bags, incubated at 30°C, and examined microscopically at frequent intervals for up to 21 days. Microscopic examination of the undiluted planktonic phase and the glass tiles was also carried out.

An investigation into the survival of CAC, which had not previously been introduced into a mixed community of microorganisms that were resident within the model system, was necessary to determine whether *Legionella* was able to proliferate other than via parasitization of a protozoan species. The results confirm the importance of the presence of the other bacteria on the survival of legionella (6). This is emphasized by the decline in CAC numbers when a pure culture was introduced into the model system; legionellae could not be detected after 120 h, suggesting they had been completely "washed out" of the system. These results agree with those of other authors who have found that *L. pneumophila* did not grow in experiments using sterile water as the growth medium (4, 7). However, this study has shown that CAC was growing in both the planktonic phase and the sessile phase of this model system when integrated into an existing consortium of aquatic microorganisms and could be maintained in this system for future study.

Furthermore, CAC remained avirulent when tested in the guinea pigs following recovery from the model water system. The reason(s) for the loss of virulence of CAC are as yet undetermined but may be associated with the loss of peroxidase/catalase activity (3). It has previously been suggested that the loss of virulence in this strain is probably due to more than one mutation and subsequently to more than one metabolic alteration (10). If this is the case, it seems unlikely that this attenuation could be easily reversed.

If intracellular multiplication is essential for the proliferation of *L. pneumophila* in aquatic systems, then elimination of trophozoites in the model system would prevent any further growth of legionellae, and consequently numbers would decrease due to dilution by the continuous culture medium. The elimination of protozoa from the model system did not result in a decrease in numbers of CAC in the system but rather an increase in bacterial counts including CAC. This increase was observed in both planktonic and sessile phases and is probably due to successful inhibition of grazing by the protozoal population and/or release from dead or dying trophozoites.

This study has shown that intracellular growth is not essential for the proliferation of *Legionella* within a mixed bacterial consortium of water microorganisms. Furthermore, it is not safe to assume that the absence of protozoal hosts within water systems precludes the survival and growth of legionellae. As long as there are other bacterial species present, appropriate measures should be taken to prevent *Legionella* proliferation.

## REFERENCES

1. **Brock, T. D.** 1971. Microbial growth rates in nature. *Bacteriol. Rev.* **35**:39–58.
2. **Fitzgeorge, R. B., A. Baskerville, M. G. Broster, P. Hambleton, and P. J. Dennis.** 1983. Aerosol infection of animals with strains of *Legionella pneumophila* of different virulence: comparison with intraperitoneal and intranasal route of infection. *J. Hyg. Cambridge* **90**:81–90.
3. **Jepras, R. I., R. B. Fitzgeorge, and A. Baskerville.** 1985. A comparison of virulence of two strains of *L. pneumophila* based on experimental aerosol infection of guinea pigs. *J. Hyg. Cambridge* **95**:29–38.
4. **Lee, J. V., and A. A. West.** 1991. Survival and growth of Legionella species in the environment. *Soc. Appl. Bacteriol. Symp. Ser.* **20**:121S–129S.
5. **Oleinick, N. L.** 1977. Initiation and elongation of protein synthesis in growing cells: differential inhibition by cycloheximide and emetine. *Arch. Biochem. Biophys.* **182**:171.
6. **Rogers, J., and C. W. Keevil.** 1992. Immunogold and flouroscein immunolabelling of *Legionella pneumophila* within an aquatic biofilm visualized using episcopic differential interference contrast microscopy. *Appl. Environ. Microbiol.* **58**:2326–2330.
7. **Skaliy, P., and H. V. McEachern.** 1979. Survival of Legionnaires' disease bacterium in water. *Ann. Intern. Med.* **90**:662–663.
8. **Surman, S.** 1994. The integration of an avirulent *Legionella pneumophila* into aquatic biofilms. Ph.D. thesis, University of Central Lancashire, Lancashire, United Kingdom.
9. **Tremaine, S. C., and A. L. Mills.** 1987. Inadequacy of the eukaryote inhibitor cycloheximide in studies of protozoan grazing on bacteria at the freshwater-sediment interface. *Appl. Environ. Microbiol.* **53**:8, 1969–1972.
10. **Tully, M. A., A. Williams, and R. B. Fitzgeorge.** 1992. Transposon mutagenesis in *Legionella pneumophila*. 11 mutants exhibiting impaired intracellular growth within cultured alveolar macrophages and reduced virulence *in vivo*. *Res. Microbiol.* **5**:143, 481–489.
11. **Walker, J. T., J. Rogers, and C. W. Keevil.** 1994. An investigation of the efficacy of a bromine containing biocide on an aquatic consortium of planktonic and biofilm microorganisms including *Legionella pneumophila*. *Biofouling* **8**:47–54.

# GENETIC ANALYSIS OF *LEGIONELLA PNEUMOPHILA* INTRACELLULAR MULTIPLICATION IN HUMAN AND PROTOZOAN HOSTS

Gil Segal and Howard A. Shuman

# 18

Several approaches have been taken to understand the genetic basis for intracellular multiplication by *Legionella pneumophila*. The first was based on the properties of avirulent variants that had lost the ability to replicate inside macrophages and were also defective in preventing phagosome-lysosome fusion. We reasoned that introduction of a wild-type region of the *L. pneumophila* genome that restored the ability to replicate within and kill human macrophages would provide information about the genes that were defective in the variants. A genomic library of wild-type *L. pneumophila* DNA was introduced to one of the avirulent variants, and complemented bacteria that regained the abilities to replicate intracellularly and kill host cells were identified with the aid of a plaque assay (3). The region of the *L. pneumophila* genome present in the complementing plasmid contained several genes that we referred to as *icm* (intracellular multiplication) genes (2). Using an independent ap-

proach that relied on rescue of a Thy⁻ auxotroph from thymine-less death, Berger and Isberg identified the same region and referred to one of the genes as *dotA*, for defective organelle trafficking (1).

To ask if the *icm/dotA* locus was the only set of genes required for intracellular multiplication and host cell killing, we used random transposon mutagenesis with Tn*903*dII*lacZ* to generate a large collection of independent mutants with random insertion mutations in the *L. pneumophila* genome. Among these we identified 55 mutants that lost the ability to kill HL-60-derived macrophages (6). The mutants grow as well as the wild type on bacteriologic media, indicating that their defect is specific to the intracellular lifestyle. Initially the mutants were classified into 16 hybridization groups on the basis of the genomic *Eco*RI fragment that contained the transposon. Subsequently these mutants have characterized genetically. Mapping and DNA sequence analysis indicate that the mutations define two unlinked regions of the *L. pneumophila* genome, which we refer to as region I and region II. (A description of the genomic analysis is found in chapter 19.)

To genetically characterize the *icm* genes we have (i) cloned the wild-type DNA that corresponds to the mutant loci, (ii) deter-

*Gil Segal* Department of Molecular Microbiology and Biotechnology, George S. Wise Faculty of Life Sciences, Tel-Aviv University, Ramat-Aviv, Israel.  *Howard A. Shuman* Department of Microbiology, College of Physicians & Surgeons, Columbia University, 701 West 168th Street, New York, NY 10032.

*Legionella*, Edited by Reinhard Marre et al.
© 2002 ASM Press, Washington, D.C.

mined the DNA sequence of these regions, (iii) determined the sequence of the fusion joints between the transposon and *L. pneumophila* DNA for 53 of 55 mutations, (iv) constructed mutations in open reading frames not containing a transposon insertion, (v) analyzed the phenotypes of the mutants, and (vi) conducted complementation tests for mutations in each gene to evaluate its role in intracellular multiplication and host cell killing.

## THE *icm/dot* GENE COMPLEX: TWO UNLINKED REGIONS COMPRISING 24 GENES

### Region I Comprises the *icmVWX/dotABCD* Genes

Region I corresponds to the previously identified 12-kb *Eco*RI fragment that complemented the avirulent variant (3) and was independently identified by Berger and Isberg. Eleven of the Tn*903*dII*lacZ* insertions map to this region including two in the *dotA* gene. The nine other insertions lie in three adjacent genes called *icmV, W,* and *X.* Figure 1 describes the arrangement of these genes. Results from Ralph Isberg's group indicate the presence of three other genes, *dotBCD,* 8 kb

downstream from *dotA* that are required for intracellular multiplication (12).

## Region II Is 22 kb and Encodes 18 Genes, 17 of Which Are Required for Intracellular Multiplication

As a result of sequencing and cosmid mapping we established that seven of the DNA hybridization groups are contiguous and contain 18 genes. Seven of these genes were not mutated in any of the transposon insertion mutants. Mutations in these genes were constructed by insertion of drug resistance elements in the *L. pneumophila* genome by allelic exchange. Complementation studies indicate that 17 of the 18 genes are required for intracellular multiplication and macrophage killing. Mutations in the other gene, *tphA* (for transport protein homolog) had no effect on intracellular multiplication in any host that has been tested so far. Many of these genes were also identified independently by the Isberg lab and are referred to as *dot* genes in their publications.

### The *icmTSRQPO* Cluster

This group of genes was initially identified by cloning the region corresponding to DNA hy-

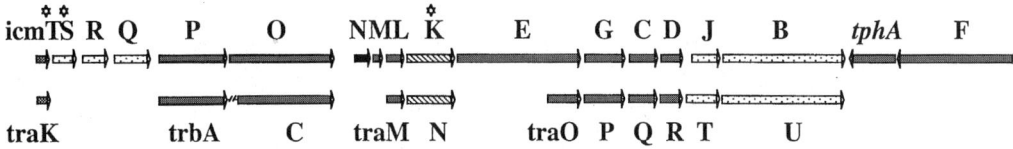

**FIGURE 1** Linkage map of the two *icm/dot* regions. Region I contains *icmVWX-dotABCD,* and region II contains *icmTSRQPONMLKEGCDJB-tphA-icmF.* Coding regions are indicated by bold arrows. The homologs from the IncI plasmid colIb-P9 are indicated under the corresponding *icm/dot* gene. Shading indicates the predicted location of the protein in the bacterial cell: ■, lipoprotein; ▦, cytoplasm; ▬, inner membrane; ▨, periplasm. The star indicates *icm* genes that were found to have homologs in *C. burnetii.*

bridization group 3 (9). The cloned DNA was sequenced (6,432 bp) and found to contain six genes, *icmT-O*. Five of these contained at least one transposon. The *icmS* gene did not contain a transposon and was mutagenized by insertion of a kanamycin resistance cassette. Strains with a mutation in the *icmS, icmR*, or *icmQ* gene retained some detectable ability to grow within and kill HL-60-derived macrophages. In contrast, mutations in the *icmT, icmP*, and *icmO* genes were completely defective in macrophage killing and intracellular multiplication. Complementation tests using plasmids with in-frame deletions of each gene indicated that the *icmTS* genes are likely to be cotranscribed, as are the *icmPO* genes. In addition, the *icmR* and *icmQ* genes are likely to be independently transcribed.

### The *icmNMLKE* Cluster

This region contained four genes (*icmNMLK*) that had not been identified from the transposon insertions (7). In contrast, the *icmE* gene was represented by several transposon mutations in groups 9, 7, and 2. The other genes were mutagenized by allele exchange with a kanamycin resistance cassette. The *icmMLKE* genes are required for growth within and killing of macrophages and amoebae. The *icmN* gene is not required for growth within or killing of HL-60-derived macrophages, but is partially required when amoebae are used as a host (11). The *icmN* gene product contains a fatty acid acylation site sequence found in lipoproteins as well as an "OmpA" box, an amino acid sequence found in several gram-negative outer membrane proteins. Complementation tests indicate that the *icmN* gene is transcribed as a single gene and that the *icmMLKE* genes are probably cotranscribed. The *icmE* gene sequence is remarkable because it encodes 42 repeats of a 10 amino acid sequence. Although the significance of the repeats is unknown at present, it suggests a highly organized repeated structural element (7).

### The *icmGCDJBF, tphA* Cluster

This region was originally identifed by complementation of an *icmB* mutation by the pMW100 plasmid, derived from a genomic library in pMMB207 (4). Mutations in *icmG* and *icmF* have only slight defects in the abilities to grow within and kill HL-60-derived macrophages, but are required for growth in amoebae (11). Mutations in the *tphA* gene result in no detectable defects in either host. This gene encodes a protein that is highly homologous to several amino acid transporters. Strains with mutations in the remaining genes are unable to grow within or kill macrophages.

### HOMOLOGY TO IncI PLASMIDS R64 AND colIb-P9 AND *COXIELLA BURNETII*

Soon after the sequence of region II was determined, several similarities to plasmid genes were noted. However, in 1998 the complete sequences of the *tra* and *trb* genes of the IncI plasmid, colIb-P9, was made available (Sampei and Mizobuchi, GenBank accession no. AB021078). When the sequences of regions I and II were used as queries in a BLAST (basic local alignment search tool) search, the sequence of the colIb-P9 plasmid was found to be highly similar to *icm* and *dot* genes in both regions I and II. As shown in Fig. 1, not only are the sequences conserved, but there is a striking match in the organization of the *icm/dot* genes and their homologs from the colIb-P9 plasmid (10). No similarity with plasmid genes was found for nine of the genes (*icmS, R, Q, N, M, F, V, W*, and *X*). When the sequence of another IncI plasmid became available (R64), the same homologies with the *icm/dot* genes were found. We interpret these homologies to indicate that the Icm and Dot products likely form a multi-subunit complex in analogy with the corresponding plasmid gene products that are known to be required for conjugal transfer. Although the imputed function of the Icm/Dot complex is related to intracellular multiplication and prevention of phagosome-lysosome fusion, the similarity of the *icm/dot* genes to the colIb-P9 transfer system provided a strong impetus to investigate the conjugation proficiency of *L. pneumophila*.

In addition to these homologies to plasmid genes, we found significant homology of three *icm* genes to partial sequences from the *C. burnetii* genome. The *icmT, S,* and *K* genes were found to have matches against three partial sequences from the *C. burnetii* genome database. Although it is difficult to understand the precise meaning of these matches, it is noteworthy that *C. burnetii* is also an intracellular pathogen of macrophages closely related to *L. pneumophila*, yet does not prevent phagosome-lysosome fusion, but rather grows in the fused phagolysosome. Both the *icmT* and *icmK* genes share homology with the IncI plasmid genes, yet *icmS* does not. This leads to the suggestion that the *C. burnetii* genome will be found to include a set of genes similar to the *icm/dot* genes. Furthermore, it would seem unlikely that the *icmS* gene is the sole determinant of intracellular fate.

## CONJUGAL ACTIVITY OF THE *icm/dot* COMPLEX

The striking homology between the *icm/dot* genes and the IncI *tra* and *trb* genes involved in conjugal DNA transfer prompted us to examine if *L. pneumophila* could conjugally transfer DNA. We found that, indeed, the mobilizable IncQ plasmid pMMB207 (derived from RSF1010) is transferred between *L. pneumophila* strains at a frequency of $10^{-3}$ per donor (7). Although transfer is absolutely dependent on the *icmR, icmT,* and *dotA* genes, mutations in other *icm* genes result in only a 50-fold decrease in transfer (10). The absence of a requirement for the majority of the *icm/dot* products may be due to the existence of additional conjugal systems in the *L. pneumophila* genome (8) (see chapters 19 and 20). The *oriT* origin of transfer of pMMB207 and the MobA relaxase protein are required for transfer. Because others have shown that the MobA protein (i) produces a single-stranded

nick at *oriT*, (ii) forms a covalent intermediate with the single strand of plasmid DNA, and (iii) is transferred to the recipient as a nucleoprotein complex with single-stranded binding protein, these results suggest that the Icm transfer apparatus, or a portion of it, can transport the same nucleoprotein complex to the recipient cell. We also have evidence that *L. pneumophila* can transfer chromosomal markers in addition to plasmids. Several strains containing Tn*903*dII*lacZ* at different locations in the genome were able to transfer the Km$^r$ phenotype of the transposon to another strain at approximately the same frequency ($10^{-6}$ per donor). This chromosome transfer activity seems not to depend on the Icm/Dot system (see chapter 20).

An indication that the conjugal activity of the Icm/Dot system may be related to its normal function came from observing the effects of the RSF1010 plasmids on the ability of the bacteria to multiply intracellularly and kill host cells. Wild-type *L. pneumophila* are approximately 100-fold less able to kill HL-60-derived macrophages and exhibit a significant intracellular growth lag if they harbor an RSF1010 plasmid. These effects are mitigated if the plasmid lacks a functional *oriT* or *mobA* gene, suggesting that an active transferable nucleoprotein complex is responsible for these effects (10). These observations suggest that the plasmid in some way diminishes the activity of the Icm/Dot complex, either by competition with endogenous substrates for the system, or by causing the formation of a conjugation-proficient, but effector transfer-deficient, complex.

## SIMILARITY TO THE *AGROBACTERIUM* SYSTEM

Because several of the *icm* genes bear homology to transfer genes of plasmids and because other systems that are known to be used for macromolecular transfer also contain genes with similarity to plasmid transfer genes, it is worthwhile to consider possible parallels between these other systems and the Icm/Dot system. The *vir* system of *Agrobacterium tumefaciens* that transfers T-DNA to plant cells, the pertussis toxin *ptl* exporter, and the *tra* conjugative system of the IncN plasmid pKM101 are closely related to one another (14). Although most of these genes do not share significant sequence similarity with the *L. pneumophila icm* genes, the overall composition and arrangements of the components suggest that the systems may share functional similarities. In the *vir, ptl,* and *tra* systems are approximately 20 components and a preponderance of proteins with transmembrane domains. However, the IcmE and DotB proteins each contain a region that shows slight similarity to VirB10 and VirB11, respectively. Each system has components with nucleotide binding sites that are thought to be required either for energization or assembly of the system. The finding that the Icm system can conjugate DNA together with its overall resemblance to these well-characterized systems reinforces the hypothesis that the Icm system may function as a transfer apparatus to deliver effector molecules specifically to the host cell in a manner that is similar to the three systems described above. The *L. pneumophila* effectors must interact with the components of the host cell that mediate phagosome-lysosome fusion.

## FUNCTION OF THE *icm/dot* COMPLEX

The earliest function of *L. pneumophila* that is critical for its survival and growth inside host cells is prevention of phagosome-lysosome fusion. It has been known for many years that avirulent mutant forms of *L. pneumophila* have lost the ability to prevent phagosome-lysosome fusion, are unable to replicate intracellularly, and do not produce disease in animals. We therefore wanted to evaluate the ability of various *icm* and *dot* mutants to prevent phagosome-lysosome fusion in macrophages. To do this, we adapted a well-known colocalization technique in which lysosomes are prelabelled with rhodamine-dextran and the bacteria are labelled using fluorescein. It has been possible to measure the degree to

which phagosomes containing different strains of *L. pneumophila* fuse with rhodamine-labelled lysosomes. This has been accomplished with the aid of the confocal laser-scanning fluorescence microscope and measuring whether there is colocalization of the green and red fluorescence signals emanating from fluorescein and rhodamine, respectively. The results of these measurements are astonishingly clear. First, 25 to 30% of the phagosomes containing wild-type, viable *L. pneumophila* colocalize with lysosomes within 30 min after infection. This proportion does not increase over the next 6 h. In the cases of all of the representative transposon-induced mutants examined in the *icmX, dotA, dotB, icmE, icmR,* and *icmB* genes, 70 to 80% of the phagosomes are colocalized with rhodamine-labelled lysosomes by 30 min (the earliest time they could be examined). This high degree of fusion was the same as that found for paraformaldehyde-killed *L. pneumophila.* Here as well, the proportion did not increase over the next 6 h, indicating that the maximum level of phagosome-lysosome fusion had been observed shortly after infection (13). A simple interpretation of these results is that the decision whether a particular phagosome is going to fuse or not fuse with lysosomes is made rapidly upon interaction of the bacteria with the host cell. Defects in any of the *icm* or *dotA* genes examined result in maximal levels of phagosome-lysosome fusion either during or immediately following uptake into the phagosome. The possibility that the unidentified "effectors" rapidly control phagosome-lysosome fusion may indicate that they are injected into the host plasma membrane or cytosol and interact directly with components that mediate organelle fusion.

## WHICH Icm PROTEINS ARE EFFECTORS AND WHICH ARE COMPONENTS OF THE TRANSFER APPARATUS?

The current model for how the Icm/Dot complex influences the intracellular fate of *L. pneumophila* postulates that there are two classes of Icm/Dot gene products. One class of proteins constitutes a "transferosome" or structure similar in composition and arrangement to the type IV secretion system used by *Agrobacterium tumefaciens, Bordetella pertussis*, and pKM101 for delivering DNA to plants, pertussis toxin to host cells, and pilus assembly and conjugation, respectively. The second class is "effector" proteins that are transferred to the host cell and that directly interact with the components of the host cell that are involved in phagosome formation and fate. An immediate challenge is to sort out which Icm/Dot components belong to each class. At the present it is tempting to focus on the nine *icm* genes that do not share homology to plasmid genes as candidates for effector genes. Several of these encode water-soluble proteins that could be transferred to the host cell cytosol. In addition, the direct demonstration of transfer of an *L. pneumophila* gene product to a host cell would be compelling evidence that the transferred protein has a function in the host. We cannot exclude the possibility that other genes encode the effectors. These may not have been identified by the forward genetic analysis if they encode redundant functions.

## HOW DO THE EFFECTORS PREVENT PHAGOSOME-LYSOSOME FUSION?

Once the effectors and components of the transfer complex are identified, the key question of how the effectors determine the fate of the phagosome will need to be addressed. Several possible mechanisms could be used to specifically interrupt the fusion of phagosomes with lysosomes. The easiest way to imagine these is in the context of the SNARE hypothesis (5). This hypothesis is based on the existence and activities of a number of different proteins that are required for fusion in several different systems ranging from synaptic vesicles fusing at nerve junctions to vacuole trafficking in *Saccharomyces*. It seems clear that integral membrane proteins containing a coiled:coil domain are responsible for pairing the compartments that are to be fused and that

several classes of cytosolic proteins regulate and/or catalyze the actual events leading to fusion. Among these are ATP-dependent proteins and small farnesylated GTP binding proteins (rabs). The distribution of $Ca^{2+}$ within different compartments may also influence fusion activity. This complexity allows several opportunities for a pathogen to influence whether fusion will take place. The assignment of specific functions to the *L. pneumophila* effector proteins will depend on their biochemical characterization.

## REFERENCES

1. **Berger, K. H., J. J. Merriam, and R. R. Isberg.** 1994. Altered intracellular targeting properties associated with mutations in the *Legionella dotA* gene. *Mol. Microbiol.* **14**:809–822.
2. **Brand, B. C., A. B. Sadosky, and H. A. Shuman.** 1994. The *Legionella pneumophila icm* locus: a set of genes required for intracellular multiplication in human macrophages. *Mol. Microbiol.* **14**:797–808.
3. **Marra, A., S. J. Blander, M. A. Horwitz, and H. A. Shuman.** 1992. Identification of a *Legionella pneumophila* locus required for intracellular multiplication in human macrophages. *Proc. Natl. Acad. Sci. USA* **89**:9607–9611.
4. **Purcell, M. W., and H. A. Shuman.** 1998. The *Legionella pneumophila icmGCDJBF* genes are required for killing of human macrophages. *Infect. Immun.* **66**:2245–2255.
5. **Rothman, J. E., and G. Warren.** 1994. Implications of the SNARE hypothesis for intracellular membrane topology and dynamics. *Curr. Biol.* **4**:220–233.
6. **Sadosky, A. B., L. A. Wiater, and H. A. Shuman.** 1993. Identification of *Legionella pneumophila* genes required for growth within and killing of human macrophages. *Infect. Immun.* **61**:5361–5373.
7. **Segal, G., M. Purcell, and H. A. Shuman.** 1998. Host cell killing and bacterial conjugation require overlapping sets of genes within a 22-kb region of the *Legionella pneumophila* genome. *Proc. Natl. Acad. Sci. USA* **95**:1669–1674.
8. **Segal, G., J. J. Russo, and H. A. Shuman.** 1999. Relationships between a new type IV secretion system and the *icm/dot* virulence system of *Legionella pneumophila*. *Mol. Microbiol.* **34**:799–809.
9. **Segal, G., and H. A. Shuman.** 1997. Characterization of a new region required for macrophage killing by *Legionella pneumophila*. *Infect. Immun.* **65**:5057–5066.

10. **Segal, G., and H. A. Shuman.** 1998. Intracellular multiplication and human macrophage killing by *Legionella pneumophila* are inhibited by conjugal components of IncQ plasmid RSF1010. *Mol. Microbiol.* **30:**197–208.

11. **Segal, G., and H. A. Shuman.** 1999. *Legionella pneumophila* utilizes the same genes to multiply within *Acanthamoeba castellanii* and human macrophages. *Infect. Immun.* **67:**2117–2124.

12. **Vogel, J. P., H. L. Andrews, S. K. Wong, and R. R. Isberg.** 1998. Conjugative transfer by the virulence system of *Legionella pneumophila.* *Science* **279:**873–876.

13. **Wiater, L. A., K. Dunn, F. R. Maxfield, and H. A. Shuman.** 1998. Early events in phagosome establishment are required for intracellular survival of *Legionella pneumophila.* *Infect. Immun.* **66:**4450–4460.

14. **Winans, S. C., D. L. Burns, and P. J. Christie.** 1996. Adaptation of the conjugal transfer system for the export of pathogenic macromolecules. *Trends Microbiol.* **4:**64–68.

# THE *LEGIONELLA PNEUMOPHILA* SEQUENCING PROJECT

Xiaoyan Qu, Irina Morozova, Minchen Chen,
Sergey Kalachikov, Gil Segal, Jing Chen, Hye Park,
Anthi Georghiou, Gifty Asamani, Marc Feder, Justin Rineer,
Joseph J. Greenberg, Curtis Goldsberry, Andrey Rzhetsky,
Stuart G. Fischer, Pieter DeJong, Peisen Zhang,
Eftihia Cayanis, Howard A. Shuman, and James J. Russo

# 19

The current work is aimed at obtaining the complete sequence of the Philadelphia 1 strain of *Legionella pneumophila*, derived from the original 1976 outbreak that established the clinical entity known as Legionnaires' disease. Previous evidence suggested the genome size of this bacterial strain was approximately 3.9 Mb, when assessed by pulsed field gel electrophoresis (4), and there have been no consistent findings of associated plasmids in the Philadelphia 1 strain. Since it has been assigned to the gamma proteobacteria on the basis of 16S RNA homology (8, 14), the legionellaceae are considered to be relatively closely related to gram-negative bacteria such as *Escherichia coli* and *Coxiella burnetii*. It is not known with certainty whether the *L. pneumophila* genome exists as a closed circular or linear molecule.

The approach that we are using to obtain the complete genomic sequence is bipartite (Fig. 1). On the one hand, the whole genome shotgun method is being used to avoid dependence for any genomic region on a single starting bacterium, which could have undergone recent damage or mutation, a potential problem with a strictly large clone-based approach. On the other hand, a bacterial artificial chromosome (BAC)-based map of the *Legionella* genome constructed from more than 200 probes and nearly 600 BAC clones (out of a starting 768 BAC library) was constructed. From this map, a tiling path of 25 BAC pairs was selected to generate additional shotgun libraries covering the length of the genome, BAC by BAC. This will minimize assembly errors associated with repetitive sequences occurring in multiple places in the genome. Other than a few M13 clones, the majority of the sequencing clones from both BAC and whole genome shotguns were plasmids, which were sequenced bidirectionally. Finally, both ends of the majority of the 768 BACs were sequenced to obtain additional anchoring probes.

To construct the BAC map, the ~30x coverage BAC library was arrayed on nylon filters and hybridized with sequences from 30 previously known *Legionella* genes, nearly 250

Xiaoyan Qu, Irina Morozova, Minchen Chen, Sergey Kalachikov, Jing Chen, Hye Park, Anthi Georghiou, Gifty Asamani, Marc Feder, Justin Rineer, Joseph P. Greenberg, Curtis Goldsberry, Andrey Rzhetsky, Stuart G. Fischer, Peisen Zhang, Eftihia Cayanis, and James J. Russo  Columbia Genome Center, Columbia University, 1150 St. Nicholas Avenue, New York, NY 10032.  Gil Segal and Howard A. Shuman  Department of Microbiology, Columbia University, 1150 St. Nicholas Avenue, New York, NY 10032. Pieter DeJong  Children's Hospital Oakland Research Institute, 747 52nd Street, Oakland, CA 94609.

*Legionella*, Edited by Reinhard Marre et al.
© 2002 ASM Press, Washington, D.C.

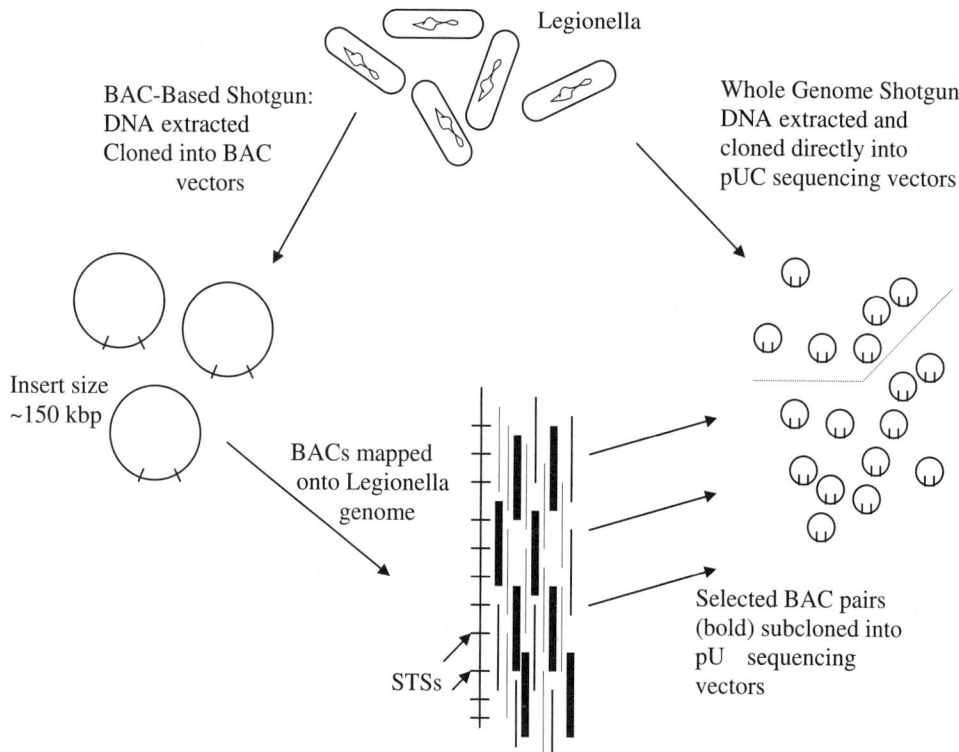

**FIGURE 1** Two-pronged sequencing approach. The method of sequencing is diagrammed in this cartoon. DNA isolated from *L. pneumophila* grown to confluence on charcoal-impregnated agar plates were either partially digested with *Eco*RI and cloned into the pBACe3.6 vector (left side of figure) or sheared by nebulization and directly cloned into the pUC19 sequencing vector (right side). In the former case, BACs were assembled by the STS mapping approach (see text for details), and BAC pairs from across the genome were individually sheared and subcloned into pUC19. Sequencing was primed from the M13–21 and reverse promoters in the pUC19 vector. BAC ends were also sequenced using T7 and SP6 promoters as extension primers. All sequences were pooled and assembled together.

random sequences from throughout the genome, and a few specific BAC insert end sequences. For each regional shotgun library, two BACs covering essentially the same area were used. The argument was that any individual BAC might display some rearrangement that occurred during the cloning operation, but that the same error would not have a high likelihood of occurring in two separate clones.

Three-eighths of the sequences were derived from the whole genome shotgun clones, and 5/8 of the sequences will come from the BAC-based shotgun clones. Following base-calling and weekly assembly using the phred/phrap tool suite (reference 7, and http://www.genome.washington.edu/UWGC/analysistools/phrap.htm), preliminary annotation of the sequences is by the gene prediction program GLIMMER, and BLAST (basic local alignment search tool) homology searches (2, 3, 6). BLAST searches are repeated regularly on old as well as new contigs, since the bacterial genome databases are expanding so rapidly. All sequences assembled into contigs are displayed on our web pages, along with graphical views of the GLIMMER and BLAST results.

## USING THE *LEGIONELLA* WEBSITE

From the outset, it has been our intention to produce a source of data for workers in the

*Legionella* and other related fields that is as informative and user friendly as feasible, given its state of flux. From the home page, which is located at http://genome3.cpmc. columbia.edu/~legion/, one can link to several types of general information using the buttons entitled "about this project," "about *Legionella*," and "personnel." The home page also includes a weekly updated indicator of the length of sequence contained within contigs and a link ("current statistics") that expands upon this information and also lists the number of single sequence reads (singlets), those not yet incorporated into contigs. We have chosen not to display singlets on the website because they are much more likely to be poor or short reads, have not been verified by overlap, and are more likely to derive from contaminating *E. coli*. Eventually, of course, any true and accurate *Legionella* singlet will merge with a contig.

As soon as two or more sequence reads join to form a longer sequence (a so-called contig), it is listed on the "contigs overview" page in approximate size order and is presented graphically on its own web page with appropriate annotation (see the example in Fig. 2). As more and more reads are appended to contigs (growth by accretion), their size, and hence their numbered position on the contigs overview page, will continuously change. To aid users in locating a contig they previously examined, contigs are identified using the name of the oldest sequence read in that contig. Thus, typing part of its name into the browser's search or find function on the contigs overview page should usually permit immediate retrieval of the contig. When two contigs coalesce, the name of the earliest contig takes precedence; in this case, it is still easy to find the new contig using one of its read names or some of its actual sequence (using the "sequence search" or "genome blast search" functions, respectively; see below). The contig overview table also provides the size and number of reads for each contig.

By clicking on the contig name, one connects to a graphical view of that contig, a highlight of our website (Fig. 2). For each contig, a large amount of information has been compiled into an easy-to-access form. All colored bars and arrows contain embedded links; mousing over them causes information to be displayed in the bottom bar of the browser window; clicking on them affects the link to the site to which they point. At the top of the page is a long blue bar representing the contig. Its current size in base pairs is shown, and by clicking on the bar, one obtains a list of all the reads that have been assembled to generate the contig. The read names usually denote the clone that has been sequenced; since all the clones have been archived, they are available to investigators upon request. Whenever the GLIMMER program has determined that there is a likely gene within the contig, this is displayed as a red arrowhead, and sized and positioned appropriately under the blue bar. Clicking on the arrowhead brings up a new window with the GLIMMER output for the entire contig. BLAST homology is shown with similarly oriented arrows (magenta if derived from the nonredundant database and green if from the protein database). Protein hits will often directly underlie the GLIMMER arrowheads, particularly when the predicted genes themselves were used to search the protein database. Mousing over such an amino acid BLAST hit will show coordinates relative to the current predicted gene. In contrast, when the entire contig is used in amino acid BLAST searches, and for all nucleotide BLAST searches, the displayed coordinates for such hits are relative to the entire contig length. In either case, clicking on the BLAST arrow brings up the NCBI (National Center for Biotechnology Information) BLAST output page with its own associated links. Thus, in addition to the alignments, one can immediately retrieve the actual GenBank entries and any associated publications. Because we use very stringent criteria for presentation of BLAST search results (*P* values <1.0E-15 for amino acid hits, <1.0E-05 for nucleotide hits), and there are page limits for the number of BLAST hits that can be displayed, we recommend the user conduct additional searches

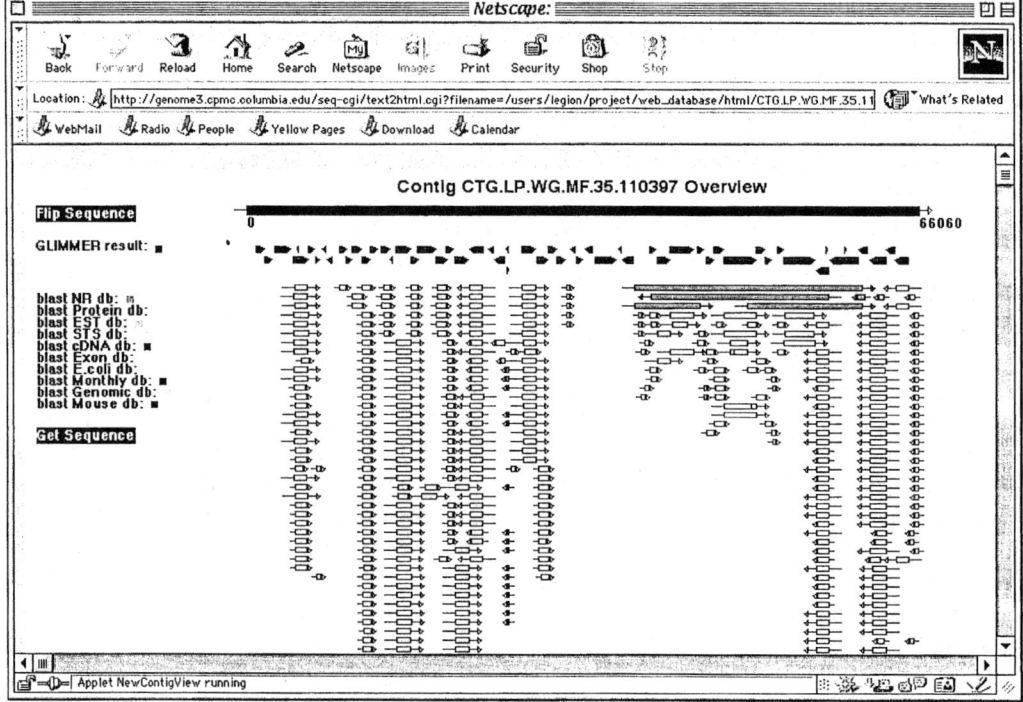

**FIGURE 2** Website contig display. Graphical representation of one of the larger contigs in the *Legionella* genome project at this time (66,060 base pairs), it contains the major region of *icm/dot* genes (grouped below approximately the third quartile and the beginning of the fourth quartile of the upper bar). Other genes within this contig include homologs to enzymes of the pentose phosphate pathway and sugar catabolism on the left side of the map, and purine ribonucleotide biosynthetic enzymes on the far right. Details on this type of image are provided in the text, and the reader is urged to explore the actual web page to better appreciate its utility and functionality.

if lower stringency or more homologs are expected. Similarly, because we are using only one program for automatic gene prediction, a few percent of false-positive or false-negative genes are bound to occur. Sometimes on the graphics pages for the larger contigs, space is too limited to present all the BLAST hits in neat registers; to ensure seeing all of those depicted, one should be sure to scroll to the bottom of the page. Two additional buttons exist on the graphics pages, "Flip Sequence" and "Get Sequence." The former redraws the contig in the opposite orientation, and the latter is a simple way to obtain the entire contig sequence in FASTA format, which can then be used conveniently for local and global database searches, codon translations, or other kinds of analysis.

From the home page, in addition to the links to general information, statistics and the contigs, additional services are provided. The "genome blast search" page allows users to use any FASTA format sequence to conduct BLAST searches (blastn, tblastx, tblastn) of our *Legionella* project sequences. Importantly, this is not restricted to contigs, but all the singlet sequences are potential search targets as well. The "sequence search" engine permits string searches of all our reads by name and date. As discussed above, this can be useful when a contig has melded with others, and its name has been subsumed by one of those. In that case, typing the "lost" name in the "sequence search" box will retrieve the new contig, within which the original sequence can be relocated. Further information on use of these services is provided on the website. Finally, we have made every effort to make our sequences publicly available as soon as they form contigs. Thus, in addition to submitting larger contigs to the Unfinished Microbial Genomes Database at NCBI, and BAC sequences to the High Throughput Genomic (HTG) division of the EMBL/GenBank/DDBJ database (links to both sites may be found on the website), users have the option of downloading current contigs, or all contigs greater than 1 kb in size, to their computers for further analysis.

## GENES OF *L. PNEUMOPHILA*

The GC content of *L. pneumophila* is ~38% over most of its length. From the genomic sequence so far (more than 85% of the sequence is currently contained in contigs greater than 1 kb), we estimate we have covered 3,000 open reading frames (ORF), about 2,000 of which are complete, and on the basis of homology to genes from other prokaryotes, we have identified more than 1,100 putative genes in *L. pneumophila*. Even using our stringent criteria, a significant number (~63%) display homology to proteins with known or putative functions; with the increasing number of completed bacterial genomes and global approaches to assessing functions of unknown proteins, this percentage is likely to increase.

In addition to those homologous to genes encoding members of most of the major metabolic pathways (e.g., synthesis of small molecules and macromolecules; enzymes of central intermediary and energy metabolism; transport and binding proteins; metabolism of DNA, transcription, translation, and protein turnover; and cell envelope proteins), there are numerous proteins involved in various cellular processes (cell division, detoxification, motility, response and transcription regulation, and protein secretion and trafficking). We have observed several putative transposases in the *L. pneumophila* Philadelphia 1 sequence,

but their precise disposition within the genome is still uncertain. Because the whole genome shotgun was supplemented with BAC-based shotguns from the beginning, many complete operons are already available. For example, one contig (36.6 kb long as of this writing) has seven members of the histidine synthesis operon near one end and 11 genes encoding flagellar structural and biosynthetic proteins (*flgB-K* and *fliC*) near the other; a second contig (46.8 kb) contains two operons with 16 additional flagellar genes (including *fliA, M, N, P, Q, R; flhB, A, F, G; motA, B, R* at one end; and *fliE-I* at the other end and with the opposite polarity). Finally, there are several well-known (e.g., the *dot/icm* system, *relA, rpoD, mip, katB, EnhA, frgA, legiolysin*) and a few new candidate genes for factors involved in the intracellular life cycle and pathogenicity of *Legionella* (including several pilus assembly proteins, putative proteases and hemolysins, an invasion associated protein [*invA/mutT* homolog], a *vacB* [RNAse R] gene, an *Agrobacterium tumefaciens virG* homolog, a homolog of *mviN*, and potential regulators of virulence genes).

## GENE COMPARISONS

The *icm/dot* genes and the *lvr/lvh* genes have been described in detail elsewhere (11–13, 15) and are highlighted in chapters 15 and 18 in this volume. Different members of these gene clusters are thought to function in conjugal DNA transfer, protein secretion, or virulence. We are analyzing these genes in a collection of *L. pneumophila* isolates and other *Legionella* species with the aim of assessing their role in these processes. Each of the genes is amplified from the Philadelphia 1 strain of *L. pneumophila*, and the product is then hybridized at low stringency to each of the other strains or species. A positive signal is tentatively assumed to represent the homologous gene; negative signals do not necessarily indicate the absence of the gene since the stringency might be too high if the genes vary considerably (a portion of the hybridization results are displayed for the *icmO* gene in Fig. 3A). For all positives,

**A**

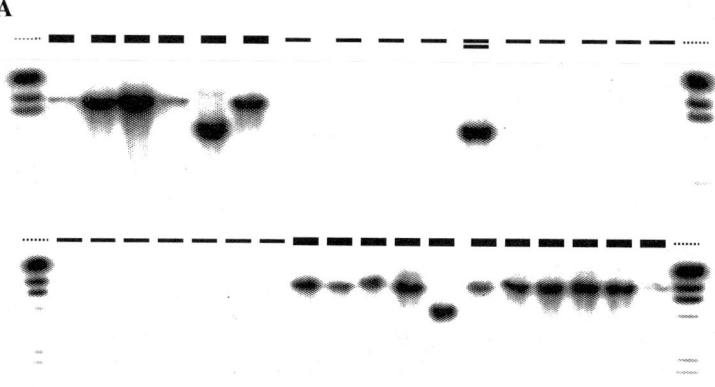

**B**

```
GATgTGGATCAGGCTGGTGAATCGGATCTCGATTCAGAAGCTTCGTTTCAATCTGGaAAAGAGGGATTAACAAAG
 D  V  D  Q  A  G  E  S  D  L  D  S  E  A  S  F  Q  S  G  K  E  G  L  T  K
GATATGGATCAGGCTGGTGAATCGGATCTCGATTCAGAAGCTTCGTTTCAATCTGGGAAAGAGGGATTAACAAAG
 D  M  D  Q  A  G  E  S  D  L  D  S  E  A  S  F  Q  S  G  K  E  G  L  T  K
GATATGGATCAGGCTGGTGAATCGGATCTCGATTCAGAAGCcTCGTaTCAATCTGGGAAAGAGGGATTAACAAAG
 D  M  D  Q  A  G  E  S  D  L  D  S  E  A  S  Y  Q  S  G  K  E  G  L  T  K
GATATGGATCAcGCTGGTGAATCGGATCTCGATTCAGAAGCTTCGTTTCAATCTGGGAAAGAGGGATTAACAAAG
 D  M  D  H  A  G  E  S  D  L  D  S  E  A  S  F  Q  S  G  K  E  G  L  T  K
GATATGGATCAGGCgGGTGAATCGGATCTCGATTCAcAAGCTTCGTaTCAATCgGGaAAAGAaGGATTAACAAgG
 D  M  D  Q  A  G  E  S  D  L  D  S  Q  A  S  Y  Q  S  G  K  E  G  L  T  R
```

**FIGURE 3** *icm* gene comparisons among legionellaceae. (A) Hybridization-based comparison of the *icmO* gene. DNA from various isolates of *L. pneumophila* (shown with bolder bars and representing 13 different serogroups) and several other species of *Legionella* (lighter bars) were digested with *Eco*RI, transferred to nylon membranes, hybridized with a probe for the *icmO* gene from the Philadelphia 1 isolate of *L. pneumophila*, and washed at reduced stringency (0.5× SSC/ 0.1% SDS). Strong hybridization signals were elicited by all the *L. pneumophila* isolates and by *Legionella hackeliae* (double black bar). (B) Sequence comparison of the *icmG* gene. A small portion of the sequence of the *icmG* homolog (near the N terminus) in different *Legionella* isolates and species. The top sequence occurs in the Bellingham 1, Bloomington 2, Chicago 8, and Concord 3 strains of *L. pneumophila*; the second pattern occurs in the 797-PA-H and another isolate in serogroup 11 of *L. pneumophila*; the middle pattern is found in Philadelphia 1, Togus 1, and Chicago 2 isolates of *L. pneumophila*; the fourth sequence is seen in the Los Angeles 1, IN-23-G1-C2 and Leiden 1 strains of *L. pneumophila*; and interestingly, the last pattern is present in *L. pneumophila*, Dallas 1, in *L. hackeliae*, Lansing 2, and in *Legionella rubrilucens*, WA-270A-C2. The less common forms of the bases are shown in small bold letters. The codons that exist in different forms and give rise to altered amino acids are also shown in bold, as are the variant amino acids themselves. Many additional base and amino acid differences that distinguish these five families exist elsewhere within the *icmG* gene coding sequence.

the PCR primers used to amplify the gene in Philadelphia 1 are then used to achieve amplification in the additional strains, again at reduced stringency. In most cases, there is correlation between PCR and hybridization positivity. Each amplifiable gene in each strain is sequenced using the same initial primers and additional walking primers as necessary to obtain full-length bidirectional coverage through the ORF. As controls, a number of housekeeping genes are being subjected to the same analysis. In very preliminary analyses, we have observed substantial sequence variation in some of the *icm/dot* genes that may correlate with the relatedness of the strains in general. For instance, in the case of the *icmG* gene, there are five variants among the *L. pneumophila* strains and two non-*pneumophila* species of *Legionella* (Fig. 3B). As this work proceeds, we will be looking for associations of gene variants with strain pathogenicity.

Having the complete sequence of *L. pneumophila* should aid many *Legionella* investigators in their work. Genes in *L. pneumophila* Philadelphia 1 can be compared with genes in other pathogenic organisms. The amino acid sequence can guide structural and functional analyses of enzymes and other proteins of the organism. We have used knockout strategies in the past to assess the function of genes discovered in the course of the sequencing project (12); this continues to be our preferred method for functional analysis. In an associated project, we are placing each newly identified gene onto microarrays for expression analysis; changes in mRNA levels at different times during the intracellular life cycle, or in amoebae versus human macrophages, may be indicative of the roles their protein products play at these various time points or under varying conditions. Finally, comparison of the *Legionella* genome and individual genes with those of the bacteria that have already been sequenced, particularly other intracellular pathogens such as *Chlamydia pneumoniae* and *trachomatis, Rickettsia prowazekii*, and *Mycobacterium tuberculosis*, should enable important information to be garnered on their various origins and evolutionary relatedness (1, 5, 9–10). Our preliminary analysis indicates, for instance, that some of the *icm/dot* genes (data not shown), and perhaps the entire *lvh/lvr* cluster (12), have been inherited by lateral transfer from other organisms.

## REFERENCES

1. **Andersson. S. G., A. Zomorodipour, J. O. Andersson, T. Sicheritz-Ponten, U. C. Alsmark, R. M. Podowski, A. K. Naslund, A. S. Eriksson, H. H. Winkler, and C. G. Kurland.** 1998. The genome sequence of *Rickettsia prowazekii* and the origin of mitochondria. *Nature* **396:**133–140.

2. **Altschul, S. F., W. Gish, W. Miller, E. W. Myers, and D. J. Lipman.** 1990. Basic local alignment search tool. *J. Mol. Biol.* **215:**403–410.

3. **Altschul, S. F., T. L. Madden, A. A. Schaffer, J. Zhang, Z. Zhang, W. Miller, and D. J. Lipman.** 1997. Gapped BLAST and PSI-BLAST: a new generation of protein database search programs. *Nucleic Acids Res.* **25:**3389–3402.

4. **Bender, L., M. Ott, R. Marre, and J. Hacker.** 1990. Genome analysis of *Legionella* spp. by orthogonal field alternation gel electrophoresis (OFAGE). *FEMS Microbiol. Lett.* **60:**253–257.

5. **Cole, S. T., R. Brosch, J. Parkhill, T. Garnier, C. Churcher, D. Harris, S. V. Gordon, K. Eiglmeier, S. Gas, C. E. Barry 3rd, F. Tekaia, K. Badcock, D. Basham, D. Brown, T. Chillingworth, R. Connor, R. Davies, K. Devlin, T. Feltwell, S. Gentles, N. Hamlin, S. Holroyd, T. Hornsby, K. Jagels, A. Krogh, J. McLean, S. Moule, L. Murphy, K. Oliver, J. Osborne, M. A. Quail, M.-A. Rajandream, J. Rogers, S. Rutter, K. Seeger, J. Skelton, R. Squares, S. Squares, J. E. Sulston, K. Taylor, S. Whitehead, and B. G. Barrell.** 1998. Deciphering the biology of *Mycobacterium tuberculosis* from the complete genome sequence. *Nature* **393:**537–544.

6. **Delcher, A. L., D. Harmon, S. Kasif, O. White, and S. L. Salzberg.** 1999. Improved microbial gene identification with GLIMMER. *Nucleic Acids Res.* **27:**4636–4641.

7. **Ewing, B., and P. Green.** 1998. Base-calling of automated sequencer traces using *Phred*. II. Error probabilities. *Genome Res.* **8:**186–194.

8. **Fry, N. K., S. Warwick, N. A. Saunders, and T. M. Embley.** 1991. The use of 16S ribosomal RNA analyses to investigate the phylogeny of the family Legionellaceae. *J. Gen. Microbiol.* **137:**1215–1222.

9. **Kalman, S., W. Mitchell, R. Marathe, C. Lammel, J. Fan, R. W. Hyman, L. Olinger, J. Grimwood, R. W. Davis, and R. S. Stephens.** 1999. Comparative genomes of *Chlamydia pneumoniae* and *C. trachomatis. Nat. Genet.* **21:**385–389.

10. **Read, T. D., R. C. Brunham, C. Shen, S. R. Gill, J. F. Heidelberg, O. White, E. K. Hickey, J. Peterson, T. Utterback, K. Berry, S. Bass, K. Linher, J. Weidman, H. Khouri, B. Craven, C. Bowman, R. Dodson, M.**

Gwinn, W. Nelson, R. DeBoy, J. Kolonay, G. McClarty, S. L. Salzberg, J. Eisen, and C. M. Fraser. 2000. Genome sequences of *Chlamydia trachomatis* MoPn and *Chlamydia pneumoniae* AR39. *Nucleic Acids Res.* **28:**1397–1406.

11. Roy, C. R. 1999. Trafficking of the *Legionella pneumophila* phagosome. *ASM News* **65:**416–421.

12. Segal, G., J. J. Russo, and H. A. Shuman. 1999. Relationships between a new type IV secretion system and the *icm/dot* virulence system of *Legionella pneumophila*. *Mol. Microbiol.* **34:**799–809.

13. Segal, G., and H. A. Shuman. 1998. How is the intracellular fate of the *Legionella pneumophila* phagosome determined? *Trends Microbiol.* **6:**253–255.

14. Tan, C. K., and L. Owens. 2000. Infectivity, transmission and 16S rRNA sequencing of a rickettsia, *Coxiella cheraxi* sp. nov., from the freshwater crayfish *Cherax quadricarinatus*. *Dis. Aquat. Organ.* **41:**115–122.

15. Vogel, J. P., and R. R. Isberg. 1999. Cell biology of *Legionella pneumophila*. *Curr. Opin. Microbiol.* **2:**30–34.

# CONJUGAL TRANSFER OF CHROMOSOMAL DNA IN *LEGIONELLA PNEUMOPHILA*

*Hiroshi Miyamoto, Hatsumi Taniguchi, Sumiyo Ishimatsu, Shin-ichi Yoshida, and Howard A. Shuman*

# 20

Conjugation is a complex process that involves the unidirectional transfer of DNA between two cells (12). One cell is the donor and encodes all the transfer functions, while the second cell serves as the recipient. During transfer, a unique site on the plasmids, the origin of transfer (*ori*T), is nicked, and the nicked strand of DNA is transferred from the donor to the recipient cells with the 5′ end associated with the nicking enzyme. In the recipient, the incoming strand is recircularized at *ori*T (to recreate a functional *ori*T) and replicated to regenerate the plasmid; thus, transconjugants become capable of acting as donors (12). If a chromosome acquires an *ori*T via integration of a conjugative element, it will become mobilizable. In *Escherichia coli*, such

strains, known as Hfr (high frequency of recombination), can transfer their chromosomes at high frequency (5). Conjugal transfer of chromosomal DNA has some different features from those of the transfer of plasmid DNA described above. Because of the large size of the chromosome and because transfer from the donor ceases at random periods during conjugation, there is a gradient of transfer, such that chromosomal markers closest to the *ori*T site are transferred most efficiently (5). It is very rare that recipients become transfer proficient, since this would require the whole chromosome to be transferred to recreate a functional *ori*T (5). For transferred chromosomal genes to be stably inherited, they must be integrated into the recipient chromosome by homologous recombination (8). In this study, we examined whether a chromosomal conjugation system exists in *Legionella pneumophila*.

## MATING EXPERIMENTS

Strain K6, which has the Km$^r$ LacZ$^+$ genes (11) transposed in the chromosome (9.4-kb *Hind*III-digested fragment) of strain Philadelphia-1, was used as one parent. Strain Chicago-2S, belonging to serogroup 6, which is a spontaneous streptomycin-resistant derivative of strain Chicago-2, was used as the

*Hiroshi Miyamoto and Hatsumi Taniguchi* Department of Microbiology, University of Occupational and Environmental Health, 1-1 Iseigaoka, Yahatanishi-ku, Kitakyushu 807-8555, Japan. *Sumiyo Ishimatsu* Department of Environmental Management 1, University of Occupational and Environmental Health, 1-1 Iseigaoka, Yahatanishi-ku, Kitakyushu 807-8555, Japan. *Shin-ichi Yoshida* Department of Bacteriology, Graduate School of Medical Sciences, Kyushu University, 3-1-1 Maidashi, Higashi-ku, Fukuoka 812-8582, Japan. *Howard A. Shuman* Department of Microbiology, College of Physicians and Surgeons, Columbia University, 701 West 168th Street, New York, NY 10032.

second parent. Recipient and donor *L. pneu-mophila* strains were harvested from buffered charcoal-yeast extract (BCYE) plates after 72 h of growth. Both strains were suspended separately in buffered yeast extract (BYE) medium and were grown overnight on a roller drum at 37°C to late-log phase. A 1.5-ml sample of the overnight cultures was centrifuged and washed with 0.5 ml of M63 medium and resuspended in 0.2 ml of M63 medium. An aliquot (10 $\mu$l) of donor and 10 $\mu$l of recipient were mixed and spotted on a BCYE plate and were incubated overnight at 37°C. The bacteria were harvested and then resuspended in 0.2 ml of M63 medium and plated, in several dilutions, on BCYE plates containing appropriate antibiotics in order to determine the number of transconjugants. In some experiments, top soft agar (0.7%) containing 0.7 mg of 5-bromo-4-chloro-3-indolyl-$\beta$-D-galacto-pyranoside (X-Gal) per ml were also used to confirm the LacZ$^+$ phenotype of the Km$^r$ recombinants. Serial dilutions of the same bacterial suspension were placed on BCYE plates containing the appropriate antibiotics to determine the number of donor and recipient cells. Conjugation frequencies were calculated as the number of transconjugants divided by the number of donor bacteria at the end of the experiment. Mating experiments between K6 (approximately 2.6 × 10$^9$ CFU) and Chicago-2S (approximately 8.5 × 10$^9$ CFU) typically yielded 10$^3$ Km$^r$ Sm$^r$ LacZ$^+$ recombinants. All recombinants tested (100/100) belonged to serogroup 6, which is the same serogroup as strain Chicago-2S. This result suggested that the donor was strain K6 and the recipient was strain Chicago-2S. The transfer frequency corresponded to about 10$^{-6}$ per donor. No Km$^r$ Sm$^r$ LacZ$^+$ colonies were obtained when only Chicago-2S was plated, and a few spontaneous Sm$^r$ mutants were obtained when K6 was plated on selective media. No recombinants were obtained when the mating experiments were carried out in BYE broth, implying that extended cell-to-cell contact or high cell density was required for efficient transfer. Recombinant formation was not affected by DNase I (10 $\mu$g/ml), and no

transfer was seen with one viable parent and one heat-killed parent before mating. No recombinants were obtained by mixing and incubating cell-free filtrates of one parent with the cells of the other parents, and no plaques were detected if filtrate from one parent was spotted onto a lawn of the other parent. These results suggested that neither transformation nor transduction were involved in the recombinant formation. The mechanism of the DNA transfer was most consistent with conjugal transfer.

## GENOTYPING OF RECOMBINANTS

To genetically examine the DNA transferred from K6 to Chicago-2S, genotyping by arbitrarily primed PCR (AP-PCR) and pulsed-field gel electrophoresis (PFGE) were performed among strains K6, Chicago-2S, and their transconjugants. Using an arbitrary primer BG2 (5′-TACATTCGAGGAC CCCTAAGTG-3′) (10), AP-PCR was carried out with 40 cycles of denaturation at 94°C for 1 min, annealing at 25°C for 1 min, and extension at 74°C for 2 min. Strains K6 and Chicago-2S produced different fingerprints from each other (Fig. 1, lanes 1 and 2). Fingerprints of transconjugants, except for those of HM1013 (Fig. 1, lane 5), were similar to that of Chicago-2S, but some new bands that were not observed in either of the parents

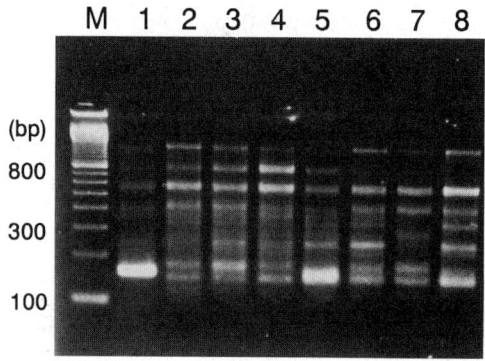

**FIGURE 1**  AP-PCR DNA fingerprints of *L. pneu-mophila* strains. Lanes: M, 100-bp ladder (Pharmacia Biotech) as a DNA size standard; 1, K6; 2, Chicago-2S; 3, HM1011; 4, HM1012; 5, HM1013; 6, HM1014; 7, HM1042; 8, HM1043.

were produced by the transconjugants (Fig. 1, lanes 6 to 8). As shown in Fig. 2, all the transconjugants exhibited identical restriction fragment polymorphism after PFGE of *Sfi*I-digested genomic DNA. The restriction fragment patterns of the transconjugants were distinct from the pattern exhibited by K6 and were similar to that exhibited by Chicago-2S (Fig. 2, lanes 3 and 8). A fragment of about 320 kb, not seen in either of the parents, was observed in all the transconjugants. These findings show that strain K6 is the donor and strain Chicago-2S is the recipient and also suggest that chromosomal genes transferred from K6 are integrated into the Chicago-2S chromosome by recombination.

## INTEGRATION OF TRANSFERRED DNA INTO A RECIPIENT CHROMOSOME

The transfer of DNA from the chromosome of strain K6 to Chicago-2S could occur by a

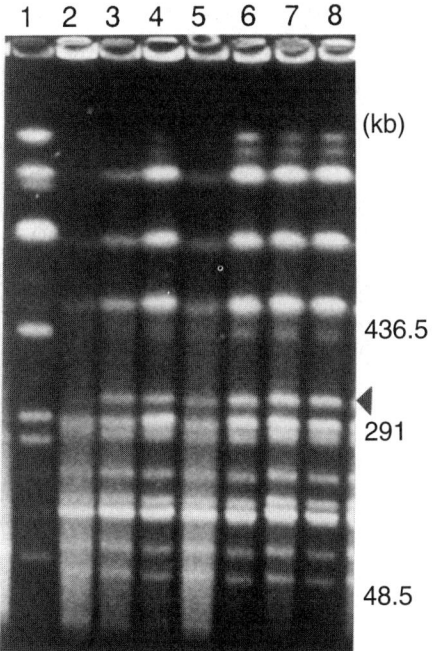

**FIGURE 2** Cleavage patterns of *Sfi*I-digested genomic DNA of *L. pneumophila* strains by PFGE. Lanes 1 to 8 show the patterns of the strains described in Fig. 1. The arrowhead indicates a band that is not observed in lanes 1 and 2. Numbers to the right of the gel represent the size of DNA in kilobases.

variety of mechanisms. After transfer of DNA from K6 to Chicago-2S, either transposition of Tn903dII*lacZ* or homologous recombination would result in the integration of the Km$^r$ and *lacZ* markers into the Chicago-2S chromosome. These two mechanisms, however, would result in very different outcomes for other genetic markers. Transposition would presumably transfer only the transposition sequences to random sites that would differ in different recombinants. Transposition is unlikely because the transposase gene does not exist in the K6 genome, since it is lost upon the initial transposition event. It is formally possible however, that the Chicago-2S strain harbors an unrecognized transposase that could conceivably result in transposition. In contrast, homologous recombination would result in the transfer of different extents of adjacent sequences in the chromosome. To confirm the presence of the K6 sequences in the Chicago-2S chromosome and to distinguish between transposition and homologous recombination, we performed Southern blot experiments with pLAW330 (11) as a probe. As shown in Fig. 3, Km$^r$ LacZ$^+$ genes were located on a 436.5-kb *Sfi*I-digested DNA fragment of strain K6. In all transconjugants tested, the genes were located on 291-kb *Sfi*I-digested DNA fragments (Fig. 3, lanes 3 to 8). This is direct evidence that chromosomal genes transferred from K6 are integrated into the chromosome of Chicago-2S by homologous recombination. A faint 436.5-kb band in the transconjugants is probably due to partial digestions, as well as faint bands observed at more than 436.5 kb in strain K6 (Fig. 3, lane 1).

The results presented here clearly show that conjugal transfer of chromosomal DNA occurs in *L. pneumophila*. This study showed that the *L. pneumophila* Philadelphia-1 chromosome itself is self-mobilizable, since extrachromosomal plasmid-like DNA had not been detected in strain Philadelphia-1 to date (1, 3, 6, our unpublished observation). This could be a result of a previous integration into the chromosome of a conjugative plasmid that has lost the ability to excise, thus resulting in an

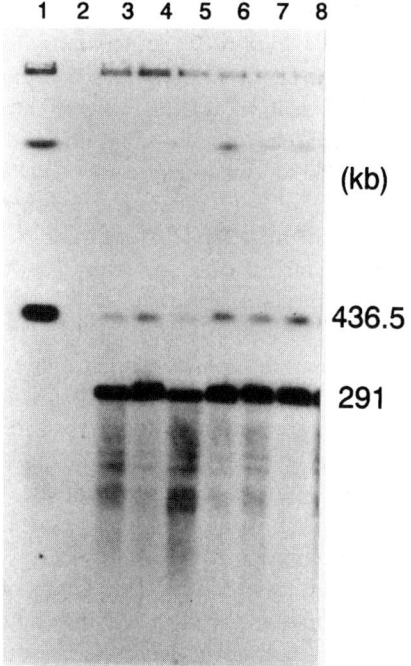

**FIGURE 3** Southern blot analysis of *Sfi*I-digested *L. pneumophila* genomic DNA separated by PFGE. Plasmid pLAW330 digested with *Hin*dIII, which does not cut within Tn903dII*lacZ*, was labeled with digoxigenin and used as a probe. Lanes 1 to 8 show the patterns of strains described in Fig. 1. Numbers to the right of the blot represent the size of DNA in kilobases.

Hfr-like chromosome (7). In *L. pneumophila* strains other than Philadelphia-1, three kinds of conjugative plasmids were reported (4, 6, 9). Although one of them, pCH1 (85-MDa plasmid), was not integrated into the chromosome of Philadelphia-1 and was unable to transfer the chromosome (6), it is unknown whether the other two plasmids, 36 MDa (4) and 36 MDa (9), are integrated into the chromosome and are able to transfer the chromosome. Dreyfus and Iglewski (2) showed that a thymine auxotroph of *L. pneumophila* was repaired by plasmid R68.45-mediated chromosomal mobilization of a prototrophic

donor strain. Therefore, if *L. pneumophila* had acquired an *ori*T by integration of these conjugative elements, it would become self-mobilizable like the Hfr of *E. coli*.

## REFERENCES

1. **Chen, G. C. C., A. Brown, and M. W. Lema.** 1986. Restriction endonuclease activities in the legionellae. *Can. J. Microbiol.* **32:**591–593.
2. **Dreyfus, L. A., and B. B. Iglewski.** 1985. Conjugation-mediated genetic exchange in *Legionella pneumophila. J. Bacteriol.* **161:**80–84.
3. **Knudson, G. B., and P. Mikesell.** 1980. A plasmid in *Legionella pneumophila. Infect. Immun.* **29:**1092–1095.
4. **Lopez, F. de.** 1993. Cloning, mapping and conjugal mobility of pLPG36, a common plasmid from *Legionella pneumophila* serogroup-1. *J. Gen. Microbiol.* **139:**3171–3175.
5. **Low, K. B.** 1987. Hfr strains of *Escherichia coli* K-12, p. 1134–1137. *In* F. C. Neidhardt (ed.), *Escherichia coli and Salmonella typhimurium.* American Society for Microbiology, Washington, D.C.
6. **Mintz, C. S., B. S. Fields, and C.-H. Zou.** 1992. Isolation and characterization of a conjugative plasmid from *Legionella pneumophila. J. Gen. Microbiol.* **138:**1379–1386.
7. **Scott, J. R., and G. G. Churchward.** 1995. Conjugative transposition. *Annu. Rev. Microbiol.* **49:**367–397.
8. **Smith, G. R.** 1991. Conjugational recombination in *E. coli:* myth and mechanisms. *Cell* **64:** 19–27.
9. **Tully, M.** 1991. A plasmid from a virulent strain of *Legionella pneumophila* confers resistance to ultraviolet light. *FEMS Microbiol. Lett.* **90:**43–48.
10. **Van Belkum, A., M. Struelens, and W. Quint.** 1993. Typing of *Legionella pneumophila* strains by polymerase chain reaction-mediated DNA fingerprinting. *J. Clin. Microbiol.* **31:**2198–2200.
11. **Wiater, L. A., A. B. Sadosky, and H. A. Shuman.** 1994. Mutagenesis of *Legionella pneumophila* using Tn903 dIII*lacZ:* identification of a growth-phase-regulated pigmentation gene. *Mol. Microbiol.* **11:**641–653.
12. **Willetts, N., and R. Skurray.** 1987. Structure and function of the F factor and mechanism of conjugation, p. 1110–1133. *In* F. C. Neidhardt (ed.), *Escherichia coli and Salmonella typhimurium.* American Society for Microbiology, Washington, D.C.

# INNATE AND ADAPTIVE IMMUNITY TO
# *LEGIONELLA PNEUMOPHILA*

*Yoshimasa Yamamoto, Thomas W. Klein,*
*Catherine Newton, and Herman Friedman*

# 21

*Legionella pneumophila* is a ubiquitous opportunistic pathogen that causes serious infection in humans, especially in immunocompromised individuals. However, this organism has many characteristics that distinguish it from other intracellular bacteria in terms of interactions with cells of the immune response, especially macrophages. For example, infection of macrophages with this bacterium results in rapid multiplication of the bacteria. There is a 100- to 1,000-fold increase in the number of these bacteria in infected macrophages in 48- to 72-h cultures of the infected macrophages (69). Such vigorous multiplication of *L. pneumophila* in macrophages is remarkable compared with the multiplication of other opportunistic bacteria. *L. pneumophila* is also very immunostimulatory as evidenced by the facts that (i) the severe symptoms of Legionnaires' disease begin abruptly and parallel those of a severe acute phase response, (ii) humans readily develop humoral and cellular immune responses to the antigens of this bacterium, and (iii) *L. pneumophila* antigens are immunostimulatory

in immune cell cultures and animal models (31). Clinical manifestations also indicate that the overall host response to *L. pneumophila* infection involves aspects of broad immunity. Although effector mechanisms of immunity against this organism in the lung are not completely understood, it has been widely accepted that development of cell-mediated immunity (CMI) in response to *L. pneumophila* plays a key role in the inhibition of bacterial growth and resolution of legionellosis.

It seems apparent that various aspects of both innate and adaptive immune responses are involved in the host defense against *L. pneumophila* infection. Adaptive immunity consists of activated T cells, cytokines such as gamma interferon (IFN-γ), and activated macrophages that restrict the growth and spread of bacteria within its intracellular environment. Innate immunity to the bacteria, on the other hand, is perhaps even more complex and includes a variety of different host cells and cytokines. Nevertheless, it is clear that the immune response to *L. pneumophila* has many features in common with other microorganisms and that the consideration of data from a variety of studies will provide greater insight into preventing and treating the disease caused by *L. pneumophila* infection in particular, as well as infections with other similar pathogens.

*Yoshimasa Yamamoto, Thomas W. Klein, Catherine Newton, and Herman Friedman* Department of Medical Microbiology and Immunology, University of South Florida College of Medicine, Tampa, FL 33612.

*Legionella*, Edited by Reinhard Marre et al.
© 2002 ASM Press, Washington, D.C.

## L. PNEUMOPHILA ANTIGENS STIMULATE VARIOUS LEVELS OF IMMUNITY

*L. pneumophila* is a gram-negative bacterium and possesses a variety of antigens usual for gram-negative bacteria, such as lipopolysaccharide (LPS), heat-shock proteins, outer-membrane proteins, flagella, and fimbria. These antigens of *L. pneumophila* are known to stimulate immune cells to produce a variety of cytokines (Fig. 1). For example, it has been shown that *L. pneumophila* LPS, which is less toxic and has lower pyrogenic effects compared with enterobacterial LPS (59, 64), stimulates macrophages to produce tumor necrosis factor (TNF) (1). On the other hand, *L. pneumophila* possesses flagella and fimbriae as cell surface structures (53). Since it has been demonstrated that flagella of gram-negative bacteria such as *Salmonella enterica* serovar Typhimurium can directly stimulate macrophages to induce a wide variety of cytokines, such as beta interleukin-1 (IL-1$\beta$), tumor necrosis factor alpha (TNF-$\alpha$), and granulocyte-macrophage colony-stimulating factor (GM-CSF) (35, 65), it is likely that *L. pneumophila* flagella may also be involved in induction of a variety of cytokines during the infection.

Sera from legionellosis patients contain antibodies to *Legionella* protein antigens such as the 58-kDa genus-specific antigen and the 11-and 25-kDa species-specific antigens (55). These antigens could be related to heat-shock protein 60 (HSP60) and the 28-kDa major outer-membrane protein antigens. HSPs, known as chaperones or stress proteins, are highly conserved proteins with important biological functions in protein biogenesis. Although these HSPs are predominantly located in intracellular compartments, recent studies demonstrated that some HSPs can be expressed on the surfaces of bacterial cells, as well as secreted extracellularly (17, 24, 49). Therefore, active involvement of HSPs in immune responses of immune cells to bacteria should be likely. In fact, bacterial HSPs are known to stimulate immune cells, including macrophages, to release cytokines (33, 48, 51). In this regard, *L. pneumophila* HSP60 has been studied for its potential to induce cytokines from macrophages. The results of studies in this laboratory indicate that *L. pneumophila* HSP60 increases cellular steady-state levels of a variety of cytokine messages, including alpha/beta interleukin-1 (IL-1$\alpha/\beta$), interleukin-6 (IL-6), TNF-$\alpha$, and GM-CSF, as well as IL-1 protein secretion of cultured macrophages in vitro, possibly through a cell surface receptor system involving a protein kinase C (PKC)-dependent signaling pathway (52). Furthermore, it has been demonstrated that HSP can participate in immune responses to bacterial infections and in development of autoimmune diseases (14). Members of the HSP60 class serve as immunodominant targets of $\alpha\beta^+$ and $\tau\delta^+$ T lymphocytes as well as stimulating antibodies during infections by many bacteria, including *L. pneumophila* (24). In particular, HSP60 has been used in attempts to induce immunological protection against infection by *L. pneumophila* (10).

In addition to these antigens, a variety of *L. pneumophila* virulence factors and other antigens have also been described (31). However, the importance of these proteins as stimulants for immunity has not been defined and therefore the role of these various immune reactivities in the immunopathogenesis of legionellosis has yet to be determined. Never-

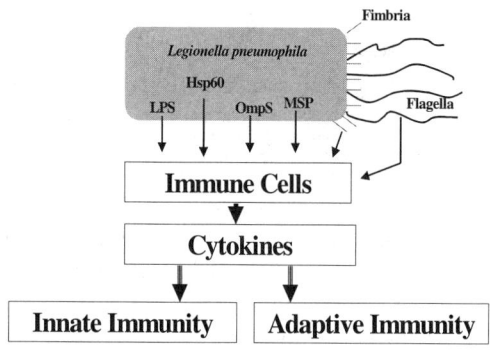

**FIGURE 1** *L. pneumophila* antigens stimulate various levels of immunity mediated by cytokines. OmpS, outer-membrane protein; MSP, major secretory protein; Hsp60, 60-kD heat-shock protein.

theless, it is clear that many *Legionella* antigens possess immunostimulatory activity for immune cells and should be involved in both innate and adaptive immunity at certain levels.

## INNATE IMMUNITY TO *L. PNEUMOPHILA* INFECTION

The course of *L. pneumophila* infection in experimental susceptible animals, such as A/J mice (69), can be divided into an early phase, during which rapid bacterial multiplication in a host cell and an inflammatory response can be observed, and a second phase beginning on the second or third day after infection with a down-regulation of the nonspecific inflammatory response and a decrease in the bacterial count in infection sites (60). The early cellular response is characterized by an interstitial inflammatory reaction consisting mainly of macrophages, B lymphocytes, and an undefined cell population, which may include natural killer (NK) cells (60). These cells probably represent a first and effective line of defense against infection as innate immunity, possibly triggered by bacterial antigens mentioned in the previous section. The induction of innate immune mechanisms includes macrophage activation by IFN-γ (3, 32, 41), protection by TNF-α (5, 34, 36, 43, 58), and the production of IL-6, IL-1, and chemokines (29, 30, 37, 40, 62, 65) from inflammatory cells mentioned above. Although the mobilization of these cytokines is generally protective, they can also induce enhanced mortality if their levels in blood and tissue become excessive (30). In the case of humans, the initial phase of Legionnaires' disease is characterized by symptoms that correspond to acute-phase cytokine mobilization (19) as observed in animal infection models.

The innate immunity to *L. pneumophila* infection limits the growth of the bacteria, which generally occurs in macrophages. Therefore, the regulation of *L. pneumophila* growth in macrophages by proinflammatory cytokines, such as TNF-α, may be a main event in the early phase of infection. However, other immune cytokines, such as IFN-

γ, which has been thought to be produced only by immune T cells and NK cells, may also be involved in innate immunity, since it was shown that macrophages produce low levels of IFN-γ (22, 47), which is involved in resistance of macrophages to bacterial infection (18). Our current studies also support an active role for endogenous IFN-γ in regulation of *L. pneumophila* growth in macrophages (K. Matsunaga, T. W. Klein, H. Friedman, and Y. Yamamoto, submitted for publication). Thus, innate immunity is not always clearly distinguished from adaptive immunity regarding mediator cytokines.

TNF-α, which is mainly produced by macrophages, is a potent cytokine and has extensive properties affecting the regulation of immunological and inflammatory cells. This cytokine has been shown to enhance the bactericidal activity of macrophages and protects against a variety of intracellular bacterial infections. The induction of TNF-α and the ability of this cytokine to control infection with *L. pneumophila* has been demonstrated (1, 4–6, 12, 34, 36). For instance, Blanchard et al. demonstrated that in addition to IFN-γ, TNF-α is produced by human peripheral blood lymphocytes in response to *L. pneumophila* antigens (6). Both IFN-γ and TNF-α augmented the killing of the bacteria by murine neutrophils treated with these cytokines. TNF-α has also been shown to be present in bronchial secretions of mice after respiratory infection with *L. pneumophila* (4). Treatment of these animals with TNF-α resulted in significant protection of the animal from *L. pneumophila* mortality, possibly via activation of neutrophil function (5). This finding agrees with the fact that TNF-α enhances the phagocytic activity and oxidative burst of human neutrophils (28, 57). Brieland et al. also demonstrated that endogenous TNF-α facilitated the resolution of in vivo *L. pneumophila* infection and this response was shown to be mediated, in part, by NO (12). Furthermore, addition of exogenous TNF-α to human peripheral monocytes inhibited the multiplication of *L. pneumophila* (2). Our current study also suggests that the endogenous TNF-$\alpha$ may be involved in the susceptibility of macrophages to *L. pneumophila* infection because anti–TNF-$\alpha$ antibody treatment of macrophages alters this susceptibility to *L. pneumophila* infection (36). Thus, these observations clearly indicate that TNF-$\alpha$ plays an important role in the innate immunity to *L. pneumophila* infection mediated by phagocytic cells, including neutrophils.

Cells other than phagocytic cells are involved in innate immunity to infection. One of these is the NK cell, which in addition to killing harmful target cells is now recognized as an important early source of cytokines. In this regard, it is of interest that the first report of cytokine induction by *L. pneumophila* antigens in nonimmune cells described the production of IFN-$\gamma$ by cultured splenocytes (7). Initially, it was believed that T cells were the sole source of the IFN-$\gamma$; however, it was shown later that NK cells also respond to *L. pneumophila* antigen stimulation by not only producing IFN-$\gamma$ but also becoming activated to kill *L. pneumophila*-infected macrophage targets (8, 9). As previously described, current studies showed that IFN-$\gamma$ is also produced by macrophages in response to bacterial stimulations. Therefore, the role of IFN-$\gamma$ in innate immunity is critical, since this cytokine shows a powerful macrophage activation to induce anti–*L. pneumophila* activity.

Chemokines, which play a critical role in mobilization and activation of various cell types to inflammatory sites, are now known to be divided into four subfamilies, such as C, CC, CXC, and CX3C chemokines, as originally defined by the spacing of the two cysteines in the conservative motif. All of these chemokines may be responsible for rapid migration of leukocytes from the bloodstream to the inflammatory site and, therefore, should work as a critical factor in innate immunity to bacterial infections. In fact, *L. pneumophila* infection of macrophages induced production of chemokines, such as macrophage inflammatory protein 1$\beta$ (MIP-1$\beta$), MIP-2, as well as KC (65, 70). Furthermore, our current studies

on chemokine induction by *L. pneumophila* infection of alveolar macrophages in vitro analyzed by the cDNA expression array technique revealed the detail of the differential chemokine induction activity between virulent vs. avirulent *L. pneumophila* (40). That is, monocyte chemotactic protein 3 (MCP-3) gene expression was significantly induced by infection with virulent *L. pneumophila* but not with avirulent bacteria. In contrast, other chemokine genes, such as MIP-1$\alpha$, were induced by both virulent and avirulent *L. pneumophila*. These results indicate that the response of the innate immunity, at least, in terms of chemokine induction to bacterial infection, may be dependent on the pathogenicity of the infecting bacteria. Such regulated response of innate immunity to bacterial pathogens may contribute to the homeostasis of the host, since overproduction of cytokine/chemokine harms tissues.

The induction mechanism of chemokines by bacterial infection is not known. In this regard, our current study found that certain chemokine inductions by bacterial infection may be regulated by the receptor/ligand group, which is distinguished from other cytokine induction systems (49). This differential regulation on chemokine vs. cytokine inductions indicates that innate immunity-related proinflammatory mediators, such as chemokines, and certain adaptive immunity-related cytokines, such as IL-1 and GM-CSF, may be regulated by different systems, including different receptors for bacteria. For instance, the attachment of *S. enterica* serovar Typhimurium or *L. pneumophila* to cultured macrophages increased the levels of mRNA for the cytokines IL-1$\beta$, IL-6, and GM-CSF, as well as for the chemokines MIP-1$\beta$, MIP-2, and KC. However, when macrophages were treated with $\alpha$-methyl-D-mannoside (AMM), a competitor of glycopeptide ligands, induction of cytokine mRNAs was inhibited, but the level of chemokine mRNAs was not (49). Analysis of cytokine GM-CSF and chemokine MIP-2 signaling pathways with protein kinase inhibitors revealed the involvement of calmodulin and myosin light-chain kinase in GM-CSF but not in MIP-2 mRNA induction. The differential regulation of cytokine versus chemokine by receptors was also supported by the study using the *Candida albicans*-macrophage interaction system (66). That is, mannose receptor of macrophages is involved in cytokine IL-1$\beta$, IL-6, and GM-CSF responses, but not in chemokine MIP-1$\beta$, MIP-2, and KC responses caused by attachment of *C. albicans* to macrophages. Thus, the differential regulation of innate vs. adaptive immunity-related cytokines/chemokines seems likely to be regulated separately with different systems (Fig. 2).

## ADAPTIVE IMMUNITY TO *L. PNEUMOPHILA* INFECTION

In general, the adaptive immunity to bacterial infections is characterized by the memory of the previous antigen stimulation, which is not necessarily the infection, and the transferable nature of the memory with lymphocytes. The antibody response to bacterial infections is one of the typical adaptive immune responses when the host has been exposed to bacterial antigens and then a heightened specific antibody response occurs after the secondary stimulation with the antigen. The role of antibodies in the resistance to infections varies between bacteria. In the case of *Legionella* infection, even though a variety of *L. pneumo-*

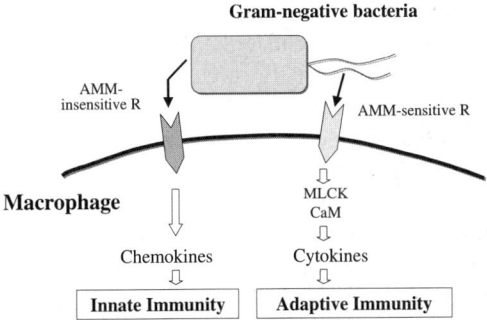

**FIGURE 2** Scheme of cytokine and chemokine induction through different receptors of macrophage by bacterial attachment. MLCK, myosin light chain kinase; CaM, calmodulin; AMM, $\alpha$-methyl-D-mannoside; R, receptor.

*phila* virulence factors and other antigens have been described, the importance of these antigens for humoral immunity in humans has not been defined. Therefore the role of these immune reactivities in the immunopathogenesis of *Legionella* infection has yet to be determined. In addition, the immunopathological role of antibodies in *Legionella* infection is not clear. However, it has been shown that antibodies to *Legionella* organisms promote uptake and replication of the bacteria in macrophages rather than promoting elimination of the bacteria (26, 27). Therefore, it is thought that the antibodies in the resistance to *Legionella* infection may be minimal or play a role as a second line of defense (11).

The role of CMI in the adaptive immunity to *Legionella* infection is known to be critical. The delayed-type hypersensitivity (DTH) reactions and CMI reactions of lymphoid cells from either immunized animals or patients who had recovered from legionellosis could be readily detected (16, 21, 45, 46, 63). For instance, peripheral blood lymphocytes from 17 subjects recovered from legionellosis and 63 control subjects were cultured with *Legionella* extracts and the proliferation responses were found significantly increased in the legionellosis group. This increase in antigen-specific lymphocyte proliferation was extended to samples from patients with acute legionellosis to determine secretion of cytokines capable of activating normal blood monocyte cultures to restrict the growth of *L. pneumophila* (25). This was strong evidence that the classic mechanisms of CMI were operating in humans and eventually it was shown that the T helper 1 (Th1) cytokine, IFN-$\gamma$, could activate monocytes to restrict *Legionella* growth (3). The extended studies regarding Th1 cytokine in the host resistance to *Legionella* infection have also been performed using animal models.

In general, mice appear to be resistant to *L. pneumophila* infection and mouse macrophages restrict the growth of this bacterium in the cultures (68, 71). However, the A/J mouse strain can support intracellular growth of *Legionella* organisms, but mortality following infection with the bacteria is only slightly greater than that of other mouse strains (69). The reason why A/J mice are moderately susceptible to *Legionella* infection has been further investigated using mice immunosuppressed by cyclosporin A treatment, which causes specific immunosuppression of T lymphocytes, and reconstituted mice with T-cell culture supernatants, which contain Th1 cytokines (67). The results indicate that lymphocytes, as well as their products, such as the Th1 cytokine IFN-γ, are critical in the host resistance probably mediated by macrophage activation to *Legionella* infection. Thus, the vital role of lymphocytes in controlling infection with *L. pneumophila* in animals is apparent.

Current studies indicate that the development of CMI to bacterial infections is dependent on the differentiation of the phenotypes of T helper cells. The functions of T helper 1 (Th1) and Th2 cells correlate well with their distinctive cytokines. For example, Th1 cytokines activate cytotoxic and inflammatory functions and, therefore, Th1 cells are recognized to be involved in cell-mediated inflammatory reactions. In contrast, Th2 cytokines are commonly found in association with strong antibody responses and therefore involved in humoral immune responses. These cytokines also cross-regulate the development of each Th phenotype. The Th1 cytokine IFN-γ selectively inhibits proliferation of Th2 cells and the Th2 cytokine IL-10 inhibits cytokine synthesis by Th1 cells. This cross-regulation may partly explain the strong biases toward Th1 or Th2 responses during infection (38). In general, the Th1 cells are more suitable for protection against intracellular pathogens, whereas extracellular pathogens are best counteracted by a combination of Th2- and Th1-type cytokines (e.g., by Th0 cells) (54).

The experimental infection model of mouse with *L. pneumophila* displayed many of the cellular and cytokine features involved in immunity similar to other intracellular bacterial infections, including the activation of Th1 cells and CMI (13, 42, 44). For example, sub-lethally infected mice with *L. pneumophila* become resistant to secondary infection with a lethal dose. The splenocytes obtained from such primed mice are sensitized and proliferate to a greater extent and produce more IFN-γ when stimulated with the bacterial antigens in vitro. Furthermore, reinfection of the primed mice induced an increase in these responses and an increase of CD4$^+$ and CD8$^+$ cells in splenic and peripheral blood T lymphocytes (44). The Th1 activity was also increased following *L. pneumophila* infection demonstrated by the detection of increased Th1 cell-related products, such as IL-12, IFN-γ, and immunoglobulin G2a, in serum as well as splenocyte cultures (42, 43, 60).

The Th1 cytokine production during *L. pneumophila* infection in humans has also currently been demonstrated (61). The significant increases of serum IFN-γ and IL-12 levels were observed during the acute phase of infection, but Th2 cytokines IL-4 and IL-10 were detected in only 1 out of 14 patients with legionellosis. Furthermore, the serum IL-12 levels remained high or increased further during the convalescent phase of infection. Thus, the relative predominance of Th1-related cellular immune responses in patients with legionellosis was evinced.

The involvement of Th2 phenotypes, as well as Th2 cytokines, such as IL-4 and IL-10, in *Legionella* infection is rather complicated. IL-4 is reported to be detrimental to the survival of infected animals because of its role in induction of Th2 cells (23, 50). However, it is known that IL-4 is detected in mice within 3 h of infection with bacteria, and the transient IL-4 does not interfere with development of Th1 responses (15, 20). In the case of *L. pneumophila* infection in the mouse model, a transient IL-4 response, both in serum as well as in ex vivo cultures of splenocytes, was detected during the early phase of infection (43, 60). IL-4 knockout mice (BALB/c-IL-4$^{tm2Nnt}$) were found to be more susceptible to *L. pneumophila* infection (43), suggesting that IL-4 had a protective role. Such a role was supported by additional findings that implied that IL-4 attenuated the mobilization of acute-phase cytokines during the early immune response. The IL-4-knockout mice had elevated levels of TNF-$\alpha$, IL-1$\beta$, and IL-6, and IL-4 treatment of *L. pneumophila*-infected macrophage cultures suppressed their production. Furthermore, treating the knockout mice with anti-TNF-$\alpha$ antibodies protected the animals from *L. pneumophila* infection (43). In addition, the IL-4-knockout mice developed a robust antigen-specific splenic IFN-$\gamma$ production and survived a secondary infection. Thus, IL-4 may play a regulatory function during the innate immune responses, such as down-regulation of acute-phase cytokines to *L. pneumophila* infection.

The control of differentiation of uncommitted T-cell precursors to Th1/Th2 is, at least partly, regulated by certain cytokines. That is, IL-4 stimulates differentiation into Th2 cells, whereas IFN-$\gamma$ and IL-12 enhance Th1 development (56). In the experimental *Legionella*-infected mouse model, as well as in humans with legionellosis, in comparison with a transient IL-4 response and weak or no IL-10 production, the levels of IFN-$\gamma$ and/or IL-12 in serum or ex vivo splenocyte cultures were maintained high during the infection or

after a secondary infection (61). Therefore, it is conceivable that the strong biases toward Th1 differentiation supported by IFN-$\gamma$ and IL-12, which are produced by macrophages and/or NK cells by stimulation with bacteria, occurred as a result during the convalescent phase of *Legionella* infection.

**CONCLUSION**

Studies in humans and animals suggest that the host response to *L. pneumophila* infection contains features of both innate and adaptive immunity (Fig. 3). Adaptive immunity consists of activated T cells, cytokines such as IFN-$\gamma$, and activated macrophages that restrict the growth and spread of bacteria within its intracellular environment. Innate immunity to *L. pneumophila*, on the other hand, is perhaps even more complex and includes a variety of different host cells and cytokines. For example, IFN-$\gamma$ is thought to be produced particularly by activated T lymphocytes; therefore, this cytokine is one of the characteristic cytokines to activate macrophages in adaptive immunity. However, current studies revealed a new role for IFN-$\gamma$ in innate immunity. That is, endogenous IFN-$\gamma$ may play a critical role in the susceptibility of macrophages to *L.*

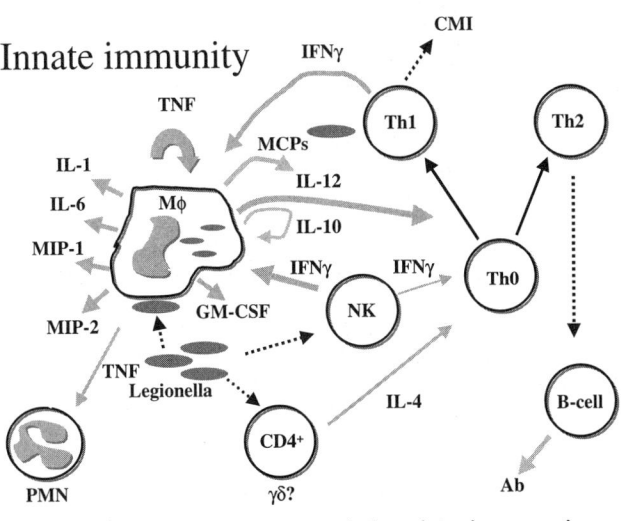

**FIGURE 3** *L. pneumophila* infection stimulates cells and cytokines of both innate and acquired immune response system. CMI, cell-mediated immunity.

*pneumophila* infection (Matsunaga et al., submitted), since macrophages can produce this cytokine, which may be enhanced by treatment with IL-12 and IL-18 (39, 47). The Th2 cytokine IL-4 is also considered a critical regulatory cytokine; besides its differentiation-promoting activity for Th2 cells, it may regulate the innate immune response to *L. pneumophila* infection. It is clear that the immune response to *L. pneumophila* has many features in common with other microbes and that the consideration of data from a variety of studies will provide greater insight into preventing and treating disease caused by *Legionella* infection in particular, as well as infections with other similar microbes.

## ACKNOWLEDGMENTS

This work was supported by grants from the National Institute of Health (AI45169, DA03646, and DA10683) and the American Lung Association of Florida.

## REFERENCES

1. **Arata, S., C. Newton, T. W. Klein, Y. Yamamoto, and H. Friedman.** 1993. *Legionella pneumophila* induced tumor necrosis factor production in permissive versus nonpermissive macrophages. *Proc. Soc. Exp. Biol. Med.* **203:**26–29.

2. **Bernard, P. M., C. Lefebre, M. Sedqui, P. Cornillet, and M. Guenoubou.** 1993. Tumor necrosis factor and *Legionella pneumophila* infection *in vitro. Infect. Immun.* **61:**4980–4983.

3. **Bhardwaj, N., T. W. Nash, and M. A. Horwitz.** 1986. Interferon-gamma-activated human monocytes inhibit the intracellular multiplication of *Legionella pneumophila. J. Immunol.* **137:**2662–2669.

4. **Blanchard, D. K., J. Y. Djeu, T. W. Klein, H. Friedman, and W. E. Stewart II.** 1987. Induction of tumor necrosis factor by *Legionella pneumophila. Infect. Immun.* **55:**433–437.

5. **Blanchard, D. K., J. Y. Djeu, T. W. Klein, H. Friedman, and W. E. Stewart II.** 1988. Protective effects of tumor necrosis factor in experimental *Legionella pneumophila* infections of mice via activation of PMN function. *J. Leukoc. Biol.* **43:**429–435.

6. **Blanchard, D. K., H. Friedman, T. W. Klein, and J. Y. Djeu.** 1989. Induction of interferon-gamma and tumor necrosis factor by *Legionella pneumophila*: augmentation of human neutrophil bactericidal activity. *J. Leukoc. Biol.* **45:**538–545.

7. **Blanchard, D. K., T. W. Klein, H. Friedman, and W. E. Stewart.** 1985. Kinetics and characterization of interferon production by murine spleen cells stimulated with *Legionella pneumophila* antigens. *Infect. Immun.* **49:**719–723.

8. **Blanchard, D. K., W. E. Stewart, T. W. Klein, H. Friedman, and J. Y. Djeu.** 1987. Cytolytic activity of human peripheral blood leukocytes against *Legionella pneumophila*-infected monocytes: characterization of the effector cell and augmentation by interleukin 2. *J. Immunol.* **139:**551–556.

9. **Blanchard, D. K., H. Friedman, W. E. Stewart, T. W. Klein, and J. Y. Djeu.** 1988. Role of gamma interferon in induction of natural killer activity by *Legionella pneumophila* in vitro and in an experimental murine infection model. *Infect. Immun.* **56:**1187–1193.

10. **Blander, S. J., and M. A. Horwitz.** 1993. Major cytoplasmic membrane protein of *Legionella pneumophila*, a genus common antigen and member of the hsp 60 family of heat shock proteins, induces protective immunity in a guinea pig model of Legionnaires' disease. *J. Clin. Invest.* **91:**717–723.

11. **Brieland, J. K., L. A. Heath, G. B. Huffnagle, D. G. Remick, M. S. McClain, M. C. Hurley, R. K. Kunkel, J. C. Fantone, and C. Engleberg.** 1996. Humoral immunity and regulation of intrapulmonary growth of *Legionella pneumophila* in the immunocompetent host. *J. Immunol.* **157:**5002–5008.

12. **Brieland, J. K., D. C. Remick, P. T. Freeman, M. C. Hurley, J. C. Fantone, and N. C. Engleberg.** 1995. In vivo regulation of replicative *Legionella pneumophila* lung infection by endogenous tumor necrosis factor alpha and nitric oxide. *Infect. Immun.* **63:**3253–3258.

13. **Brieland, J. K., D. G. Remick, M. L. LeGendre, N. C. Engleberg, and J. C. Fantone.** 1998. In vivo regulation of replicative *Legionella pneumophila* lung infection by endogenous interleukin-12. *Infect. Immun.* **66:**65–69.

14. **Cohen, I. R., and D. B. Young.** 1991. Autoimmunity, microbial immunity and the immunological homunculus. *Immunol. Today* **12:**105–110.

15. **Collins, H. L., U. E. Schaible, and S. H. Kaufmann.** 1998. Early IL-4 induction in bone marrow lymphoid precursor cells by mycobacterial lipoarabinomannan. *J. Immunol.* **161:**5546–5554.

16. **Davis, G. S., W. C. Winn, D. W. Gump, and H. N. Beaty.** 1983. The kinetics of early inflammatory events during experimental pneu-

monia due to *Legionella pneumophila* in guinea pigs. *J. Infect. Dis.* **148:**823–835.

17. **Ensgraber, M., and M. Loos.** 1992. A 66-kilodalton heat shock protein of *Salmonella typhimurium* is responsible for binding of the bacterium to intestinal mucus. *Infect. Immun.* **60:**3072–3078.

18. **Fenton, M. J., M. W. Vermeulen, S. Kim, M. Burdick, R. M. Strieter, and H. Kornfeld.** 1997. Induction of gamma interferon production in human alveolar macrophages by Mycobacterium tuberculosis. *Infect. Immun.* **65:** 5149–5156.

19. **Finegold, S. M.** 1988. Legionnaires' disease— still with us. *N. Engl. J. Med.* **318:**571–573.

20. **Flesch, I. E., A. Wandersee, and S. H. Kaufmann.** 1997. IL-4 secretion by CD4+ NK1+ T cells induces monocyte chemoattractant protein-1 in early listeriosis. *J. Immunol.* **159:**7–10.

21. **Friedman, H., R. Widen, T. Klein, L. Searls, and K. Cabrian.** 1984. *Legionella pneumophila*-induced blastogenesis of murine lymphoid cells in vitro. *Infect. Immun.* **43:**314–319.

22. **Fultz, M. J., S. A. Barber, C. W. Dieffenbach, and S. N. Vogel.** 1993. Induction of IFN-gamma in macrophages by lipopolysaccharide. *Int. Immunol.* **5:**1383–1392.

23. **Haak-Frendscho, M., J. F. Brown, Y. Iizawa, R. D. Wagner, and C. J. Czuprynski.** 1992. Administration of anti-IL-4 monoclonal antibody 11B11 increases the resistance of mice to *Listeria monocytogenes* infection. *J. Immunol.* **148:**3978–3985.

24. **Hoffman, P. S., L. Houston, and C. A. Butler.** 1990. *Legionella pneumophila* htpAB heat shock operon: nucleotide sequence and expression of the 60-kilodalton antigen in *L. pneumophila*-infected HeLa cells. *Infect. Immun.* **58:**3380–3387.

25. **Horwitz, M. A.** 1983. Cell-mediated immunity in Legionnaires' disease. *J. Clin. Invest.* **71:**1686–1697.

26. **Horwitz, M. A., and S. C. Silverstein.** 1981. Interaction of the legionnaires' disease bacterium (*Legionella pneumophila*) with human phagocytes. II. Antibody promotes binding of *L. pneumophila* to monocytes but does not inhibit intracellular multiplication. *J. Exp. Med.* **153:**398–406.

27. **Johnson, W., E. Pesanti, and J. Elliott.** 1979. Serospecificity and opsonic activity of antisera to *Legionella pneumophila. Infect. Immun.* **26:**698–704.

28. **Klebanoff, S. J., M. A. Vadas, J. M. Harlan, L. H. Sparks, J. R. Gamble, J. M. Agosti, and A. M. Waltersdorph.** 1986. Stimulation of neutrophils by tumor necrosis factor. *J. Immunol.* **136:**4220–4225.

29. **Klein, T. W., C. A. Newton, D. K. Blanchard, R. Widen, and H. Friedman.** 1987.

30. **Klein, T. W., C. Newton, R. Widen, and H. Friedman.** 1993. Delta 9-tetrahydrocannabinol injection induces cytokine-mediated mortality of mice infected with *Legionella pneumophila. J. Pharmacol. Exp. Ther.* **267:**635–640.

31. **Klein, T. W., C. Newton, Y. Yamamoto, and H. Friedman.** 1999. Immune responses to Legionella, p. 149–166. *In* L. J. Paradise, H. Friedman, and M. Bendinelli (ed.), *Opportunistic Bacteria and Immunity.* Plenum Press, New York, N.Y.

32. **Klein, T. W., Y. Yamamoto, H. K. Brown, and H. Friedman.** 1991. Interferon-gamma induced resistance to *Legionella pneumophila* in susceptible A/J mouse macrophages. *J. Leukoc. Biol.* **49:**98–103.

33. **Kol, A., T. Bourcier, A. H. Lichtman, and P. Libby.** 1999. Chlamydial and human heat shock protein 60s activate human vascular endothelium, smooth muscle cells, and macrophages. *J. Clin. Invest.* **103:**571–577.

34. **Matsiota-Bernard, P., C. Lefebre, M. Sedqui, P. Cornillet, and M. Guenounou.** 1993. Involvement of tumor necrosis factor alpha in intracellular multiplication of *Legionella pneumophila* in human monocytes. *Infect. Immun.* **61:**4980–4983.

35. **McDermott, P. F., F. Ciacci-Woolwine, J. A. Snipes, and S. B. Mizel.** 2000. High-affinity interaction between gram-negative flagellin and a cell surface polypeptide results in human monocyte activation. *Infect. Immun.* **68:** 5525–5529.

36. **McHugh, S. L., C. A. Newton, Y. Yamamoto, T. W. Klein, and H. Friedman.** 2000. Tumor necrosis factor induces resistance of macrophages to *Legionella pneumophila* infection. *Proc. Soc. Exp. Biol. Med.* **224:**191–196.

37. **McHugh, S. L., Y. Yamamoto, T. W. Klein, and H. Friedman.** 2000. Murine macrophages differentially produce proinflammatory cytokines after infection with virulent vs. avirulent *Legionella pneumophila. J. Leukoc. Biol.* **67:**863–868.

38. **Mosmann, T. R., and S. Sad.** 1996. The expanding universe of T-cell subsets: Th1, Th2 and more. *Immunol. Today* **17:**138–146.

39. **Munder, M., M. Mallo, K. Eichmann, and M. Modolell.** 1998. Murine macrophages secrete interferon gamma upon combined stimulation with interleukin (IL)-12 and IL-18: A novel pathway of autocrine macrophage activation. *J. Exp. Med.* **187:**2103–2108.

Induction of interleukin 1 by *Legionella pneumophila* antigens in mouse macrophage and human mononuclear leukocyte cultures. *Zentralbl. Bakteriol. Mikrobiol. Hyg. A* **265:**462–471.

40. Nakachi, N., K. Matsunaga, T. W. Klein, H. Friedman, and Y. Yamamoto. 2000. Differential effects of virulent versus avirulent *Legionella pneumophila* on chemokine gene expression in murine alveolar macrophages determined by cDNA expression array technique. *Infect. Immun.* **68:**6069–6072.

41. Nash, T. W., D. M. Libby, and M. A. Horwitz. 1988. IFN-gamma-activated human alveolar macrophages inhibit the intracellular multiplication of *Legionella pneumophila. J. Immunol.* **140:**3978–3981.

42. Newton, C. A., T. W. Klein, and H. Friedman. 1994. Secondary immunity to *Legionella pneumophila* and Th1 activity are suppressed by delta-9-tetrahydrocannabinol injection. *Infect. Immun.* **62:**4015–4020.

43. Newton, C., S. McHugh, R. Widen, N. Nakachi, T. Klein, and H. Friedman. 2000. Induction of interleukin-4 (IL-4) by *Legionella pneumophila* infection in BALB/c mice and regulation of tumor necrosis factor alpha, IL-6, and IL-1beta. *Infect. Immun.* **68:**5234–5240.

44. Newton, C. A., R. Widen, H. Friedman, and T. W. Klein. 1995. Lymphocyte subset changes following primary and secondary infection of mice with *Legionella pneumophila. Immunol. Infect. Dis.* **5:**18–26.

45. Plouffe, J. F., and I. M. Baird. 1981. Lymphocyte transformation to *Legionella pneumophila. J. Clin. Lab. Immunol.* **5:**149–152.

46. Plouffe, J. F., and I. M. Baird. 1982. Lymphocyte blastogenic responses to *L. pneumophila* in acute Legionellosis. *J. Clin. Lab. Immunol.* **7:**43–44.

47. Puddu, P., L. Fantuzzi, P. Borghi, B. Varano, G. Rainaldi, E. Guillemard, W. Malorni, P. Nicaise, S. F. Wolf, F. Belardelli, and S. Gessani. 1997. IL-12 induces IFN-gamma expression and secretion in mouse peritoneal macrophages. *J. Immunol.* **159:**3490–3497.

48. Ratnakar, P., S. P. Rao, and A. Catanzaro. 1996. Isolation and characterization of a 70 kDa protein from *Mycobacterium avium. Microb. Pathog.* **21:**471–486.

49. Raulston, J. E., T. R. Paul, S. T. Knight, and P. B. Wyrick. 1998. Localization of *Chlamydia trachomatis* heat shock proteins 60 and 70 during infection of a human endometrial epithelial cell line in vitro. *Infect. Immun.* **66:**2323–2329.

50. Reiner, S. L., and R. M. Locksley. 1995. The regulation of immunity to *Leishmania major. Annu. Rev. Immunol.* **13:**151–177.

51. Retzlaff, C., Y. Yamamoto, P. S. Hoffman, H. Friedman, and T. W. Klein. 1994. Bacterial heat shock proteins directly induce cytokine mRNA and interleukin-1 secretion in macrophage cultures. *Infect. Immun.* **62:**5689–5693.

52. Retzlaff, C., Y. Yamamoto, S. Okubo, P. S. Hoffman, H. Friedman, and T. W. Klein. 1996. *Legionella pneumophila* heat-shock protein-induced increase of interleukin-1 beta mRNA involves protein kinase C signaling in macrophages. *Immunology* **89:**281–288.

53. Rodgers, F. G., P. W. Greaves, A. D. Macrae, and M. J. Lewis. 1980. Electron microscopic evidence of flagella and pili on *Legionella pneumophila. J. Clin. Pathol.* **33:**1184–1188.

54. Romagnani, S. 1997. The Th1/Th2 paradigm. *Immunol. Today* **18:**263–266.

55. Sampson, J. S., B. B. Plikaytis, and H. W. Wilkinson. 1986. Immunologic response of patients with legionellosis against major protein-containing antigens of *Legionella pneumophila* serogroup 1 as shown by immunoblot analysis. *J. Clin. Microbiol.* **23:**92–99.

56. Seder, R. A., and W. E. Paul. 1994. Acquisition of lymphokine-producing phenotype by CD4+ T cells. *Annu. Rev. Immunol.* **12:**635–673.

57. Shalaby, M. R., B. B. Aggarwal, E. Rinderknecht, L. P. Svedersky, B. S. Finkle, and M. A. Palladino. 1985. Activation of human polymorphonuclear neutrophil functions by interferon-gamma and tumor necrosis factors. *J. Immunol.* **135:**2069–2073.

58. Skerrett, S. J., G. J. Bagby, R. A. Schmidt, and S. Nelson. 1997. Antibody-mediated depletion of tumor necrosis factor-alpha impairs pulmonary host defenses to *Legionella pneumophila. J. Infect. Dis.* **176:**1019–1028.

59. Sonesson, A., E. Jantzen, K. Bryn, L. Larsson, and J. Eng. 1989. Chemical composition of a lipopolysaccharide from *Legionella pneumophila. Arch. Microbiol.* **153:**72–78.

60. Susa, M., B. Ticac, T. Rukavina, M. Doric, and R. Marre. 1998. *Legionella pneumophila* infection in intratracheally inoculated T cell-depleted or -nondepleted A/J mice. *J. Immunol.* **160:**316–321.

61. Tateda, K., T. Matsumoto, Y. Ishii, N. Furuya, A. Ohno, S. Miyazaki, and K. Yamaguchi. 1998. Serum cytokines in patients with *Legionella pneumonia*: relative predominance of Th1-type cytokines. *Clin. Diagn. Lab. Immunol.* **5:**401–403.

62. Widen, R. H., T. W. Klein, C. A. Newton, and H. Friedman. 1989. Induction of interleukin 1 by *Legionella pneumophila* in murine peritoneal macrophage cultures. *Proc. Soc. Exp. Biol. Med.* **191:**304–308.

63. Widen, R., I. Lee, T. Klein, and H. Friedman. 1983. Blastogenic responsiveness of spleen cells from guinea pigs sensitized to *Legionella pneumophila* antigens. *Proc. Soc. Exp. Biol. Med.* **173:**547–552.

64. **Wong, K. H., C. W. Moss, D. H. Hochstein, R. J. Arko, and W. O. Schalla.** 1979. "Endotoxicity" of the Legionnaires' disease bacterium. *Ann. Intern. Med.* **90:**624–627.

65. **Yamamoto, Y., T. W. Klein, and H. Friedman.** 1996. Induction of cytokine granulocyte-macrophage colony-stimulating factor and chemokine macrophage inflammatory protein 2 mRNAs in macrophages by *Legionella pneumophila* or *Salmonella typhimurium* attachment requires different ligand-receptor systems. *Infect. Immun.* **64:**3062–3068.

66. **Yamamoto, Y., T. W. Klein, and H. Friedman.** 1997. Involvement of mannose receptor in cytokine interleukin-1beta (IL-1beta), IL-6, and granulocyte-macrophage colony-stimulating factor responses, but not in chemokine macrophage inflammatory protein 1beta (MIP-1beta), MIP-2, and KC responses, caused by attachment of *Candida albicans* to macrophages. *Infect. Immun.* **65:**1077–1082.

67. **Yamamoto, Y., T. W. Klein, C. Newton, and H. Friedman.** 1992. Differing macrophage and lymphocyte roles in resistance to *Legionella pneumophila* infection. *J. Immunol.* **148:**584–589.

68. **Yamamoto, Y., T. W. Klein, C. A. Newton, R. Widen, and H. Friedman.** 1987. Differential growth of *Legionella pneumophila* in guinea pig versus mouse macrophage cultures. *Infect. Immun.* **55:**1369–1374.

69. **Yamamoto, Y., T. W. Klein, C. Newton, R. Widen, and H. Friedman.** 1988. Growth of *Legionella pneumophila* in thioglycolate-elicited peritoneal macrophages from A/J mice. *Infect. Immun.* **56:**370–375.

70. **Yamamoto, Y., C. Retzlaff, P. He, T. W. Klein, and H. Friedman.** 1995. Quantitative reverse transcription-PCR analysis of *Legionella pneumophila*-induced cytokine mRNA in different macrophage populations by high-performance liquid chromatography. *Clin. Diagn. Lab. Immunol.* **2:**18–24.

71. **Yoshida, S., and Y. Mizuguchi.** 1986. Multiplication of *Legionella pneumophila* Philadelphia-1 in cultured peritoneal macrophages and its correlation to susceptibility of animals. *Can. J. Microbiol.* **32:**438–442.

# LEGIONELLA PNEUMOPHILA AND INTERLEUKIN-12 PRODUCTION: IN VITRO INFECTION MODEL

*Kazuto Matsunaga, Thomas W. Klein, Catherine Newton, Herman Friedman, and Yoshimasa Yamamoto*

# 22

The mechanism by which *Legionella pneumophila* infection of the lung is controlled is not yet clear, but the activation of macrophages to suppress intracellular bacterial growth is thought to be an essential effector mechanism of cell-mediated immunity (CMI) in the resolution of legionellosis (9). In this regard, it is conceivable that Th1 cells, which are essential for the development of CMI, may play a pivotal role in the defense against *L. pneumophila* infection. Interleukin-12 (IL-12), one of the key cytokines in regulating the development of Th1 response (12), is a heterodimeric cytokine composed of two disulfide-linked p35 and p40 subunits. Both subunits have to be expressed within the same cell to produce biologically active p70 heterodimer (6). It has been shown that p40 mRNA accumulation is up-regulated in the cells producing IL-12, whereas p35 mRNA is constitutively expressed in various cells (5). Previous studies have demonstrated that IL-12 is critical for resolution of some replicative intracellular pathogens, including *Leishmania major* (7, 8),

*Mycobacterium tuberculosis* (4), and *L. pneumophila* (2). Furthermore, it was shown that the Th1 cytokine, gamma interferon (IFN-$\gamma$), could activate macrophages to inhibit *L. pneumophila* growth (10). Therefore, regulation of IL-12 production may eventually regulate, at least somewhat, the outcome of *L. pneumophila* infection.

The production of IL-12 by monocytes/macrophages is induced by exposing responsive cells to a variety of microbial products such as lipopolysaccharide (LPS). On the other hand, the production of IL-12 is regulated by multiple mechanisms; these include cytokines, chemoattractants, and activation-induced deactivation pathways (1, 12). Furthermore, some intracellular pathogens have been shown to suppress macrophage IL-12 production. For example, the interaction of *Leishmania* (7) and human immunodeficiency virus (HIV) (3) with macrophages and monocytes results in a marked decrease in IL-12 production. Therefore, it seems likely that the suppression of IL-12 production may be exploited by these intracellular pathogens as a way to escape from cell-mediated immunity.

In vitro virulent-*L. pneumophila* infection of A/J mouse peritoneal macrophages (thioglycollate elicited) showed minimal induction of IL-12 and, furthermore, induced an inhibition

*Kazuto Matsunaga, Thomas W. Klein, Catherine Newton, Herman Friedman, and Yoshimasa Yamamoto* Department of Medical Microbiology and Immunology, University of South Florida College of Medicine, Tampa, FL 33612-4799.

*Legionella*, Edited by Reinhard Marre et al.
© 2002 ASM Press, Washington, D.C.

of IL-12 production of macrophages in response to LPS. In contrast, avirulent, as well as UV-killed, *L. pneumophila* showed a nominal IL-12 induction and did not affect the production of IL-12 induced by LPS. As shown in Table 1, both avirulent (obtained by multiple passages of virulent bacteria [14]) and UV-killed *L. pneumophila* induced a significant level of IL-12 protein. However, virulent bacteria did not induce any significant amounts of IL-12, even with a higher infection ratio such as 100 bacteria per macrophage. Furthermore, infection of macrophages with virulent bacteria caused a marked down-regulation of the LPS-induced IL-12 production in a dose-dependent manner. On the other hand, neither avirulent nor killed bacteria showed any down-regulation of LPS-induced IL-12 production. These results clearly indicate that IL-12 suppression is dependent on *L. pneumophila* virulency and its viability in the macrophages. Whether IL-12 was suppressed in a selective fashion by *L. pneumophila* infection was examined by determination of other cytokine productions. As seen in Table 2, the virulent *L. pneumophila* infection induced a marked production of alpha interleukin-1 (IL-1α) and IL-10. Furthermore, the production of IL-1α, IL-6, and

IL-10 induced by LPS was not affected by the infection. From these results, it is obvious that the suppression of cytokines by *L. pneumophila* infection was selective for IL-12. The results also indicate that the suppression of IL-12 production by *L. pneumophila* infection is not the result of a generalized failure of macrophage function. The data also indicate that the suppression may not be dependent upon *L. pneumophila*-induced IL-10, which is known to suppress IL-12 production in the presence of LPS (1), because *L. pneumophila* infection did not enhance the production of IL-10 induced by LPS but did enhance suppression of IL-12 production.

The suppression of IL-12 by *L. pneumophila* infection may be occurring at the level of gene transcription. The analysis of the steady-state levels of IL-12 p35 and IL-12 p40 mRNA determined by reverse transcriptase-PCR (RT-PCR) showed that *L. pneumophila* infection induced the suppression of mRNA accumulation for the IL-12 p40 gene in response to LPS stimulation, but not the IL-12 p35 gene, which was constitutive in all macrophages treated (data not shown). In addition, the virulent *L. pneumophila* infection induced mRNA accumulation for monocyte chemotactic protein (MCP)-1, which is also known

**TABLE 1**  Effect of *L. pneumophila* infection of macrophages on the protein levels of IL-12 p40/p70 production induced by LPS

| Treatment (infectivity ratio)[a] | IL-12 p40/p70 (ng/ml)[b] | |
|---|---|---|
| | LPS (−) | LPS (+)[c] (% of control) |
| Control | 0.27 + 0.18 | 30.73 ± 3.04 (100) |
| LP-V (1:1) | 1.24 ± 0.23 | 24.34 ± 5.40 (79 ± 18) |
| LP-V (10:1) | 1.47 ± 0.24 | 8.58 ± 0.58 (28 ± 2)★★ |
| LP-V (100:1) | 2.07 ± 0.51 | 5.29 ± 0.60 (17 ± 3)★★ |
| LP-Av (10:1) | 4.57 ± 0.76★ | 31.41 ± 3.96 (102 ± 13) |
| UV-killed LP-V (10:1) | 13.21 ± 2.67★ | 32.16 ± 2.23 (105 ± 7) |

[a] Macrophages were infected with virulent- (LP-V), avirulent- (LP-Av), or UV-killed virulent-*L. pneumophila* for 60 min and then nonphagocytized bacteria were washed out. The macrophages were then incubated for further 24 h. The infectivity ratios (bacteria per cell) are shown in the parentheses.
[b] The amount of IL-12 p40/p70 protein in the culture supernatants obtained at 24 h after infection was measured by ELISA. Results are expressed as mean ± SD for three independent experiments. ★, $P < 0.05$ compared with noninfected control group; ★★, $P < 0.05$ compared with LPS-stimulated control group.
[c] Macrophage monolayers were treated with 1 μg of *E. coli* LPS per ml.

**TABLE 2** Effect of virulent *L. pneumophila* (LP-V) infection of macrophages on the protein levels of IL-1$\alpha$, IL-6, and IL-10 production induced by LPS

| Treatment | IL-1$\alpha$ (ng/ml)[a] | | IL-6 (ng/ml)[a] | | IL-10 (pg/ml)[a] | |
|---|---|---|---|---|---|---|
| | LPS (−) | LPS (+) | LPS (−) | LPS (+) | LPS (−) | LPS (+) |
| Control | 0.06 ± 0.04 | 5.08 ± 0.61 | 0.19 ± 0.18 | 29.59 ± 5.21 | 65.7 ± 24.0 | 493.3 ± 92.1 |
| Lp-V | 4.34 ± 0.15 | 5.35 ± 0.29 | 1.25 ± 0.53 | 27.85 ± 2.04 | 312.8 ± 88.2 | 504.2 ± 71.2 |

[a] The amount of indicated cytokine proteins in the culture supernatants obtained at 24 h after infection was measured by ELISA. Results are expressed as mean ± SD for three independent experiments.

to suppress IL-12 production (1) in response to LPS stimulation at 24 h after infection. These results indicate that *L. pneumophila*-suppressed IL-12 production induced by LPS is at the level of message accumulation. This is consistent with a prior report of the IL-12 suppression by *Leishmania* (7). However, IL-12 suppression by HIV is known to associate with decreased mRNA accumulation for both p35 and p40 (3). Therefore, mechanisms of IL-12 suppression by infection may depend on the pathogen used.

Since *L. pneumophila* infection enhanced the accumulation of MCP-1 mRNA in response to LPS stimulation, the MCP-1 protein level in macrophage cultures infected with *L. pneumophila* in the presence of LPS was measured by enzyme-linked immunosorbent assay (ELISA) (data not shown). *L. pneumophila* infection induced production of MCP-1 protein and up-regulated the LPS-induced production of MCP-1 protein regardless of the virulence of *L. pneumophila* and its viability in the macrophages. Therefore, it seems unlikely that MCP-1 induced by infection may play a significant role in down-regulation of IL-12 by infection because IL-12 inhibition was dependent on the virulence and viability of *L. pneumophila*. To rule out a possible involvement of MCP-1 in the suppression of IL-12 by infection, we further determined the MCP-1 concentration necessary for IL-12 suppression in this system. In the dose-response study concerning the suppression of IL-12 protein by MCP-1, pretreatment with MCP-1 at concentrations induced by virulent bacteria did not suppress the LPS-induced IL-12 production (data not shown). Even though there were no neutralization experiments of MCP-1 by antibody in this study due to lack of commercially available antibodies, these results indicate that the MCP-1 may not be involved in the suppression of LPS-induced IL-12 by *L. pneumophila* infection.

The experimental mouse infection with *L. pneumophila* resulted in certain levels of IL-12 (2). Since IL-12 production is regulated by multiple mechanisms, including cytokines produced by other cells, it can be speculated that the suppressed IL-12 by infection may be overcome by other systems in vivo, such as the host defense system. This speculation may be supported by the fact that the infected animals tested were eventually cured. In addition, the systemic administration of exogenous IL-12 increases host resistance to several intracellular pathogens (8, 11, 13). Nevertheless, it is obvious that virulent *L. pneumophila* selectively suppresses IL-12 production induced by LPS from macrophages in vitro. Although the mechanism of suppression is not yet clear, the suppression of IL-12 production may be exploited by *L. pneumophila* as a way to escape from cell-mediated immunity.

### ACKNOWLEDGMENTS

This work was supported by grants from the National Institute of Allergy and Infectious Diseases (AI45169) and the American Lung Association of Florida.

### REFERENCES

1. **Braun, M. C., E. Lahey, and B. L. Kelsall.** 2000. Selective suppression of IL-12 production by chemoattractants. *J. Immunol.* **164:**3009–3017.

2. **Brieland, J. K., D. G. Remick, M. L. Legendre, N. C. Engleberg, and J. C. Fantone.** 1998. In vivo regulation of replicative *Legionella pneumophila* lung infection by endogenous interleukin-12. *Infect. Immun.* **66:**65–69.

3. **Chehimi, J., S. E. Starr, I. Frank, A. D'Andrea, X. Ma, R. R. McGregor, J. Sennelier, and G. Trinchieri.** 1994. Impaired interleukin 12 production in human immunodeficiency virus-infected patients. *J. Exp. Med.* **179:**1361–1366.

4. **Cooper, A. M., A. D. Roberts, E. R. Rhoades, J. E. Callahan, D. M. Getzv, and I. M. Orme.** 1995. The role of interleukin-12 in acquired immunity to *Mycobacterium tuberculosis* infection. *Immunology* **84:**423–432.

5. **D'Andrea, A., M. Rengaraju, N. M. Valiante, J. Chehimi, M. Kubin, M. Aste, S. H. Chan, M. Kobayashi, D. Young, E. Nickbarg, R. Chizzonite, S. F. Wolf, and G. Trinchieri.** 1992. Production of natural killer cell stimulatory factor (NKSF/IL-12) by peripheral blood mononuclear cells. *J. Exp. Med.* **176:**1387–1398.

6. **Gubler, U., A. Chua, D. S. Schoenhaut, C. M. Dwyer, W. McComas, R. Motyka, N. Nabavi, A. G. Wolitzky, P. M. Quinn, P. C. Familletti, and M. C. Gately.** 1991. Coexpression of two distinct genes is required to generate secreted bioactive cytotoxic lymphocyte maturation factor. *Proc. Natl. Acad. Sci. USA* **88:**4143–4147.

7. **Gui-Jie, F., H. S. Goodridge, M. M. Harnet, X. Wei, A. V. Nikolaev, A. P. Higson, and F. Liew.** 1999. Extracellular signal-related kinase (ERK) and p38 mitogen-activated protein (MAP) kinases differentially regulate the lipopolysaccharide-mediated induction of inducible nitric oxide synthase and IL-12 in macrophages: *Leishmania* phosphoglycans subvert macrophage IL-12 production by targetting ERK MAP kinase. *J. Immunol.* **163:**6403–6412.

8. **Heinzel, F. P., D. S. Schoenhaut, R. M. Rerco, L. E. Rosser, and M. C. Gately.** 1993. Recombinant interleukin-12 cures mice infected with *Leishmania major. J. Exp. Med.* **177:**1505–1512.

9. **Klein, T. W., C. Newton, Y. Yamamoto, and H. Friedman.** 1999. Immune responses to Legionella, p. 149–166. *In* L. J. Paradise, H. Friedman, and M. Bendinelli (ed.), *Opportunistic Intracellular Bacteria and Immunity.* Plenum Press, New York, N.Y.

10. **Nash, T. W., D. M. Libby, and D. M. Horwitz.** 1988. IFN-γ activated human alveolar macrophages inhibit the intracellular multiplication of *Legionella pneumophila. J. Immunol.* **140:**3978–3981.

11. **Sypek, J. P., C. L. Chung, S. E. H. Mayor, J. M. Subramanyam, S. J. Goldman, D. S. Sieburth, S. F. Wolf, and R. G. Schaub.** 1993. Resolution of cutaneous leishmaniasis: interleukin-12 initiates a protective T helper type 1 immune response. *J. Exp. Med.* **177:**1797–1802.

12. **Trinchieri, G.** 1993. Interleukin-12 and its role in the generation of Th1 cells. *Immunol. Today* **14:**335–337.

13. **Wagner, R. D., H. Steinberg, J. F. Brown, and C. J. Czuprynski.** 1994. Recombinant interleukin-12 enhances resistance of mice to *Listeria monocytogenes* infection. *Microb. Pathog.* **17:**175–186.

14. **Yamamoto, Y., T. W. Klein, and H. Friedman.** 1993. *Legionella pneumophila* virulence conserved after multiple single-colony passage on agar. *Curr. Microbiol.* **27:**241–245.

# DIFFERENTIAL CYTOKINE RESPONSE FOLLOWING CHALLENGE OF A/J MICE WITH VIRULENT OR AVIRULENT *LEGIONELLA PNEUMOPHILA*

*Antonella Torosantucci, Paola Chiani, Maria Luisa Ricci, and Maddalena Castellani Pastoris*

# 23

*Legionella pneumophila* causes a severe atypical pneumonia in humans, the so-called Legionnaires' disease. Although the disease mostly occurs in immunocompromised subjects, several virulence factors of *Legionella* have been described that confer to the microorganism an intrinsic aggressive potential (5, 9). Mechanisms underlying the pathogenic action of *L. pneumophila*, however, are not completely understood, mostly due to the lack of suitable animal models mimicking the human disease.

The ability of this pathogen to replicate in host macrophages is considered a major virulence trait. For this reason, the susceptibility to the experimental infection with *L. pneumophila* observed in guinea pigs and in selected mouse strains has been generally explained by the permissiveness of macrophages of these animals for *Legionella* invasion and intracellular replication in vitro, as reported, for instance, for elicited peritoneal macrophages from susceptible A/J mice (2, 11, 12). However, in this mouse strain, the extent of the intracellular survival of *L. pneumophila* and its limited

in vivo multiplication do not justify the lethal effect exerted by the experimental inoculation of the microorganism.

In a previous study, we described the differential lethality of a flagellated, virulent strain of *L. pneumophila* (VIR+) and of an aflagellated, avirulent spontaneous mutant (VIR−) when inoculated intraperitoneally (i.p.) in suckling CD1 mice (4). We also observed that only the lethal VIR+ strain could induce tumor necrosis factor alpha (TNF-$\alpha$) gene expression by peritoneal exudate cells (PECs) of challenged mice (4). Although TNF-$\alpha$ induction is generally considered a protective response against *Legionella* infections (3), this cytokine is also a major mediator in septic shock, and its local or systemic production has been associated with a wide variety of inflammatory and neoplastic diseases (1, 10). It was therefore of interest to determine whether, in *Legionella*-permissive A/J mice, the differential induction by VIR+ and VIR− *Legionella* strains of the in vivo release of TNF-$\alpha$ and of other potentially harmful proinflammatory cytokines was related to the differential lethality exerted by the two strains.

To this aim, we injected i.p. A/J mice with VIR+ or VIR− *Legionella* cells and monitored the survival of the animals, the clearance of *Legionella* from PECs, and the release of

*Antonella Torosantucci, Paola Chiani, Maria Luisa Ricci, and Maddalena Castellani Pastoris* Laboratorio di Batteriologia e Micologia Medica, Istituto Superiore di Sanità, 00161 Rome, Italy.

*Legionella*, Edited by Reinhard Marre et al.
© 2002 ASM Press, Washington, D.C.

TNF-α and other proinflammatory cytokines (beta interleukin-1 [IL-1β], interleukin-6 [IL-6]) in the peritoneal cavity and in sera of challenged animals. In some experiments, A/J mice were also pretreated with IL-10 or with anticytokine antibodies to investigate more precisely the role of the cytokines released by *Legionella* inoculation in causing the death of the animals.

Female A/J mice, 4 to 6 weeks old, were obtained from Charles River, Italy, and used within 15 days of their arrival. *L. pneumophila* serogroup 6, VIR+ strain was isolated from a fatal case of Legionnaires' disease, while strain VIR− was a spontaneous, aflagellated mutant originated from this latter strain and shown to be avirulent in guinea pigs as well as in CD1 suckling mice (4). Both strains were kept at −80°C as a suspension in skim milk.

For animal inoculation, *Legionella* cells grown 48 to 72 h on buffered charcoal-yeast extract (BCYE) agar plates (Oxoid, Italy) were resuspended in pyrogen-free saline, adjusted at the desired cell density by comparison with a McFarland opacity standard, and injected i.p. Inoculum size, as specified in single experiments, was determined by CFU counts. In selected experiments, mice were pretreated with human recombinant IL-10 (≥98% purity, kindly provided by M. Cignitti, Istituto Superiore di Sanità, Rome, Italy), which is fully bioactive in mice, or with neutralizing rabbit anti-mouse TNF-α serum (100 µl/mouse) or rat anti-mouse IL-6 antibodies (100 µg/mouse) (Genzyme). At different times after *Legionella* inoculation, the animals were sacrificed by cervical dislocation and the peritoneal cavity was washed with 1 ml of RPMI 1640 medium (Gibco-BRL). Peritoneal washings were centrifuged and cytokine (IL-1β, IL-6, and TNF-α) levels in cell-free supernatants were measured by enzyme-linked immunosorbent assay (ELISA) (R&D System). PECs in the pellet were washed with saline and lysed by resuspension in double-distilled water (ddH$_2$O) for 30 min; the number of PEC-associated, viable *Legionella* cells was determined by standard CFU counts on BCYE

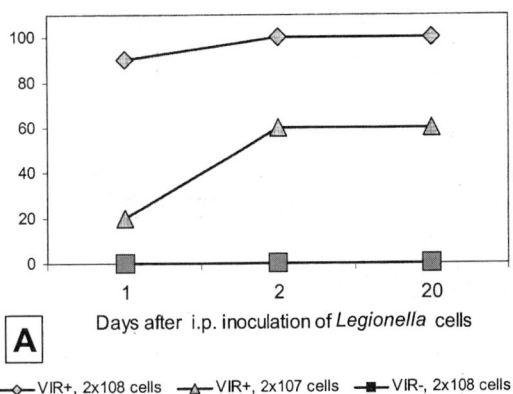

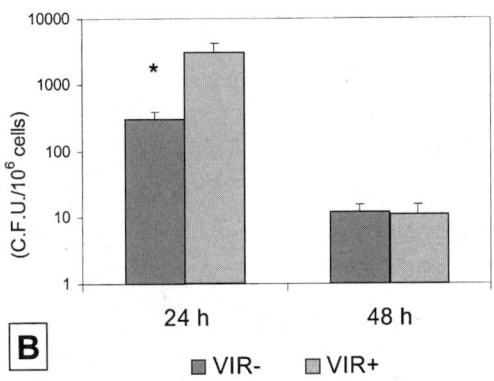

**FIGURE 1** Mortality of A/J mice and recovery of PEC-associated viable *L. pneumophila* cells after an i.p. challenge with VIR+ or VIR− strain. (A) Differential lethality of VIR+ and VIR− *L. pneumophila* strain for A/J mice. Groups of 12 mice were inoculated i.p. at day 0 with the indicated dose of *Legionella* cells, VIR+ or VIR− strain. Data represent cumulative percent mortality of animals at the indicated day postchallenge. (B) Recovery of *Legionella* cells from PECs of A/J mice injected i.p. with VIR+ or VIR− strain. Mice were given 2 × 10$^7$ to 3 × 10$^7$ bacterial cells. *Legionella* CFU in PECs were enumerated, as described in the text, at the indicated time postinoculation. Values are expressed as means ± standard error of the individual CFU counts measured in four mice from two independent experiments. The asterisk marks a statistically significant difference ($P < 0.05$, Student's *t* test, two tailed) with respect to values measured for the VIR+ strain.

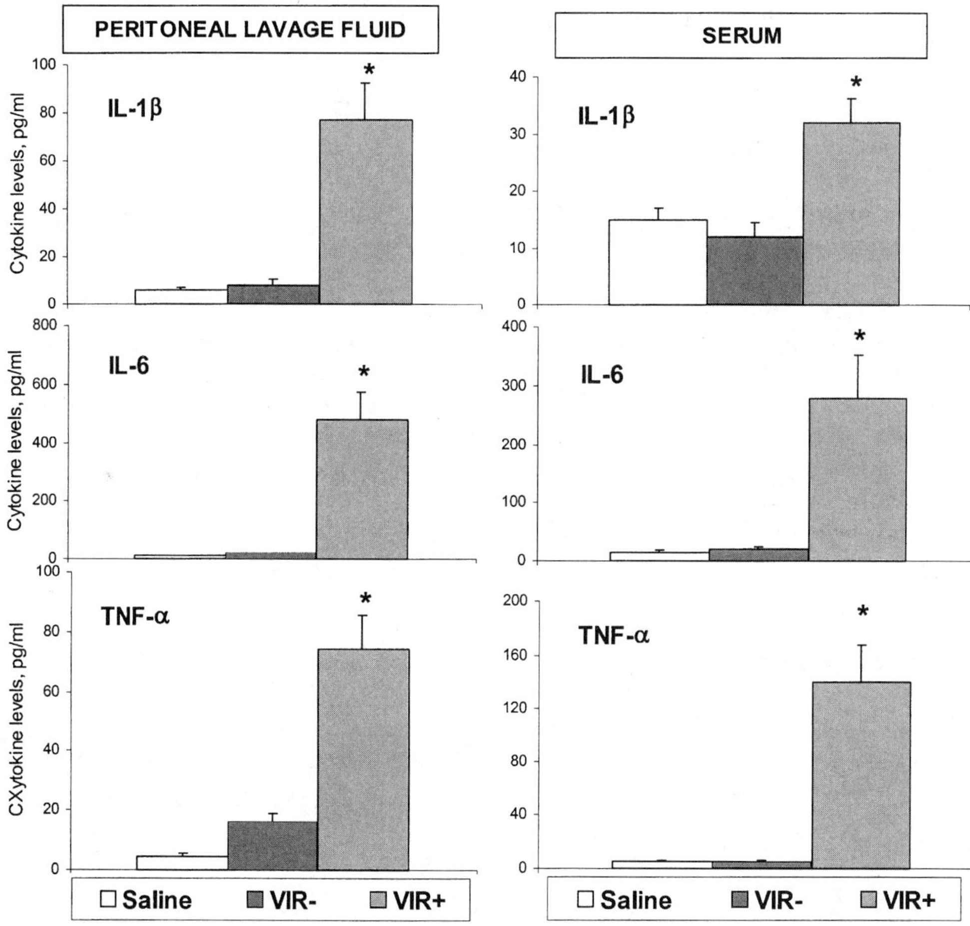

**FIGURE 2** Release of proinflammatory cytokines in the peritoneal cavity and in serum of VIR+ or VIR− challenged mice. Mice were injected i.p. with saline (control) or with $2 \times 10^7$ to $5 \times 10^7$ cells of the indicated *L. pneumophila* strain. Twenty-four hours after the bacterial challenge, cytokine levels in individual peritoneal lavage fluids (eight mice for each experimental group) and in serum (four mice for each experimental group) were measured by ELISA. Values respresent mean cytokine concentrations ± standard error measured in mice from each experimental group. The asterisks indicate a statistically significant difference ($P < 0.01$; Mann-Whitney U test, two tailed) with respect to saline-injected, control mice.

agar. Samples of serum collected from animals by retroorbital puncture were also evaluated for cytokine content as described above.

We found that the i.p. inoculation of virulent *Legionella* cells from the VIR+ strain was rapidly lethal for A/J mice, since 100 and 60% of the animals acutely died within 2 days following the challenge with $2 \times 10^8$ or $2 \times 10^7$ bacterial cells, respectively (Fig. 1A). Con-

versely, all inoculated animals survived a challenge with $2 \times 10^8$ cells from VIR− strain (Fig. 1A). The lethal/nonlethal outcome of the bacterial challenge was unrelated to the in vivo replication of *Legionella* in PECs. Although more numerous *Legionella* cells were recovered from PECs of mice inoculated with the VIR+ strain, both VIR+ and VIR− strains were rapidly cleared from the peritoneal cavity so that only a negligible number of bacterial cells were recovered from PECs 48 h postchallenge (Fig. 1B).

The inoculation of sublethal doses of VIR+ cells reproducibly induced, when measured 24 h postchallenge, a sharp and statistically significant rise of IL-1$\beta$, IL-6, and TNF-$\alpha$ levels in the peritoneal cavity and in serum (Fig. 2). No rise of proinflammatory cytokine levels was seen following the inoculation of A/J mice with nonlethal VIR− cells (Fig. 2). Differential lipopolysaccharide (LPS) expression was not responsible for the differential cytokine induction by the two strains that contained an equivalent amount of LPS, as judged by *Limulus* amoebocyte lysate (LAL) test dosage (4). A nonlethal challenge with the VIR+ strain, both as live cells in resistant CD1 mice, or as heat-inactivated cells in A/J mice, similarly failed to induce local or systemic proinflammatory cytokine release (data not shown). Since proinflammatory cytokine release was closely associated with a fatal outcome of the bacterial challenge, we investigated whether cytokine neutralization could totally or partially rescue A/J mice from the lethal effects exerted by virulent legionellae. We used both Il-10, an antinflammatory cytokine that potently inhibits IL-1$\beta$, IL-6,

and TNF-$\alpha$ release (6, 7), and specific, neutralizing anti-TNF-$\alpha$ or anti-IL-6 antibodies. Results from these experiments, reported in Table 1, suggested a role for the proinflammatory cytokines (in particular for TNF-$\alpha$) in mediating the lethal effect exerted by the VIR+ strain. Both wide-range cytokine inhibition by IL-10 and selective TNF-$\alpha$ neutralization with anti-TNF-$\alpha$ antibodies significantly prolonged the mean survival times of lethally challenged mice. In particular, by TNF-$\alpha$ neutralization, 3 of 12 mice definitively survived the *Legionella* challenge, while in the untreated group, 12 of 12 mice died within 48 h postchallenge. Conversely, no significantly protective effect could be achieved by IL-6 neutralization.

These data demonstrate that distinct *L. pneumophila* strains might be characterized by a differential ability of inducing the release of TNF-$\alpha$, IL-1$\beta$, and IL-6, upon i.p. inoculation in *Legionella*-susceptible A/J mice. Induction of high levels of these acute-phase cytokines in the peritoneal cavity and in serum is a distinctive feature of a virulent *L. pneumophila* strain and is strictly associated with the death of challenged animals, while being unrelated to the replication of legionellae in mice PECs. The precise nature of mutation(s) oc-

**TABLE 1** Effect of the treatment with IL-10 or with anti-mouse TNF-$\alpha$ or IL-6 antibodies on the course of a lethal *L. pneumophila* VIR+ challenge[a]

| Experiment and treatment | No. of mice dead/total no. at: | | | | MST[b] (days) | P[c] |
|---|---|---|---|---|---|---|
| | 24 h | 36 h | 48 h | 15 days | | |
| Experiment 1 | | | | | | |
| None | 7/12 | 8/12 | 12/12 | | 1.3 | |
| Anti-TNF-$\alpha$ serum | 1/12 | 2/12 | 9/12 | 9/12 | 5.1 | <0.025 |
| Anti-IL-6 antibody | 1/6 | 3/6 | 5/6 | 5/6 | 3.8 | NS |
| Experiment 2 | | | | | | |
| None | 11/12 | 11/12 | 12/12 | | 1.1 | |
| IL-10, 100 $\mu$g | 0/6 | 0/6 | 6/6 | | 2.0 | <0.025 |
| IL-10, 10 $\mu$g | 2/6 | 2/6 | 6/6 | | 1.5 | NS |

[a] Mice were injected i.p. with $10^8$ bacterial cells. Animals treated with anticytokine antibodies received one dose at the time of the bacterial challenge and two further doses 5 and 24 h later. IL-10, at the indicated doses, was administered at the time of the bacterial challenge.
[b] MST, mean survival times.
[c] P, probability, as evaluted by Mann–Whitney U test, two tailed, comparing survival times of the animals treated with anticytokine antibodies or with IL-10 with those of untreated controls; NS, not significant.

curring in the VIR− strain, which leads to its inability for TNF-$\alpha$ stimulation and to non-lethality in this model of infection, is presently unknown. As a major difference with respect to the parental VIR+ strain, the VIR− strain lacks flagellum. Involvement of flagellum expression in modulating bacterial phagocytosis and cytokine production by murine macrophages, as well as production of virulence-related factors (DotA, Mip) by this mutant, are currently under study. These observations suggest that the lethal effect of the bacterial challenge, in this animal model, relies on the selective ability by the virulent *Legionella* cells of stimulating an intense local and systemic release of proinflammatory cytokines. Unchecked TNF-$\alpha$ production upon i.v. *Legionella* inoculation has recently been reported as the causative factor in the death of *Legionella* replication-unpermissive BALB/c mice (8). Accordingly, the protection afforded by IL-10 treatment or TNF-$\alpha$ neutralization in our model also indicates that the release of TNF-$\alpha$, a well-known toxic shock-related cytokine, plays a major role in mediating the lethal effects of the virulent legionellae. Therefore induction of proinflammatory cytokines, in particular TNF-$\alpha$, besides being an important factor facilitating the resolution of *L. pneumophila* infections, might also be regarded as a possible contributory factor to the pathogenic action of virulent *L. pneumophila* strains.

## REFERENCES

1. **Beutler, B., and A. Cerami.** 1986. Cachectin and tumor necrosis factor as two sides of the same biological coin. *Nature* **320:**584–588.
2. **Brieland, J., P. Freeman, R. Kunkel, C. Chrisp, M. Hurley, J. Fantone, and C. Engleberg.** 1994. Replicative *Legionella pneumophila* lung infection in intratracheally inoculated A/J mice. *Am. J. Pathol.* **145:**1537–1546.
3. **Brieland, J. K., D. G. Remick, P. T. Freeman, M. C. Hurley, J. C. Fantone, and N. C. Engleberg.** 1995. In vivo regulation of replicative *Legionella pneumophila* lung infection by endogenous tumor necrosis factor alpha and nitric oxide. *Infect. Immun.* **63:**3253–3258.
4. **Castellani Pastoris, M., E. Proietti, C. Mauri, P. Chiani, and A. Cassone.** 1997. Suckling CD1 mice as an animal model for studies of *Legionella pneumophila* virulence. *J. Med. Microbiol.* **46:**647–655.
5. **Cianciotto, N., B. I. Eisenstein, C. Engleberg, and H. Shuman.** 1989. Genetics and molecular pathogenesis of *Legionella pneumophila*, an intracellular parasite of macrophages. *Mol. Biol. Med.* **6:**409–424.
6. **Fiorentino, D., A. Zlotnik, T. Mosmann, M. Howard, and A. O'Garra.** 1991. IL-10 inhibits cytokine production by activated macrophages. *J. Immunol.* **147:**3815–3822.
7. **Gerard, C., C. Bruyns, A. Marchant, D. Abramowicz, P. Vandenabeele, A. Delvaux, W. Fiers, M. Goldman, and T. Velu.** 1993. Interleukin-10 reduces the release of tumor necrosis factor and prevents lethality in experimental endotoxemia. *J. Exp. Med.* **177:**1205–1208.
8. **Newton, C., S. McHugh, R. Widen, N. Nakachi, T. Klein, and H. Friedman.** 2000. Induction of interleukin-4 (IL-4) by *Legionella pneumophila* infection in BALB/c mice and regulation of tumor necrosis factor alpha, IL-6 and IL-1$\beta$. *Infect. Immun.* **68:**5234–5240.
9. **Swanson, M. S., and Hammer, B. K.** 2000. *Legionella pneumophila* pathogenesis: a fateful journey from amoeba to macrophages. *Annu. Rev. Microbiol.* **54:**567–613.
10. **Tracey, K. J., Y. Fong, D. G. Hesse, K. R. Manogue, A. T. Lee, G. C. Kuo, S. F. Lowry, and A. Cerami.** 1987. Anti-cachectin/TNF monoclonal antibodies prevent septic shock during lethal bacteraemia. *Nature* **330:**662–664.
11. **Yamamoto, Y., T. W. Klein, C. A. Newton, R. Widen, and H. Friedman.** 1988. Growth of *Legionella pneumophila* in thioglycollate-elicited macrophages from A/J mice. *Infect. Immun.* **56:**370–375.
12. **Yoshida, S., and Y. Mizuguchi.** 1986. Multiplication of *Legionella pneumophila* Philadelphia 1 in cultured peritoneal macrophages and its correlation to susceptibility of animals. *Can. J. Microbiol.* **32:**438–442.

# PROTECTION AGAINST LETHAL CHALLENGE BY *LEGIONELLA PNEUMOPHILA* IN A/J MICE FOLLOWING IMMUNIZATION WITH FLAGELLA

*Maria Luisa Ricci, Antonella Torosantucci,*
*Lucilla Baldassarri, Paola Chiani, Antonella Pinto,*
*and Maddalena Castellani Pastoris*

# 24

Bacterial flagella are complex organelles that have been shown to be highly immunogenic, inducing strong protection in several animal studies (12, 13). In particular it has been reported that passive transfer of antibodies directed against the flagellum of the gram-negative microorganism *Pseudomonas aeruginosa* protects mice against a subsequent lethal infection of this microorganism (7). More than 40 genes are involved in the synthesis and functions of flagella in *Escherichia coli* and *Salmonella enterica* serovar Typhimurium (10, 11). Their preservation and role in chemotaxis and motility are probably important in the pathogenic activity of the microorganisms. However, flagella are known to be involved in the clearance of bacteria from tissues (9). *Legionella pneumophila* possesses a single polar or subpolar flagellum with a 47-kDa filament subunit (8). The expression of flagellum has been suggested to coregulate virulence factors (3, 4). It has also been reported that flagella may contribute to the rapid spread of infection by *L. pneumophila* in the lungs (6). However, we observed that susceptible A/J mice inoculated with a suspension of *L. pneumophila* intact flagella survived a lethal challenge by a virulent *L. pneumophila* strain. In this study, we investigated the role of the flagellum in the observed protection from legionella infection.

First, the minimal lethal dose (MLD) of two different strains of *L. pneumophila* was determined by infecting intraperitoneally (i.p.) female A/J mice, aged 4 to 6 weeks, with different doses of an *L. pneumophila* serogroup 6 strain of human origin (VIR+), or from the *L. pneumophila* serogroup 1 Corby strain. The MLD was approximately $5 \times 10^7$ CFU for both strains. A nonflagellated spontaneous mutant of the VIR+ strain, which was avirulent in previous studies on guinea pigs and suckling mice (VIR−) (5), was also used in the study.

A flagellar preparation was performed from a 6-day culture of the flagellated VIR+ strain on buffered charcoal-yeast extract (BCYE; Oxoid, Italy) agar plates at 36°C, in humidified atmosphere and 2.5% $CO_2$. Bacteria were harvested by flooding each plate with 5 ml of sterile pyrogen-free distilled water and then maintained at room temperature for 30 min. The flagella were mechanically separated from

*Maria Luisa Ricci, Antonella Torosantucci, Paola Chiani, Antonella Pinto, and Maddalena Castellani Pastoris* Laboratorio di Batteriologia e Micologia Medica, Istituto Superiore di Sanità, 00161 Rome, Italy. *Lucilla Baldassarri* Laboratorio di Ultrastrutture, Istituto Superiore di Sanità, 00161 Rome, Italy.

*Legionella*, Edited by Reinhard Marre et al.
© 2002 ASM Press, Washington, D.C.

bacterial cells by passage through a 27-gauge needle. Bacteria were removed by centrifugation at 5,500 × $g$ for 20 min, followed by centrifugation at 12,400 × $g$ for 20 min. Flagella were obtained by ultracentrifugation (180,000 × $g$ for 30 min) of the resulting supernatant, resuspended in sterile pyrogen-free distilled water, and further centrifuged with a Millipore Ultrafree unit containing Biomax 100K NMWL membrane, cut off of 100 kDa (Millipore, Italy) to eliminate low-molecular-weight contaminant proteins.

The same procedure was performed with a suspension of the nonflagellated mutant (VIR−) containing approximately the same number of legionellae/volume as the flagellated strain to prepare a control sham-flagellar extract. The flagellar preparation and sham flagellar extract were stored at −20°C. Protein determination for both preparations was performed by the Coomassie blue Bio-Rad protein assay. The absence of contamination by gross bacterial debris was verified in the two preparations by transmission electron microscopy. The presence of lipopolysaccharides (LPS) was checked by the method of the *Limulus* amoebocyte lysate (LAL) test (sensitivity = $\lambda$ 0.125 Endotoxin Units/ml).

Mouse protection studies were carried out by injecting i.p. groups of A/J mice (weekly, three times) with the flagellar preparation (500 $\mu$l containing 10 $\mu$g of protein) or with an equal volume of the sham-flagellar extract. Control mice were injected with pyrogen-free saline. Immunized, sham-immunized, and control mice were challenged i.p. 4 days after the last immunization with a lethal dose of the VIR+ *L. pneumophila* serogroup 6 strain or the virulent *L. pneumophila* serogroup 1 Corby strain (approximately 5 × 10^7 CFU/mouse for both strains). Mice were observed for signs of illness and for survival for 15 days.

As shown in Table 1, immunization with flagella afforded a significant protection in mice against a lethal challenge with the homologus VIR+ strain. In flagella-immunized mice, no mortality was observed, compared with 100% mortality of similarly challenged

**TABLE 1** Mortality of A/J mice immunized with flagellar or sham-flagellar preparations after a lethal challenge with virulent *L. pneumophila*[a]

| Treatment | No. of mice dead/total no. | Median survival time (days) |
|---|---|---|
| Immunization with flagella | 0/14 | >14 |
| Immunization with sham flagella preparation | 14/14 | 2 |
| Control | 14/14 | 2 |

[a] A lethal dose (5 × 10^7 CFU/mouse) of virulent legionellae was given i.p. 5 days after the third immunization. Data represent the cumulative results of three independent experiments.

mice immunized with the sham-flagellar preparation or unimmunized control mice. Immunization of mice with the flagellar preparation from VIR+ *L. pneumophila* serogroup 6 strain also induced protection across a different serogroup of *L. pneumophila*. In fact, immunized mice lethally challenged with *L. pneumophila* serogroup 1 Corby strain showed an 80% survival and a median survival time (MST) of >15 days with respect to 0% survival and an MST of 1 day of control unimmunized mice.

Involvement of humoral immune responses in the protective effect due to flagellar immunization was investigated, also considering that flagella are present in most *Legionella* species and serogroups, and their composition is common in all of them (2, 8). To assess whether resistance to lethal challenge could be achieved by passive transfer of flagellar antibodies, rabbit and mouse antiflagella immunesera were prepared. Two New Zealand White rabbits were immunized with the partially purified flagellar preparation. Briefly, an emulsion of flagellum suspension (100 $\mu$l containing 80 $\mu$g of protein) and an equal amount of incomplete Freund's adjuvant were inoculated subcutaneously in two sites in the scapular region of the back. After 45 days the rabbits were injected intravenously with 500 $\mu$l of the flagellum suspension, and 1 week later the procedure was repeated. Fifteen days after the last immunization, rabbits were bled and immunesera were pooled and filtered through a 0.22-$\mu$m-pore-size membrane (Millipore, Italy). Mouse antiserum was obtained from A/J mice by i.p. immunization with the flagellum suspension (500 $\mu$l containing 10 $\mu$g protein) once a week for 5 weeks. Six days after the last immunization, mice were bled and the sera were collected, pooled, and filtered. Rabbit and mouse immunesera were absorbed with a suspension of the nonflagellated mutant VIR− (37°C for 2 h and 4°C overnight) to remove possible cross-reactive nonflagellar antibodies. The mixture was then centrifuged at 6,000 × $g$ for 15 min and the supernatant collected. This procedure was repeated three times, and the final adsorbed serum was filtered and stored at −20°C. Specificity of the adsorbed sera for flagella was evaluated by immunofluorescence and by immunogold electron microscopy on the flagellated and the nonflagellated *Legionella* strains (1). A clear positive reaction was observed by both methods with the flagellated strain but not with the nonflagellated strain (data not shown). Groups of five A/J mice were injected i.p. with inactivated (56°C for 30 min, to remove complement activity) mouse (ELISA titer 50,000; 300 $\mu$l/mouse) or rabbit (ELISA titer 64,000; 500 $\mu$l/mouse) hyperimmune antiflagellar serum, or with nonimmune rabbit or murine sera (ELISA titer <100) or sterile pyrogen-free saline as controls. Four hours after treatment, mice were challenged with a lethal dose (5 × 10$^7$ CFU/mouse) of the VIR+ legionella strain.

No significant differences in mortality rates or in MST were observed in mice pretreated with murine or rabbit hyperimmune antiflagellum serum, with respect to mice treated with nonimmune sera as evaluated by Student's $t$ test (Fig. 1). Surprisingly, mice inoculated with murine nonimmune serum partially survived lethal challenge. Nevertheless comparing survival of mice treated with nonimmune murine serum and mice inoculated with pyrogen-free saline, the difference was statistically significant ($P = 0.04$). On the basis of these results it could be speculated that

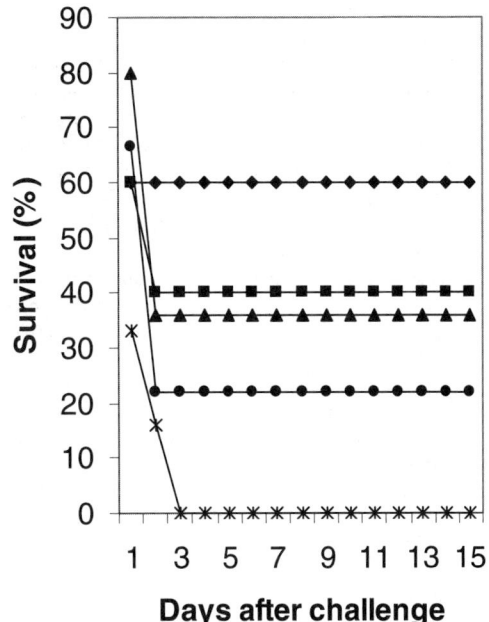

**FIGURE 1** Survival of A/J mice treated with murine or rabbit immunesera after challenge with *L. pneumophila* VIR+ strain. ♦, mouse antiflagellum serum; ■, mouse nonimmune serum; ▲, rabbit antiflagellum serum; ●, rabbit nonimmune serum; ∗, sterile, pyrogen-free saline.

in murine serum are present unidentified factors that induce a partially protective response in mice.

In conclusion, these preliminary results indicate that vaccination of A/J mice with highly immunogenic flagella preparations from *L. pneumophila* confers a significant degree of protection against a lethal i.p. challenge with the microorganism. However, humoral immunity appears not to be involved in mediating protection, since passive transfer of antiflagellum antibodies did not abolish or reduce mortality in *Legionella*-challenged mice.

Mechanisms underlying the protection and the role of cell-mediated immunity are currently being investigated.

**REFERENCES**
1. **Baldassarri, L., G. Donelli, A. Gelosia, M. C. Voglino, A. W. Simpson, and G. D.**

**Christensen.** 1996. Purification and characterization of the staphylococcal slime-associated antigen and its occurrence among *Staphylococcus epidermidis* clinical isolates. *Infect. Immun.* **177:** 2460–2468.

2. **Bornstein, N., D. Marmet, M. H. Dumaine, M. Surgot, and J. Fleurette.** 1991. Detection of flagella in 278 *Legionella* strains by latex reagent sensitized with antiflagellum immunoglobulins. *J. Clin. Microbiol.* **29:**953–956.

3. **Bosshardt, S. C., R. F. Benson, and B. S. Fields.** 1997. Flagella are a positive predictor for virulence in *Legionella. Microb. Pathog.* **23:**107–112.

4. **Byrne, B., and M. S. Swanson.** 1998. Expression of *Legionella pneumophila* virulence traits in response to growth conditions. *Infect. Immun.* **66:**3029–3034.

5. **Castellani Pastoris, M., E. Proietti, C. Mauri, P. Chiani, and A. Cassone.** 1997. Suckling CD1 mice as an animal model for studies of *Legionella pneumophila* virulence. *J. Med. Microbiol.* **46:**647–655.

6. **Chandler, F. W., B. M. Thomason, and G. A. Hebert.** 1980. Flagella on Legionnaries' disease bacteria in the human lung. *Ann. Intern. Med.* **93:**715–716.

7. **Drake, D., and T. C. Montie.** 1987. Protection against *Pseudomonas aeruginosa* infection by passive transfer of anti-flagellar serum. *Can. J. Microbiol.* **33:**755–763.

8. **Elliot, J. A, and W. Johnson.** 1981. *Legionella pneumophila* serogroups 1, 2 and 3. *Infect. Immun.* **33:**602–610.

9. **Feldman, M., R. Bryan, S. Rajan, L. Sheffler, S. Brunnet, H. Tang, and A. Prince.** 1998. Role of flagella in pathogenesis of *Pseudomonas aeruginosa* pulmonary infection. *Infect. Immun.* **66:**43–51.

10. **Jones, C. J., and S. Aizawa.** 1991. The bacterial flagellum and flagellar motor: structure, assembly and function. *Adv. Microb. Physiol.* **32:** 110–171.

11. **Macnab, R. M.** 1992. Genetics and biogenesis of bacterial flagella. *Annu. Rev. Genet.* **26:**131–158.

12. **Nossal, G. J. V., G. L. Ada, and C. M. Austin.** 1964. Antigens in immunity II. Immunogenic properties of flagella, polimerized flagellin and flagellin in the primary response. *Aust. J. Exp. Biol. Med. Sci.* **42:**283–294.

13. **Parish, C. R.** 1996. Immune deviation: a historical perspective. *Immunol. Cell. Biol.* **74:**449–456.

# *LEGIONELLA* AND PROTOZOA

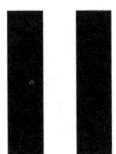

# THE SOCIAL LIFE OF LEGIONELLAE

*Barry S. Fields*

# 25

Until the last quarter of the 20th century, bacteria were assumed to lead a primarily asocial existence (5). Legionellae were first identified in 1977, at a time when microbiologists were beginning to focus upon mechanisms of bacterial interaction, both within the bacterial population and between the bacteria and host cells. Therefore, the study of *Legionella* can be considered a paradigm for these changing concepts in microbiology.

Legionellae were initially characterized by criteria typically used to describe an autonomous unicellular organism. Initial studies focused upon identification of their staining properties, ultrastructure, and biochemical and physical requirements for growth (11). These early studies accomplished the compulsory task of taxonomic classification of these bacteria, but did little to elucidate their complex ecology. Bacteria of the genus *Legionella* were described as gram-negative, aerobic, and rod shaped with one or more polar or lateral flagella (3). They use amino acids as their carbon and energy sources and do not oxidize or ferment carbohydrates. The uncommon nutritional requirements of these bacteria appeared to be remarkable for a bacterium that was readily isolated from a number of freshwater environments. This observation, combined with the the knowledge that the bacterium multiplied intracellularly in human tissue, resulted in landmark studies describing the ability of *L. pneumophila* to multiply intracellularly in freshwater protozoa (13). This observation has resulted in a new precept in microbiology: bacteria commonly parasitize protozoa and can utilize the same process to infect humans.

## INTERACTION WITH A HOST CELL

Prior to the widespread use of molecular techniques, the pathogenesis of intracellular bacteria was characterized through analysis using a variety of invasion assays. At that time, legionella was being characterized in invasion assays involving two very different host organisms: humans and protozoa. Initial work by Horwitz showed that *L. pneumophila* multiplied intracellularly in human macrophages by avoiding phagosome-lysosome fusion (10). This capability was regarded as central to the pathogenesis of the bacterium while similar observations regarding the invasion of protozoa were considered to be primarily of ecological significance.

*Barry S. Fields*    Centers for Disease Control and Prevention, Atlanta, Georgia 30333.

*Legionella*, Edited by Reinhard Marre et al.
© 2002 ASM Press, Washington, D.C.

Studies conducted in the last 10 years have shown that the pathogenesis and ecology of legionellae are inherently related (6). It is now established that the abilities of legionellae to infect mammalian and protozoan cells are related using common genes and gene products. Several genetic loci have been shown to be essential for the bacteria to infect both types of organisms, including the *mip* gene and the *dot/icm* loci (2, 4, 14). However, other genes, such as *mil*, are critical for the infection of a mammalian host but are not necessary for the infection of certain protozoa (9). Recent work by Abu Kwaik suggests that there may be genes that are required for the infection of certain species of protozoa but not others (8). Therefore important information has been gained by focusing on interactions that lead to the development of disease (pathogenesis) and the total spectrum of the bacteria's interaction with other organisms (ecology). However, we are far from realizing the complete ecological profile of legionellae. Currently, 42 species comprise 64 distinct serogroups in the genus *Legionella* (1, 12). Of these 42 species, only a few have been evaluated for their ability to infect various eukaryotic species. No systematic study of potential protozoan hosts has been conducted and the host range of most species of legionellae are unknown. *L. pneumophila* has been documented to multiply in 14 species of amoebae, 2 species of ciliates, and 1 slime mold (6, 7). A more complete ecological profile of legionellae will provide the scientific basis for selecting the most appropriate host for pathogenesis studies as well as studies to identify procedures to control amplification of the bacteria in certain environments.

## INTERACTION WITH THE MICROBIAL COMMUNITY

Analysis of bacterial group behavior represents the most recent facet in the study of the ecology of legionellae. In building water systems, legionellae are most frequently detected in biofilms of plumbing fixtures and heating, ventilating, and air-conditioning (HVAC) equipment. Although it is generally accepted that legionellae primarily exist within biofilms, only a limited number of studies have attempted to characterize the bacteria's interaction within these complex ecosystems (15). The *Legionella*/biofilm studies that have been conducted employ naturally occurring microbial communities, making it difficult to identify all organisms present and their contribution to the survival and multiplication of legionellae. Biofilm matrices are known to provide shelter and a gradient of nutrients. The complex nutrients available with biofilms have led some researchers to propose that the biofilm might allow the survival and multiplication of legionellae outside a host cell. This concept is certainly plausible; most facultative intracellular bacteria are known to multiply extracellularly in some environments. However, to date, the only documented extracellular growth of legionellae has occurred on laboratory medium (6). If legionellae can multiply extracellularly within biofilms, the study and characterization of this phenomenon could have tremendous impact on control strategies for the prevention of legionellosis.

## THE BIOFILM MODEL

The majority of the remaining text will focus on research designed to determine whether legionellae can colonize and grow within potable water biofilms with and without the association of amoebae. The biofilm used in this research was constructed from preselected heterotrophic bacteria and amoebae to allow better characterization of the interaction of these organisms. This model biofilm used a rotating disk reactor at a retention time of 6.7 h to grow biofilms on stainless-steel coupons (12a).

Rotating disk reactors (Center for Biofilm Engineering, Bozeman, Mont.) containing stainless-steel coupons were used for all experiments. The disk reactors were placed in a water bath to hold the temperature at 30°C.

Mixing was provided by a digitally controlled mixing plate placed underneath the water bath. Figure 1 shows the system setup. Initially, reactors were operated in batch mode to establish the biofilms on the steel substrata. The medium used was R2A broth. Following the period of batch growth, the system was then operated as an open system with dechlorinated tap water at a flow rate of 1 ml/min (retention time of 6.7 h) for 24 h for the duration of the experiment, approximately 21 days.

Each reactor was inoculated with the following heterotrophic bacteria: ATCC 7700 *Pseudomonas aeruginosa*, DMDS Lab no. 92-08-28a *Klebsiella pneumoniae*, and CDC-65 *Flavobacterium*-like organism. Cultures were stored at −70°C, transferred to R2A plates and re-

suspended to a concentration equal to a 0.5 McFarland standard. One milliliter of each cell suspension was used to inoculate each reactor to a final concentration of approximately $5 \times 10^5$/ml.

*L. pneumophila* strain RI-243-GFP containing the plasmid pANT4, which expresses green fluorescent protein (GFP) from a tac promoter, was used for all experiments. The plasmid backbone is RSF1010 and contains ampicillin and kanamycin markers. The strain was stored as a suspension in defibrinated rabbit blood in a liquid nitrogen (−120°C) freezer. Four days before the isolate was needed, the strain was cultured onto buffered charcoal-yeast extract (BCYE) media with kanamycin and incubated at 36°C with 2.5% $CO_2$. After the 4 days, the isolate was re-

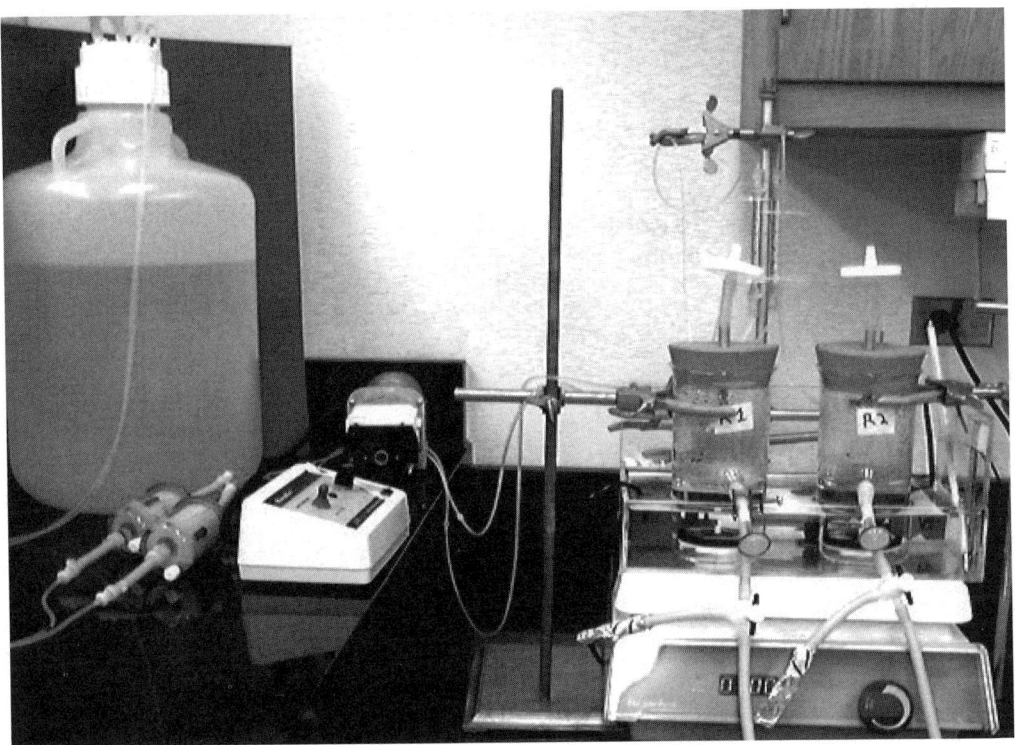

**FIGURE 1** Photograph of the biofilm reactors. Reactors are submerged in a 30°C water bath and operated as an open system with dechlorinated tap water at a flow rate of 1 ml/min (retention time of 6.7 h) for 24 h for the duration of the experiment.

suspended in sterile $H_2O$ and diluted to the desired concentration. One milliliter of a suspension of *Legionella* was added to each reactor for a final concentration of approximately $5 \times 10^5$/ml.

Experiments including amoebae used *Hartmannella vermiformis* strain CDC-19. Amoeba stocks were kept in axenic growth medium at 35°C without $CO_2$, and subcultured twice weekly into T75 cell culture flasks. Flasks were tapped on a solid surface to dislodge *H. vermiformis* from the growth surface, transferred to 50-ml conical tubes, centrifuged to pellet the amoebae, and resuspended in phosphate buffer saline. Reactors were inoculated with *H. vermiformis* to obtain a final concentration of $10^4$/ml. The base biofilm was considered to be at steady state after 7 days and was composed of *P. aeruginosa*, *K. pneumoniae*, and the *Flavobacterium*-like organism isolated from a water sample containing legionellae.

Coupons were removed from the reactors, placed into 10 ml of phosphate buffer water, sonicated for three 30-s cycles of sonicating and vortexing, homogenized for 1 min, and then spread plated on R2A medium for quantification of the base biofilm organisms. For the recovery of *Hartmannella*, 100 $\mu$l from several dilutions were plated onto nonnutritive agar that had been spread with viable *Escherichia coli*. Plates were read at 3 and 7 days for the presence or absence of *Hartmannella* at the dilution plated. For the recovery of *Legionella*, the supernate from processing the coupons was acid-treated, filtered, resuspended, and plated onto plates of BCYE agar supplemented with glycine, polymyxin B, vancomycin, and anisomycin.

Base biofilm densities of $10^7$ to $10^8$ CFUs per coupon (0.4 in$^2$) were consistently recovered from the reactors prior to the inoculation of *Hartmannella* and/or *Legionella*. Following the addition of *Hartmannella*, there was an approximately 1 log increase in the number of amoebae and a concomitant decrease in the number of heterotrophic bacteria to a concentration of approximately $10^5$ CFU/coupon (Fig. 2). These changes appear to reflect the effects of the amoebae actively feeding on the bacterial population. Figure 3 shows a scanning electron micrograph of *Hartmannella* feeding on the bacterial biofilm after 1 day. The amoebae and heterotrophic bacteria populations appeared to stabilize at these concentrations after 3 to 4 days and remained constant through the remainder of the experiment. This pattern of stabilization was consistent and occurred in experiments with or without the addition of *L. pneumophila* (Fig. 2 and 4).

A strain of *L. pneumophila* constitutively expressing GFP was used to visualize these bacteria within the biofilm. No microcolonies of *L. pneumophila* were detected in the biofilm and the bacteria that were observed were frequently single filamentous forms. *L. pneumophila* persisted in the biofilm for the duration of the experiments, both in the presence of amoeba, and without the addition of amoebae (Fig. 2 and 4). However, in the presence of the amoeba, *L. pneumophila* could be detected in both the biofilm and the bulk (planktonic) phase of the reactor while, in the absence of amoebae, *L. pneumophila* could be detected only in the biofilm phase. In addition, the *L. pneumophila* concentration in the biofilm phase was approximately 1,000-fold higher in experiments in which the amoebae were added. These findings demonstrated that *L. pneumophila* did multiply in the presence of the amoebae and could persist in both the planktonic and biofilm phases. In the absence of amoebae, *L. pneumophila* still persisted in the biofilm phase throughout the experiment. Because the reactor volume was replaced every 6.7 h with fresh medium and the *L. pneumophila* continued to persist in the biofilm, it was possible that they were exhibiting a low level of extracellular growth. Additional testing based upon loss of the GFP-containing plasmid was used to determine the amount of multiplication of *L. pneumophila* in these systems.

## MEASURING MULTIPLICATION OF *L. PNEUMOPHILA* IN THE BIOFILM

*L. pneumophila* RI-243-GFP will shed the GFP-containing plasmid when grown in the

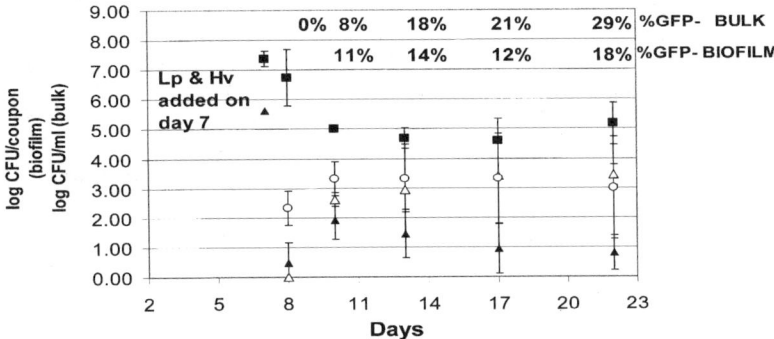

**FIGURE 2** Bacterial concentration in the biofilm reactors in the presence of *H. vermiformis*. The percentage of *L. pneumophila* RI-243-GFP that has lost fluorescence due to the absence of selective pressure is shown as %GFP−. Coupons from separate reactor experiments were processed for each data point presented in all graphs. Error bars indicate the standard deviation for $n = 3$. Symbols: ■, *P. aeruginosa*, *K. pneumoniae*, and *Flavobacterium* spp. in biofilm; △, *L. pneumophila* in biofilm; ○, *H. vermiformis* in biofilm; ▲, *L. pneumophila* in bulk liquids. Abbreviations: Lp, *L. pneumophila*; Hv, *H. vermiformis*.

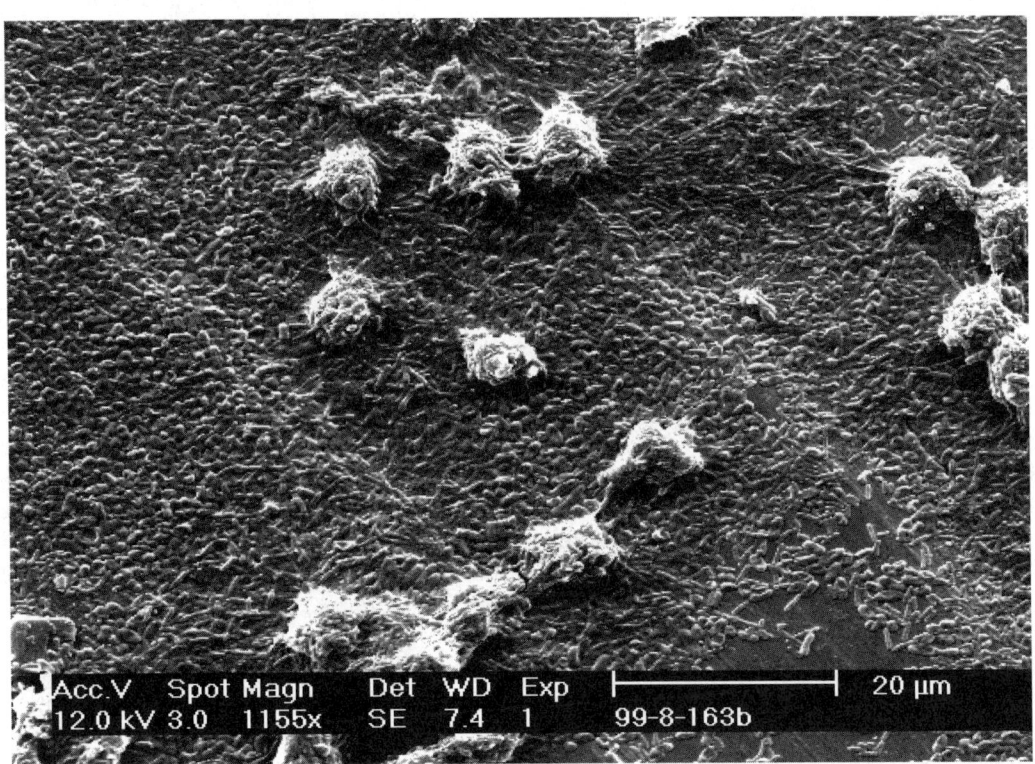

**FIGURE 3** Scanning electron micrograph showing *H. vermiformis* trophozoites feeding on the biofilm of heterotrophic bacteria on a stainless-steel coupon. Magnification, ×1,155.

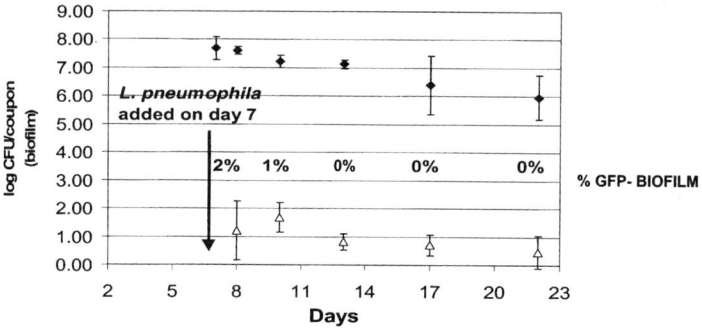

**FIGURE 4**   Bacterial concentration in the biofilm reactors in the absence of *H. vermiformis*. The percentage of *L. pneumophila* RI-243-GFP that has lost fluorescence due to the absence of selective pressure is shown as %GFP−. Coupons from separate reactor experiments were processed for each data point presented in all graphs. Error bars indicate the standard deviation for *n* = 3. Symbols: ◆, *P. aeruginosa, K. pneumoniae,* and *Flavobacterium* spp. in biofilm; △, *L. pneumophila* in biofilm.

absence of selective pressure with kanamycin. Although loss of such plasmids/fluorescence has hampered other biofilm studies using GFP-producing strains, we used the fact that loss of the plasmid/fluorescence occurs at a uniform rate to measure growth of *L. pneumophila* in the biofilm reactor. Preliminary experiments were conducted to determine what percentage of CFU lose fluorescence in multiplying RI-243-GFP in the absence of selective pressure. This was accomplished by plating a coculture of RI-243-GFP grown in *H. vermiformis* over a 7-day period and exposing these agar plates to UV light to determine the number of fluorescent colonies. Data indicated that strain RI-243-GFP loses fluorescence at a rate of 5% of the CFU per log of growth when grown in coculture with *H. vermiformis* (data not shown). When *L. pneumophila* RI-243-GFP was incubated for the same 7-day period in axenic medium without the amoeba, there was no loss of fluorescence. Therefore, the percentage of nonfluorescent GFP colonies cultured from the biofilm experiments were used to determine the amount of growth of *L. pneumophila* in the biofilm reactor.

This method of measuring growth was applied to biofilm experiments with and without *H. vermiformis*. The number of fluorescent

(GFP+) and nonfluorescent (GFP−) colonies were determined for all *L. pneumophila* CFU isolated from the biofilm experiments. These counts are shown as percent GFP− on Fig. 2 and 4. Although *L. pneumophila* persisted in the biofilm without amoebae, only a few GFP− colonies were detected at 1 and 3 days postinoculation and no GFP− colonies were detected for the remainder of the experiment. This indicates that *L. pneumophila* was not multiplying in the biofilm in the absence of amoebae. In experiments with amoebae added, the percent GFP− colonies increased throughout the 14-day period. The percent GFP− reached 18% in the biofilm itself and 29% in the bulk (planktonic) phase. These data suggest that the *L. pneumophila* increased approximately 6 logs during the 14-day period. In addition, these experiments confirm a long-standing supposition that the majority of the multiplying bacteria are shed into the planktonic phase.

This biofilm reactor was used to develop a reproducible, steady-state bacterial biofilm on nonsupplemented potable water. The addition of *H. vermiformis* to the reactor resulted in a reproducible equilibrium between the amoeba and heterotrophic bacteria. *L. pneumophila* associated with and persisted in these biofilms with and without *H. vermiformis* for a period of 14 days after inoculation. *L. pneumophila* cells did not appear to develop microcolonies in the biofilm reactors. Growth measurement studies indicated that *L. pneumophila* did not multiply within this biofilm in the absence of amoebae. *L. pneumophila* did multiply in the biofilm and planktonic phase in the presence of *H. vermiformis*, and the majority of these bacteria appear to be shed into the planktonic phase. In this model, it appears that *L. pneumophila* is not capable of extracellular growth. However, this model biofilm was constructed of five preselected organisms and certainly does not represent the many potentially diverse biofilms that may support the growth of legionellae in the environment. Additional studies are need to determine if legionellae possess a means to multiply independent of a host cell within biofilms.

## FUTURE DIRECTIONS

Researchers have only begun to characterize the interaction of legionellae with the microbial community. While it appears clear that legionellae are common inhabitants of biofilms, the significance of biofilms to the multiplication and distribution of legionellae remains unknown. Controlling legionellae within biofilms may lead to the most effective control measures to prevent legionellosis. Institutions that have experienced outbreaks of legionellosis are all too aware of how tenacious legionellae can be within building water biofilms. Application of advances in cell signaling, quorum sensing, and bacterial chemotaxis to the study of legionellae in biofilms will lead to a better understanding of the ecology of these bacteria and to more efficient mechanisms to control this disease. To date, autoinducers of quorum sensing have not been identified in legionellae. However, these studies are quite preliminary and it is doubtful that legionella are dormant asocial bacteria within these microbial communities.

## ACKNOWLEDGMENTS

I gratefully acknowledge the contributions of the members of CDC Biofilm Labortory, Division of Healthcare and Quality Promotion, Rodney Donlan, Ricardo Murga, Terri Forster, and Janice Carr.

## REFERENCES

1. **Benson, R. F., and B. S. Fields.** 1998. Classification of the genus *Legionella. Semin. Respir. Infect.* **13:**90–99.
2. **Berger, K. H., and R. R. Isberg.** 1993. Two distinct defects in intracellular growth complemented by a single genetic locus in *Legionella pneumophila. Mol. Microbiol.* **7:**7–19.
3. **Brenner, D. J., J. C. Feeley, and R. E. Weaver.** 1984. Family VII. *Legionellaceae*, p. 279. *In* N. R. Krieg and J. G. Holt (ed.), *Bergey's Manual of Systematic Bacteriology*, vol. 1. Williams & Wilkins, Baltimore, Md.
4. **Cianciotto, N. P., B. I. Eisenstein, C. H. Mody, G. B. Toews, and N. C. Engleberg.** 1989. A *Legionella pneumophila* gene encoding a species-specific surface protein potentiates initiation of intracellular infection. *Infect. Immun.* **57:**1255–1262.
5. **Dunny, G. M., and S. C. Winans.** 1999. Bacterial life: neither lonely nor boring, p. 1–5. *In* G. M. Dunny and S. C. Winans (ed.), *Cell-Cell Signaling.* ASM Press, Washington, D.C.
6. **Fields, B. S.** 1996. The molecular ecology of Legionellae. *Trends Microbiol.* **4:**286–290.
7. **Hagele, S., R. Kohler, H. Merkert, M. Schleicher, J. Hacker, and M. Steinert.** 2000. *Dictostelium discoideum*: a new host model system for intracellular pathogens of the genus *Legionella. Cell. Microbiol.* **2:**165–171.
8. **Harb, O. S., C. Cenkataraman, B. J. Haack, L. Y. Gao, and Y. Abu Kwaik.** 1998. Heterogeneity in the attachment and uptake mechanisms of the Legionnaires' disease bacterium, *Legionella pneumophila*, by protozoan hosts. *Appl. Environ. Microbiol.* **64:**126–132.
9. **Harb, O. S., and Y. Abu Kwaik.** 2000. Characterization of a macrophage-specific infectivity locus (*milA*) of *Legionella pneumophila. Infect. Immun.* **68:**368–376.
10. **Horwitz, M. A., and S. C. Silverstein.** 1983. Formation of a novel phagosome by the Legionnaires' disease (*Legionella pneumophila*) in human monocytes. *J. Exp. Med.* **158:**1319–1331.
11. **Isenberg, H. D.** 1979. Microbiology of Legionnaires' disease bacterium. *Ann. Intern. Med.* **90:**502–505.
12. **Lo Presti, F., S. Riffard, H. Meugnier, M. Reyrolle, Y. Lasne, P. A. D. Grimont, F. Grimont, F. Vandenesch, J. Etienne, J. Fleurette, and J. Freney.** 1999. *Legionella taurinensis* sp. nov., a new species antigenically similar to *Legionella spiritensis. Int. J. Syst. Bacteriol.* **49:**397–403.

12a. Murga, R., T. S. Forster, E. Brown, J. M. Pruckler, B. S. Fields, and R. M. Donlan. The role of biofilms in the survival of *Legionella pneumophila* in a model potable water system. *Microbiology,* in press.

13. Rowbotham, T. J. 1980. Preliminary report on the pathogenicity of *Legionella pneumophila* for freshwater and soil amoebae. *J. Clin. Pathol.* **33:** 1179–1183.

14. Segal, G., and H. A. Shuman. 1998. How is the intracellular fate of the *Legionella pneumophila* phagosome determined? *Trends Microbiol.* **6:**253–255.

15. Walker, J. T., J. Rogers, and C. W. Keevil. 1994. An investigation of the efficacy of bromine containing biocide on an aquatic consortium of planktonic and biofilm micro-organisms including *Legionella pneumophila*. *Biofouling* **8:**47–54.

# PORE FORMATION-MEDIATED EGRESS FROM MAMMALIAN AND PROTOZOAN CELLS BY *LEGIONELLA PNEUMOPHILA*

O. A. Terry Alli, Maëlle Molmoret, and Yousef Abu Kwaik

# 26

The Legionnaires' disease bacterium, *Legionella pneumophila*, is one of the common etiologic agents of bacterial pneumonia. In the aquatic environment, *L. pneumophila* is a parasite of at least 15 species of amoebae and ciliated protozoa (11). Intracellular replication of *L. pneumophila* within protozoa plays a major role in bacterial ecology and pathogenesis (3, 11).

Upon transmission to the human host, *L. pneumophila* invades alveolar macrophages and possibly epithelial cells (1). After entry into the host cell, the bacteria modulate the biogenesis of their vacuole into a niche (6) that evades maturation along the "default" endosomal-lysosomal degradation pathway (13) and is subsequently surrounded by the rough endoplasmic reticulum (2, 12). Formation of this replicative niche is controlled by a type IV-like secretion machinery, designated Dot/Icm (16). The bacteria replicate in this idiosyncratic niche, and this intracellular replication in the alveoli is the hallmark of Legionnaires' disease (1). Infections of mammalian and protozoan cells by *L. pneumophila* share a number

of similarities but differ in several attributes. Following entry into both host cells, *L. pneumophila* replicates within a ribosome-studded phagosome that does not fuse to lysosomes (11).

A fundamental step in the pathogenic cycle of intracellular pathogens is their ability to lyse and egress the host cell after termination of intracellular replication, to infect other cells within the same host, or to be transmitted to a new susceptible host. The mechanisms of killing of the host cell and release of intracellular bacteria after termination of intracellular replication are not known for *L. pneumophila* or any other vacuolar intracellular pathogen. It has been presumed that the physical and metabolic burden on the host cell by a large number of intracellular bacteria is sufficient to kill the host cell by nonspecific means.

## MUTANTS OF *L. PNEUMOPHILA* DEFECTIVE IN CYTOLYSIS AND EGRESS FROM MAMMALIAN CELLS

We have previously identified the protozoa and macrophage infectivity (*pmi*) and macrophage infectivity loci (*mil*) mutants of *L. pneumophila* that are defective in both cytotoxicity and intracellular replication, and the degree of both defects are correlated (9, 10). During our screening of the miniTn*10*::kan mutant library

O. A. Terry Alli, Maëlle Molmoret, and Yousef Abu Kwaik Department of Microbiology and Immunology, University of Kentucky Chandler Medical Center, Lexington, KY 40536-0084.

*Legionella*, Edited by Reinhard Marre et al.
© 2002 ASM Press, Washington, D.C.

(~5,000 clones) of *L. pneumophila* (9, 10) for the *pmi* and *mil* mutants, we discovered 5 mutants (GP247, GL208, GN229, GP263, and GR159) that were severely defective in their cytotoxicity but replicated similar to the parental strain AA100 within U937 macrophages and type I alveolar epithelial cells (Fig. 1A and B, and data not shown) (4). All the intracellular bacteria belonging to the parental strain were released into the tissue culture medium within 24 to 48 h postinfection (Fig. 1C and D and data not shown). In contrast, despite the prolific intracellular replication of the five mutants, they were "trapped" within and failed to egress from macrophages and epithelial cells during the 48-h infection, and the majority of the infected cells remained viable and intact (Fig. 1C and D and data not shown) (4). Phase-contrast images of the infection showed that the AA100-infected cells underwent complete cytolysis within 24 to 48 h postinfection, concomitant with termination of intracellular replication, while cells infected by the mutants were intact during this period (data not shown). Therefore, the defective loci in the mutants were designated *rib* (for release of intracellular bacteria) (4). However, after 72 h postinfection, viability of the cells infected by the mutants declined gradually and the bacteria were subsequently released (see below) (4).

## THE *rib* MUTANTS ARE DEFECTIVE IN THE PORE-FORMING TOXIN/PORE-FORMING ACTIVITY

We have recently proposed a model of biphasic death of mammalian cells by *L. pneumophila* initiated by caspase-3-dependent apoptosis followed by necrosis (7), which is probably mediated by the pore-forming toxin (14). We confirmed the ability of the mutants to induce apoptosis, similar to the parental strain. The *rib* mutants were next examined for the pore-forming activity, using two different strategies (14). In contrast to the wild-type strain, all five *rib* mutants were completely defective in contact-dependent lysis of sheep red blood cells (SRBCs) (4). Heat-killed bacteria, a *dotA* mutant, or bacterial culture supernatants did not cause hemolysis of SRBCs (data not shown). In the second strategy, we examined permeability of the plasma membrane of macrophages and epithelial cells to propidium iodide (PI, molecular mass 668) upon infection with a multiplicity of infection (MOI) of 500. In contrast to the

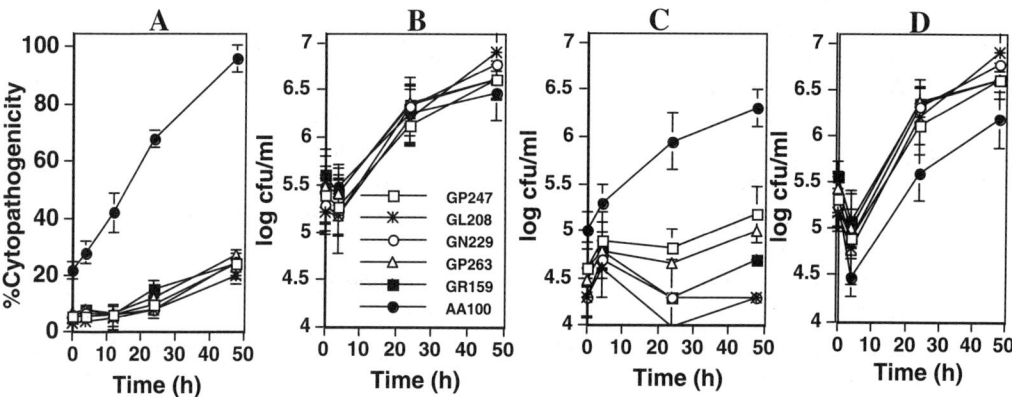

**FIGURE 1** The *L. pneumophila* mutants are defective in killing and exiting U937 macrophages, but not in intracellular replication. (A) Cytopathogenicity to infected cells (MOI 5) was determined by Alamar blue assays and compared with that of the noninfected cells. (B) Growth kinetics within U937 macrophages, where the indicated number of bacteria is the combined numbers of intracellular bacteria and the ones that were released into the supernatant. (C) The bacteria that were released into the tissue culture medium. (D) The number of intracellular bacteria. Values are the mean of triplicate samples, and error bars represent standard deviations. Reprinted from reference 4 with permission.

parental strain, all five *rib* mutants were severely defective in pore formation in macrophages and epithelial cells (4). No alteration in permeability to PI was detected when the cells were incubated with heat-killed bacteria, bacterial culture supernatants, or supernatants of AA100-infected cells obtained 3 h postinfection (4). Taken together, the data indicated that the five *rib* mutants were defective in expression of the pore-forming toxin and pore-forming activity (14).

## THE Rib TOXIN IS NOT REQUIRED FOR INTRACELLULAR TRAFFICKING

Several *dot/icm* mutants that are targeted into lysosomes are defective in intracellular replication and are also defective in the pore-forming activity (14). Thus, it has been proposed that the pore-forming activity is required for export of effector molecules that are required for evasion of lysosomal fusion (14). It is important to note that these *dot/icm* mutants are defective in components of the Dot/Icm secretion apparatus, and thus their defect in the pore-forming activity may be due to a defect in a Dot/Icm-mediated export of the molecules responsible for the pore-forming activity as well as molecules responsible for evasion of lysosomal fusion. Another class of *dot/icm* mutants that are defective in trafficking and intracellular replication, but retain the pore-forming activity, has also been isolated (18). On the basis of the phenotypes of these mutants, it has been concluded that the pore-forming activity is not sufficient for phagosomal trafficking, but that the pore may be a vehicle to deliver effector molecules into the host cell cytoplasm (18). However, these observations do not exclude a role for the pore-forming activity in phagosomal trafficking.

The *rib* mutants constitute a novel class of mutants that are defective in the pore-forming activity but not in intracellular replication (4). Therefore, we examined whether the pore-forming activity is required for intracellular trafficking. Confocal laser scanning microscopy showed that similar to strain AA100, the *rib* mutants did not colocalize with the late endosomal/lysosomal marker Lamp-1 at 2 to 4 h postinfection (data not shown) (4). In contrast, heat-killed *L. pneumophila*, or a *dot*A mutant, used as controls, exhibited predominant colocalization with Lamp-1 (data not shown). Taken together, these data showed that the *rib* mutants exhibited normal trafficking and prolific intracellular replication despite their defect in the pore-forming activity. Therefore, if the pore-forming activity is required to export bacterium-derived effector molecules into the host cell cytoplasm (18), the exported molecules play no detectable role in the intracellular replication. Importantly, our data clearly show that the pore-forming activity is not required for evasion of acquisition of Lamp-1, or intracellular replication. However, our data do not exclude the presence of another "less cytotoxic" pore utilized by *L. pneumophila* to export effector molecules required for phagosomal trafficking and intracellular replication.

The infection of U937 macrophages by one of the mutants was examined at the ultrastructural level. At 24 h postinfection, at least 50% of the cells in the AA100-infected monolayers were lysed, and the remaining cells exhibited necrotic morphology (Fig. 2). At 48 h postinfection, >95% of the AA100-infected cells were lysed and the remaining cells exhibited severe signs of necrosis (Fig. 2). In contrast, the mutant-infected cells were still intact at 48 h postinfection and were not necrotic, but apoptotic nuclei with condensed chromatin were readily detectable (Fig. 2) (4). These data were consistent with the substantial intracellular replication by the mutants and the defect in cytolysis of macrophages. The data further confirmed that the mutants are not defective in induction of apoptosis but are defective in induction of necrosis.

## THE *rib* MUTANTS ARE DEFECTIVE IN ACUTE CYTOTOXIC LETHALITY TO MICE

Pulmonary histopathology of Legionnaires' disease patients and *L. pneumophila*-infected experimental animals is characterized by extensive lysis of inflammatory cells and necrosis of the alveolar epithelium, which has been

## 24 h        48 h

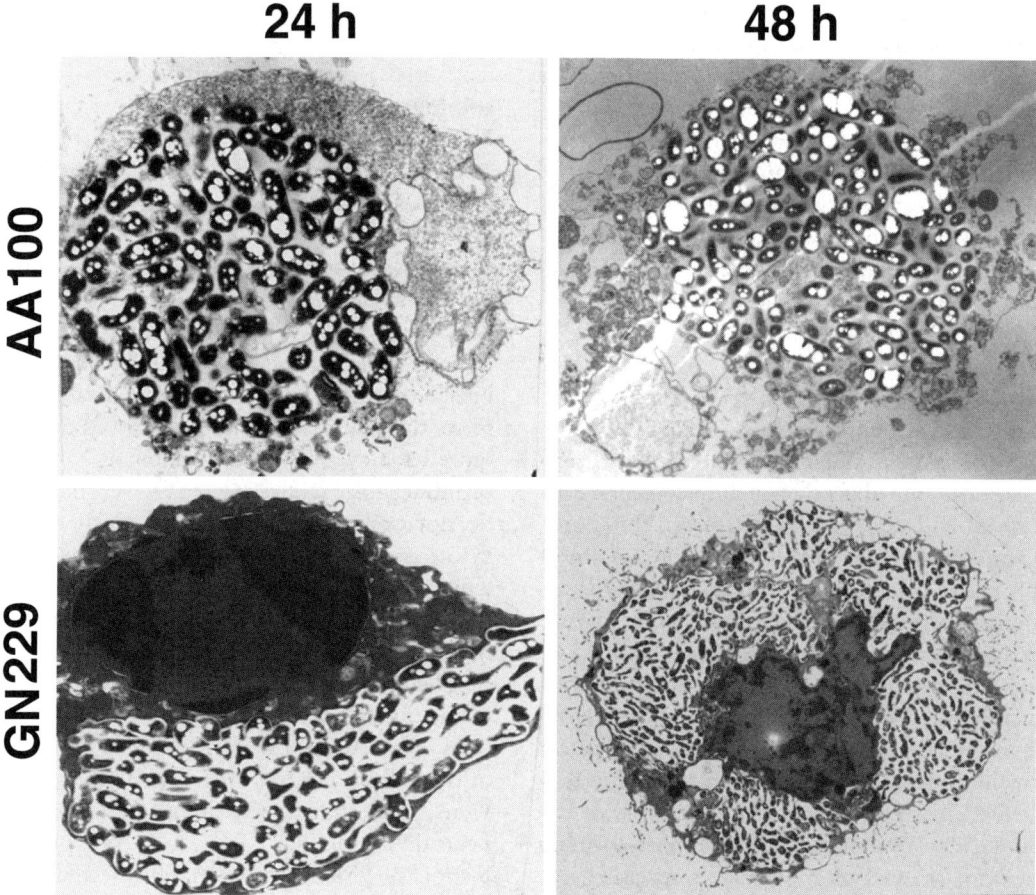

**FIGURE 2** The *rib* mutants defect in cytolysis of the host cell is due to a defect in necrosis-mediated killing. Representative transmission electron micrographs of infected U937 macrophages at 24 h and 48 h postinfection by the wild-type strain AA100 and the GN229 mutant. Magnifications are ×7,000 and ×5,000 for the 24-h and 48-h infections, respectively. Reprinted from reference 4 with permission.

proposed to be mediated by a cytotoxin (17). In addition, intratracheal inoculation of A/J mice with >10⁸ CFU of *L. pneumophila* results in bacterial growth-independent acute death (i.e., within 48 h) that is thought to be mediated by a cytotoxin. Intratracheal inoculation of A/J mice with 2.7 × 10⁹ or 2.7 × 10⁸ CFU (5 mice each) of the parental strain resulted in 100 and 60% death, respectively, within 24 to 48 h (4). In contrast, all 5 GN229-infected animals survived a similar dose, similar to animals infected by heat-killed AA100. Moreover, when 10 mice were infected by 4 × 10⁹ CFU of the parental strain

or the GN229 mutant, all 10 of the AA100-infected animals died within 24 to 48 h, but all 10 of the GN229-infected animals survived for the 7-day observation period (4). These data showed that the pore-forming activity played a major role in acute lethality and in the pathophysiology of Legionnaires' disease.

## PORE FORMATION-MEDIATED EGRESS FROM *ACANTHAMOEBA POLYPHAGA* BY *L. PNEUMOPHILA*

The pore-forming activity of *L. pneumophila* mediates cytolysis of macrophages and alveolar epithelial cells (4, 14), and the *rib* mutants of

*L. pneumophila* that are defective in expression of the pore-forming activity are defective in killing and egress from mammalian cells (4). Therefore, we utilized the *rib* mutants to examine whether the pore-forming activity of *L. pneumophila* is similarly required for necrotic killing and subsequent egress from the protozoan host *A. polyphaga*.

Necrotic killing of *A. polyphaga* by *L. pneumophila* was examined for the wild-type strain AA100 and for two distinct *rib* mutants, GP247 and GN229 (4). The monolayers were infected by strains of *L. pneumophila* at an MOI of 1 and pelleted to allow bacteria-cell contact. The data showed that the wild-type strain killed the majority (~70%) of the cells by 24 h postinfection, that all of the monolayers were destroyed by 48 h postinfection, and that intracellular bacteria were released into the supernatant (Fig. 3) (8). In contrast, killing of *A. polyphaga* by the GP247 and GN229 mutants was less than 5% by 48 h postinfection, despite their prolific intracellular replication (Fig. 3) (8). These data were consistent with PI staining of the infected cells, which showed that <3% of the GP247-infected cells were permeable to PI at 24 h postinfection. In contrast, at least 25% of the viable cells (60% of the cells have already lysed by this time) infected by the wild-type strain were PI positive (8).

Confocal laser scanning microscopy of infected *A. polyphaga* at an MOI of 1 confirmed that the GN229 mutant bacteria replicated within the protozoan cells. However, in contrast to the wild-type strain that replicated within almost all of the cells in the monolayer and lysed ~60% of the infected cells by 24 h postinfection, the mutant replicated in only ~15% of the cells, and the monolayers were intact with no detectable lysis of cells. Taken together, our data indicated that expression of the pore-forming activity was not required for intracellular replication but was required for necrotic killing of *A. polyphaga* and subsequent release of the intracellular bacteria.

To confirm the roles played by the pore-forming activity in necrotic killing of *A.* *polyphaga* and subsequent release of the intracellular bacteria, we examined infections at an MOI of 500, for the following two reasons. First, infection at this MOI may ensure that most of the cells were infected by *L. pneumophila* and may allow better examination of whether the *rib* mutants were defective in exiting the protozoan host. Second, it has been shown that extracellular *L. pneumophila* induces rapid necrotic killing of mammalian cells within 20 to 180 min at an MOI of 500 (14). At 4 h postinfection, there was no detectable staining with PI. By 12 and 24 h postinfection, 41 and 100% of the AA100-infected cells, respectively, were killed (8). In contrast, approximately 5 and 15% of the *rib* mutant-infected cells were killed at 12 and 24 h postinfection, respectively (8). The data suggested that, in contrast to the rapid pore-forming toxin-mediated necrotic killing of mammalian cells by extracellular *L. pneumophila* at high MOI, necrotic killing of *A. polyphaga* is mostly mediated by intracellular bacteria. It is possible that the pore-forming activity of *L. pneumophila* is not translocated or is not properly assembled in the outer leaflet of the plasma membrane of the protozoan cells. The ability of intracellular bacteria to lyse the protozoan host from within suggests that the pore-forming activity is properly translocated and assembled by the intracellular bacteria in the inner phagosomal and, subsequently, inner plasma membrane. This difference in the mechanism of necrotic killing of protozoan cells may illustrate an adaptation of *L. pneumophila* to intracellular parasitism within this unicellular protozoan host to avoid premature lysis of neighboring uninfected cells when large numbers of toxin-expressing bacteria are released and are searching for a new "niche" for intracellular replication.

Defect of the *rib* mutants in necrotic killing of *A. polyphaga* was not due to the defect in invasion and intracellular replication (8). At 24 h postinfection at an MOI of 1, cells harbored large numbers of intracellular bacteria. When infections were carried out at an MOI of 500 to allow infection of most cells, at 4 h

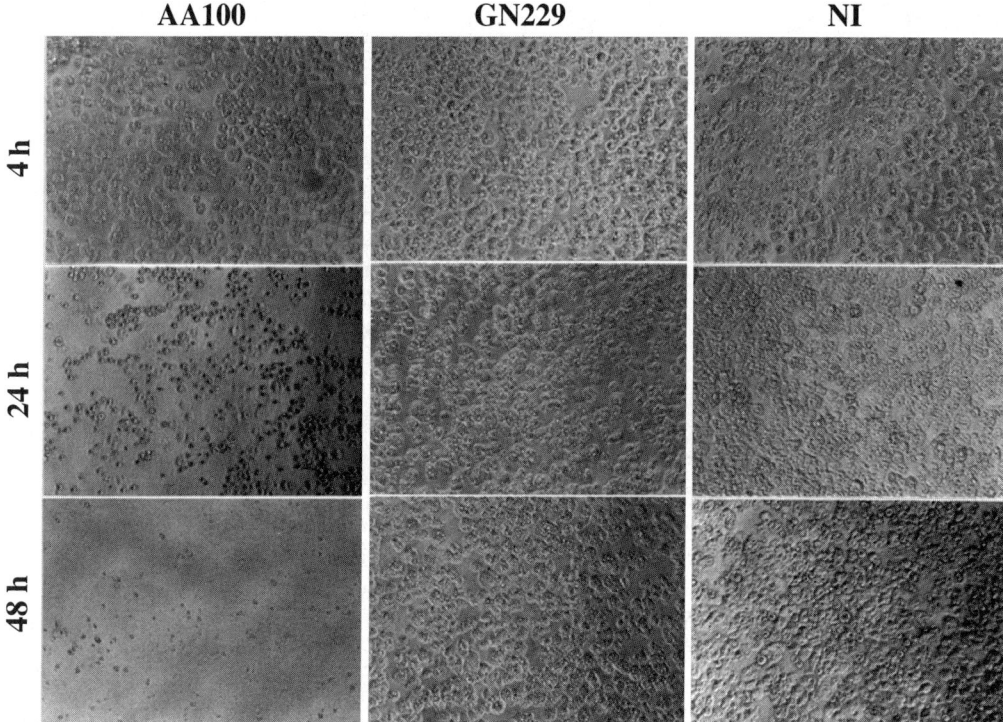

**AA100**  **GN229**  **NI**

4 h

24 h

48 h

**FIGURE 3** Representative phase contrast images of *A. polyphaga* infected by the wild-type strain AA100 or the GN229 mutant of *L. pneumophila*, and compared with noninfected (NI) cells. Infections were performed at an MOI of 1, exactly as described in the Fig. 5 legend. Phase contrast images at 4, 24, and 48 h postinfection are shown. Similar results to the GN229 mutant were also obtained for the GP247 mutant (data not shown). Reprinted from reference 8 with copyright permission from Blackwell Sciences.

postinfection cells harbored small numbers of bacteria (8). All the protozoan cells contained large numbers of the mutant bacteria at 24 h postinfection, similar to that of the wild-type strain. Examination by confocal laser scanning microscopy showed that the majority of the strain AA100-infected cells were lysed at 24 h postinfection, and only few cells in the monolayer remained and harbored large numbers of intracellular bacteria. In contrast, although *A. polyphaga* contained large numbers of the *rib* mutant bacteria, the monolayers remained intact during the first 24 h postinfection. Importantly, examination of the intracellular growth kinetics showed that there were at least 10-fold more AA100 bacteria at 24 h, compared with the *rib* mutants (8). This difference is likely due to failure of the mutants

in exiting the host cell during this period, while secondary infections have already occurred by the AA100 strain following their first round of infection and release of the intracellular bacteria. Interestingly, compared with complete lysis of the AA100-infected monolayers by 48 h postinfection, the *rib* mutants-infected monolayers remained intact during the entire course of the infection for up to 4 days postinfection (Fig. 4).

Importantly, the sizes of the phagosomes harboring the *rib* mutant bacteria were condensed after 72 h postinfection (8). This reduction in the size of the phagosomes was even more dramatic at 96 h postinfection. At these time points, intact individual bacteria were not visible (as detected by the polyclonal antiserum), suggesting bacterial degradation

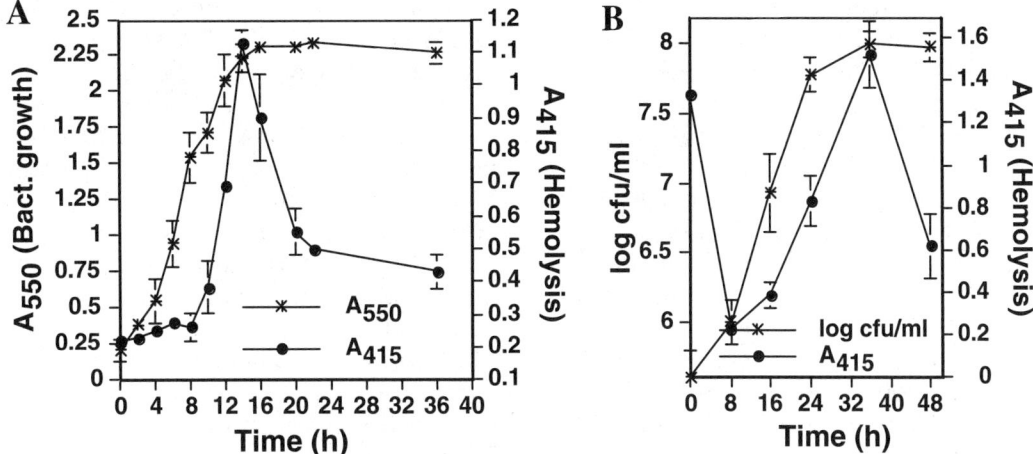

**FIGURE 4** Growth phase–dependent expression of the pore-forming activity by *L. pneumophila*, in vitro and intracellularly. Contact-dependent hemolysis of SRBCs by in vitro-grown *L. pneumophila* (A) or intracellular bacteria, isolated from U937 macrophages (B). Infection of the cells in panel B was performed using in vitro-grown bacteria that reached their maximal growth and hemolysis (14 h in panel A). At the indicated time points, the bacterial growth was determined by the absorbance at 550 nm ($A_{550}$) in panel A or by the CFU in panel B (left $y$ axis), and hemolytic activity was determined (right $y$ axis) using equivalent numbers of bacteria at all time points. Values are the mean of triplicate samples, and error bars represent standard deviations. Bact., bacterial. Reprinted from reference 4 with permission.

within *A. polyphaga*. This was consistent with the growth kinetics, which showed that the CFU declined after their peak at 48 h postinfection (8), suggesting that the mutant bacteria gradually lost viability within *A. polyphaga*. Taken together, the data confirmed that expression of the pore-forming activity by *L. pneumophila* was required for necrotic killing of *A. polyphaga* and subsequent release of intracellular bacteria. Our data indicated that the pore-forming activity is the only mechanism by which *L. pneumophila* kills and egresses from the protozoan host.

## TEMPORAL EXPRESSION OF THE PORE-FORMING ACTIVITY

We hypothesized that due to the potency of the pore-forming toxin/pore-forming activity to disrupt biological membranes and to cause necrosis and cytolysis of the host cell, its expression by intracellular bacteria is incompatible with the viability of the host cell, which is essential for intracellular bacterial proliferation. Therefore, we examined the kinetics of

expression of the pore-forming activity by in vitro-grown and intracellular bacteria at several stages of growth, using contact-dependent hemolysis of SRBCs. Our data showed that expression of the pore-forming toxin/pore-forming activity by *L. pneumophila* grown in vitro and within macrophages was completely repressed during exponential growth, but was temporally activated to a maximal level upon entry into the postexponential phase, and declined rapidly afterward (Fig. 4) (4). Although the infecting bacteria were competent for pore formation ($t_0$, Fig. 4), this capacity was abolished within 4 to 8 h of invasion (early exponential phase) (Fig. 4). Our data showed that the growth transition of intracellular *L. pneumophila* into the postexponential phase was associated with expression of the pore-forming toxin/pore-forming activity.

## CONCLUDING REMARKS

The mechanisms by which *L. pneumophila* or other vacuolar intracellular pathogens lyse and egress the host cell after its exploitation for intracellular proliferation are not known. In contrast to all previously isolated mutants of *L. pneumophila*, the *rib* mutants are not defective in modulating the biogenesis of their vacuole, nor in intracellular replication, but are defective in the pore-forming activity. The *rib* mutants are defective in expression of the pore-forming toxin/pore-forming activity, which is only expressed upon termination of replication. Our studies provide the first example of a fascinating strategy by which a vacuolar intracellular pathogen regulates cytolysis of the host cell to ensure maximal exploitation for intracellular proliferation. During intracellular replication, *L. pneumophila* undergoes a dramatic phenotypic modulation, but the signals that trigger this modulation are not known. The signal that triggers expression of the pore-forming toxin by intracellular bacteria is also not known but starvation (5), quorum sensing, or deterioration of cellular processes may contribute. It is intriguing that other vacuolar intracellular pathogens, such as *Mycobacterium tuberculosis, Mycobacterium haemophilum, Salmonella, Leishmania,* and *Chlamydia* also exhibit contact-mediated hemolysis or cytotoxicity, but its role in pathogenesis is

not known (4). Interestingly, the pore-forming activity of *Leishmania* is triggered to a maximal level upon entry into the stationary phase of growth (15), and has been proposed to play a role in egress of the parasites from the host cell. It is, therefore, possible that temporal pore formation-mediated cytolysis of the host cell is a strategy utilized by other vacuolar intracellular pathogens to kill and egress the spent host cell after exploitation for intracellular proliferation.

Our data are consistent with the recent model that we have proposed by which *L. pneumophila* kills mammalian cells through two independent mechanisms manifested in two phases (Fig. 5) (7). During early stages of the infection, *L. pneumophila* induces apoptosis in the host cell in a dose-dependent but growth phase-independent fashion (7). In contrast, expression of the pore-forming toxin/pore-forming activity is completely repressed during exponential replication, but is temporally expressed upon entering into the postexponential phase. We speculate that upon termination of intracellular replication, the bacteria exhibit the contact-dependent pore formation in the phagosomal membrane that results in its dis-

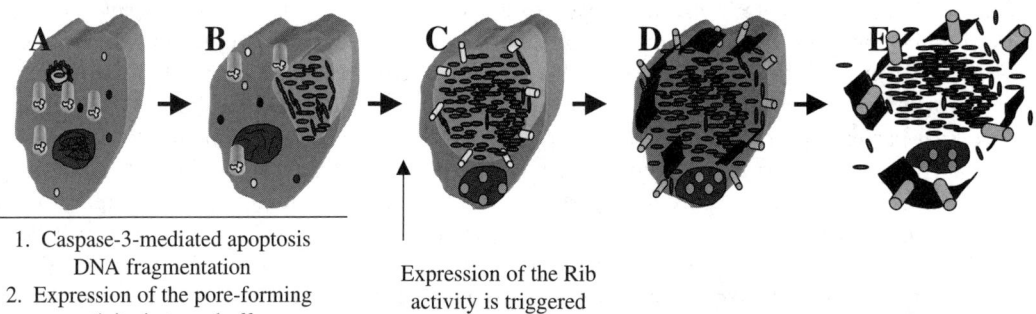

1. Caspase-3-mediated apoptosis
   DNA fragmentation
2. Expression of the pore-forming
   activity is turned off

Expression of the Rib
activity is triggered

**FIGURE 5** A model of growth phase-dependent cytolysis of mammalian cells by *L. pneumophila* upon termination of intracellular bacterial replication to egress from the spent host cell. During early stages of formation of the mitochondria and RER-surrounded phagosome (A) and during exponential intracellular replication (B) expression of the Rib toxin is turned off, but caspase-3-mediated apoptosis is triggered. Upon transition to the postexponential phase of growth, the Rib toxin activity is triggered, which results in insertions of pores in the phagosomal membrane first (C), leading to its disruption (D); see Fig. 1 for the absence of a recognizable phagosomal membrane. This is followed by insertions of the pores in the plasma membrane (E), leading to osmotic lysis of the cell and release of the intracellular bacteria. Reprinted from reference 4 with permission. The same model applies to protozoa with the exception of the absence of apoptosis.

ruption, followed by access of the bacteria to the cytoplasm and subsequent contact-dependent pore formation in organelles and in the plasma membrane, followed by osmotic cytolysis of the host cell (Fig. 5). In contrast, pore formation-mediated cytolysis upon termination of intracellular replication is the major mechanism by which *L. pneumophila* egresses from the protozoan host (Fig. 5).

## REFERENCES

1. **Abu Kwaik, Y.** 1998. Fatal attraction of mammalian cells to *Legionella pneumophila*. *Mol. Microbiol.* **30:**689–696.
2. **Abu Kwaik, Y.** 1996. The phagosome containing *Legionella pneumophila* within the protozoan *Hartmanella vermiformis* is surrounded by the rough endoplasmic reticulum. *Appl. Environ. Microbiol.* **62:**2022–2028.
3. **Abu Kwaik, Y., L.-Y. Gao, B. J. Stone, C. Venkataraman, and O. S. Harb.** 1998. Invasion of protozoa by *Legionella pneumophila* and its role in bacterial ecology and pathogenesis. *Appl. Environ. Microbiol.* **64:**3127–3133.
4. **Alli, O. A. T., L.-Y. Gao, L. L. Pedersen, S. Zink, M. Radulic, M. Doric, and Y. Abu Kwaik.** 2000. Temporal pore formation-mediated egress from macrophages and alveolar epithelial cells by *Legionella pneumophila. Infect. Immun.* **68:**6431–6440.
5. **Byrne, B., and M. S. Swanson.** 1998. Expression of *Legionella pneumophila* virulence traits in response to growth conditions. *Infect. Immun.* **66:**3029–3034.
6. **Clemens, D. L., and M. A. Horwitz.** 1995. Characterization of the *Mycobacterium tuberculosis* phagosome and evidence that phagolysosomal maturation is inhibited. *J. Exp. Med.* **181:**257–270.
7. **Gao, L.-Y., and Y. Abu Kwaik.** 1999. Activation of caspase-3 in *Legionella pneumophila*-induced apoptosis in macrophages. *Infect. Immun.* **67:**4886–4894.
8. **Gao, L.-Y., and Y. Abu Kwaik.** 2000. The mechanism of killing and exiting the protozoan host *Acanthamoeba polyphaga* by *Legionella pneumophila. Environ. Microbiol.* **2:**79–90.
9. **Gao, L.-Y., O. S. Harb, and Y. Abu Kwaik.** 1998. Identification of macrophage-specific infectivity loci (*mil*) of *Legionella pneumophila* that are not required for infectivity of protozoa. *Infect. Immun.* **66:**883–892.
10. **Gao, L.-Y., O. S. Harb, and Y. Abu Kwaik.** 1997. Utilization of similar mechanisms by *Legionella pneumophila* to parasitize two evolutionarily distant hosts, mammalian and protozoan cells. *Infect. Immun.* **65:**4738–4746.
11. **Harb, O. S., L.-Y. Gao, and Y. Abu Kwaik.** 2000. From protozoa to mammalian cells: a new paradigm in the life cycle of intracellular bacterial pathogens. *Environ. Microbiol.* **2:**251–265.
12. **Horwitz, M. A.** 1983. Formation of a novel phagosome by the Legionnaires' disease bacterium (*Legionella pneumophila*) in human monocytes. *J. Exp. Med.* **158:**1319–1331.
13. **Horwitz, M. A.** 1983. The Legionnaires' disease bacterium (*Legionella pneumophila*) inhibits phagosome-lysosome fusion in human monocytes. *J. Exp. Med.* **158:**2108–2126.
14. **Kirby, J. E., J. P. Vogel, H. L. Andrews, and R. R. Isberg.** 1998. Evidence for pore-forming ability by *Legionella pneumophila. Mol. Microbiol.* **27:**323–336.
15. **Noronha, F. S., F. J. Ramalho-Pinto, and M. F. Horta.** 1996. Cytolytic activity in the genus *Leishmania*: involvement of a putative pore-forming protein. *Infect. Immun.* **64:**3975–3982.
16. **Segal, G., and H. A. Shuman.** 1998. How is the intracellular fate of the *Legionella pneumophila* phagosome determined. *Trends Microbiol.* **6:**253–255.
17. **Winn, W. C., F. L. Glavin, D. P. Perl, J. L. Keller, T. L. Andres, T. M. Brown, C. M. Coffin, J. E. Sensecqua, L. N. Roman, and J. E. Craighead.** 1978. The pathology of Legionnaires' disease: fourteen fatal cases from the 1977 outbreak in Vermont. *Arch. Pathol. Lab. Med.* **102:**344–350.
18. **Zuckman, D. M., J. B. Hung, and C. R. Roy.** 1999. Pore-forming activity is not sufficient for *Legionella pneumophila* phagosome trafficking and intracellular replication. *Mol. Microbiol.* **32:**990–1001.

# SELECTION OF SIGNATURE-TAGGED *LEGIONELLA PNEUMOPHILA* MUTANTS IN *ACANTHAMOEBA CASTELLANII*

*Lucy S. Tompkins, Andrea Polesky, Julianna Ross, and Stanley Falkow*

# 27

*Legionella pneumophila* is a facultative intracellular bacillus that causes nosocomial and community-acquired pneumonia and, rarely, extrapulmonary infections in humans. Pneumonia occurs primarily in individuals with compromised immune systems or with pulmonary disease, and thus should be considered an opportunistic pathogen (13). Freshwater, including potable water supplies, is thought to be the primary environmental reservoir of infection. In water sources implicated in epidemics of Legionnaires' disease, *Legionella* is found replicating within free living amoebae, linking amoeba to the transmission of Legionnaires' disease (6). In amoeba, *L. pneumophila* resides within a phagosome, and virulent strains prevent phagosome-lysosome fusion (2). Replication occurs, followed by lysis of the infected cell. These events also occur in human macrophages (14), the target cell for replication in human infection.

Many genes involved in entry and replication of *L. pneumophila* in macrophages in vitro have been identified (8, 18), but fewer genes involved in entry and replication in amoeba have been previously determined (10, 11). Although there are superficial similarities between the behavior of *L. pneumophila* in amoebae versus macrophages, it is likely that different genes may also be necessary for growth in one or the other target cell. For example, *L. pneumophila* grown in amoebae express different morphology and staining characteristics compared with those grown on agar. Also, amoeba-grown *L. pneumophila* invades macrophage cell lines and induces coiling phagocytosis at greater frequency than that grown on agar (3, 4). These data suggest that *L. pneumophila* genes that may be important in human infection are activated within amoeba. Thus, it is important to identify genes important for entry, survival, and replication within amoeba.

We utilized signature-tagged mutagenesis, a negative-selection technique developed by Hensel et al. (12), to screen for genes important for *L. pneumophila* entry and replication within host cells. Signature-tagged mutagenesis employs uniquely tagged transposons that are used to randomly mutagenize a bacterial chromosome and create a library. Pools of mutants, rather than individual clones, are then screened in host cells. Thus, this is a

*Lucy S. Tompkins, Julianna Ross, and Stanley Falkow* Department of Microbiology and Immunology, Sherman Fairchild Science Building, Stanford University School of Medicine, Stanford, CA 94305. *Andrea Polesky* Tuberculosis Clinic, Santa Clara Valley Health and Hospitals, 976 Lenzen Avenue, San Jose, CA 95126.

*Legionella*, Edited by Reinhard Marre et al.
© 2002 ASM Press, Washington, D.C.

negative-selection strategy whereby mutants deficient in entry or replication gene functions will not be isolated from the output pool recovered from the host cells. The output pool is compared with the input pool via filter hybridization. Those clones missing from the output are therefore potentially avirulent and are saved for further analysis.

A library of 700 mutant clones created by signature-tagged mutagenesis was screened using this negative-selection strategy in *Acanthamoeba castellanii*, a free-living amoeba that may serve as an environmental reservoir of legionellae. Twelve mutants were reproducibly absent from filter hybridizations. These mutants were then retested individually in *A. castellanii*. Six mutants, STM-1 to STM-6, were different from the wild-type control (Fig. 1A and B). An avirulent mutant, the salt-resistant mutant (Salt$^R$), isolated by serial passage on buffered charcoal-yeast extract alpha-morpholinepropanesulfonic acid (BCYEα-MOPS) agar with 125 mM NaCl, was included for comparison. Two steps, entry of and intracellular replication within host cells, were studied for each mutant. The efficiency of invasion was studied by incubating *L. pneumophila* strains grown to postexponential phase with *A. castellanii*, using gentamicin to kill extracellular organisms and then determining remaining intracellular CFU (arrows on Fig. 1A and B). Follow-up time points represent intracellular replication. Figure 1A and B shows that three mutants (STM-3, -5, and -6) had a significant defect in entry and all six mutants had a replication defect in *A. castellanii* (Fig. 1A and B). Reduction in invasion frequency was not related to a defect in attachment since those mutants with defects in invasion were able to attach to *A. castellanii* cells (17).

The six mutant strains isolated from, and shown to be defective in, *A. castellanii* were then screened in several different host cells, including *Hartmanella vermiformis*, a free-living amoeba linked to clinical infections with *L. pneumophila* (6), phorbol myristate acetate (PMA)-differentiated U-937 cells (20), a macrophage-like transformed cell line, and

human macrophages derived from peripheral blood mononuclear cells (PBMCs). In addition, salt sensitivity, response to growth in different media, and the ability to make flagella were examined for STM-1 to STM-6.

The interaction of the mutants with *H. vermiformis* was similar to that of *A. castellanii*. STM-3, -5, and -6 invaded significantly less well than the wild type. STM-2, -3, -5, and -6 had a replication defect in *H. vermiformis* (Fig. 1C and D). However, compared with *A. castellanii*, the growth of STM-1 and STM-4 in *H. vermiformis* was not significantly different than the wild type. Two of the mutants, STM-2 and STM-5, had invasion deficits of greater magnitude in *H. vermiformis* than in *A. castellanii* (Fig. 1A to D) and this was shown to be secondary to a change in the *L. pneumophila* growth media, from BCYEα-MOPS to BCYEα-*N*-(2-acetamido)-2-aminoethanesulfonic acid (ACES) (BYEα-MOPS media is made with 2 g of MOPS, 2 g of α-ketoglutaric acid, 15 g of yeast extract, 2 g of KOH, 0.4 g of L-cysteine, and 0.025 g of ferric pyrophosphate per liter, pH 6.9. BCYEα-MOPS agar is made with 2 g of activated charcoal and 15 g of Bacto agar per liter added to BYEα-MOPS media. BYEα-ACES is made with 10 g of ACES, 0.77 g of α-ketoglutaric acid, 10 g of yeast extract, 2.6 g of KOH, 0.4 g of L-cysteine, and 0.025 g of ferric pyrophosphate per liter, pH 6.9) (17), prior to invasion (see below and Fig. 3B).

The behavior of the mutants was also examined in human macrophages derived from PBMCs and in PMA-differentiated U-937 cells. In macrophages derived from PBMCs, STM-1 and STM-4 entered and replicated as well as the wild type. STM-2 and STM-5 entered much less efficiently than, but replicated to the same extent as, the wild type. STM-3 and STM-6, which also had invasion defects, did not replicate once inside PBMCs (Fig. 2A and B). In contrast, all of the mutants replicated within PMA-differentiated U-937 cells, indicating that U-937 cells are deficient in killing *L. pneumophila* compared with freshly isolated macrophages (Fig. 2C and D). This

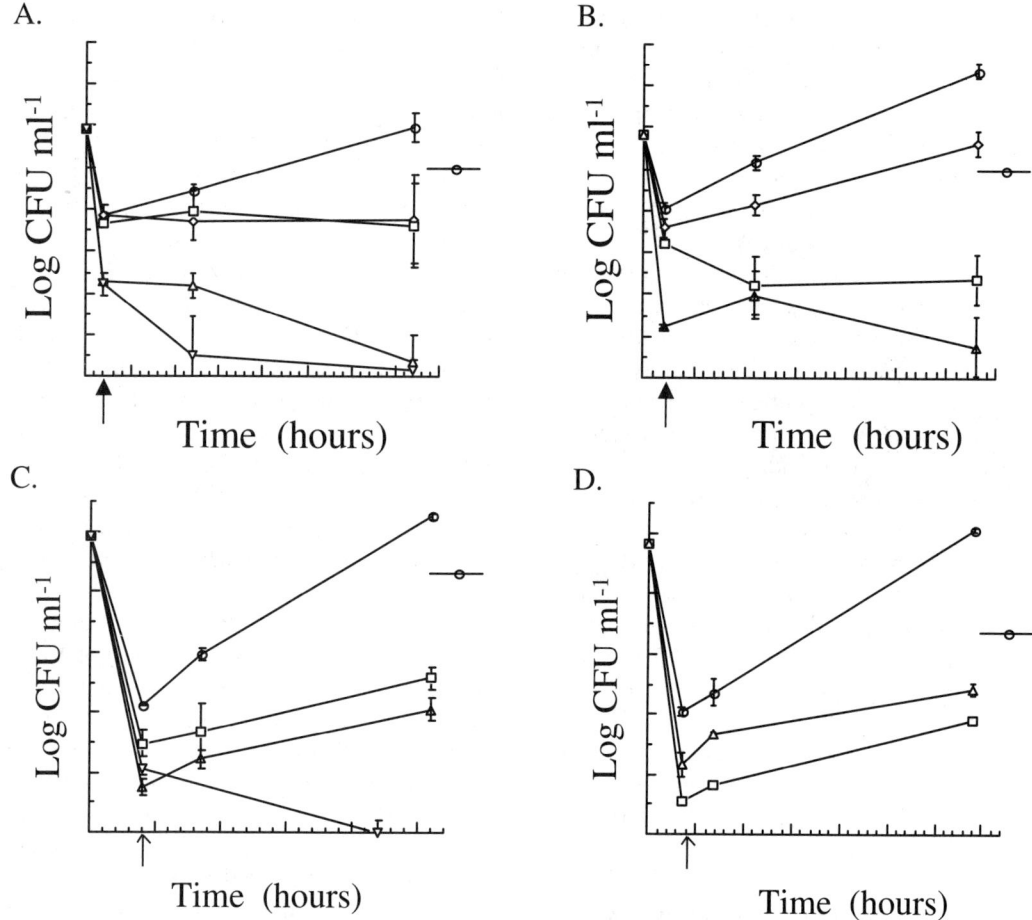

**FIGURE 1** Invasion and intracellular growth of *L. pneumophila* strains in *A. castellanii* and *H. vermiformis* at 37°C. After growth to postexponential phase in BYEα-MOPS, wild-type *L. pneumophila*, Salt[R], STM-1, -2 and -3 (A) and STM-4, -5 and -6 (B) were incubated for 2 h with *A. castellanii*. After growth in BYEα-ACES, wild-type *L. pneumophila*, Salt[R], STM-2 and -3 (C), and STM-5 and -6 (D) were incubated with *H. vermiformis* for 2 h. The initial time point ($T = 0$ h) is the log CFU ml$^{-1}$ of input bacteria. The arrow at $T = 4$ h, after 2 h gentamicin killing of extracellular bacteria, represents invasion. Subsequent time points represent intracellular replication. Reprinted from *Infection and Immunity* (17) with permission of the publisher.

suggests that results obtained in U-937 cells may be misleading in mutants that are partially defective.

Salt resistance is a phenotype associated with loss of virulence in macrophages and in the animal model of infection (18). By growing mutant strains to postexponential phase and comparing CFU on BCYEα-agar with 125 mM NaCl to CFU on BCYEα-agar without NaCl, salt resistance can be determined. STM-6 was as salt resistant as the control salt resistant strain and STM-4 was partially salt resistant.

Interestingly, as part of the invasion and intracellular growth experiments, we noted that *L. pneumophila* grown to postexponential phase is 10- to 100-fold more invasive when grown in BYEα-ACES media versus BYEα-

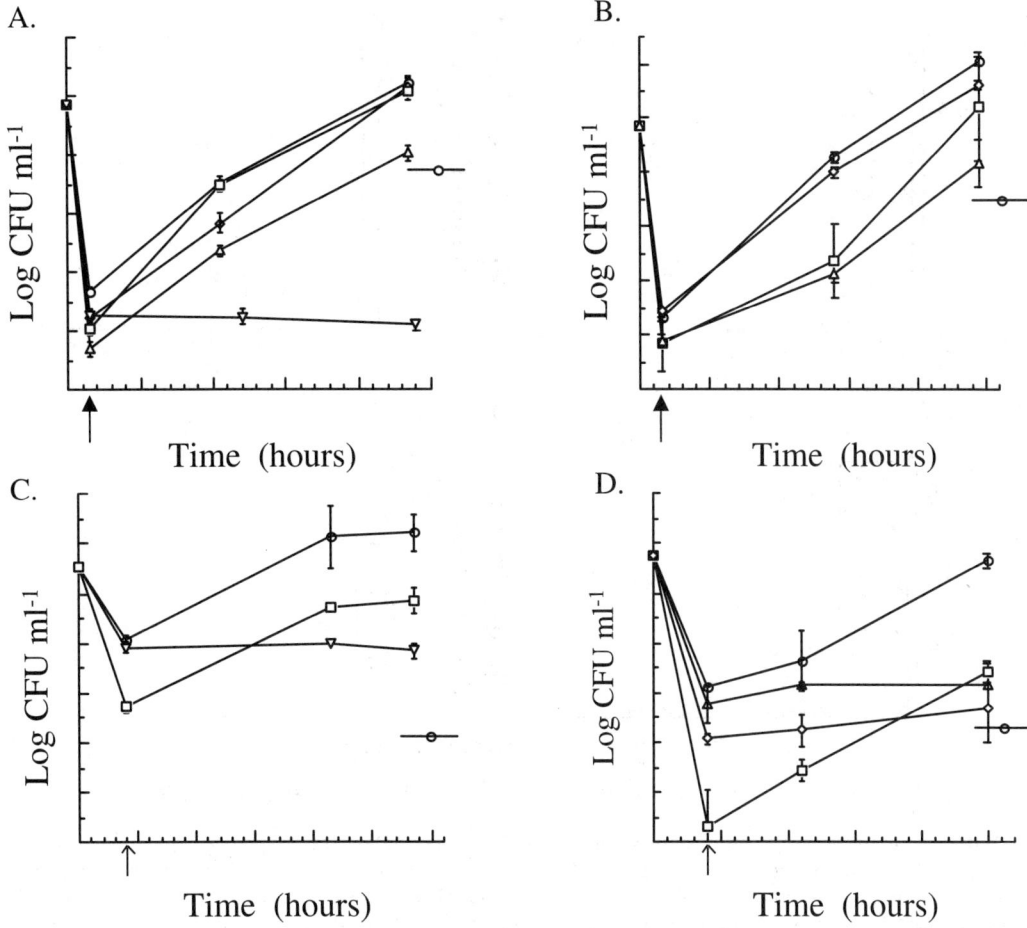

**FIGURE 2** Invasion and intracellular growth of *L. pneumophila* strains in PBMC-derived macrophages and PMA-differentiated U-937 cells at 37°C. After growth to postexponential phase in BYEα-ACES, wild-type *L. pneumophila*, Salt$^R$, and STM-2 (A) and STM-3, -5, and -6 (B) were incubated with PBMC-derived macrophages for 2 h. After growth to postexponential phase in BYEα-MOPS, wild-type *L. pneumophila*, the salt resistant mutant, STM-1, -2, and -3 (C) and STM-4, -5, and -6 (D) were incubated with PMA-differentiated U-937 cells for 1 h. The initial time point ($T = 0$ h) is the log CFU ml$^{-1}$ of input bacteria. The arrow represents invasion. Subsequent time points represent intracellular replication. Reprinted from *Infection and Immunity* (17) with permission of the publisher.

MOPS media, depending on the host cell tested (Fig. 3A) (17). The two media contain a different buffer and different amounts of yeast extract and α-ketoglutarate. On the other hand, the invasion frequencies of STM-2, -3, and -5 were not enhanced in BYEα-ACES (Fig. 3B), suggesting that BYEα-ACES broth activates a pathway in *L. pneumophila*

that enhances the ability of the wild type to invade multiple cell types and that the mutations in STM-2, -3, and −5 interfere with this pathway. STM-6, in comparison, has a broth-independent phenotype invasion. As described below, the broth-dependent phenotype is probably related to impaired production of flagella.

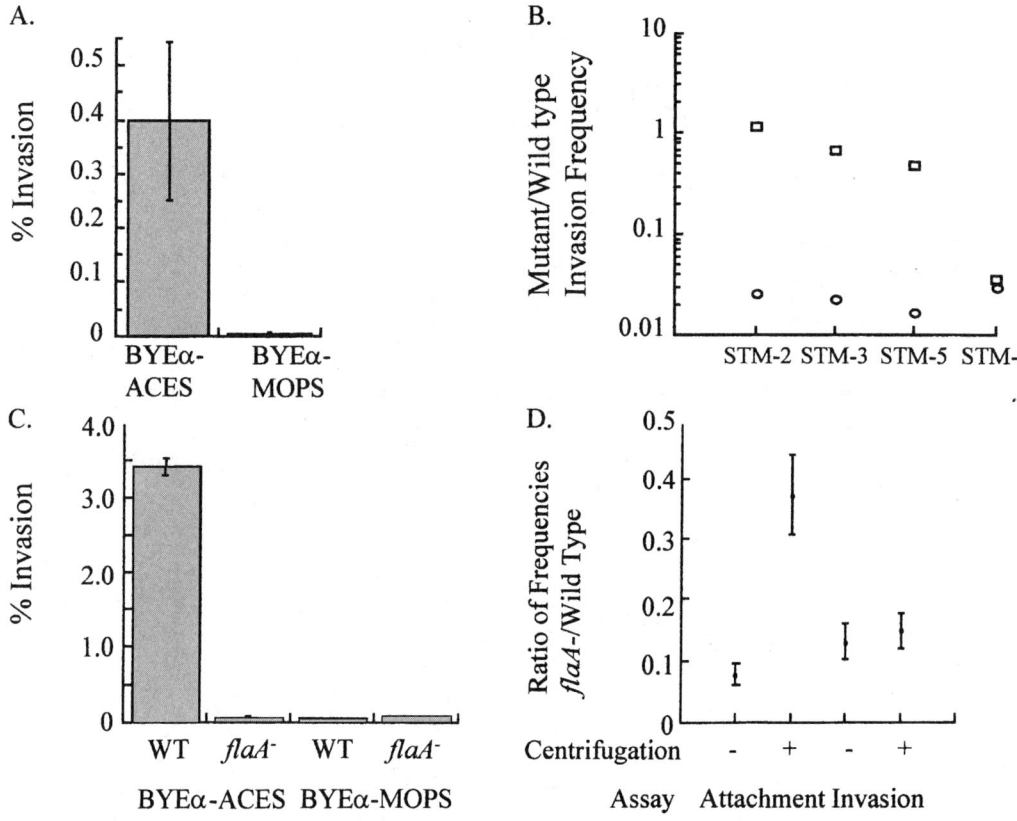

**FIGURE 3** Comparison of invasion and attachment frequencies. Comparison of wild-type *L. pneumophila* invasion of *H. vermiformis* after growth in BYEα-ACES or BYEα-MOPS broths (A). Ratio of mutant to wild-type invasion frequencies in *H. vermiformis*, after growth in BYEα-ACES broth (circle) and in BYEα-MOPS broth (square) (B). Comparison of wild-type and *flaA L. pneumophila* invasion of *A. castellanii* after growth in BYEα-ACES or BYEα-MOPS broths (C). Ratio of *flaA* to wild-type attachment and invasion frequencies with or without centrifugation of bacteria onto *A. castellanii* (D). Parts of this figure reprinted from *Infection and Immunity* (17) with permission of the publisher.

Many mutant *L. pneumophila* strains that lack flagella have been shown to be less virulent, suggesting that flagella production may be coregulated with other virulence factors (1). The role of flagellin, however, in *L. pneumophila* pathogenicity is not completely defined. We looked at the expression of flagella by Western blot for STM-1 to STM-6 and the flagellar structure by negative staining electron microscopy for mutants expressing less flagella. Surprisingly, three of the mutants, STM-2, STM-3, and STM-5, had either abnormal amounts of flagella (STM-2) or no normal flagellar structure (STM-3 and -5).

To further understand the role of flagella in these mutants, the conditions under which flagella were made were explored and a disruption of the *flaA* structural gene was made. Wild-type *L. pneumophila* starts to produce flagella during the postexponential phase in BYEα-ACES, but not until the stationary phase in BYEα-MOPS. As expected, the *flaA* mutant had no flagella by negative staining electron microscopy. Of note, the *flaA* mutant also had the BYEα-ACES invasion defect (Fig. 3C), which could be complemented with a plasmid containing the *flaA* gene. Together these observations suggest that under conditions where flagella are made, invasion is enhanced.

To look more closely at the role that flagella play in invasion, we asked whether centrifugation of the *flaA* mutant onto host cells increased attachment and invasion frequencies to wild-type levels. Attachment is measured by allowing *L. pneumophila* to bind to *A. castellanii* for 30 min in the presence of cyclohexamide, which prevents bacterial uptake by the amoeba, and extensively washing (17). As can be seen in Fig. 3D, the attachment deficit of *flaA* bacteria can be partially overcome by centrifugation, but the invasion deficit of the *flaA* mutant cannot be overcome by spinning the bacteria down on to host cells (Fig. 3D), suggesting that flagella have a more complex role in entry than just getting the bacteria to the host cell.

DNA sequence analysis of the *L. pneumophila* region flanking the transposon insertion from each of the mutants revealed that three genes were homologues of known genes in other bacterial species (Table 1). STM-1 has homology to *ccmF* of *Pseudomonas fluorescens*; STM-2 is homologous to *flrC* of *Vibrio cholera*, a transcriptional activator of a two-component regulatory system that regulates flagella biosynthesis (16); and STM-6 is homologous to *traA* of Rhizobium sp. NGR234 (7). TraA is involved in conjugal transfer of DNA. Two genes, STM-3 and STM-5, are known *L. pneumophila* genes (*lspK* and *aroB*, respectively) (5, 10). *lspK* encodes a component of the type II secretion system, while *aroB* is involved in aromatic amino acid biosynthesis. STM-4 has an unknown function.

STM-1 has a mutation in a gene with homology to a cytochrome c-type biogenesis gene. The function of cytochrome-c biogenesis proteins in *L. pneumophila* is unknown. The growth defect of this mutant was observed only in *A. castellanii* suggesting that the intracellular milieu may be different from *H. vermiformis*.

STM-2 has a mutation in a gene homologous to a transcriptional regulator of flagellar synthesis. This mutant has an amoeba-

**TABLE 1** Summary of the STM phenotypes

| Mutant strain | Salt resistant | Normal flagella present | Invasion defect[b] | | Replication defect | | |
| --- | --- | --- | --- | --- | --- | --- | --- |
| | | | BYEα-MOPS (amoeba) | BYEα-ACES (amoeba and PBMCs) | *A. castellanii* | *H. vermiformis* | PBMC-derived macrophages |
| STM-1 | | Yes[a] | | | + | | |
| STM-2 | | Decreased amount | | | + + | | |
| STM-3 | | No | +[c] | + + | + + | + + | |
| STM-4 | ±/− | Yes[a] | | + + | + + | | + |
| STM-5 | | No | + | + | + | + + | |
| STM-6 | + | Yes | | | | | + |

[a] Normal amounts of flagella present, but flagella not examined by electron microscopy.
[b] 10-fold or greater difference from wild type.
[c] *Acanthamoeba castellanii* only.

**TABLE 2** Sequence similarities of *L. pneumophila* genes identified by signature-tagged mutagenesis

| Mutant strain | Homologous gene/organism | Putative function | % Identities/% positives/amino acid length[a] | Score/E value[a] |
|---|---|---|---|---|
| STM-1 | *camF/Pseudomonas fluorescens* | Cytochrome C biogenesis | 46/56/213 | 159/4e$^{-38}$ |
| STM-2 | *flrC/Vibrio cholera* | Transcriptional activator of a two-component regulatory system that regulates flagella biosynthesis | 60/74/258 | 280/1e$^{-74}$ |
| STM-3 | *lspK/Legionella pneumophila* | Type II secretion system structural protein | | |
| STM-4 | Unknown; 207 nucleotides | | | |
| STM-5 | *aroB/Legionella pneumophila* | Aromatic amino acid biosynthesis | | |
| STM-6 | *traA/Rhizobium sp. NGR234* | Protein involved in conjugal transfer | 36/56/271 | 166/1e$^{-39}$ |

[a] The values are taken from a Basic Local Alignment Search Tool (BLAST) for amino acid comparison (blastx program) (3). The amino acid length refers to a contiguous length of sequence similarity. Reprinted from *Infection and Immunity* (17) with permission of the publisher.

dependent replication defect and a BYEα-ACES-dependent defect in entry. About 20% of STM-2 bacteria produce flagella when grown under conditions where the majority of wild-type bacteria also express flagella. The structure of the flagella on the mutant is normal.

The transposon insertion in STM-3 occurs within the *lspK* gene, part of the larger *lspFGHIJK* operon encoding a type II secretory system (10). Investigators have also shown that a deletion in the *lspGH* genes leads to a mutant with impaired replication in *A. castellanii* but not in HL-60 cells, a macrophage-like cell line (10). We also noted that STM-3 has a more subtle phenotype in U-937 cells than in amoeba.

STM-5 contains a mutation in the *aroB* gene of *L. pneumophila*. This mutation was also isolated by Edelstein et al. (5) by screening signature-tagged mutants in the guinea pig pneumonia model using a library that overlapped with ours. The homologous gene in *Salmonella enterica* serovar Typhimurium is linked to virulence since mutants are attenuated in their ability to kill mice (9). Possibly this is because mutations within the aromatic amino acid synthesis pathway reduce the ability of bacteria to obtain these essential nutrients or appropriate precursors. Perhaps amino acid precursors are limiting in *A. castellanii* and *H. vermiformis*, thus preventing replication of STM-5, but are not limiting in PBMCs. We have not yet determined whether the lack of flagella on the STM-5 mutant is due to the mutation in *aroB*, is a polar effect, or is caused by another impaired regulatory pathway.

The STM-6 transposon insertion is located in a gene with similarity to *traA*, a conjugal transfer protein gene (7). This gene is not located within the previously isolated *dot/icm* or *lvh* locus that encode putative proteins with similarity to the Tra/Trb proteins of the plasmid *collb-P9* and the *vir* secretion system of *Agrobacterium tumifaciens* (*lvh* locus), a type IV secretion system involved in DNA transfer (19). In *L. pneumophila*, the *dot/icm*-encoded secretory system is needed for pore formation and for proper trafficking of virulent *L. pneumophila* (15, 19). STM-6 is salt-resistant and is unable to replicate within PBMC-derived macrophages, as are many of the *dot* and *icm* mutant strains (18). However, STM-6 has a mutation in a gene not known to be in the *dot/icm* regions. These results suggest that salt resistance may not be exclusively linked to the *dot/icm* loci.

In summary, we characterized signature-tagged transposon mutants of *L. pneumophila* in *A. castellanii, H. vermiformis*, PBMC-derived macrophages, and PMA-differentiated U-937 cells to identify genes linked to entry and/or intracellular replication. Two mutants, STM-1 and STM-4, appeared to be deficient in *A. castellanii* alone, and two other mutants, STM-2 and STM-5, led to intracellular replication defects that were observed in both *A. castellanii* and *H. vermiformis*. Two mutants, STM-3 and STM-6, were unable to replicate in amoeba and in PBMC-derived macrophages and are therefore more likely to have a more global role in virulence. Although we did find one gene, *aroB*, also identified by screening an overlapping library in the guinea pig model of infection, we did not find genes in the *dot/icm* loci. This is probably related to the small number of clones screened. Furthermore, we showed that the production of flagella enhances invasion under growth conditions where flagella are produced and to a great extent this explains why growth of wild-type *L. pneumophila* in BYEα-ACES broth leads to improved invasion. The behavior of the mutants in the two species of free-living amoeba and human-derived PBMCs is summarized in Table 2. The use of free-living amoeba that serve as a natural hosts for replication in the environment to select for strains that are decreased in virulence has been a productive strategy to identify a previously unknown locus, to confirm the contribution of two known *L. pneumophila* genes, and to identify three homologues in other bacterial species.

## REFERENCES

1. **Bosshardt, S. C., R. F. Benson, and B. S. Fields.** 1997. Flagella are a positive predictor for virulence in *Legionella*. *Microb. Pathog.* **23**:107–112.
2. **Bozue, J. A., and W. Johnson.** 1996. Interaction of *Legionella pneumophila* with *Acanthamoeba castellanii*: uptake by coiling phagocytosis and inhibition of phagosome-lysosome fusion. *Infect. Immun.* **64**:668–673.
3. **Cirillo, J. D., S. L. Cirillo, L. Yan, L. E. Bermudez, S. Falkow, and L. S. Tompkins.** 1999. Intracellular growth in *Acanthamoeba castellanii* affects monocyte entry mechanisms and enhances virulence of *Legionella pneumophila*. *Infect. Immun.* **67**:4427–4434.
4. **Cirillo, J. D., S. Falkow, and L. S. Tompkins.** 1994. Growth of *Legionella pneumophila* in *Acanthamoeba castellanii* enhances invasion. *Infect. Immun.* **62**:3254–3261.
5. **Edelstein, P. H., M. A. Edelstein, F. Higa, and S. Falkow.** 1999. Discovery of virulence genes of *Legionella pneumophila* by using signature tagged mutagenesis in a guinea pig pneumonia model. *Proc. Natl. Acad. Sci. USA* **96**:8190–8195.
6. **Fields, B. S., G. N. Sanden, J. M. Barbaree, W. E. Morrill, R. M. Wadowsky, E. H. White, and J. C. Feeley.** 1989. Intracellular multiplication of *Legionella pneumophila* in amoebae isolated from hospital hot water tanks. *Curr. Microbiol.* **18**:131–137.
7. **Freiberg, C., R. Fellay, A. Bairoch, W. J. Broughton, A. Rosenthal, and X. Perret.** 1997. Molecular basis of symbiosis between *Rhizobium* and legumes. *Nature* **387**:394–401.
8. **Gao, L. Y., O. S. Harb, and Y. A. Kwaik.** 1998. Identification of macrophage-specific infectivity loci (*mil*) of *Legionella pneumophila* that are not required for infectivity of protozoa. *Infect. Immun.* **66**:883–892.
9. **Gunel-Ozcan, A., K. A. Brown, A. G. Allen, and D. J. Maskell.** 1997. *Salmonella typhimurium aroB* mutants are attenuated in BALB/c mice. *Microb. Pathog.* **23**:311–316.
10. **Hales, L. M., and H. A. Shuman.** 1999. *Legionella pneumophila* contains a type II general secretion pathway required for growth in amoebae as well as for secretion of the Msp protease. *Infect. Immun.* **67**:3662–3666.
11. **Hales, L. M., and H. A. Shuman.** 1999. The *Legionella pneumophila rpoS* gene is required for growth within *Acanthamoeba castellanii*. *J. Bacteriol.* **181**:4879–4889.
12. **Hensel, M., J. E. Shea, C. Gleeson, M. D. Jones, E. Dalton, and D. W. Holden.** 1995. Simultaneous identification of bacterial virulence genes by negative selection. *Science* **269**:400–403.
13. **Hoge, C. W., and R. F. Brieman.** 1991. Advances in the epidemiology and control of *Legionella* infections. *Epidemiol. Rev.* **13**:329–340.

14. **Isberg, R. R.** 1994. Intracellular trafficking of *Legionella pneumophila* within phagocytic cells, p. 263–278. *In* V. L. Miller, J. B. Kaper, D. A. Portnoy, and R. R. Isberg (ed.), *Molecular Genetics of Bacterial Pathogenesis.* ASM Press, Washington, D.C.

15. **Kirby, J. E., and R. R. Isberg.** 1998. Legionnaires' disease: the pore macrophage and the legion of terror within. *Trends Microbiol.* **6:**256–258.

16. **Klose, K. E., and J. J. Mekalanos.** 1998. Distinct roles of an alternative sigma factor during both free-swimming and colonizing phases of the *Vibrio cholerae* pathogenic cycle. *Mol. Microbiol.* **28:**501–520.

17. **Polesky, A. H., J. T. Ross, S. Falkow, and L. S. Tompkins.** 2001. Identification of *Legionella pneumophila* genes important for infection of amoebas by signature-tagged mutagenesis. *Infect. Immun.* **69:**977–987.

18. **Sadosky, A. B., L. A. Wiater, and H. A. Shuman.** 1993. Identification of *Legionella pneumophila* genes required for growth within and killing of human macrophages. *Infect. Immun.* **61:**5361–5373.

19. **Segal, G., and H. A. Shuman.** 1998. How is the intracellular fate of the *Legionella pneumophila* phagosome determined? *Trends Microbiol.* **6:**253–255.

20. **Sundstrom, C., and K. Nilsson.** 1976. Establishment and characterization of a human histiocytic lymphoma cell line (U-937). *Int. J. Cancer* **17:**565–577.

# INTERACTION OF *LEGIONELLA PNEUMOPHILA* WITH *DICTYOSTELIUM DISCOIDEUM*

M. Steinert, S. Hägele, C. Skriwan, D. Grimm,
M. Fajardo, K. Heuner, M. Schleicher, U. Hentschel,
W. Ludwig, R. Marre, and J. Hacker

# 28

Several pathogens exhibit a considerable host range. *Legionella pneumophila*, for example, can infect various protozoa species, experimentally inoculated guinea pigs, and human macrophages, as well as epithelial cells (7, 9, 20). This suggests that there are common infection strategies regardless of the host (8). In addition, it has become apparent that certain aspects of the host defense are highly conserved during evolution (13, 17). Therefore important insights into *Legionella*-host interactions are expected from the use of well-characterized host models (3). One such model system is the haploid amoeba *Dictyostelium discoideum*. Vegetative cells of *Dictyostelium* feed on bacteria and upon starvation aggregate and differentiate into pluricellular fruiting bodies (16). Beside its amenability to

*M. Steinert, S. Hägele, C. Skriwan, D. Grimm, M. Fajardo, K. Heuner, U. Hentschel, and J. Hacker* Institut für Molekulare Infektionsbiologie, Universität Würzburg, Röntgenring 11, D-97070 Würzburg, Germany.  *M. Schleicher* Institut für Zellbiologie, Ludwig-Maximilians-Universität, Schillerstrasse 42, D-80336 München, Germany.  *W. Ludwig* Lehrstuhl für Mikrobiologie, Technische Universität München, Am Hochanger 4, D-85350 Freising, Germany.  *R. Marre* Abteilung für Medizinische Mikrobiologie und Hygiene, Robert-Koch-Strasse 8, D-89081 Ulm, Germany.

genetic manipulation, *D. discoideum* expresses highly conserved cellular markers, and cell signaling pathways are well characterized. Moreover, the complete genome sequence will be available in the year 2002.

## ESTABLISHMENT OF THE *DICTYOSTELIUM* MODEL SYSTEM

To evaluate whether *D. discoideum* is a suitable model system for studying *Legionella* pathogenicity, we compared the intracellular growth of different *Legionella* species in *Dictyostelium* with the established host model system *Acanthamoeba castellanii* (Table 1). We found that virulent *Legionella* species including *L. pneumophila* Corby, LLAP10, and *Sarcobium lyticum* are able to grow intracellularly in single-cell stages of *D. discoideum* and that infection results in host cell lysis. After 96 h of coculture, the inoculum of $10^3$ cells/ml of these strains increased 150- to 1,500-fold, as measured by CFU. The increasing numbers of bacteria were the result of intracellular replication, since they were unable to grow in the cell culture medium. The avirulent strain *Legionella erythra* exhibited decreasing counts in *D. discoideum*. These results showed that the infection process parallels the infection of freshwater amoebae and macrophages (11).

*Legionella*, Edited by Reinhard Marre et al.
© 2002 ASM Press, Washington, D.C.

**TABLE 1** Intracellular growth of *Legionella* in *Dictyostelium discoideum* and *Acanthamoeba castellanii*[a]

| Strain (reference) | Phenotype | Intracellular growth in: | |
|---|---|---|---|
| | | *D. discoideum* | *A. castellanii* |
| *L. pneumophila* Corby (21) | Patient isolate | Yes | Yes |
| *L. pneumophila* Corby KH3 (14) | FlaA-negative mutant | Attenuated | Attenuated |
| *L. pneumophila* Corby-1 (21) | Mip-negative mutant | Attenuated | Attenuated |
| *L. pneumophila* (*ligA*-) (6) | *ligA*-negative mutant | Avirulent | Avirulent |
| *L. erythra* (11) | Avirulent | Avirulent | Avirulent |
| LLAP10 (11) | Legionella-like amoebal pathogen | Yes | Yes |
| *Sarcobium lyticum* (11) | Obligate intracellular parasite of amoebae | Yes | Yes |

[a] Abbreviations: FlaA, flagellin major subunit; Mip, macrophage infectivity potentiator; *ligA*, *Legionella pneumophila* infectivity gene A. For infection of *D. discoideum* and *A. castellanii* 5 × 10⁵ host cells/ml were infected with 10³ legionellae. After 0, 24, 48, 72, and 96 h of incubation, the bacterial numbers of CFU were determined by plating.

## SUBCELLULAR ANALYSIS OF INFECTION AND TESTING OF MUTANTS

The subcellular analysis of the infection indicates that *Legionella* grows within membrane-bound vesicles of *Dictyostelium* (Fig. 1). In addition, the bacteria inhibit the fusion of phagosomes and lysosomes in this particular host system. Colocalization studies with green fluorescent protein (GFP)-tagged bacteria and antibodies directed against specific lysosomal markers (DdLIMP) revealed that the bacteria inhibit the phagolysosome fusion. These data suggest that the replicative phagosome in *Dictyostelium* exhibits important features characteristc for *Legionella* infections (11, 18).

Testing of various well-established *Legionella* mutants and their corresponding complementants in infection assays showed that *Dictyostelium* is a representative model system. *L. pneumophila* mutants that are unable to grow in amoebae and macrophages are also unable to grow in *Dictyostelium* (Table 1). The FlaA- and the Mip-negative mutant of *L. pneumophila* Corby revealed moderate growth defects and the *ligA*-negative mutant was severely impaired to grow intracellularly (5, 6, 12, 14, 15, 21). To examine host functions required for growth we also investigated defined *Dictyostelium* mutants. The infection of mutated host cells revealed that the profilin-minus phenotype had a slight positive effect on bacterial growth when compared with *Dictyostelium* wild-type cells. This observation is consistent with the finding that profilin-minus cells have a higher rate of phagocytosis (11).

## DETECTION OF *DICTYOSTELIUM* IN THE ENVIRONMENT

Due to the occurrence of *Legionella* in wet soils and the fact that *Dictyostelium* feeds on bacteria by phagocytosis, it is conceivable that *Dictyostelium* represents a natural reservoir of *Legionella*. Therefore we surveyed the occurrence of *Dictyostelium* and other well-established host organisms in *Legionella*-positive environmental samples by culture and in situ hybridization with a fluorescence-labeled 16S rRNA probe that specifically detects *L. pneumophila* and two eukaryotic 18S rRNA probes that specifically detect *Dictyostelium* (DICT2) and *Hartmannella* (HART498) (Table 2) (10). Isolation and morphological characterization of potential host protozoa revealed that the genera *Acanthamoeba*, *Echinamoeba*, *Hartmannella*, *Platyamoeba*, *Saccamoeba*, *Thecamoeba*, and *Vexillifera* were present in various *Legionella*-positive water habitats. In situ hybridization confirmed the results of the morphological identification of environmental *Hartmannella* isolates. In addition, we were able to use amoeba-specific 18S rRNA probes and *Legionella*-specific 16S probes simultaneously to monitor the infection of *Hartmannella vermiformis* with *L. pneumophila* in vitro. They hybridized with the target strains and no cross-reactions with other

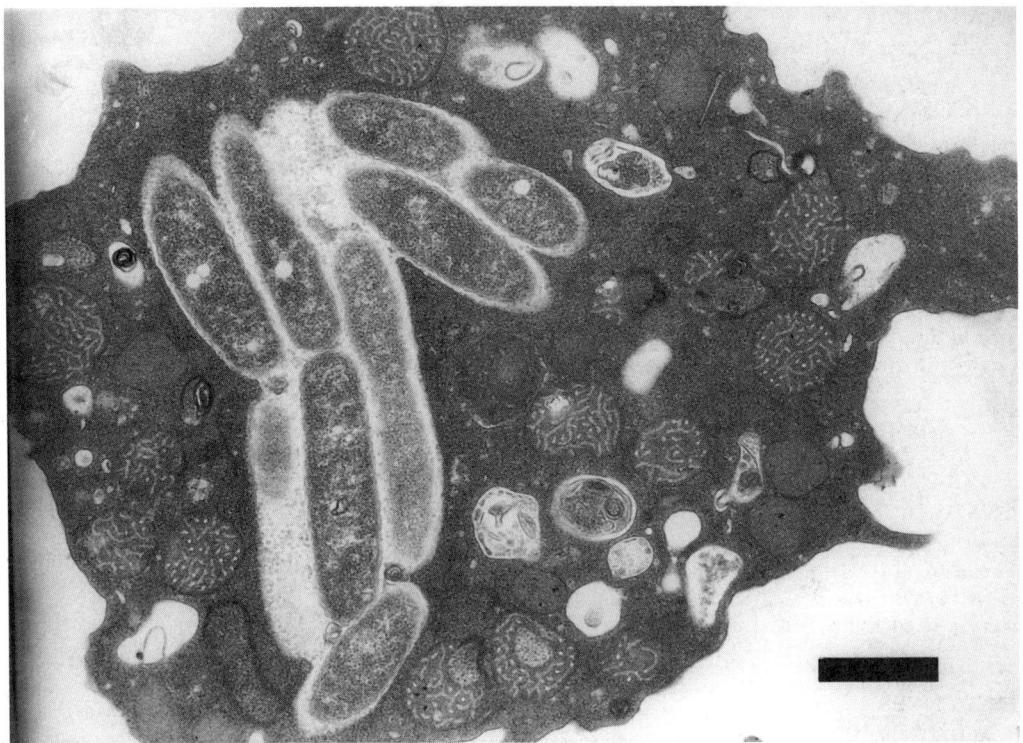

**FIGURE 1** Transmission electron micrograph of *L. pneumophila* within a single vacuole of *D. discoideum* after 48 h of coincubation. Bar, 1 μm.

strains were observed. The natural interaction of *Legionella* and *Dictyostelium* in the environment, however, remains to be confirmed. Since we were able to detect *Dictyostelium* in soil samples, future studies may show a colocalization with *Legionella* in these habitats.

## CONCLUSION

New methods to limit or prevent growth of *Legionella* within protozoan or human host cells will be based on the understanding of the factors that promote intracellular survival and growth (1, 2, 4). Insights are expected from

**TABLE 2** Identification of *Legionella* spp., *Dictyostelium* spp., and *Hartmannella* spp. by fluorescence-labeled rRNA probes[a]

| Samples | Hybridization with rRNA probe | | |
|---|---|---|---|
| | LEG705[b] | DICT2[c] | HART498[c] |
| *D. discoideum*-*Legionella* coculture | + | + | − |
| *Hartmannella* spp.-*Legionella* coculture | + | − | + |
| Water samples[d] | + | − | + |
| Soil sample | − | + | n.d. |

[a] The genus-specific probes have been developed on the basis of a comparative sequence analysis (ARB software environment for sequence data).
[b] Genus-specific 16S rRNA probe.
[c] Genus-specific 18S rRNA probe. n.d., not done.
[d] River and fountain water.

systems where both bacterial and host factors can be manipulated (11, 19). Since the *Dictyostelium-Legionella* interaction allows a two-sided genetic approach, our future strategies will rely on genetic mutational analysis of the pathogen and the host. Available molecular tools to manipulate the host are transformation with integrating and nonintegrating eukaryotic vectors, homologous recombination, antisense techniques, and restriction enzyme mediated integration (REMI). The application of these methods should allow the elucidation of the interaction of bacterial virulence factors with specific host targets.

## ACKNOWLEDGMENTS

This work was supported by grants from the Bavarian Ministry of Environmental Protection, the Bayerische Forschungsstiftung, and the Deutsche Forschungsgemeinschaft (DFG).

## REFERENCES

1. **Abu Kwaik, Y.** 1998. Fatal attraction of mammalian cells to *Legionella pneumophila*. *Mol. Microbiol.* **30:**689–695.
2. **Abu Kwaik, Y., L.-Y. Gao, B. J. Stone, C. Venkataraman, and O. S. Harb.** 1998. Invasion of protozoa by *Legionella pneumophila* and its role in bacterial ecology and pathogenesis. *Appl. Environ. Microbiol.* **64:**3127–3133.
3. **Beckers, M. C., S. Yoshida, K. Morgan, E. Skamene, and P. Gros.** 1995. Natural resistance to infection with *Legionella pneumophila*: chromosomal localization of the *lgn*1 susceptibility gene. *Mamm. Genome* **6:**540–545.
4. **Coers, J., C. Monahan, and C. R. Roy.** 1999. Modulation of phagosome biogenesis by *Legionella pneumophila* creates an organelle permissive for intracellular growth. *Nature Cell Biol.* **1:**451–453.
5. **Dietrich, C., K. Heuner, B. Brand, J. Hacker, and M. Steinert.** 2001. Flagellum of *Legionella pneumophila* positively affects the early phase of infection of eukaryotic host cells. *Infect. Immun.* **69:**2116–2122.
6. **Fettes, P. S., M. Susa, J. Hacker, and R. Marre.** 2000. Characterization of the *Legionella pneumophila* gene *ligA*. *Int. J. Med. Microbiol.* **290:**239–250.
7. **Fields, B.** 1996. The molecular ecology of legionellae. *Trends Microbiol.* **7:**286–290.
8. **Finlay, B. B.** 1999. Bacterial disease in divers hosts. *Cell* **96:**315–318.
9. **Gao, L. Y., O. S. Harb, and Y. Abu Kwaik.** 1997. Utilization of similar mechanisms by *Legionella pneumophila* to parasitize two evolutionary distant hosts, mammalian and protozoan cells. *Infect. Immun.* **65:**4738–4746.
10. **Grimm, D., H. Merkert, W. Ludwig, K. H. Schleifer, J. Hacker, and B. C. Brand.** 1998. Specific detection of *Legionella pneumophila*: construction of a new 16S rRNA-targeted oligonucleotide probe. *Appl. Environ. Microbiol.* **64:**2686–2690.
11. **Hägele, S., R. Köhler, H. Merkert, M. Schleicher, J. Hacker, and M. Steinert.** 2000. *Dictyostelium discoideum*: a new host model system for intracellular pathogens of the genus *Legionella*. *Cell. Microbiol.* **2:**165–171.
12. **Helbig, J. H., P. C. Lück, M. Steinert, E. Jacobs, and M. Witt.** 2001. Immunlocalization of Mip protein of extracellularly and intracellularly grown *Legionella pneumophila*. *Lett. Appl. Microbiol.* **32:**83–88.
13. **Hentschel, U., M. Steinert, and J. Hacker.** 2000. Common molecular mechanisms of symbiosis and pathogenesis. *Trends Microbiol.* **8:**226–231.
14. **Heuner K., B. C. Brand, and J. Hacker.** 1999. The expression of the flagellum of *Legionella pneumophila* is modulated by different environmental factors. *FEMS Microbiol. Lett.* **175:**69–77.
15. **Köhler, R., A. Bubert, W. Goebel, M. Steinert, J. Hacker, and B. Bubert.** 2000. Expression and use of the green fluorescent protein as a reporter system in *Legionella pneumophila*. *Mol. Gen. Genet.* **262:**1060–1069.
16. **Mutzel, R.** 1995. Molecular biology, growth and development of the cellular slime mold *Dictyostelium discoideum*. *Experientia* **51:**1103–1109.
17. **Steinert, M., U. Hentschel, and J. Hacker.** 2000. Symbiosis and pathogenesis: evolution of the microbe-host interaction. *Naturwissenschaften* **87:**1–11.
18. **Solomon, J. M., A. Rupper, J. A. Cardelli, and R. R. Isberg.** 2000. Intracellular growth of *Legionella pneumophila* in *Dictyostelium discoideum*, a system for genetic analysis of host-pathogen interactions. *Infect. Immun.* **68:**2939–2947.
19. **Solomon, J. M., and R. R. Isberg.** 2000. Growth of *Legionella pneumophila* in *Dictyostelium discoideum*: a novel system for genetic analysis of host-pathogen interactions. *Trends Microbiol.* **8:**478–480.
20. **Swanson, M. S., and B. K. Hammer.** 2000. *Legionella pneumophila* pathogenesis: a fateful journey from amoebae to macrophages. *Annu. Rev. Microbiol.* **54:**567–613.
21. **Wintermeyer, E., B. Ludwig, M. Steinert, B. Schmidt, G. Fischer, and J. Hacker.** 1995. Influence of site specifically altered Mip proteins on intracellular survival of *Legionella pneumophila* in eukaryotic cells. *Infect. Immun.* **63:**4576–4583.

# CHARACTERIZATION OF A 16-KILODALTON SPECIES-SPECIFIC PROTEIN OF *LEGIONELLA PNEUMOPHILA* PROMOTING UPTAKE IN AMOEBAE

*Christine Steudel, Jürgen Herbert Helbig, and Paul Christian Lück*

# 29

*Legionella pneumophila* is the major agent responsible for Legionnaires' disease. To identify proteins that participate in the interaction of *Legionella* and its host, we screened a genomic library of *L. pneumophila* strain Corby with anti-Corby antiserum. Briefly, rabbits were immunized with heat inactivated (15 min at 70°C) *L. pneumophila* strain Corby grown on solid medium. Immunization was done by intravenous (i.v.) injections, each $3 \times 10^8$ CFU without adjunvants, on days 1, 4, 7, 10, and 45, and serum was collected at day 55. To reduce cross-reactivity, the collected serum was absorbed to total cells of *Escherichia coli* DH5$\alpha$ harboring plasmid pUC19 either inactivated by heat or by formalin treatment. Construction of the genomic library was done according to Heuner et al. (5) with minor modifications. Chromosomal DNA of *L. pneumophila* strain Corby was partially digested with *Sau*3AI. Fragments of 1.0 to 4.0 kb were ligated into the *Bam*HI restriction site of vector pUC19 and transformed into *E. coli* DH5$\alpha$. Replicates of recombinant clones were screened for reactivity with anti-Corby antiserum by immuno colony dot assays and reactive clones were further analyzed by Western blotting.

One recombinant clone expressed a protein with an apparent molecular mass of 16 kDa. This protein was designated protein P16. By sequence analysis, the corresponding open reading frame of 411 bp encoding a protein of 136 amino acids was identified (AC Z97066). The predicted molecular mass of 15.7 kDa was in good agreement with the size of protein P16 determined by sodium dodecyl sulfate-polyacrylamide gel electrophoresis (SDS-PAGE) analysis. Databank searches revealed no significant homology to previously published bacterial or eukaryotic genes and proteins.

To facilitate protein isolation, an N-terminal 6xhisTag protein of P16 was constructed. The gene encoding P16 was amplified by PCR. Primers (P16P/5' GCG GGC CTG CAG CAT ATT CTT TTT GTA TTG TGA 3'; P16B/5' CGA CCG GAT CCA GTA AAA AAT CTA TCT T '3) were chosen to amplify the open reading frame without a start and stop codon and additional restriction sites for *Bam*HI and *Pst*I. After cloning in vector pQE30 (QIAGEN GmbH, Hilden, Germany), the resulting

*Christine Steudel, Jürgen Herbert Helbig, and Christian Paul Lück* Institut für Medizinische Mikrobiologie und Hygiene, TU Dresden, Fiedlerstr. 42, D-01307 Dresden, Germany.

*Legionella*, Edited by Reinhard Marre et al.

plasmid was transformed into *E. coli* M15 (pREP4). Expression was done for 5 h after induction with 2 mM isopropyl-$\beta$-D-thiogalactopyranoside (IPTG) in selective Luria-Bertani (LB) broth (ampicillin 200 $\mu$g ml$^{-1}$, kanamycin 25 $\mu$g ml$^{-1}$) supplemented with 2% glucose. Purification was performed using Ni$^{2+}$-chelate affinity chromatography under denaturing conditions.

By using the recombinant N-terminal 6xHisTag protein of P16 for immunization of BALB/c mice, seven monoclonal antibodies (MAb 61/1 to MAb 61/7) specific against protein P16 were prepared in our laboratory according to protocols described elsewhere (4).

To investigate the distribution of *p16*-related sequences in the genus *Legionella*, Southern blot hybridizations with an internal *p16*-specific probe were performed according to standard techniques. Specific signals were found in all serotype strains of *L. pneumophila* (*n* = 15) under high-stringency conditions. Even under low-stringency conditions, no signals were detected for the non-*L. pneumophila* *Legionella* species tested: *L. adelaidensis, L. birminghamensis, L. oakridgensis, L. feelei,* and *L. micdadei.* PCR reactions using *p16*-specific primers (p16colo/5′-ATT GTG ATT TTT GTT CGT TGG TTA-3′; p16coup/5′-GCC ACG CTC GCT TTG ATA-3′), which amplify an internal 370-bp fragment of *p16*, showed similar results. Additionally the same strains were tested by whole-cell enzyme-linked immunosorbent assay (ELISA) tests with the P16-specific monoclonal antibodies for the presence of P16-related proteins. Furthermore, total cell extracts of various bacteria (*n* = 17) not belonging to the genus *Legionella* were separated by SDS-PAGE and screened by Western blot analysis with MAb 61/1. The non-*L. pneumophila* *Legionella* strains gave negative results in whole cell ELISA tests and no signals were found testing the various bacteria. Taken together, the results confirmed the findings on the DNA level. P16-related proteins and *p16* sequences were present exclusively in strains belonging to *L. pneumophila*.

To analyze whether transcription of *p16* is constitutively or regulated under in vitro conditions, reverse transcriptase-PCR (RT-PCR) reactions were performed using Ready-To-Go RT-PCR Beads (Pharmacia Biotech, Freiburg, Germany) in single-step reactions according to the suppliers' instructions. Total RNA was isolated by using TRIZOL (GibcoBRL, Eggenstein, Germany) according to the manufacturers' instructions from *L. pneumophila* strain Corby cultures grown in broth at variable temperatures (37°C, 30°C, and room temperature) for 8, 24, and 48 h. Per reaction, 60 ng of total RNA treated with DNase I was used as a template. *p16*-specific primers (p16colo/5′-ATT GTG ATT TTT GTT CGT TGG TTA-3′; p16coup/5′-GC C ACG CTC GCT TTG ATA-3′) were chosen to generate a product of 370 bp. To control for the amount of RNA in the reaction, the constitutively expressed *mip* gene of *L. pneumophila* (2) was simultaneously subjected to the RT-PCR reaction. The data (not presented) indicated that neither temperature nor growth phase had any influence on the transcription of gene *p16*. These results showed that *p16* is expressed constitutively like *mip* under in vitro conditions.

To determine the size of the *p16* transcript, a Northern blot of total RNA was screened with a radioactively labelled 370-bp *p16*-specific probe. Total RNA was isolated from in vitro-grown *L. pneumophila* strain Corby at 37°C, separated onto a 1.2% agarose-0.66 M formaldehyde gel, and transferred to a positively charged nylon membrane (QIAGEN GmbH). Hybridization and signal detection were done under high-stringency conditions according to standard techniques (8). A *p16*-specific transcript of approximately 0.520 kb was detected (data not shown). The length of the transcript corresponds to the coding region of *p16*, indicating that the gene is transcribed as a monocistronic unit.

Additionally the expression of P16 antigen was investigated by indirect ELISA with MAb 61/1. To see whether intracellular growth has any influence on the expression of P16, the expression of antigen of *L. pneumophila* cultivated (16 h) in broth (extracellular) was compared with expression of antigen of *L. pneumophila* grown (16 h) in *Acanthamoeba castellanii* (intracellular). The results (Fig. 1) indicated that protein P16 is present in similar amounts extracellularly and intracellularly. To start with functional studies we constructed an isogenic knockout mutant. First, the P16 coding gene and flanking sequences were cloned as a 3.3-kb *Sph*I fragment into pUC19. A kanamycin resistance cassette was then introduced in the open reading frame of *p16* to disrupt the gene by using the GPS-1 genome priming system (New England Biolabs, Schalbach/Taunus, Germany). Subsequently, the resulting 5-kb *p16::npt-Sph*I insert was subcloned into the *sac*B–positive vector pBOC20 (1) and transferred into *L. pneumophila* strain Corby by electroporation. Colonies growing on solid medium supplemented with kanamycin and

sucrose were chosen as potential mutants and further analyzed. For one of the mutants, designated *L. pneumophila* strain Corby CP7, allelic exchange was confirmed on the one hand genetically by Southern hybridization and by sequencing the disrupted gene locus, and on the other hand on the protein level. Characterization on the protein level was done by screening whole bacteria with MAb 61/1 as dot blot. The mutant showed the expected reaction type—loss of reactivity with the P16-specific monoclonal antibody. To complement the P16-negative phenotype, the wild-type allele of *p16* was amplified by PCR with primers E2331 (5′-ATG ATG GAA TTC GTT TGG ACT ATC GCC TGT ATG TCT ACG-3′) and X5334 (5′-ATG ATG TCT AGA TGC CAA TCG CAA TCG ACT AAC GTA ATT-3′) and cloned into the MCS of pBC KS +/− (Stratagene Europe, Amsterdam, Netherlands), conferring

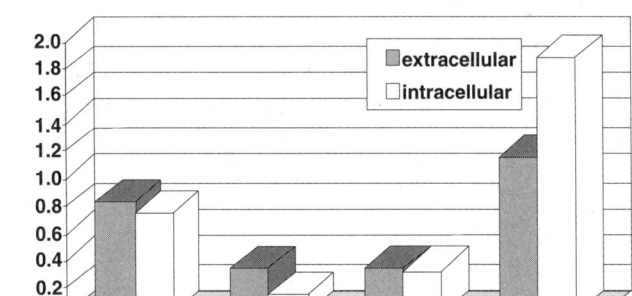

**FIGURE 1** Comparison of the expression of *Legionella* antigen in extracellular and intracellular cultures analyzed by indirect ELISA with monoclonal antibodies. Expression of antigen was measured for *L. pneumophila* strain Corby cultured in broth (extracellular) and in *A. castellanii* (intracellular) each for 16 h. The amounts of legionellae used in the indirect ELISA were approximately $5 \times 10^6$ per well, as determined by plating broth and intra-amoebal-grown bacteria on buffered charcoal-yeast extract (BYCE) agar. Monoclonal antibodies used for detection were Mab 22/1 specific for Mip, which is expressed constitutively (4); MAb 39/1 (6) specific for Hsp60, a protein synthesized primarily under extracellular (6) conditions; MAb 61/1 specific for P16; and one antibody specific for OmpM (6), a protein present especially under intracellular conditions. OD 492 nm, optical density at 492 nm.

resistance to chloramphenicol. The resulting plasmid pCS-31 was introduced into the knockout strain by electroporation and selection for Cat CFU. Complementation was confirmed genetically by Southern hybridization and on the protein level for the presence of P16 screened with the specific monoclonal antibody. By comparing growth on the solid medium it was determined that *p16* is not essential for growth of *L. pneumophila* and that genetic manipulations did not generate additional effects that influenced growth or colony morphology.

To investigate the importance of *L. pneumophila* P16 for attachment, uptake, and/or intracellular growth in its different host cells, infection assays were performed in differentiated U937 cells and in *A. castellanii*. Growth, maintenance, and differentiation of cells were carried out as described elsewhere (3, 7). Infections were performed in 48-well cell culture plates in six repeats at a multiplicity of infection of 100. After 2 h of incubation, remaining extracellular bacteria were killed by gentamicin treatment (80 $\mu$g ml$^{-1}$) for an additional 60 min. Gentamicin was removed by washing the cells three times with antibiotic-free medium. This was defined to be the zero time point of the infection, and further incubation was performed for several time periods.

At the end of each period the supernatants were stored per well and the cells lysed. Lysates were combined with supernatants and dilutions plated to determine the number of CFU. First we measured the ability of the isogenic knockout mutant to replicate within the macrophage-like cell line U937. The results (data not presented) showed that the knockout mutant entered macrophages and replicated to the same degree as the wild-type strain Corby. In contrast to the macrophage model system in the protozoan host model system *A. castellanii*, the mutant strain showed a delay in replication (Fig. 2). By calculating the initial attachment/uptake it was shown that only 2% compared with the wild type was recovered at the zero time point of infection. The rate of intracellular replication up to 24 h postinfection was found to be similar. The wild-type phenotype was restored in the complemented mutant. From these results we speculate that the surface-exposed 16-kDa protein promotes the attachment/initial uptake and might act as an adhesin in the receptor-mediated uptake mechanism in amoebae. Further infection assays with other known *Legionella* natural hosts will show whether the described locus *p16* might be responsible for the broad host spectrum of *L. pneumophila* in contrast to the other species of *Legionella*.

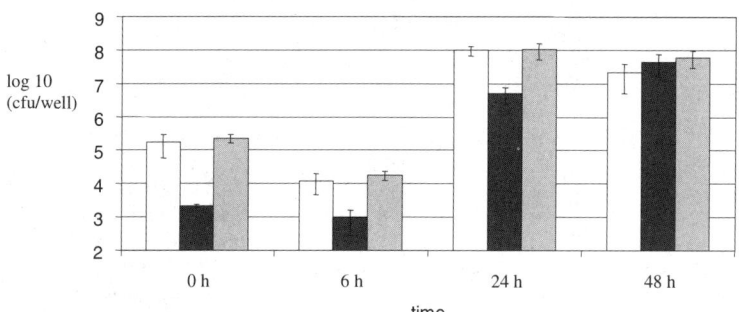

**FIGURE 2** Growth of *L. pneumophila* strains in *A. castellanii* cells: comparison between wild-type Corby, isogeneic *p16* knockout mutant CP7, and complemented mutant CP7 (pCS-31). Infection assays were performed with a multiplicity of infection of 100. The number of intracellular bacteria was determined at indicated time points postinfection. Each value represents the mean colony count of six samples and error bars indicate standard deviation. □, wild type; ■, knockout mutant; ▨, complemented mutant.

## REFERENCES

1. **Abu Kwaik, Y., and L. L. Pederson.** 1996. The use of differential display-PCR to isolate and characterize a *Legionella pneumophila* locus induced during the intracellular infection of macrophages. *Mol. Microbiol.* **21:**543–556.

2. **Abu Kwaik, Y., and N. C. Engleberg.** 1994. Cloning and molecular characterization of a *Legionella pneumophila* gene induced by intracellular infection and by various *in vitro* stress conditions. *Mol. Microbiol.* **13:**243–251.

3. **Abu Kwaik, Y., B. L. Eisenstein, and N. C. Engleberg.** 1993. Phenotypic modulation by *Legionella pneumophila* upon infection of macrophages. *Infect. Immun.* **61:**1320–1329.

4. **Helbig, J. H., B. Ludwig, P. C. Lück, A. Groh, W. Witzleb, and J. Hacker.** 1995. Monoclonal antibodies to *Legionella* Mip proteins recognize genus- and species-specific epitopes. *Clin. Diagn. Lab. Immunol.* **2:**160–165.

5. **Heuner, K., L. Bender-Beck, B. C. Brand, P. C. Lück, K. H. Mann, R. Marre, M. Ott, and J. Hacker.** 1995. Cloning and genetic characterization of the flagellum subunit gene (*fla*A) of *Legionella pneumophila* serogroup 1. *Infect. Immun.* **63:**2499–2507.

6. **Lück, P.C., J. W. Schmitt, A. Hengerer, and J. H. Helbig.** 1998. Subinhibitory concentrations of antimicrobial agents reduce the uptake of *Legionella pneumophila* into *Acanthamoeba castellanii* and U937 cells by altering the expression of virulence-associated antigens. *Antimicrob. Agents Chemother.* **42:**2870–2876.

7. **Moffat, J. F., and L. S. Tompkins.** 1992. A quantitative model of intracellular growth of *Legionella pneumophila* in *Acanthamoeba castellanii*. *Infect. Immun.* **60:**296–301.

8. **Sambrook, J., E. F. Fritsch, and T. Maniatis.** 1989. *Molecular Cloning: a Laboratory Manual*, 2nd ed. Cold Spring Harbor Laboratory Press, Cold Spring Harbor, N.Y.

# IMPACT OF AMOEBAE, BACTERIA, AND *TETRAHYMENA* ON *LEGIONELLA PNEUMOPHILA* MULTIPLICATION AND DISTRIBUTION IN AN AQUATIC ENVIRONMENT

*Tamera McNealy, Anthony L. Newsome,*
*Rebecca A. Johnson, and Sharon G. Berk*

# 30

Laboratory studies have clearly demonstrated the ability of *Legionella pneumophila* to use amoebae as a host cell for intracellular replication (1, 3). In vitro studies showed also that *L. pneumophila* can multiply within the protozoan *Tetrahymena pyriformis* and it can produce respirable-sized vesicles containing numerous *Legionella* (2, 3). These laboratory studies often have described the singular addition of *Legionella* cells (usually at a multiplicity of infection [MOI] of 10:1 to 200:1) to protozoa host cells suspended in various types of media and the subsequent increased recovery of bacteria CFU. In more natural settings, however, *L. pneumophila* occurs in conjunction with many different bacterial and protozoan species (4). Here the MOI could be substantially less than that observed in laboratory studies. Furthermore, non-*Legionella* species of bacteria could impact or diminish the ability of *Legionella* bacteria to contact and infect potential protozoan host cells.

In this investigation there were several objectives. The first objective was to define a minimum MOI beyond that which was previously described. A second objective was to determine if the presence of non-*Legionella* species of bacteria would influence the recovery of *L. pneumophila* CFU during replication and lysis of amoebae host cells. It was observed that *L. pneumophila* replication within amoebae (at an MOI as little as 0.001:1) lysed monolayers of amoebae in 96 to 144 h when amoebae were suspended in spring water in the presence of non-*Legionella* species of bacteria. Thus, a subsequent third objective was to document the impact of adding the free-swimming ciliate *Tetrahymena* to the amplified number of *Legionella* after they had lysed the population of amoebae host cells. For this, the cells were suspended in water from a cooling tower to more closely approximate events that could occur in natural settings. Completion of these objectives provide novel insight into events that could occur in aquatic environments such as cooling towers and natural bodies of water.

*Tamera McNealy* Klinikum Mannheim, Urologisches Labor, ZMF, Haus 8, Ebene 4N, Theodor Kutzer Ufer, 1-3, 68135 Mannheim, Germany. *Anthony L. Newsome* Department of Biology, Box 60, Middle Tennessee State University, Murfreesboro, TN 37132. *Rebecca A. Johnson and Sharon G. Berk* Center for the Management, Utilization and Protection of Water Resources, Tennessee Technological University, Cookeville, TN 38505.

*Legionella*, Edited by Reinhard Marre et al.
© 2002 ASM Press, Washington, D.C.

## MAINTENANCE OF BACTERIA AND PROTOZOA AND INFECTION OF AMOEBAE WITH *L. PNEUMOPHILA*

*Legionella pneumophila* strain AA100 was cultured on buffered charcoal-yeast extract (BCYE) agar at 37°C. *Escherichia coli, Pseudomonas fluorescens, Serratia marcescens,* and *Micrococcus luteus* were cultured on Trypticase soy agar (TSA) at 37°C. The amoeba, *Acanthamoeba polyphaga* (ATCC 30461), was maintained by continuous passage in Trypticase soy broth (TSB) at 25°C in 25-cm² tissue culture flasks. A *Tetrahymena* sp. originally isolated from a cooling tower was maintained axenically in plate count broth medium. Spring water (Carolina Biological, Burlington, N.C.), which is commonly used for the maintenance of protozoa, was heat sterilized prior to use in cocultures. Agar-grown *L. pneumophila* were suspended in the water for use in coculture experiments. The optical density (OD) of bacterial suspensions was determined at 660 nm and subsequently 10-fold serial dilutions were made in sterile spring water and plated onto BCYE agar to establish a correlation between OD and CFU/ml. Monolayers of amoebae (72 h old) in TSB were dislodged by sharp taps and harvested by centrifugation at 400 × *g*. Amoebae were then washed and suspended in sterile spring water and the cell concentration determined by haemocytometer counts. Approximately 0.5 ml containing 10⁶ amoebae was placed in duplicate wells of a multiwell tissue culture dish. *L. pneumophila* from 72-h-old BCYE agar cultures were suspended in spring water and added to amoebae at multiplicity of infections (ratio of bacteria to amoebae or MOI) of 100:1, 10:1, 1:1, 0.1:1, 0.01:1, and 0.001:1. Total volume of each well was brought to 3 ml with the addition of spring water. Cultures with the different MOIs were incubated for 96 h at 30°C. At an MOI of 0.001:1 however, the incubation period was increased to 144 h. The number of CFU was determined by 10-fold serial dilutions (in sterile spring water) of 100-μl aliquots from the wells and plating 100 μl of the

dilutions onto BCYE agar at time zero, 96 h, and 144 h. Plates were incubated at 37°C.

## ADDITION OF EXOGENOUS BACTERIA AND ADDITION OF *TETRAHYMENA* TO AMOEBAE/ *LEGIONELLA* COCULTURES

The non-*Legionella* (exogenous bacteria) bacteria species, *E. coli, P. fluorescens, S. marcescens,* and *M. luteus* were suspended in spring water. Bacterial concentrations (CFU/ml) of the suspension were determined by spectrophotometric analysis and dilution plating. Subsequently, bacteria were inactivated by UV irradiation. *Legionella*/amoebae cocultures were prepared, as previously described, at an MOI of 0.001:1. The UV-inactivated bacteria were added to the cocultures at an MOI of 100:1. Cocultures were incubated at 30°C for 144 h. The number of *L. pneumophila* (CFU) on BCYE agar was determined, as previously described, at time zero, 96 h, and 144 h. The *Tetrahymena* sp. was also added to amoebae/ *Legionella* cocultures after 72 h of incubation at 30°C. Control suspensions composed of *Tetrahymena* and *L. pneumophila* alone also were established. All cultures in cooling tower water were performed in triplicate and incubated at 30°C. Subsequently, the cultures with *Tetrahymena* sp. were examined microscopically for the production of released phagosomes (vesicles) containing *Legionella*. The respiratory indicator 2-(4-iodophenyl)-3-(4-nitrophenyl)-5-phenyltetrazolium chloride (INT, Eastman Kodak, Rochester, N.Y.) was used at a final concentration of 0.05% to test for viability of bacteria within the released vesicle.

## IMPACT OF MULTIPLICITY OF INFECTION ON *LEGIONELLA* INFECTION OF *ACANTHAMOEBA*

*L. pneumophila* was added to *Acanthamoeba polyphaga* at different MOIs (ratio of bacteria to amoeba) to evaluate its impact on recoverable CFU. Results are summarized in Table 1. As the MOI was sequentially reduced from 100:1 to eventually 0.001:1, a dramatic in-

**TABLE 1**  Multiplication of *L. pneumophila* in *A. polyphaga* incubated in spring water at 30°C

| Ratio (MOI)[a] bacteria/amoebae | CFU/ml at time: | | Average increase (fold) |
|---|---|---|---|
| | 0 h | 96 h | |
| 100/1 | $1.57 \times 10^8 \pm 2.45 \times 10^7$ | $2.20 \times 10^8 \pm 4.00 \times 10^7$ | $1.40 \pm 0.04$ |
| 1.0/1 | $1.49 \times 10^6 \pm 1.50 \times 10^4$ | $3.80 \times 10^7 \pm 2.50 \times 10^6$ | $25.95 \pm 1.95$ |
| 0.1/1 | $1.60 \times 10^5 \pm 1.80 \times 10^4$ | $7.65 \times 10^7 \pm 6.50 \times 10^6$ | $4.79 \times 10^2 \pm 13.50$ |
| 0.01/1 | $1.12 \times 10^4 \pm 6.50 \times 10^2$ | $2.20 \times 10^7 \pm 1.55 \times 10^6$ | $1.98 \times 10^3 \pm 2.55 \times 10^2$ |
| 0.001/1[b] | $1.15 \times 10^3 \pm 6.00 \times 10^1$ | $1.79 \times 10^6 \pm 3.00 \times 10^4$ | $1.56 \times 10^3 \pm 1.07 \times 10^2$ |

[a] Each MOI was performed in duplicate.
[b] CFU/ml (time 144 h), $2.06 \times 10^7 \pm 8.5 \times 10^5$; fold increase, $1.79 \times 10^4 \pm 1.11 \times 10^3$.

crease in *L. pneumophila* CFU/ml was observed. After 96 h, the CFU began to stabilize and this was a reflection of *Legionella*-mediated lysis of the amoebae host cells due to intracellular replication. At 0.001:1 MOI, the number of *L. pneumophila* in amoebae and the percentage of infected amoebae (data not shown) increased in conjunction with the recovery of CFU/ml. At 144 h, all amoebae trophozoites were lysed as a result of *Legionella* intracellular replication.

## ADDITION OF EXOGENOUS BACTERIA

When *P. fluorescens*, *S. marcescens*, *E. coli*, or *M. luteus* were added at a $10^5$-fold-higher concentration than *L. pneumophila*, the recovery of *L. pneumophila* was not diminished. After 144 h in the presence of these exogenous bacteria, the recovery of *L. pneumophila* CFU/ml was equivalent to that observed in control cocultures with amoebae and only *L. pneumophila*. No *Legionella* growth-supporting activity was present (data not shown) in the absence of amoebae (*L. pneumophila* and inactivated exogenous bacteria only).

## IMPACT OF *TETRAHYMENA* ADDITION TO *LEGIONELLA/ AMOEBA* COCULTURES

When the *Tetrahymena* sp. was added 72 h after the amoebae/*Legionella* cocultures were established, numerous vesicles were present within 24 h after addition of the ciliates (Fig. 1A and B). It was not possible to enumerate the tightly packed bacteria within the vesicles. On the basis of the vesicle size (approximately 5 μm in diameter) however, they could con-

tain more than 100 bacteria. In addition, the reaction with INT showed that the *Legionella* were viable (Fig. 1C). The number of vesicles per ciliate ranged from 3.3 in one experiment to as much as 20 per ciliate in another run of the experiment. No vesicles were observed in the hemocytometer grids of samples from experiments of amoebae/*Legionella* cocultures alone or when the ciliates were incubated with *Legionella* in the absence of amoebae.

## CONCLUDING REMARKS

Results of this study provide insight into interactions that may occur in aquatic environments, and some events have not previously been documented in laboratory studies. First, it is likely that the MOI does not appear to be a critical requirement in initiating an infection in amoebae. A remarkable feature in the sequential reduction of the MOI (from 100:1 to 0.001:1) was that it did not diminish the ability of *L. pneumophila* to infect, multiply within, and ultimately lyse the population of amoebae host cells. This, however, may not establish the lowest possible effective MOI. It does suggest a highly efficient infection mechanism and intracellular replication process that operated in spring water and cooling tower water.

At an *L. pneumophila* MOI of 0.001:1, the addition of a gram-positive bacterium or a variety of gram-negative non-*Legionella* species of bacteria had little effect on the recovery of *Legionella* CFU. The MOI of the non-*Legionella* bacteria was $10^5$ greater than that of *L. pneumophila*. If amoebae infection by *L. pneumophila* was the result of inadvertent con-

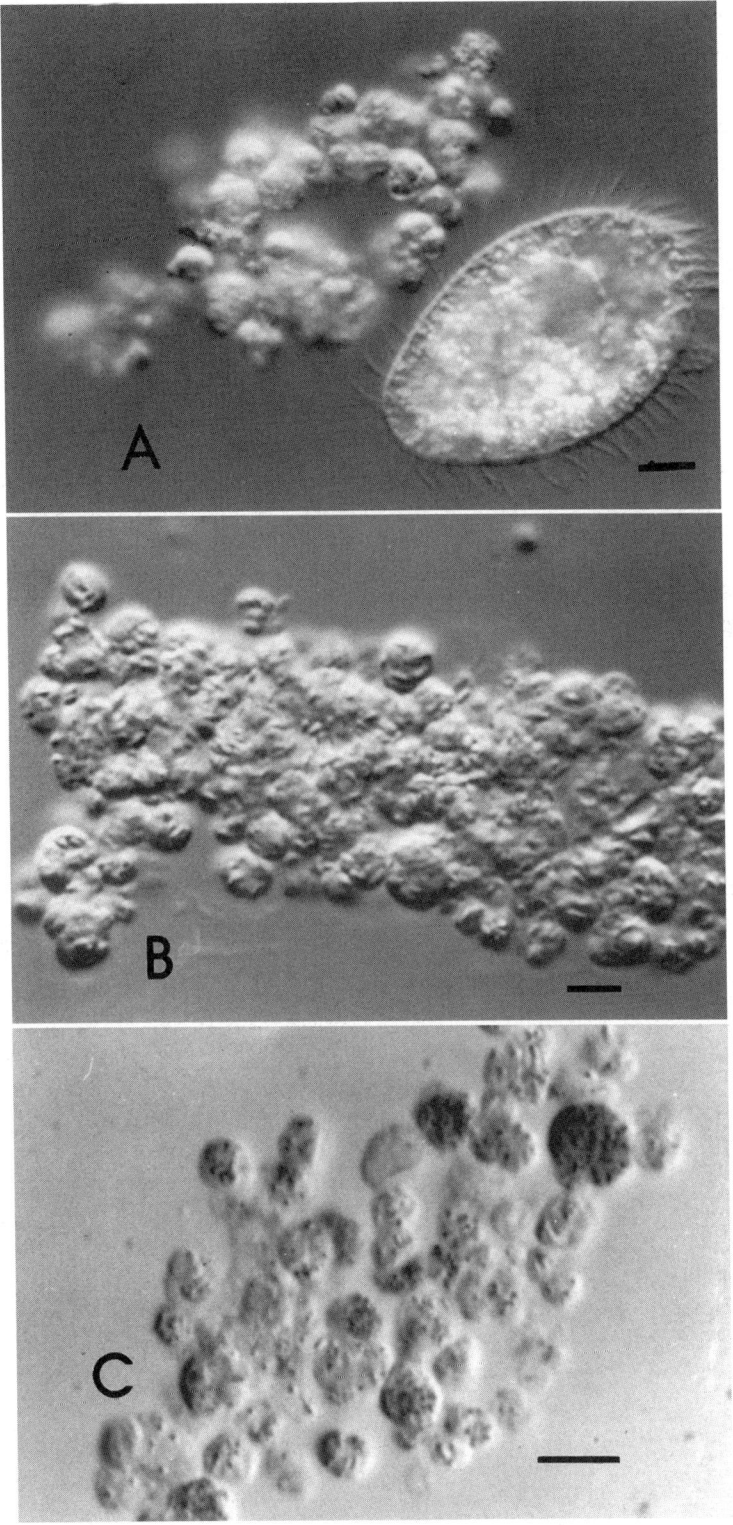

**FIGURE 1** (A) The ciliate, *Tetrahymena*, next to a cluster of expelled food vacuoles (vesicles). Bar, 5.0 μm. (B) Large clusters of loosely attached vesicles released from *Tetrahymena* after 24 h in coculture with amoebae and *L. pneumophila*. Bar, 5.0 μm. (C) Vesicles containing viable *L. pneumophila* as determined by reduction of INT, which resulted in a dark-colored product within respiring bacteria. Bar, 5.0 μm.

tact and subsequent phagocytosis, an inhibitory effect might have been expected since addition of exogenous bacteria would likewise result in increased inadvertent contact with phagocytosis, and thus diminish potential contact and uptake of virulent *L. pneumophila*. The results suggest *L. pneumophila* enter amoebae through a mechanism that is distinct from simple contact phagocytosis. A more likely conclusion is that *L. pneumophila* is able to attach and infect amoebae via a specific mechanism that is highly efficient in spring water and cooling tower water.

The presence of a specific uptake mechanism has been suggested by studies showing that *L. pneumophila* uptake by *A. polyphaga* was partially mediated by a galactose/*N*-acetylgalactosamine lectin, and additional receptors may be involved (5, 6). *L. pneumophila* invasive-defective mutants were severely defective in attachment to *A. polyphaga*. In addition, distinct pili (designated competence- and adherence-associated pili) appear to be important in attachment to protozoan cells (10).

The addition of a $10^5$ greater number of UV-killed *L. pneumophila* (at an MOI of 0.001:1) did not diminish recovery of *Legionella* CFU. This suggests nonviable *Legionella* cells failed to inhibit specific uptake and subsequent intracellular replication of virulent cells. The inability of nonviable *Legionella* to diminish intracellular replication suggests these cells were unable to saturate sites that would be associated with an uptake or internalization mechanism. A likely conclusion is that viable cells have features that actively promote their uptake by free-living amoebae species such as *Acanthamoeba*. The inability of UV-inactivated *L. pneumophila* (at an MOI of 100:1) to have a lytic effect on amoebae suggested they were destroyed as a direct result of *Legionella* intracellular replication rather than due to the presence of a bacteria-associated toxin or toxin-like effect. The AA100 strain of *L. pneumophila* was a clinical isolate and has frequently been used in amoebae/*Legionella* interaction studies (1, 5).

The time required for lysis and eventual destruction of all the susceptible *Acanthamoeba* host cells was at most 144 h for the lowest MOI (0.001:1) evaluated. Lysis of amoebae monolayers was more rapid at the greater MOIs. This rapid destruction of host cells followed by release of the bacteria suggests that in naturally occurring environments, *L. pneumophila* may actually spend a minor portion of the bacterial lifespan in amoebae although it may use them for intracellular replication. After lysis and release from amoebae, *Legionella* likely become part of the planktonic flora or incorporated into biofilms in the surrounding area. The incorporation of extracellular *Legionella* into biofilms has been documented in laboratory studies (8, 9, 11).

Typically, the distribution of *Legionella* in aquatic habitats has been based on the occurrence of bacteria in the planktonic zone. In the planktonic setting, amoebae may play a lesser role because studies suggest attachment to a surface is necessary for amoebae ingestion or feeding on particulate matter. In aquatic environments, and particularly in planktonic zones, amoebae can be outcompeted by free-swimming protozoa (7). Thus if *Legionella* are in suspension in aquatic environments, the role of free-swimming protozoa such as *Tetrahymena* is particularly relevant.

The subsequent production of *Legionella*-filled vacuoles by *Tetrahymena* demonstrates a phenomenon wherein the presence of protozoa from different phyla cooperatively influence both the number and apportion of *L. pneumophila* in a laboratory-derived aquatic environment. Similar events may occur in natural and human-made aquatic environments. In our investigation, the production of *Legionella*-filled vesicles by *Tetrahymena* occurred only in the presence of amoebae, which amplified the number of *Legionella* bacteria, athough a low MOI of 0.001 was used to establish the coculture. As a direct result of *L. pneumophila* amplification, amoebae lysed, liberating the bacteria, which were then concentrated into vesicles by the *Tetrahymena* sp. The production of *Legionella*-filled vesicles has previously been reported in *Acanthamoeba* spp. only when a much higher (30 to 10,000) MOI was initially used (2).

A conclusion reached in this study is that *L. pneumophila* can initiate infection in amoebae at an MOI considerably lower than often used in laboratory studies. Extraneous bacteria do not diminish the recovery of the *Legionella* CFU. A second conclusion is that when *L. pneumophila* cell numbers are amplified by multiplication within amoebae, which are ultimately destroyed, the presence of free-swimming ciliates such as *Tetrahymena* can further influence the distribution of *Legionella* by concentrating planktonic forms into free-floating vesicles. Of additional importance was that these events were demonstrated to occur in spring water or water from a cooling tower. Thus, it is likely the results and conclusions are not a reflection of using cells suspended in various types of laboratory media or salt solutions.

## REFERENCES

1. **Abu Kwaik, Y., L.-Y. Gao, B. J. Stone, C. Venkataraman, and O. S. Harb.** 1998. Invasion of protozoa by *Legionella pneumophila* and its role in bacterial ecology and pathogenesis. *Appl. Environ. Microbiol.* **64:**3127–3133.
2. **Berk, S. B., R. S. Ting, G. W. Turner, and R. J. Ashburn.** 1998. Production of respirable vesicles containing live *Legionella pneumophila* cells by two *Acanthamoeba* spp. *Appl. Environ. Microbiol.* **64:**279–286.
3. **Fields, B. S.** 1993. *Legionella* and protozoa: interactions of a pathogen and its natural host, p. 437–441. *In* J. M. Barbaree, R. F. Breiman, and A. P. Dufour (ed.), *Legionella: Current Status and Emerging Perspectives.* American Society of Microbiology, Washington, D.C.
4. **Fliermans, C. B.** 1996. Ecology of *Legionella*: from data to knowledge with a little wisdom. *Microb. Ecol.* **32:**203–228.
5. **Harb, O. S., L.-Y. Gao, and Y. Abu Kwaik.** 2000. From protozoa to mammalian cells: a new paradigm in the life cycle of intracellular bacterial pathogens. *Environ. Microbiol.* **2:**251–265.
6. **Harb, O. S., C. Venkataraman, B. J. Haack, L.-Y. Gao, and Y. Abu Kwaik.** 1998. Heterogenity in the attachment and uptake mechanisms of the Legionnaires' disease bacterium, *Legionella pneumophila*, by protozoan hosts. *Appl. Environ. Microbiol.* **64:**126–132.
7. **Rodriguez-Zaragoza, S.** 1994. Ecology of free-living amoebae. *Crit. Rev. Microbiol.* **20:**225–241.
8. **Rogers, J., A. B. Dowsett, P. J. Dennis, J. V. Lee, and C. W. Keevil.** 1994. Influence of temperature and plumbing material selection on biofilm formation and growth of *Legionella pneumophila* in a model potable water system containing complex microbial flora. *Appl. Environ. Microbiol.* **60:**1585–1592.
9. **Rogers, J., A. P. Dowsett, P. J. Dennis, J. V. Lee, and C. W. Keevil.** 1994. Influence of plumbing material on biofilm formation and growth of *Legionella pneumophila* in potable water systems. *Appl. Environ. Microbiol.* **60:**1842–1851.
10. **Stone, B. J., and Y. Abu Kwaik.** 1998. Expression of multiple pili by *Legionella pneumophila*: identification and characterization of a type IV pilin gene and its role in adherence to mammalian and protozoan cells. *Infect. Immun.* **66:**1768–1775.
11. **Wright, J. B., I. Ruseska, M. A. Athar, S. Corbett, and J. W. Coserton.** 1989. *Legionella pneumophila* grows adherent to surfaces in vitro and in situ. *Infect. Control Hosp. Epidemiol.* **10:**408–415.

# BIOFILM FORMATION AND MULTIPLICATION OF *LEGIONELLA* ON SYNTHETIC PIPE MATERIALS IN CONTACT WITH TREATED WATER UNDER STATIC AND DYNAMIC CONDITIONS

*Dick van der Kooij, Harm R. Veenendaal,
Nellie P. G. Slaats, and Dick Vonk*

# 31

Biofilms and sediments in plumbing systems are potential niches for the multiplication of *Legionella* when water temperatures are between 25 and 45°C. Protozoa grazing on the biofilm may serve as hosts for *Legionella* (3, 5), but it has been suggested that multiplication of *Legionella* may also occur in biofilms, outside protozoa (2). Biofilm formation depends on the supply of biodegradable compounds to microorganisms attached to the water-exposed surfaces. Such biodegradable compounds may originate from the water, from the material, or from both sources. The growth-promoting properties of certain materials for *Legionella* have clearly been demonstrated in practice and in laboratory experiments (1, 4, 6).

Copper is the predominant pipe material used in domestic plumbing systems in The Netherlands. An increasing variety of synthetic pipe materials is available for use in such systems and may be used as an alternative for copper. A concern regarding the use of synthetic pipe materials is their effect on biofilm formation and growth of *Legionella*. The growth-promoting properties of 10 selected synthetic materials, as well as copper and stainless steel, were tested in static (batch) experiments at 25°C and also in a dynamic (flowthrough) test at ambient temperature simulating flow conditions in a household-plumbing system. The study objectives were (i) to compare the microbial growth-promoting properties of various synthetic materials with those of copper and stainless steel under static and dynamic test conditions, (ii) to determine the effect of the materials on the multiplication of *Legionella*, and (iii) to evaluate the materials on the basis of the obtained results.

## SYNTHETIC MATERIALS

Synthetic materials were selected on the basis of polymer type and present application. The following types of synthetic materials were tested: polyethylene (crosslinked) (PE-X), polypropylene (PP), polybuthylene (PB), and chlorinated PVC (PVC-C). Metals (copper and stainless steel [SS]) were included for comparison. Glass and silicone tubing (SIL) were used as controls.

*Dick van der Kooij, Harm R. Veenendaal, and Nellie P. G. Slaats* Kiwa N.V. Research and Consultancy, PO Box 1072, 3430 BB Nieuwegein, The Netherlands. *Dick Vonk* Ministry of Housing, Spatial Planning and the Environment, PO Box 30945, 2500 GX The Hague, The Netherlands.

*Legionella*, Edited by Reinhard Marre et al.
© 2002 ASM Press, Washington, D.C.

## BIOMASS PRODUCTION POTENTIAL (BPP) OF MATERIALS

Pieces (each about 8 cm$^2$) of the materials were rinsed with drinking water and incubated at 25°C in 600 ml slow sand filtrate (SSF) at a surface-to-volume ratio of 0.15 cm$^{-1}$. Filtered (1.2 $\mu$m) river water (1 ml) was added to each flask to ensure the presence of a wide variety of microorganisms in the test water. The flasks were also inoculated with a mixed culture including *Legionella*, originating from a plumbing system and maintained in tap water containing pieces of natural rubber. Duplicate flasks were incubated at 25°C. Concentrations of attached biomass ("biofilm") and suspended biomass were assessed using adenosine triphosphate (ATP) analysis after 7, 14, 28, 56, 84, and 112 days of incubation. Biofilm was released with a series (6 × 2 min) of low-energy sonications in autoclaved SSF prior to ATP analysis (7). The BPP value was calculated as the average value of the sum of the concentration of attached biomass and the concentration of suspended biomass, expressed as pg of ATP/cm$^2$ of material, after 56, 84, and 112 days of incubation. This BPP value equals the sum of the biofilm formation potential (BFP, pg of ATP/cm$^2$), which is the average value of the attached biomass concentration and the suspended biomass production (SBP, pg of ATP/cm$^2$), which is calculated from the average value of the concentration of suspended biomass. Hence, BPP = BFP + SBP.

## REFERENCE SYSTEM

Hydraulic conditions prevailing in domestic systems were simulated in the reference system. Pipes (internal diameter, ~13 mm; length, 5 m) of the various materials were connected with a central supply, which was switched on and off at intervals typical for domestic water use, resulting in a total flow for each pipe of 130 liters in a 24-h period. Locally available drinking water (groundwater derived, no disinfectant residual) was used as the supply (temperature, 18°C). The system was inoculated with a volume of the mixed

culture, including *Legionella*, at the start of the test and again after 2 weeks and run for a period of 112 days.

## BIOFILM FORMATION RATE OF WATER

The biofilm formation rate (BFR) (pg of ATP/cm$^2$/day) of tap water was assessed with a biofilm monitor, which consists of a vertically placed glass column containing glass cylinders on top of each other (8). The flow rate in the monitor is 0.2 m/s. Glass cylinders are taken from the column at regular intervals and the concentration of attached biomass is assessed with ATP analysis. The BFR value is calculated from the linear increase of the biomass concentration with time.

## *LEGIONELLA*

*Legionella* was enumerated in water and in the biofilm (after sonication) using buffered charcoal-yeast extract agar medium, incubated at 37°C for 7 days. Typical colonies were counted and confirmed on buffered charcoal-yeast extract medium without cysteine. The *Legionella* growth potential (LegGP) (CFU/cm$^2$) of the materials in the BPP test was calculated from the concentrations of *Legionella* in water and in biofilm after 56, 84, and 112 days of incubation of the flasks with the material samples (see BPP).

## RESULTS

### Static Test

The biofilm concentration on the materials rapidly increased in time, reaching maximum concentrations within 1 to 2 weeks with most materials (Fig. 1). Growth occurred more slowly on copper and from the observed increase of the biofilm concentration as a function of time, maximum BFR values of 4.0 and 8.5 pg of ATP/cm$^2$/day were calculated. BPP values ranged from <100 pg of ATP/cm$^2$ for glass (control) and stainless steel (SS) to about 1,800 pg of ATP/cm$^2$ for PE-X-based materials and higher for silicone tubing (control). The relative standard deviations of the BPP

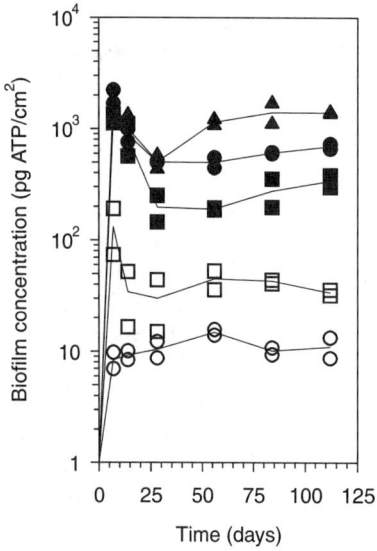

**FIGURE 1** Attached biomass concentrations (biofilm) as a function of time on various materials incubated in slow sand filtrate at 25°C (static test). Samples were taken in duplicate from one flask. Symbols: ○, glass; □, stainless steel; ■, PVC-C; ●, PP; ▲, PE-Xa.

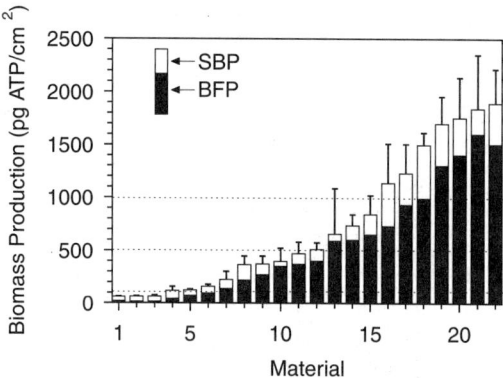

**FIGURE 2** Biomass production potential (pg of ATP/cm²) values (with upper limit of the standard deviation) of the selected materials calculated from the biomass concentrations on samples (in duplicate) of the materials and in the water on days 56, 84, and 112. BPP is the sum of the biofilm formation potential (BFP) and the suspended biomass production (SBP); see text. Materials: 1, 2, 3, glass; 4, 5, 6, SS; 7, PVC-C; 8, PB; 9, PVC-C; 10, copper; 11, PP; 12, PE-Xc; 13, copper; 14, PP; 15, PB; 16, PE-Xc; 17, SIL; 18, 19, PE-Xa; 20, SIL; 21, PE-Xb; 22, SIL.

values on average were about 20%. BFP values were >80% of BPP values for most materials, except for glass, SS, and SIL (Fig. 2). *Legionella* multiplied in the presence of all materials and the LegGP values ranged from about 100 CFU/cm² for glass to about 2 × 10⁴ CFU/cm² for PE-X-based materials (Fig. 3). *Legionella* in the biofilm was the major fraction of the LegGP value for PVC-C, PB, and a few of the PE-X-based materials, but attached growth was very limited (<6%) with silicone tubing.

## Biofilm Formation in Reference System and in Biofilm Monitor

Average biofilm concentrations on the materials in the dynamic test ranged from 80 pg of ATP/cm² (PVC-C) to 250 pg of ATP/cm² (copper). *Legionella* was not observed in the reference system. The biofilm concentration on glass rings in the biofilm monitor supplied with the same tap water at a constant flow increased linearly with time (BFR value: 4.5 ± 0.6 pg of ATP/cm²/day) and reached 600

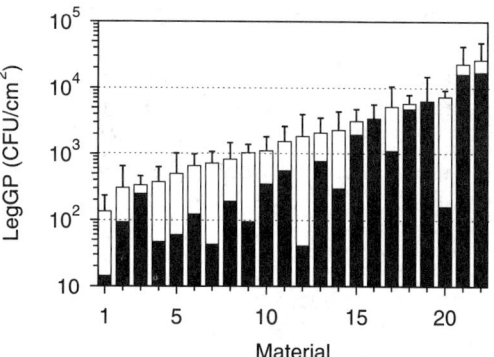

**FIGURE 3** LegGP (CFU/cm²) of selected materials tested at 25°C in the static test, calculated from the *Legionella* concentrations on material pieces and in the water on days 56, 84, and 112; see text. The upper limit of the standard deviation is indicated. The open segments of the columns represent the fraction of suspended *Legionella*, the filled part represents attached growth. Materials: 1, 2, glass; 3, PVC-C; 4, SS; 5, glass; 6, PE-Xa; 7, Sil; 8, SS; 9, copper; 10, SS; 11, PE-Xc; 12, Sil; 13, copper; 14, PP; 15, PB; 16, PVC-C; 17, PE-Xc; 18, PB; 19, PP; 20, Sil; 21, PE-Xa; 22, PE-Xb.

pg of ATP/cm$^2$ after 150 days. Thus, biofilm accumulation in the biofilm monitor exceeded biofilm formation on the materials in the reference system.

## DISCUSSION

Copper released from the pipes in domestic plumbing systems contributes significantly (60%) to the copper content of the sludge obtained from sewage treatment plants, hampering its use for agricultural purposes. For this reason, certain synthetic materials may be preferred for use in plumbing systems. Most of these materials clearly stimulated biomass production and growth of *Legionella* in the static test, thus confirming earlier reports (4, 6). The biofilm formation on copper was likely related to the presence of some oil on the pipe surface. The highest LegGP values were observed with PE-X-based materials, which also had relatively high BPP values. LegGP values correlated significantly with BPP values, but some test results did not fit with the calculated relationship (Fig. 4). In these cases the development of the autochthonous population may have been less favorable for the growth of *Legionella* at an incubation temperature (25°C), which is relatively low for *Legionella* (4). The observations with the reference system indicate that the various materials had little impact on the bacteriological quality of water at frequent use in a relatively small system at a temperature below 20°C. Biofilm concentrations on the materials were even lower than on glass in the biofilm monitor. The following explanation may be given for this phenomenon: the supply of the reference system with biodegradable compounds present in the water is a small fraction (2%) of the supply of the biofilm monitor with a constant flow of 0.2 m/s. Furthermore, in the reference system, periods of stagnancy were frequently interrupted by short periods (of about 30 s) with a relatively high flow rate (about 0.7 m/s). Microorganisms multiplying under stagnant conditions are flushed from the pipe wall and biofilm formation is limited. The results of the static test reveal that materials may affect biofilm formation at long periods of stagnation and a temperature of 25°C. However, in practice also, water contributes to biofilm formation. Therefore, data about biofilm concentrations and *Legionella* in plumbing systems are needed to enable a quantitative evaluation of the BPP and BFP values as observed for the various materials in the static test.

## ACKNOWLEDGMENT

This study was conducted on behalf of the Ministry of Housing, Spatial Planning and the Environment, project no. 9712.0030.

## REFERENCES

1. **Colbourne, J. S., D. J. Pratt., M. G. Smith, S. P. Fisher–Hoch, and D. Harper.** 1984. Water fittings as sources of *Legionella pneumophila* in a hospital plumbing system. *Lancet* **i:**210–213.
2. **Desai, R., C. Welsh, M. Summy, M. Farone, and A. L. Newsome.** 1999. The potential of in situ hybridisation and an immunogold assay to identify *Legionella* associations with other microorganisms. *J. Microbiol. Methods* **37:**155–164.
3. **Kwaik, Y. A., L. Y. Gao, B. J. Stone, C. Venkataraman, and O. S. Harb.** 1998. Invasion of protozoa by *Legionella pneumophila* and its role in bacterial ecology and pathogenesis. *Appl. Environ. Microbiol.* **64:**3127–3133.
4. **Rogers, J., A. B. Dowsett, P. J. Dennis, and C. W. Keevil.** 1994. Influence of plumbing materials on biofilm formation and growth of *Le-*

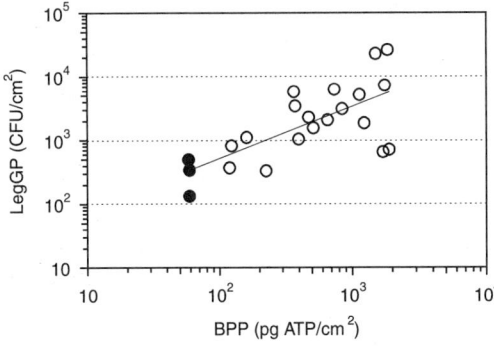

**FIGURE 4** Relationship between BPP and the LegGP in the batch test at 25°C. Black dots, glass controls. The relationship is given by log (LegGP) = 0.81 log BPP + 1.1 (r$^2$ = 0.48; $P < 0.01$).

*gionella pneumophila* in potable water systems. *Appl. Environ. Microbiol.* **60:**1842–1851.

5. **Rowbotham, T. J.** 1980. Preliminary report on the pathogenicity of *Legionella pneumophila* for freshwater and soil amoeba. *J. Clin. Pathol.* **33:** 1179–1183.

6. **Schoenen, D., R. Schulze-Röbbecke, and N. Schirdewahn.** 1988. Microbial contamination of water by materials of pipes and hoses. 2nd communication: growth of *Legionella pneumophila*. *Zentralbl. Bakteriol. Hyg.* **B186:**326–332.

7. **Van der Kooij, D., and H. R. Veenendaal.** 1993. Assessment of the biofilm formation potential of synthetic materials in contact with drinking water during distribution, p. 1395–1407. *In Proc. AWWA Wat. Qual. Technol. Conf.* American Water Works Association, Denver, Colo.

8. **Van der Kooij, D., H. R. Veenendaal, C. Baars-Lorist, D. W. van der Klift, and Y. C. Drost.** 1995. Biofilm formation on surfaces of glass and teflon exposed to treated water. *Water Res.* **29:**1655–1662.

# CLINICAL PRESENTATION, LABORATORY DIAGNOSIS, AND THERAPY

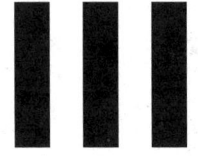

# CHEMOTHERAPY OF LEGIONNAIRES' DISEASE WITH MACROLIDE OR QUINOLONE ANTIMICROBIAL AGENTS

*Paul H. Edelstein*

# 32

Erythromycin was chosen as the treatment of choice for Legionnaires' disease on the basis of retrospective analysis of the 1976 Philadelphia epidemic (12). Erythromycin effectiveness was attributed to its intracellular activity. However, it soon became apparent that many severely ill and immunocompromised patients responded slowly to erythromycin and that relapses sometimes occurred, requiring long courses of chemotherapy (13). Effective antimicrobial chemotherapy of Legionnaires' disease is driven primarily by the location of *Legionella pneumophila* inside cells, primarily alveolar macrophages. This intracellular location of the bacterium protects it from extracellular antibacterial factors such as antibody, complement, and antimicrobial agents that are not found within the cell itself. Determining optimal chemotherapy for Legionnaires' disease by conducting truly informative clinical trials is generally of little use since the disease is uncommon and because the fatality rates in most community-acquired cases are relatively low. This means that predictions of effective therapy have to depend on the results of in vitro and experimental animal model studies.

Results of these studies make it highly likely that the optimal therapy of Legionnaires' disease should be with the newer quinolone and azalide antimicrobial agents, especially in patients with severe disease, or those with compromised cellular immune systems. Erythromycin and tetracycline therapy should be confined to those with less severe disease, and no longer constitute the therapies of choice in hospitalized or immunocompromised patients.

## THE IMPORTANCE OF *L. PNEUMOPHILA* CELL BIOLOGY

The location and physiologic state of *L. pneumophila* within the cell are key determinants of the efficacy of antimicrobial therapy. After its phagocytosis by macrophages, the bacterium resides within a ribosomal-studded phagosome that is blocked from maturation to a late endosome (16). Experimental studies show that only about 20 to 25% of such phagosomes are fused with cellular lysosomes. There is now good, but still preliminary, evidence that later in the bacterial-cell cycle, dramatic changes occur in the bacterial phenotype and in the nature of the bacterial phagosome (15, 16). These changes occur before

*Paul H. Edelstein*  Department of Pathology and Laboratory Medicine, University of Pennsylvania Medical Center, Philadelphia, PA 19104.

*Legionella*, Edited by Reinhard Marre et al.
© 2002 ASM Press, Washington, D.C.

the bacterium is released from the cell, at which time a new host cell is found and the cycle begins again. The bacterium becomes smaller and rapidly motile and undergoes a number of physiologic changes, including the development of resistance to antimicrobial agents normally active against the bacterium (1). The phagosome itself matures into a late endosome and fuses with lysosomes.

*L. pneumophila* intracellular behavior and physiologic state is important because only antimicrobial agents that are found in the same intracellular compartment as the bacterium can be effective against the organism. For effective chemotherapy to occur there must be colocalization of the bacterium and antimicrobial agents, and the antimicrobial agent must retain bioactivity against the bacterium. Thus simply knowing the intracellular concentrating ability of the antimicrobial agent cannot be used to predict efficacy, since the agent may be concentrated in a noncolocalized cellular compartment, or it may be colocalized but only with loss of activity. In addition, the kinetics and reversibility of intracellular bacterial inhibition/killing by the antimicrobial agent must be important, as is the cell-cycle-dependent antimicrobial resistance of the bacterium.

The antimicrobial agents that are most active against intracellular *L. pneumophila* are those that are concentrated within cellular lysosomes; these include macrolide/azalide and quinolone drugs (17). The $\beta$-lactam drugs are instead found in the cytosol, probably the main reason why they are ineffective in the treatment of Legionnaires' disease. It is of interest that aminoglycoside antimicrobial agents are found in the lysosomal compartments, but accumulate very slowly within the cell, perhaps explaining why these agents are ineffective in the treatment of the disease.

Exactly how the lysosomally distributed intracellular antimicrobial agents become colocalized with the bacteria is not known. During the early intracellular growth phase of the bacterium, about 25% of bacterium-containing phagosomes fuse with lysosomes. It may be

these 25% of the bacterial population that are affected by the antimicrobial agents. Later in the cell cycle the majority of phagosomes fuse with lysosomes, giving a second chance for antimicrobial agent-bacterial interaction. However, it is also probably at this stage when the bacterium is relatively resistant to antimicrobial agents; bacterial growth is still inhibited at this stage, which may be enough to tip the balance in favor of the host. Since it is unlikely that bacterial growth within the cells is synchronized, it is probable that there is a very complex interaction between the bacteria and the antimicrobial agents. Regardless, as demonstrated in the guinea pig model, the very effective antimicrobial agents effectively reduce bacterial lung concentrations within the lung, over a period of several days (6, 10).

## RELATIVE INTRACELLULAR ACTIVITIES OF ANTIMICROBIAL AGENTS

Incubation of antimicrobial agents with cells infected by *L. pneumophila* can be used to determine the intracellular activity of the drug. The greatest data exist for human monocyte-derived macrophages and guinea pig alveolar macrophages. Results of assays using these cell types has been shown to correlate very well with animal model results, as well as with what is known about drug efficacy in humans with Legionnaires' disease (3). It is unknown if the use of other cell types, especially continuous cell lines, correlates with primary macrophage studies. A recent study highlighted this, showing that use of two different cell lines gave different results in the determination of antimicrobial activity against *L. pneumophila* (14). Antimicrobial agent activity against *L. pneumophila* can be divided into three categories: inactive, inhibitory, and bactericidal. The reversibility of activity of the latter two categories is assessed by observing bacterial growth after washout of the agent from the tissue culture well.

Erythromycin is only inhibitory in its activity against intracellular *L. pneumophila*, and this inhibition can be easily and rapidly reversed after removal of the drug from the tissue culture well (3). This relatively poor drug activity occurs over a broad range of antibiotic concentration and cannot be overcome by concentrations as high as 5 $\mu$g/ml. In contrast, azithromycin is bactericidal or inhibitory in its activity, depending on test strain, even at concentrations as low as 0.25 $\mu$g/ml (8). Azithromycin activity is slowly reversible after drug washout, taking about 3 to 4 days for regrowth to occur. At higher extracellular concentrations (1 $\mu$g/ml), azithromycin is bactericidal regardless of test strain, and this effect is either very slowly reversible or completely irreversible, again dependent on test strain, for at least 4 days after drug washout. The very slowly reversible activity of azithromycin is probably due to its very high intracellular concentrations and slow drug efflux after extracellular drug removal. Clarithromycin is generally no more active than erythromycin in the cell infection model (7). Thus within the macrolide/azalide group, azithromycin intracellular activity is far superior to that of either clarithromycin or erythromycin.

Several new ketolide compounds have good activity against *L. pneumophila* in the intracellular infection model. Telithromycin (HMR3647) is as about as active as erythromycin in the intracellular infection model, while ABT-773 is substantially more active than erythromycin or clarithromycin, and almost as active as azithromycin (7).

Most licensed quinolone antimicrobial agents are more active against intracellular *L. pneumophila* than is erythromycin. In particular, levofloxacin, trovafloxacin, and sparfloxacin are all quite active in the intracellular infection model (9–11). Ciprofloxacin is slightly less active than is levofloxacin. These agents are bactericidal in their activity, which is concentration dependent. In the United States, trovafloxacin is the most active currently licensed and available quinolone agent. However, because of the potential for severe liver toxicity this drug should probably not be used for the treatment of Legionnaires' disease. Levofloxacin is highly active against the bacterium, usually being about as active as azithromycin.

## ANTIMICROBIAL EFFICACY IN THE GUINEA PIG MODEL OF *L. PNEUMOPHILA* PNEUMONIA

The guinea pig model of *L. pneumophila* pneumonia is a very reliable predictor of drug efficacy for the treatment of Legionnaires' disease (5). Data available from the model include bacterial clearance rates, crude mortality, weight and temperature responses, and tissue histopathology. This model can easily discriminate between those drugs that are reversibly inhibitory and those that are bactericidal in the cell culture model when responses other than mortality are considered. In this model, erythromycin therapy results in survival rates that are the same for azithromycin or active quinolone antimicrobial agents. However, 5 to 7 days after the end of erythromycin therapy, a significant number of animals have persistent *L. pneumophila* bacteria in their lungs, and extensive residual lung inflammation. This is in contrast to the findings with azithromycin, in which residual lung bacteria are unusual, and for which residual lung inflammation is markedly less than in the erythromycin-treated animals. The same differences can be observed between erythromycin and levofloxacin therapy, although the degree of lung inflammation and residual bacterial counts are intermediate between azithromycin and erythromycin treatments. The dramatic reduction in lung inflammation in azithromycin-treated animals may be due to antiinflammatory properties of the drug that are separate from its effects on the intracellular *L. pneumophila* bacteria.

## HUMAN STUDIES

No adequately powered prospective comparative studies of the treatment of Legionnaires' disease have been published or presumably performed (3, 4). A number of obstacles have prevented such studies, including the great cost of diagnostic testing for Legionnaires' disease, the relative rarity of the disease, and the usually low mortality in most community-acquired cases of the disease. A battery of diagnostic tests for Legionnaires' disease usually costs more than $500, especially when the administrative and logistic costs of conducting a study by FDA guidelines are included. Since only about 1 to 2% of adults with pneumonia requiring hospitalization have Legionnaires' disease, and since there are no good clinical discriminative indicators of the disease, many hundreds of patients with pneumonia have to be screened to find only a handful of cases. Study of several hundred cases of community-acquired Legionnaires' disease is required to accurately determine differential antimicrobial agent activity. This means that at least 10,000 patients with community-acquired pneumonia need to be studied to determine relative antimicrobial efficacies for Legionnaires' disease, requiring a study budget of at least $5,000,000, and a multiyear, multinational study.

A number of small uncontrolled, or underpowered controlled studies of the treatment of Legionnaires' disease exist. Since in most studies the expected outcome is good, with overall fatality rates of <10% and cure rates >80%, it is difficult to interpret the existing studies as anything but anecdotal. These studies have shown that small numbers of patients with Legionnaires' disease have responded adequately to erythromycin, tetracycline, azithromycin, dirithromycin, clarithromycin, pefloxacin, ciprofloxacin, grepafloxacin, sparfloxacin, trovafloxacin, and levofloxacin. One retrospective study appears to show that pefloxacin therapy may be superior to erythromycin therapy for very severe Legionnaires' disease, which would correlate with the superior activity of pefloxacin in animal and cell models of infection (2).

In the absence of adequately sized human studies, decisions about potential antimicrobial efficacy for Legionnaires' disease must be made on the basis of experimental animal and cell culture studies. As noted above, erythromycin is relatively poorly active against *L. pneumophila* in cell culture and animal model studies. The superior drugs are azithromycin, levofloxacin, and some of the newer quinolone antimicrobial agents. There are in addition a number of quinolone antimicrobial agents possessing extraordinary activity against *L. pneumophila* in these model systems. Unfortunately all of the extraordinarily active quinolone agents, such as sparfloxacin and trovafloxacin, have associated significant toxicity, prohibiting their use.

The clinical implications of use of antimicrobial agents with experimental activity superior to erythromycin are unknown. Here considerations of risk versus potential benefit are key. Erythromycin, while usually a nontoxic agent, has considerable gastrointestinal toxicity, such that up to 50% of outpatients never complete a prescribed dose of the drug. In addition, erythromycin can cause serious cardiac arrhythmias, venous irritation, transient deafness, and hepatitis. The toxicity profile of azithromycin or levofloxacin is not more severe than that of erythromycin, and in fact these drugs may be tolerated better than erythromycin by many patients. In balance, the theoretical benefit of either azithromycin or levofloxacin far outweighs the potential risks of giving these drugs rather than erythromycin. The only reason to give erythromycin for Legionnaires' disease is an economic one, except for those patients who have significant side effects caused by both azithromycin or levofloxacin. Ciprofloxacin is a reasonable alternative to levofloxacin for use in regions where neither azithromycin or levofloxacin are available.

## THERAPY RECOMMENDATIONS

Recommendations for therapy are based on the severity of pneumonia and immunocompromise of the patient (Table 1). This is because the fatality rate is higher in those with more severe pneumonia and in those who are immunocompromised. Since previously healthy patients with mild Legionnaires' disease not requiring hospitalization will likely do well with any of the specific therapies, the main considerations are cost and patient tolerance of the drug. Severely ill patients probably need intravenously administered antimicrobial agents, at least for the first sev-

**TABLE 1** Preferred therapy for Legionnaires' disease

| Clinical condition | 1st Choices | Dosage[a] | 2nd Choices | Dosage[a] |
|---|---|---|---|---|
| Mild pneumonia, not immunocompromised, outpatient | Erythromycin | 500 mg 4×/d for 14 to 21 d | | |
| | OR Doxycycline | 200 mg load, then 100 mg 2×/d for 14 to 21 d | | |
| | OR Azithromycin | 500 mg 1×/d for 3 to 5 d | | |
| | OR Levofloxacin | 500 mg 1×/d for 7 to 10 d | | |
| | OR Ciprofloxacin | 500 mg 2×/d for 7 to 10 d | | |
| | OR Clarithromycin | 500 mg 2×/d for 14 to 21 d | | |
| Hospitalized with pneumonia or immunocompromised | Azithromycin | 500 mg 1×/d for 7 to 10 d | Ciprofloxacin | 750 mg 2×/d for 14 d |
| | OR Levofloxacin | 500 mg 1×/d for 10 to 14 d | Erythromycin PLUS Rifampin | 750 to 1,000 mg 4×/d for 21 d 600 mg 2×/d for 5 d |

[a] Dosage adjustments have to be made for renal insufficiency for some of these drugs. Therapy duration may need to be considerably longer for patients with lung abscesses, empyema, endocarditis, or extrathoracic infection. d, day.

eral days of therapy. Since some of the more active drugs are not available in parenteral form in some countries, erythromycin is retained as a second choice for severely ill patients, in combination with rifampin. There is little good evidence that addition of rifampin is beneficial for those receiving azithromycin, levofloxacin, or ciprofloxacin, and there is potential for undesirable toxicities or side effects from addition of rifampin.

## REFERENCES

1. **Barker, J., H. Scaife, and M. R. Brown.** 1995. Intraphagocytic growth induces an antibiotic-resistant phenotype of *Legionella pneumophila. Antimicrob. Agents Chemother.* **39:**2684–2688.

2. **Dournon, E., C. Mayaud, M. Wolff, B. Schlemmer, D. Samuel, J. P. Sollet, and P. Levasseur-Rajagopalan.** 1990. Comparison of the activity of three antibiotic regimens in severe Legionnaires' disease. *J. Antimicrob. Chemother.* **26**(Suppl. B)**:**129–139.

3. **Edelstein, P. H.** 1995. Antimicrobial chemotherapy for legionnaires' disease: a review. *Clin. Infect. Dis.* **21:**S265–S276.

4. **Edelstein, P. H.** 1998. Antimicrobial chemotherapy for Legionnaires disease: time for a change. *Ann. Intern. Med.* **129:**328–330.

5. **Edelstein, P. H.** 1999. The guinea-pig model of Legionnaires' disease, p. 303–314. *In* O. Zak and M. A. Sande (ed.), *Handbook of Animal Models of Infection.* Academic Press, London, United Kingdom.

6. **Edelstein, P. H., K. Calarco, and V. K. Yasui.** 1984. Antimicrobial therapy of experimentally induced Legionnaires' disease in guinea pigs. *Am. Rev. Respir. Dis.* **130:**849–856.

7. **Edelstein, P. H., and M. A. Edelstein.** 1999. In vitro activity of the ketolide HMR 3647 (RU 6647) for Legionella spp., its pharmacokinetics in guinea pigs, and use of the drug to treat guinea pigs with Legionella pneumophila pneumonia. *Antimicrob. Agents Chemother.* **43:**90–95.

8. **Edelstein, P. H., and M. A. C. Edelstein.** 1991. In vitro activity of azithromycin against

clinical isolates of *Legionella* species. *Antimicrob. Agents Chemother.* **35:**180–181.

9. **Edelstein, P. H., M. A. C. Edelstein, K. H. Lehr, and J. Ren.** 1996. In-vitro activity of levofloxacin against clinical isolates of *Legionella* spp, its pharmacokinetics in guinea pigs, and use in experimental *Legionella pneumophila* pneumonia. *J. Antimicrob. Chemother.* **37:**117–126.

10. **Edelstein, P. H., M. A. C. Edelstein, J. J. Ren, R. Polzer, and R. P. Gladue.** 1996. Activity of trovafloxacin (cp-99,219) against *Legionella* isolates: in-vitro activity, intracellular accumulation and killing in macrophages, and pharmacokinetics and treatment of guinea-pig with *L. pneumophila* pneumonia. *Antimicrob. Agents Chemother.* **40:**314–319.

11. **Edelstein, P. H., M. A. C. Edelstein, J. Weidenfeld, and M. B. Dorr.** 1990. In vitro activity of sparfloxacin (CI-978; AT-4140) for clinical *Legionella* isolates, pharmacokinetics in guinea pigs, and use to treat guinea pigs with *L. pneumophila* pneumonia. *Antimicrob. Agents Chemother.* **34:**2122–2127.

12. **Fraser, D. W., T. R. Tsai, W. Orenstein, W. E. Parkin, H. J. Beecham, R. G. Sharrar, J. Harris, G. F. Mallison, S. M. Martin, J. E.** McDade, C. C. Shepard, and P. S. Brachman. 1977. Legionnaires' disease: description of an epidemic of pneumonia. *N. Engl. J. Med.* **297:**1189–1197.

13. **Kirby, B. D., K. M. Snyder, R. D. Meyer, and S. M. Finegold.** 1980. Legionnaires' disease: report of sixty-five nosocomially acquired cases and review of the literature. *Medicine* (Baltimore) **59:**188–205.

14. **Kunishima, H., H. Takemura, H. Yamamoto, K. Kanemitsu, and J. Shimada.** 2000. Evaluation of the activity of antimicrobial agents against *Legionella pneumophila* multiplying in human monocytic cell line, THP-1, and an alveolar cell line, A549. *J. Infect. Chemother.* **6:**206–210.

15. **Sturgill-Koszycki, S., and M. S. Swanson.** 2000. *Legionella pneumophila* replication vacuoles mature into acidic, endocytic organelles. *J. Exp. Med.* **192:**1261–1272.

16. **Swanson, M. S., and B. K. Hammer.** 2000. *Legionella pneumophila* pathogenesis: a fateful journey from amoebae to macrophages. *Annu. Rev. Microbiol.* **54:**567–613.

17. **Tulkens, P. M.** 1991. Intracellular distribution and activity of antibiotics. *Eur. J. Clin. Microbiol. Infect. Dis.* **10:**100–106.

# CLINICAL VALIDATION
## OF DIAGNOSIS OF
## *LEGIONELLA* INFECTIONS

*Anneke van der Zee, Harold Verbakel,*
*Caroline de Jong, Raymond Pot, Marcel Peeters,*
*Joop Schellekens, and Anneke Bergmans*

# 33

*Legionella pneumophila* is the etiologic agent of Legionnaires' disease, which is a very serious illness with pneumonia and a mortality of 15 to 20% (1, 4). In addition to *L. pneumophila*, more than 40 other *Legionella* spp. are known (here designated non-*L. pneumophila* species), of which several species have been shown to be pathogenic for humans (3).

A rapid diagnosis is highly important since legionellosis has a poor prognosis when treatment starts late. To improve diagnosis of *Legionella* infections, we designed a novel PCR to specifically amplify all *Legionella* DNA. Discrimination between *L. pneumophila* and non-*L. pneumophila* species was established by means of specific probes.

The performance of the PCR was compared with those of culture, serology, and urine antigen detection in patients suspected to suffer from legionellosis.

The *Legionella* species-specific primer set included LEG1 and LEG2; they were derived

from the 16S rRNA gene and used to amplify a 200-bp DNA fragment. Specific probes LPN and LSPP were used for discrimination of, respectively, *L. pneumophila* and non-*L. pneumophila* species (Fig. 1). To be able to detect inhibition of amplification, an internal control was added to each reaction resulting in amplification of a 150-bp DNA fragment when no inhibition was present in the clinical sample.

Besides PCR, serology, culture, and urine antigen detection was performed. Serology was carried out by measuring agglutinating antibodies of *L. pneumophila* in serial dilutions of acute and reconvalescent serum (2). Culturing was done on buffered charcoal-yeast extract agar plates. Urine antigen detection was performed with Binax enzyme immunoassay.

## SENSITIVITY AND SPECIFICITY OF PCR

The sensitivity of PCR was determined by spiking bacteria in negative clinical material. The lower detection limit was found to be at least 0.1 CFU (Fig. 2). The specificity of the PCR was investigated using a range of different bacteria, among which were *Pseudomonas aeruginosa*, *Acinetobacter baumannii*, and *Lactobacillus casei*, which are most closely related to

*Anneke van der Zee, Harold Verbakel, Caroline de Jong, Raymond Pot, Marcel Peeters, and Anneke Bergmans* Laboratory of Molecular Microbiology, St. Elisabeth Hospital, P.O. Box 747, 5000AS Tilburg, The Netherlands. *Joop Schellekens* National Institute of Public Health and Environment, P.O. Box 1, 3720 BA Bilthoven, The Netherlands.

*Legionella*, Edited by Reinhard Marre et al.
© 2002 ASM Press, Washington, D.C.

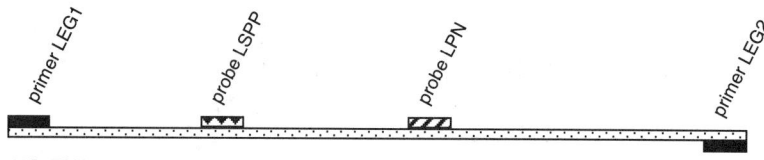

16S rRNA gene

**FIGURE 1** Schematic presentation of the PCR/probe procedure. LEG1: 5'-TACCTACCCTTGACATACAGTG-3', LEG2: 5'-CTTCCTCCGGTTTGTCAC-3', LPN-B: 5'-ATGTGATGGTGGGGACTCT 3', LSPP-B: 5'-CGTAACGAGCGCAACCC-3'.

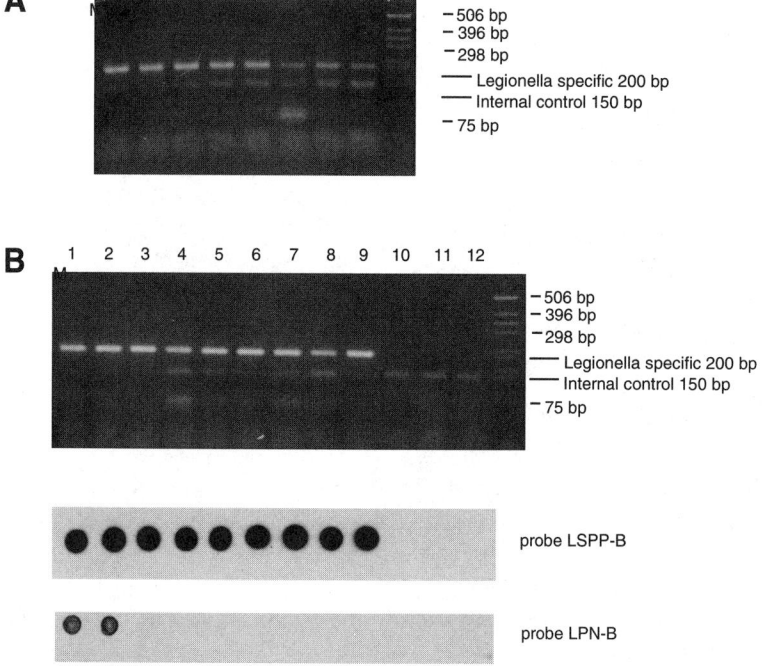

**FIGURE 2** (A) The sensitivity of PCR detection of non-*L. pneumophila*. Two-fold dilutions of bacterial cells were used in PCR after processing in addition to internal control. Lanes 1 to 8 correspond to a range of 10 to .08 *L. pneumophila* cells per reaction. The sizes of amplified fragments are indicated on the right. Below, PCR products are hybridized to probe LPN-B. (B) The specificity of the PCR detection of non-*L. pneumophila*. PCR was performed on the equivalent of 100 cells of two different clinical isolates of *L. pneumophila* (lanes 1, 2), *L. tucsoniensis* (lane 3), *L. birminghamiensis* (lane 4), *L. haekeliae* (lane 5), *L. brunensis* (lane 6), *L. jordanis* (lane 7), *L. jamestowniensis* (lane 8), *L. bozemannii* (lane 9), *Acinetobacter baumannii* (lane 10), *Lactobacillus casei* (lane 11), and *Pseudomonas aeruginosa* (lane 12). Below, PCR products are hybridized to probe LSPP-B at 60°C, and to probe LPN-B at 61°C.

*Legionella.* None of these bacteria yielded a positive result in PCR (Fig. 2).

## CLINICAL PERFORMANCE OF PCR

A total of 208 samples from 208 patients clinically suspected of legionellosis were subjected to the *Legionella* PCR/probe procedure. Samples consisted of sputum or bronchalveolar lavage. A total of 79 of the 208 samples (38%) were positive in the *Legionella* PCR: in 32 (15%) samples, the amplified product only hybridized with the *Legionella* genus probe but did not hybridize with the probe specific for *L. pneumophila*; in 47 cases (23%), the amplified product hybridized also with the *L. pneumophila*-specific probe.

## THE VALUE OF PCR DETECTION OF L. PNEUMOPHILA

In 34 of 208 patients, the maximum diagnostic effort had been done, i.e., PCR/probe, culture, urine antigen assay, and serology in reconvalescence serum.

Comparison of results of PCR, serology, culture, and urine antigen detection revealed that PCR-based detection of *L. pneumophila*, and serology in reconvalescent serum, yielded 2.8-fold more positives than *Legionella* culture. The number of urine antigen positives was slightly lower but comparable with the number of PCR and serology positives. When diagnostic methods were pairwise compared with PCR in larger patient groups ($n = 176$, $n = 77$, and $n = 45$ for culture, urine antigens, and serology, respectively), similar results were found.

Relative sensitivities of diagnostic methods were calculated as follows: The relative sensitivity of an assay was defined as the percentage positives in patients in whom at least two of three other assays were positive (Table 1). The relative specificity of an assay was defined as the percentage negatives in patients in whom all other three assays were negative. The relative sensitivity of the PCR/probe assay resembles that of serology in reconvalescence serum (92%). The relative sensitivity of urine antigen detection and culture were respectively 85 and 26%.

Relative specificities are 100% for culture and urine antigen tests, and 94% for the PCR/probe assay and serology in reconvalescence serum.

## PCR DETECTION OF NON-L. PNEUMOPHILA SPECIES

A total of 32 of the 208 samples were non-*L. pneumophila*-positive. Five PCR products were sequenced and identified as *L. dumoffii*, *L. jamestowniensis*, *L. worsliensis*, LLAP1, and LLAP6. In all 32 cases, culture and urine antigen detection were negative. In seven cases, serology in reconvalesence serum had been done, and four patients were positive. One patient was confirmed with a positive DFA test for *Legionella*, and nine patients had strongly indicative clinical symptoms.

## DISCUSSION

PCR may provide an important contribution to an early diagnosis of legionellosis. PCR is the only method suitable to diagnose non-*L. pneumophila* infections. Since 40% of PCR-positive samples were non-*L. pneumophila*, the clinical relevancy of non-*L. pneumophila* infections should be further investigated. Future

**TABLE 1** Relative sensitivities and specificities of diagnostic methods

| Test | No. (%) positive | Relative sensitivity (%) (no. positive/no. positive in ≥ 2 other assays) | Relative specificity (%) (no. negative/ no. negative in 3 other assays) |
|---|---|---|---|
| PCR | 15 (44) | 92 (12/13) | 94 (17/18) |
| Culture | 4 (12) | 26 (4/17) | 100 (17/17) |
| Urine antigen detection | 13 (38) | 85 (11/13) | 100 (17/17) |
| Serology in reconvalescence serum | 15 (44) | 92 (12/13) | 94 (17/18) |

studies could include sequencing of non-*L. pneumophila* PCR products to get an impression of the distribution of *Legionella* species in patient samples.

## REFERENCES

1. **Ching, W. T. W., and R. D. Meyer.** 1987. *Legionella* infections. *Infect. Dis. Clin. N. Am.* **1:** 595–614.

2. **Harrison, T. G., and A. G. Taylor.** 1988. The diagnosis of legionnaires' disease by estimation of antibody levels, p. 113–136. *In* T. G. Harrison and A. G. Taylor (ed.), *A Laboratory Manual for Legionella.* John Wiley & Sons Ltd., New York, N.Y.

3. **Marston, B., J. F. Plouffe, R. F. Breiman, T. M. File, Jr., R. F. Benson, M. Moyenudden, W. L. Thacker, K.-H. Wong, S. Skelton, B. Hackman, S. J. Salstrom, J. M. Barbaree, and the Community-Based Pneumonia Incidence Study Group.** 1993. Preliminary findings of a community-based pneumonia incidence study, p. 36–37. *In* J. M. Barbaree, R. F. Breiman, and A. P. Dufour (ed.), *Legionella: Current Status and Emerging Perspectives.* American Society for Microbiology, Washington, D.C.

4. **Plouffe, J. F., T. M. File, R. F. Breiman, B. A. Hackman, S. J. Salstrom, B. J. Marston, B. S. Fields, and the Community-Based Pneumonia Incidence Study Group.** 1995. Reevaluation of the definition of Legionaires disease: use of the urinary antigen assay. *Clin. Infect. Dis.* **20:**1286–1291.

# *LEGIONELLA* PNEUMONIA: THREE CASES IN AN ONCOLOGICAL HOSPITAL

Margherita Giglio, Marco Scuri,
Rita Passerini, and Maria Teresa Sandri

# 34

*Legionella pneumophila* is known as an important cause of nosocomial pneumonia (8). The hospitalized population is at high risk of acquiring legionellosis, and this is especially true for patients with impaired immunity (7). In fact, many nosocomial outbreaks have been described all over the world (2, 9), and in most of the cases the hospital hot water distribution system was colonized (5).

Our hospital is a referral center for oncological care with 200 beds. In January 1999, the first case of pneumonia caused by *L. pneumophila* was diagnosed. The patient was a 47-year-old woman with malignant non-Hodgkin lymphoma, hospitalized for more than 10 days, treated with high-dose chemotherapy. During treatment she developed a pneumonia, with a positive urinary *Legionella* antigen test (Biotest enzyme immunoassay urinary *Legionella* antigen). Despite therapy with macrolides and fluoroquinolones, the patient died from respiratory failure 1 week after the diagnosis.

Immediately after the detection of the first case of *Legionella* pneumonia, the water distribution system was sampled in several sites, including the shower in the patient's room, the intake from the municipal water supply, the water storage tank, and some distant outlets. Sampling from the air-conditioning system was also performed. Environmental and patient-care measures were adopted in response to this first case: the measures consisted of substituting all the shower heads and the tap nebulizers in all the hospital bathrooms, keeping elevated (58°C) hot water temperatures at the outlet, and using sterile water to fill in and rinse all the nebulization devices and nasogastric tubes. Moreover, an active surveillance (by looking for *Legionella* soluble antigen) in both patients and staff was instituted.

To isolate the microorganism, the water samples were concentrated by filtration and inoculated onto buffered charcoal-yeast extract supplemented with alpha-ketoglutarate, with and without antimicrobial agent (4). Subtyping was performed with the Oxoid antisera. *L. pneumophila* subtype 2-14 was isolated from all the water samples, except those from the incoming municipal water supply, while the samples of the air-conditioning system were negative.

To eradicate the microorganism from the hot water distribution system, we planned a

*Margherita Giglio* European Institute of Oncology, Milan, Italy. *Marco Scuri* Technical Service, European Institute of Oncology, Milan, Italy. *Rita Passerini and Maria Teresa Sandri* Deptartment of Pathology and Laboratory Medicine, European Institute of Oncology, Milan, Italy.

*Legionella*, Edited by Reinhard Marre et al.
© 2002 ASM Press, Washington, D.C.

decontamination with the superheat and flush method (6). This was the only procedure we could follow because our Institute is provided with its own drained water depuration system (hence we are not connected to the municipal drainage) precluding a hyperchlorination method. In the meantime, in March 1999, a second case was diagnosed, again by the detection of the soluble antigen in the patient's urine. The patient was a 59-year-old woman with high-risk breast carcinoma being treated with high-dose chemotherapy. A therapy with macrolides and fluoroquinolones was effective in curing the patient.

By the beginning of April 1999, the first decontamination of the water system was performed and was followed by three additional interventions in June 1999, February 2000, and November 2000, with various results (Fig. 1). After each intervention, the water system was monitored for *Legionella* for an extended time to check the water concentration of the microorganism and to prevent the recurrence of nosocomial transmission. It can be seen, however, that decontamination was only effective in the short term; after a few months the water system was colonized again. Accordingly, the control of *Legionella* contamination on a long-term basis requires other measures.

A key point to emphasize is that the control of nosocomial Legionnaires' disease in large institutions is difficult and requires the strict cooperation of professionals with different areas of expertise, including maintenance and infection control staff, nurses, and physicians. Our experience documents that the awareness of the problem and the coordination of multiple efforts are crucial in at least limiting the risk of outbreaks.

It is also remarkable that the diagnosis has always been performed by the detection of the urinary *Legionella* antigen, although the colonizing subtype was of the serogroup 2-14.

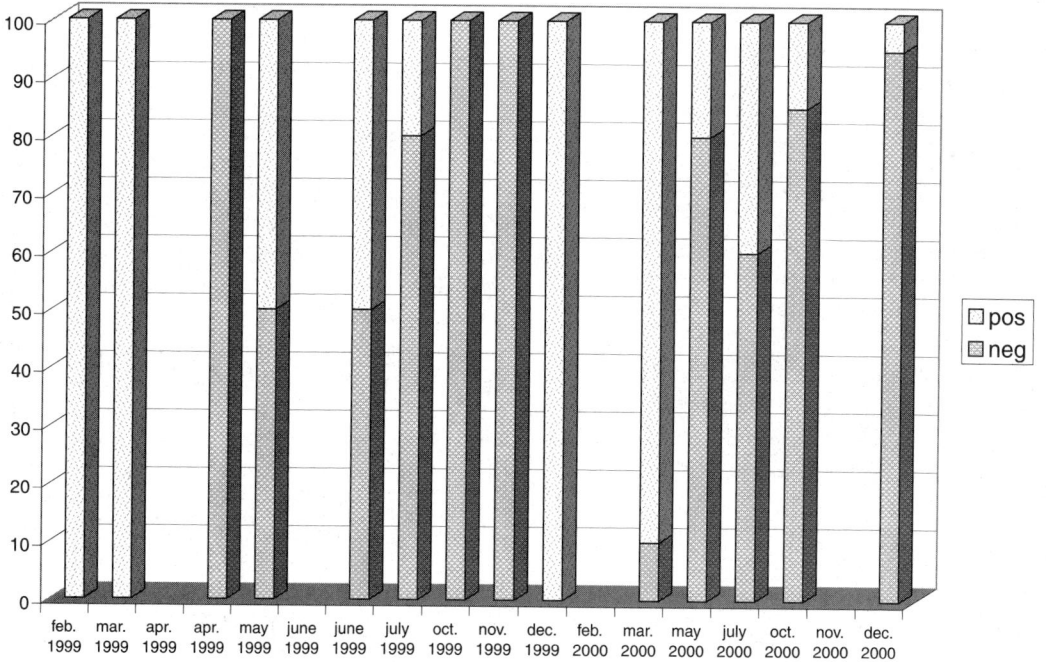

**FIGURE 1** Percentage of positive results in water distribution system samples.

This confirms the value of the enzyme immunoassay in diagnosing infection caused by non-serogroup 1 *Legionella*, as previously reported (3).

Despite the decontamination, the strict environmental monitoring, and the measures adopted, at the beginning of November 2000 a third case was detected. The patient was a 54-year-old man with multiple myeloma who was admitted on October 14 for a severe renal failure (creatinine, 891.9 $\mu$mol/liter). He had received appropriate chemotherapy and his general condition was improving, but at the end of the month, he developed *Legionella* pneumonia, as documented by a positive urinary *Legionella* antigen. Despite macrolide and fluoroquinolone treatment, the patient died 5 days later. The flush and heat decontamination method is not effective in eradicating *L. pneumophila* from the hot water distribution system, and it is therefore mandatory to keep surveillance measures for early diagnosis and prompt treatment of possible new cases (1). Major causes of decontamination failure may be both the complexity of the hot water distribution system whereby it can be difficult to reach all the distal tubes, and the kind of patients in our hospital who are susceptible to infection even at low concentrations of *Legionella*.

## REFERENCES

1. **Ezzeddine, H., C. Van Ossel, M. Delmee, and C. Wauters.** 1989. *Legionella* spp. in a hospital hot water system: effect of control measures. *J. Hosp. Infect.* **13**:121–131.
2. **Fallon, R. J.** 1980. Nosocomial infection with *Legionella pneumophila. J. Hosp. Infect.* **1**:299–305.
3. **Harrison, T., S. Uldum, S. Alexiou-Daniel, J. Bangsborg, S. Bernander, V. Drasar, J. Etienne, J. Helbig, D. Lindsay, I. Lochman, T. Marquez, F. de Ory, I. Tartakovskii, G. Wewalka, and F. Fehrenbach.** 1998. A multicenter evaluation of the Biotest legionella urinary antigen EIA. *Clin. Microbiol. Infect.* **4**:359–365.
4. **Kusnetov, J. M., H. R. Jousimiens Somer, A. I. Nevalainen, and P. J. Martikainen.** 1994. Isolation of *Legionella* from water samples using various culture methods. *J. Appl. Bacteriol.* **76**:155–162.
5. **Lepine, L. A., D. B. Jernigan, J. C. Butler, J. M. Pruckler, R. F. Benson, G. Kim, J. L. Hadler, M. L. Cartter, and B. S. Fields.** 1998. A recurrent outbreak of nosocomial Legionnaires' disease detected by urinary antigen testing: evidence for long-term colonization of a hospital plumbing system. *Infect. Control Hosp. Epidemiol.* **19**:905–910.
6. **Muraca, P. V., V. Yu, and A. Goetz.** 1990. Disinfection of water distribution systems for legionella: a review of application procedures and methodologies. *Infect. Control Hosp. Epidemiol.* **11**:79–88.
7. **Pedro Botet, M. L., M. Sabria-Leal, N. Sopena, J. M. Manterola, J. Morera, R. Blavia, E. Padilla, L. Matas, and J. M. Gimeno.** 1998. Role of immunosuppression in the evolution of legionnaires' disease. *Clin. Infect. Dis.* **26**:14–19.
8. **Stout, J. E., and V. L. Yu.** 1997. Legionellosis. *N. Engl. J. Med.* **337**:682–687.
9. **Vincent-Houdek, M., H. L. Muytjens, G. P. Bongaerts, and R. J. Van Ketel.** 1993. *Legionella* monitoring: a continuing story of nosocomial infection prevention. *J. Hosp. Infect.* **25**:117–124.

# HUMAN LEUKOCYTE ANTIGEN TYPING IN *LEGIONELLA*-POSITIVE TRANSPLANT PATIENTS

Marcela Jaresova, Nina Bendukidze, Eva Ivaskova,
Ilja Striz, Ivo Hlozanek, Milan Hatala,
Pavel Totusek, and Zdenek Kocmoud

## 35

Since the original description of *Legionella* in 1976, the frequency of unexpected outbreaks of legionellosis accompanied by a high mortality rate has been gradually increasing. *Legionella* is considered to be a very important infectious agent, causing an atypical pneumonia. It is well known that total mortality by *Legionella pneumophila* usually reaches 19% (5), but mortality of nearly 80% can be expected in immunosuppressed persons (7). The detection of *L. pneumophila* infection was routinely established in our laboratories after the outbreak of nosocomial Legionnaires' disease (*L. pneumophila* serogroup 3) at Transplant Center of the Institute for Clinical and Experimental Medicine in 1998. The aim of the current study was to compare HLA (human leukocyte antigen) frequency and HLA haplotype frequency in *Legionella*-positive patients with frequencies in healthy individuals from a local panel (control group).

Sputum, bronchoalveolar lavage (BAL), or urine obtained from 114 patients after solid organ (heart, kidney, liver, pancreas) transplantation were examined for the presence of *Legionella* by using the culture method (sputum, BAL), and the direct fluorescent-antibody assay method (sputum, BAL), and by the detection of urinary antigen (urine) during the 4 months after transplantation. PCR (sputum, BAL) was used in only five cases. All examined patients developed either pneumonia, febrility, or diarrhea.

A buffered charcoal-yeast extract medium (OXOID) was the culture method used in parallel with BMPA and GVPC selective supplements. *Legionella* serotypes were determined by using microagglutination test (National *Legionella* Reference Laboratory, Vyskov, V. Drasar). The monoclonal antibody of MONOFLUO *L. pneumophila* IFA Test Kit (Sanofi-Pasteur, Redmond, Calif.) was used for the direct fluorescent-antibody assay method. The urinary antigen was detected by using *Legionella* Urin Antigen enzyme immunoassay (Biotest, Dreieich, Germany). PCR was performed at The National Institute of Public Health, Prague (D. Hulinska) as semi-nested PCR by using Lmip primers (9) and

*Marcela Jaresova* Department of Clinical Immunology, Institute for Clinical and Experimental Medicine, Prague 4, 140 21, Czech Republic. *Nina Bendukidze, Eva Ivaskova, and Ilja Striz* Department of Immunology, Institute for Clinical and Experimental Medicine, Prague 4, 140 21, Czech Republic. *Ivo Hlozanek, Milan Hatala, and Pavel Totusek* Clinical Laboratories, Institute for Clinical and Experimental Medicine, Prague 4, 140 21, Czech Republic. *Zdenek Kocmoud* Department of Hygienic Microbiology, Regional Centre of Hygiene, Ceske Budejovice, 370 71, Czech Republic.

*Legionella*, Edited by Reinhard Marre et al.
© 2002 ASM Press, Washington, D.C.

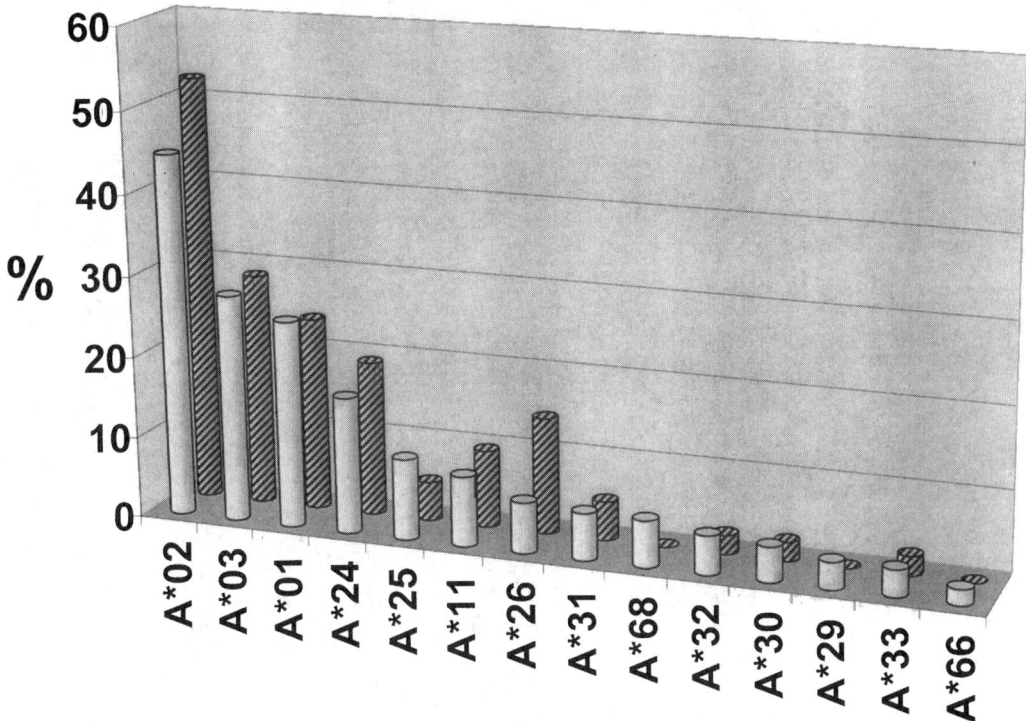

**FIGURE 1** HLA-A antigen frequency. ▨, control group; ▨, *Legionella*-positive patients.

M-Mix QIAGEN. Isolation of DNA was done using the salt-out method or QIAamp Tissue Kit QIAGEN.

HLA class I was typed in blood of 42 (42 of 114) *Legionella*-positive patients after heart, kidney, liver, or pancreas transplantation and in 205 healthy subjects (control group, local panel) by microlymphocytotoxic test or by PCR-SSP using Dynal kits (2). HLA class II was typed by PCR-SSOP (reverse hybridization) using INNO-LIPA kits or PCR-SSP with Dynal kits (2).

The test for comparison of a relative frequency (*Legionella*-positive patients) with the underlying parameter (control group) was used to rate statistically significant differences for antigen frequency. Software Arlequin (11) was used to calculate genetic frequencies of antigens and haplotypes and to rate differences in frequencies between both groups.

All patients after transplantation were treated with ciprofloxacin starting the first day after surgery. Despite this treatment, pneumonia, diarrhea, or febrility occurred in some patients. *Legionella* infection was found by DFA in 73 (73 of 114) cases, by PCR in 4 (4 of 5) cases, and by culture in 2 (2 of 114) cases only. *L. pneumophila* serogroup 3 was determined in both positive cultures. On the other hand, detection of urinary antigen was negative in all 114 cases.

Differences were found in HLA-A antigen frequencies (Fig. 1) and HLA-B antigen frequencies (Fig. 2) between *Legionella*-positive patients and a control group. Differences were statistically significant for antigens A★26, B★13, and B★39 (Table 1).

We did not detect any differences in HLA class II antigen frequencies in these groups. Differences in HLA A-B haplotypes and HLA

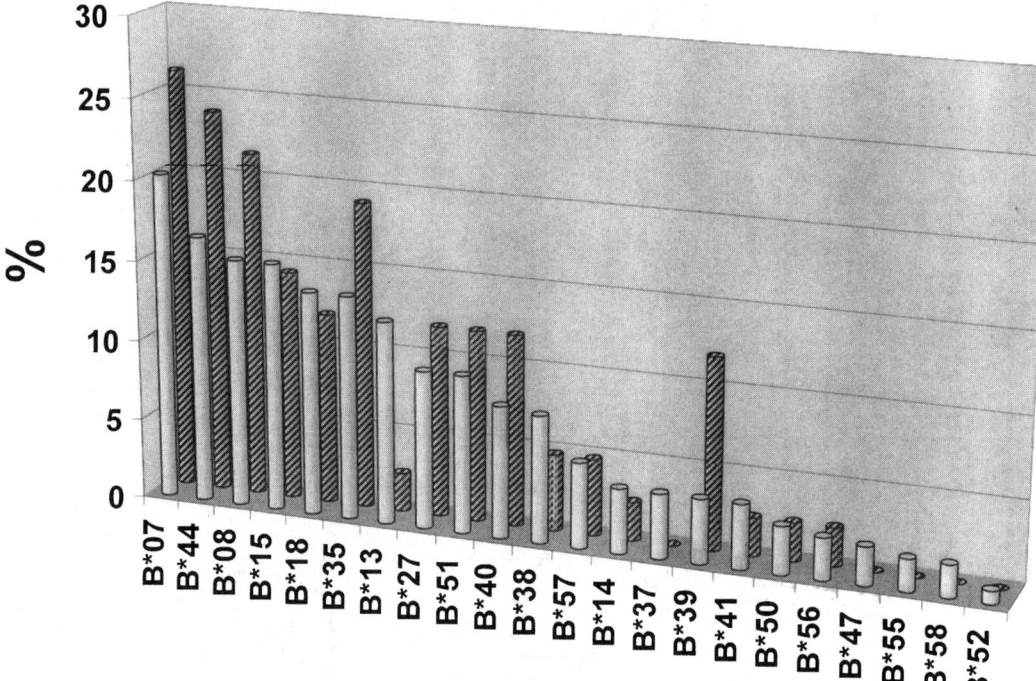

**FIGURE 2** HLA-B antigen frequency. ▨, control group; ▨, *Legionella*-positive patients.

A-B-DR haplotypes were not statistically significant between healthy individuals and *Legionella*-positive patients ($P > 0.05$).

Several published reports suggest that natural resistance or susceptibility to infection with *Legionella* might be genetically determined. Multiplication of *L. pneumophila* in macrophages of guinea pigs and inbred mice revealed that murine macrophages from most inbred strains are nonpermissive to intracellular replication of *Legionella* (1) and that the permissiveness is controlled by the single autosomal gene designated *lgn1* and mapped in to Chr 13, the nonpermissiveness having been dominant over permissiveness. This portion of mouse Chr 13 is homologous to the distal portion of human Chr5 (5q11-5q13), suggesting a possible location of a human LGN1 homolog (4). Analysis of genetically determined resistance to *Legionella* infection (4) indicates that in the human genome, a human version of the *lgn1* gene can be identified.

The association between some diseases, e.g., infection with *Mycobacterium tuberculosis*

**TABLE 1** Comparison of antigen frequency: the test for comparison of a relative frequency with the underlying parameter

| HLA antigen | Antigen frequency (%) | | P value | Statistically significant |
| --- | --- | --- | --- | --- |
| | Control group (n = 205) | *Legionella*-positive patients (n = 42) | | |
| A★26 | 6.24 | 14.28 | 0.0401 | Yes |
| B★13 | 12.60 | 2.38 | 0.0478 | Yes |
| B★39 | 4.00 | 11.90 | 0.0128 | Yes |

(10), *Mycobacterium avium* complex (8), *Neisseria meningitidis* (6), and *Chlamydia trachomatis* (3), and the HLA complex has already been described.

We found statistically significant differences in HLA class I antigen frequencies between *Legionella*-positive patients and a control group. The higher frequency of HLA-A★26 and HLA-B★39 and lower frequency of HLA-B★13 were detected in *Legionella*-positive patients. The genotype frequencies of these antigens were also significantly different.

Our data suggest that HLA-A★26 and HLA-B★39 antigens might play a role in susceptibility to *L. pneumophila* infection. On the other hand, the antigen HLA-B★13 might affect the resistance to infection with this bacterium.

However, no significant difference in HLA class II antigens and the frequencies of haplotypes HLA A-B and HLA A-B-DR was found between both defined groups. The susceptibility to infection by *L. pneumophila* might be associated with the HLA complex.

## ACKNOWLEDGMENT

This work was supported by GACR no. 310/01/0095.

## REFERENCES

1. **Beckers, M. C., S. Yoshida, K. Morgan, E. Skamene, and P. Gros**. 1995. Natural resistance to infection with *Legionella pneumophila*: chromosomal localization of the Lgn1 susceptibility gene. *Mamm. Genome* **6**:540–545.
2. **Bendukidze, N., I. Hana, and E. Ivaskova**. 1998. Molecular typing of HLA class I and class II for a transplantation programme. *Bone Marrow Transplant.* **4**:31–33.
3. **Cohen, C. R., S. S. Sinei, E. A. Bukusi, J. J. Bwayo, K. K. Holmes, and R. C. Brunham**. 2000. Human leucocyte antigen class II DQ alleles associated with Chlamydia trachomatis tubal infertility. *Obstet. Gynecol.* **95**:72–77.
4. **Dietrich, W. F., D. M. Damron, R. R. Isberg, E. S. Lander, and M. S. Swanson**. 1995. Lgn1, a gene that determines susceptibility to *Legionella pneumophila*, maps to mouse chromosome 13. *Genomics* **26**:443–450.
5. **England, A. C., D. W. Fraser, B. B. Plikaytis, T. F. Tsai, G. Storch, and C. V. Broome**. 1981. Sporadic legionellosis in the United States: the first thousand cases. *Ann. Intern. Med.* **94**:1263–1270.
6. **Holub, M., J. Hobstova, J. Prazak, and P. Pudil**. 1998. Association of class I HLA antigens with invasive meningococcal disease. *Cas Lek Cesk.* **137**:598–600.
7. **Kirby, B. D., K. M. Snyder, R. D. Meyer, and S. M. Finegold**. 1980. Legionnaires' disease: report of sixty-five nosocomially acquired cases and review of the literature. *Medicine* **59**:188–205.
8. **LeBlanc, S. B., E. G. Naik, L. Jacobson, and R. A. Kaslow**. 2000. Association of DRB1★1501 with disseminated Mycobacterium avium complex infection in North American AIDS patients. *Tissue Antigens* **55**:17–23.
9. **Mahbubani, M. H., A. K. Bej, R. Miller, L. Haff, J. DiCesare, and R. M. Atlas**. 1990. Detection of *Legionella* with polymerase chain reaction and gene probe methods. *Mol. Cell. Probes* **4**:175–187.
10. **Rajalingam, R., N. K. Mehra, S. Neolia, R. C. Jain, and J. N. Pande**. 1997. HLA class I profile in Asian Indian patients with pulmonary tuberculosis. *Indian J. Exp. Biol.* **35**:1055–1059.
11. **Schneider, S., J.-M. Kueffer, D. Roessli, and L. Excoffier**. 1997. *A Software for Population Genetic Data Analysis*. Genetics and Biometry Laboratory, University of Geneva, Geneva, Switzerland.

# LEGIONELLA SEROGROUP AND SUBGROUP DISTRIBUTION AMONG PATIENTS WITH LEGIONNAIRES' DISEASE IN DENMARK

*Søren A. Uldum and Jürgen H. Helbig*

# 36

From January 1994 to June 2000, legionellae were isolated by culture from 195 patients with Legionnaires' disease in Denmark. This represents more than 30% of all laboratory-proven cases in this period (4). In this survey we present the serogroup and subgroup distribution of the isolates stratified according to where the patients acquired the infection: in the community (in Denmark) or during hospitalization or during traveling abroad. One patient counts only once, although more than one isolate was obtained from some patients, but we have never isolated more than one serogroup (probably the same strain) from a patient.

The non-*Legionella pneumophila* species of the isolates was determined to species-serogroup with inhouse polyclonal rabbit antisera. All *L. pneumophila* isolates were determined to serogroup and all *L. pneumophila* serogroup 1 isolates were determined to subgroup with the Dresden panel of monoclonal antibodies (1).

Since Legionnaires' disease is a mandatory notifiable disease in Denmark, clinical and epidemiological information was obtained from the notifications for most of the patients. Additional information was obtained from the relevant hospital departments for almost all patients.

## PATIENTS

Of the195 patients, 71 (36.4%) were females and 124 (63.6%) were males. The median age for all patients was 59 years (range, 20 to 92 years); for females the median age was 65 years (range, 20 to 86 years); and for males, 54 years (range, 32 to 92 years). For 24 of the patients, no information was available about dispositions or their health conditions before the infection. Of the remaining 171 patients, 50 (29.2%) were healthy before the infection (group A), 25 (14.6%) were generally healthy but had a smoking/alcohol/drug use or abuse problem (group B), 49 (28.6%) of the patients had an underlying chronic lung/heart/circulatory disease or diabetes, in some instances combined with cigarette smoking or alcohol abuse (group C), 26 (15.2%) of the patients were severely ill and immunocompromised before the infection (e.g., cancer, leukemia, and human immunodeficiency virus patients or those with recent organ transplants) (group

*Søren A. Uldum* Department of Respiratory Infections, Meningitis and STIs, Statens Serum Institut, DK-2300 Copenhagen S, Denmark. *Jürgen H. Helbig* Institute of Medical Microbiology and Hygiene, Technical University Dresden, D-01307 Dresden, Germany.

*Legionella*, Edited by Reinhard Marre et al.
© 2002 ASM Press, Washington, D.C.

E), and 21 (12.3%) of the patients had other physical or mental diseases or disorders (group D). The number of smokers or alcohol abusers is probably higher than recorded. At least 37 (19%) of the 195 patients died with or as a consequence of the infection. Among healthy and generally healthy patients (groups A and B), 49 (65.3%) cases were caused by *L. pneumophila* serogroup 1 subgroup Pontiac. Among the patients with an underlying health condition (groups C, D, and E), 68 (70.8%) cases were caused by non-Pontiac serogroup 1 subgroups or other *L. pneumophila* serogroups or other *Legionella* species.

## SEROGROUP AND SUBGROUP DISTRIBUTION AMONG PATIENT CATEGORIES

Isolates from 190 patients were *L. pneumophila* of which 185 could be assigned to a definitive serogroup or subgroup. Five isolates were non-*L. pneumophila*: one was *L. micdadei*, two were *L. bozemanii*, and two were *L. longbeachae*. Of all the strains, 111 (57%) were *L. pneumophila* serogroup 1, of which 83 (75%) were subgroups belonging to the Pontiac subgroup (Philadelphia, Knoxville, Benidorm, or Allentown/France—all reactive with monoclonal antibody 3/1 of the Dresden panel), and 28 (25%) were non-Pontiac subgroups (OLDA/Oxford or Bellingham). A total of 174 of the patients (all known; Table 1) could be placed in one of the categories: community acquired, 96 cases (55%); hospital acquired, 39 cases (22%); or travel associated, 39 cases (22%), of which 30 patients were from groups A and B. For the remaining 21 patients, there was no or insufficient information (not known; Table 1). The data are presented in Table 1 and graphically summarized in Fig. 1.

## CONCLUSIONS

*L. pneumophila* serogroup 1 subgroups were the most common cause of culture-confirmed Legionnaires' disease in Denmark. However, the serogroup caused only 57% of all cases in Denmark (Pontiac subgroups only 42.6%), which is a lower number than reported from other European countries (5) and the United States (3). For cases where the infection was acquired in Denmark, only 39.7% (69 of 174) of cases were caused by *L. pneumophila* serogroup 1 (Pontiac subgroups only 27.6%). *L. pneumophila* serogroup 3 was a relatively common cause of community-acquired and nosocomial Legionnaires' disease in Denmark, accounting for 20% of all culture-confirmed cases. In Europe, only 4.5% of all culture-confirmed cases were caused by serogroup 3 in 1999 (5). Almost all cases of Legionnaires' disease acquired during traveling abroad were caused by *L. pneumophila* serogroup 1 (95%), with subgroup Pontiac accounting for 90% of the cases (mostly healthy persons). In contrast, non-serogroup 1 serogroups caused more than 70% of the culture-confirmed nosocomial cases, with subgroup Pontiac accounting for only 7.7% of the cases. A high proportion of non-serogroup 1 cases among nosocomial cases have been reported previously (2), but not as high as reported here.

## DISCUSSION

There could be more than one explanation for why the serogroup distribution of legionellae in Danish patients differs from that reported from other countries. One explanation could be that non-serogroup 1 (and non-Pontiac) infection is underdiagnosed in many countries. Denmark has one of the highest reported incidences of Legionnaires' disease in Europe (5) and one of the highest rates of culture-confirmed cases—approximately 30% compared with a European average of 16.8% in 1999 (5). This could partly be explained by the use of PCR at the central reference laboratory at Statens Serum Institut (see chapter 40) and at some local hospitals in Denmark, as a routine method (followed by culture of positive samples) for diagnosing Legionnaires' disease. The sensitivities of the commercially available *Legionella* urinary antigen tests for serogroups other than serogroup 1 is low and is also lower for serogroup 1 non-Pontiac subgroups than for Pontiac subgroups (see chapter 37). It is therefore important to supplement

**TABLE 1** Serogroup and subgroup distribution of clinical isolates of legionellae[a]

| Isolated serogroup/subgroup | No. (%) of patients in the following category: | | | | | |
|---|---|---|---|---|---|---|
| | All | Not known | All known | Community | Hospital | Travel |
| *L. pneumophila* | | | | | | |
| Serogroup 1 Pontiac | 83 (43) | 0 (0) | 83 (48) | 45 (47) | 3 (7.7) | 35 (90) |
| Serogroup 1 non-Pontiac | 28 (14) | 5 (24) | 23 (13) | 13 (14) | 8 (21) | 2 (5.1) |
| Serogroup 2 | 1 (0.5) | 0 (0) | 1 (0.6) | 0 (0) | 1 (2.6) | 0 (0) |
| Serogroup 3 | 39 (20) | 5 (24) | 34 (20) | 25 (26) | 7 (18) | 2 (5.1) |
| Serogroup 4 | 6 (3.1) | 0 (0) | 6 (3.4) | 5 (5.2) | 1 (2.6) | 0 (0) |
| Serogroup 5 | 10 (5.1) | 3 (14) | 7 (4) | 1 (1) | 6 (15) | 0 (0) |
| Serogroup 6 | 15 (7.7) | 2 (9.5) | 13 (7.5) | 3 (3.1) | 10 (26) | 0 (0) |
| Serogroup 8 | 1 (0.5) | 1 (4.8) | 0 (0) | 0 (0) | 0 (0) | 0 (0) |
| Serogroup 10 | 2 (1) | 0 (0) | 2 (1.1) | 1 (1) | 1 (2.6) | 0 (0) |
| Serogroup not known | 5 (2.6) | 3 (14) | 0 (0) | 1 (1) | 1 (2.6) | 0 (0) |
| *L. micdadei* | 1 (0.5) | 1 (4.8) | 1 (0.6) | 0 (0) | 0 (0) | 0 (0) |
| *L. bozemanii* | 2 (1) | 1 (4.8) | 2 (1.1) | 1 (1) | 0 (0) | 0 (0) |
| *L. longbeachae* | 2 (1) | 0 (0) | 2 (1.1) | 1 (1) | 1 (2.6) | 0 (0) |
| Total | 195 (100) | 21 (100) | 174 (100) | 96 (100) | 39 (100) | 39 (100) |

[a] For most patients with culture-confirmed Legionnaires' disease (all known), it was known where they acquired the infection: in the community, during hospitalization, or during traveling abroad.

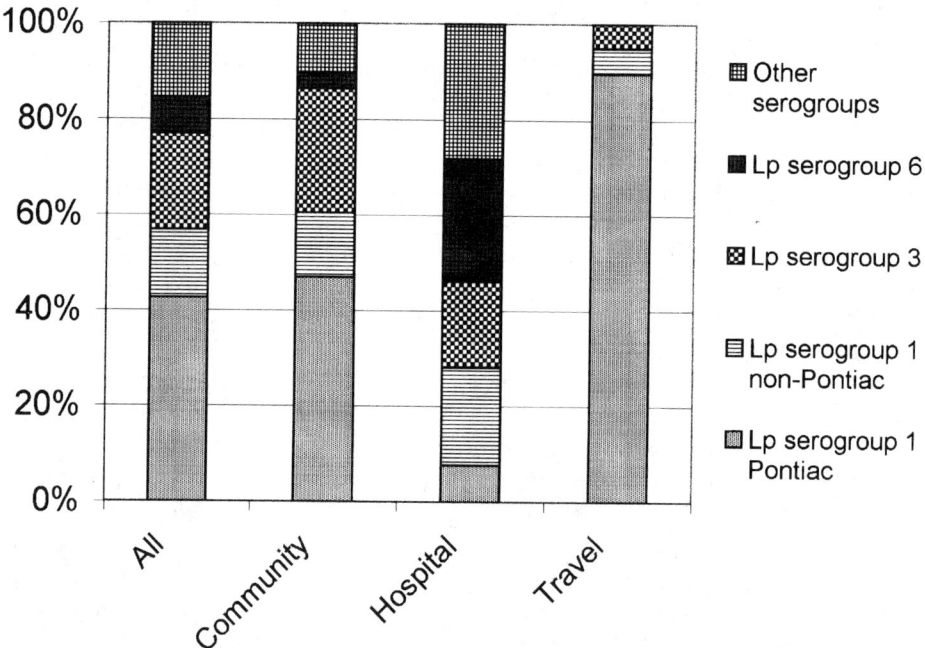

**FIGURE 1** Subgroup and serogroup distribution of clinical isolates of legionellae according to category of infection (figures from Table 1). The group "Other serogroups" contains all non-serogroup 1, 3, and 6 *L. pneumophila* serogroups and non-*L. pneumophila* species. Lp, *L. pneumophila*.

the use of *Legionella* urinary antigen assays in the diagnosis of Legionnaires' disease with other methods such as PCR and culture, particularly for the groups of patients with underlying disease and for those who are infected during hospitalization.

## REFERENCES

1. **Helbig, J. H., J. B. Kurtz, M. C. Pastoris, C. Pelaz, and P. C. Lück.** 1997. Antigenic lipopolysaccharide components of Legionella pneumophila recognized by monoclonal antibodies: possibilities and limitations for division of the species into serogroups. *J. Clin. Microbiol.* **35:**2841–2845.

2. **Joseph, C. A., J. M. Watson, T. G. Harrison, and C. L. Bartlett.** 1994. Nosocomial Legionnaires' disease in England and Wales, 1980–92. *Epidemiol. Infect.* **112:**329–345.

3. **Marston, B. J., H. B. Lipman, and R. F. Breiman.** 1994. Surveillance for Legionnaires' disease. Risk factors for morbidity and mortality. *Arch. Intern. Med.* **154:**2417–2422.

4. **Uldum, S., and S. Bang.** 2000. *Legionella infections 1998.* EPI-NEWS, No. 2. Statens Serum Institut, Copenhagen, Denmark.

5. **World Health Organization.** 2000. Legionnaires' disease, Europe, 1999. *Wkly. Epidemiol. Rec.* **43:**347–352.

# DETECTION OF *LEGIONELLA PNEUMOPHILA* ANTIGEN IN URINE SAMPLES: RECOGNITION OF SEROGROUPS AND MONOCLONAL SUBGROUPS

*Jürgen H. Helbig, Søren A. Uldum, P. Christian Lück, and Timothy G. Harrison*

# 37

The detection of *Legionella* antigen in urine samples is the most powerful method for diagnosing legionellosis in the early stage of illness, and it is therefore important for making therapeutic decisions. With respect to *Legionella pneumophila* serogroup 1, the assays are reported to have a sensitivity of 80 to 93% for culture-proven cases (1, 3, 9–11). However, the sensitivity is noticeably lower if cases proven by serology are taken into account (3, 10). Representative data for the sensitivity for non-serogroup 1 infections are rare. Recently, Benson et al. (2) used both Binax *Legionella* Urinary Antigen enzyme immunoassay (EIA) and Biotest *Legionella* Urin Antigen EIA in a small series of patients to detect antigenuria in 26 cases proven by isolation of *L. pneumophila* non-serogroup 1. They found sensitivities of 35% (Binax EIA) and 46% (Biotest-EIA). The present study compared the usefulness of urinary antigen detection for diagnosing Legion-

naires' disease caused by *L. pneumophila* serogroup 1 of different monoclonal subgroups in addition to cases caused by other serogroups.

A total of 152 urine samples from 152 patients with culture-proven legionellosis were tested. Group A consisted of 119 specimens from patients with Legionnaires' disease confirmed by isolation of *L. pneumophila* serogroup 1, subdivided into groups A1 to A4 (Table 1) on the basis of monoclonal antibody (MAb) subgrouping of the isolates (see below). Group B consisted of specimens from 31 culture-proven cases, in which *L. pneumophila* serogroup 2 (2 patients), serogroup 3 (17 patients), serogroup 4 (3 patients), serogroup 5 (2 patients), serogroup 6 (6 patients), serogroup 10 (one patient), serogroup 13 (one patient), and one untypeable strain (not serogroups 1 to 15) had been isolated.

Urine samples were tested simultaneously using Binax *Legionella* Urinary EIA (Binax, Portland, Maine) and Biotest *Legionella* Urin Antigen EIA (Biotest, Dreieich, Germany). All samples were tested without any concentration steps. The tests and the calculation of the results were performed according to the manufacturers' instructions.

Serogrouping of *L. pneumophila* using MAbs was performed as described by Helbig

*Jürgen H. Helbig and Christian P. Lück*  Institute of Medical Microbiology and Hygiene, Technical University Dresden, D-01307 Dresden, Germany.  *Søren A. Uldum* Department of Respiratory Infections, Meningitis and STIs, Statens Serum Institute, Dk-2300 Copenhagen, Denmark.  *Timothy G. Harrison* Respiratory and Systemic Infection Laboratory, PHLS Central Public Health Laboratory, London NW9 5HAT, United Kingdom.

*Legionella*, Edited by Reinhard Marre et al.
© 2002 ASM Press, Washington, D.C.

**TABLE 1**  Urinary antigen detection in specimens from culture-proven legionellosis

| Patient group | Legionellosis confirmed by isolation of *L. pneumophila* | No. of specimens positive/no. tested (% positive) | |
|---|---|---|---|
| | | Binax EIA | Biotest EIA |
| A1 | Serogroup 1, MAb 3/1 positive[a] | 71/73 (97.3) | 87/91 (95.6) |
| A2 | Serogroup 1, monoclonal subgroup OLDA/Oxford | 5/6 (83.3) | 4/8 (50) |
| A3 | Serogroup 1, monoclonal subgroup Bellingham | 5/8 (62.5) | 5/9 (55.6) |
| A4 | Serogroup 1, monoclonal subgroup not known | 10/11 (90.9) | 11/11 (100) |
| A (1 to 4) | Serogroup 1, all monoclonal subgroups | 91/98 (92.9) | 106/119 (89.1) |
| B | Non-serogroup 1 | 3/24 (12.5) | 11/33 (33.3) |
| A + B | All serogroups | 94/122 (77.0) | 117/152 (77.0) |

[a] Strains belong to monoclonal subgroups Philadelphia, Allentown, Benidorm, France, Knoxville.

et al. (5). For the division of *L. pneumophila* serogroup 1 isolates into monoclonal subgroups, MAbs 8/5, 3/1, 8/4, 20/1, and 10/6 (6), or/and MAb 2, MAb 3, W32, and 33G2 (7) were used. Using these MAbs, the division according to the international standard scheme by Joly et al. (7) into the subgroups Philadelphia, Allentown/France, Benidorm, Knoxville, OLDA/Oxford, and Bellingham was possible.

Ninety-one of our 152 culture-proven infections were caused by strains having the virulence-associated epitope recognized by the MAb 3/1 (6) and MAb 2 (4, 7), respectively. These strains belong to the monoclonal subgroups Philadelphia, Allentown, Benidorm, Knoxville, or France. The sensitivities of both Binax and Biotest EIA for culture-proven cases caused by these subgroups are more than 95% (Table 1). The incidence of legionellosis caused by other monoclonal subgroups is much lower. We have found only eight cases due to OLDA/Oxford-like strains and nine cases due to Bellingham-like ones. Compared with infections caused by MAb 3/1-positive strains, the sensitivity of Biotest EIA for the OLDA/Oxford was significantly reduced ($P < 0.0001$). By contrast, this difference was not obtained for Binax EIA (Table 1). With respect to legionellosis caused by Bellingham-like strains, the sensitivities of both assays were approximately 60%, again significantly less ($P < 0.0002$) than for cases caused by MAb 3/1-positive strains.

*L. pneumophila* strains that did not belong to serogroup 1 were isolated from 33 patients. All of the urine specimens were tested using Biotest EIA and 24 of them by Binax EIA. Binax EIA is marketed by the manufacturer as a kit for detection of *L. pneumophila* serogroup 1, but in three cases we were able to detect antigenuria. Using Biotest EIA, which is marketed as recognizing all serogroups, the sensitivity was higher ($P = 0.071$) but was still far short of the sensitivity obtained for serogroup 1 infections (Table 1).

Diagnosis by detection of urinary antigen has increased in recent years. As a consequence, Plouffe et al. (10) proposed that the international case definition for definitive Legionnaires' disease be expanded to include positive urinary assays. Taking all cases of legionellosis into account, we have found a sensitivity of 77% for both Binax EIA and Biotest EIA. This is in good agreement with other studies (1, 3, 9, 11). In addition, we have demonstrated in this study that the sensitivities for infections caused by MAb 3/1- and MAb 2-positive strains are much higher, exceeding 95%; thus, urinary antigen detection is the best method for diagnosing community-acquired as well as travel-associated cases. On the other hand, diagnosing infections caused by other *L. pneumophila* serogroups and serogroup 1 strains that do not have the virulence-associated epitope is inadequate using these kits. Therefore, it remains an open question as to whether or not infections caused by strains not belonging to the MAb 3/1- or MAb 2-positive strains are really as rare as many studies report, or if these infections are significantly underdiagnosed due to the low sensitivity of current urinary tests. Diagnosis of such infections has especially far-reaching implications for nosocomially acquired legionellosis, which is significantly more often caused by strains belonging to monoclonal subgroups OLDA/Oxford and Bellingham or to serogroups 2 to 15 than are community-acquired infections (8).

## ACKNOWLEDGMENTS

We thank Ines Wolf, Nita Doshi, and Ilse Kjaerulff for excellent technical assistance.

## REFERENCES

1. **Aguero-Rosenfeld, M. E., and P. H. Edelstein.** 1988. Retrospective evaluation of the Du Pont radioimmunoassay kit for detection of *Legionella pneumophila* serogroup 1 antigenuria in humans. *J. Clin. Microbiol.* **26:**1775–1778.

2. **Benson, R. F., P. W. Tang, and B. S. Fields.** 2000. Evaluation of the Binax and Biotest urinary antigen kits for the detection of Legionnaires' disease due to multiple serogroups and species of *Legionella*. *J. Clin. Microbiol.* **38:**2763–2765.

3. **Dominguez, J. A., N. Gali, P. Pedroso, A. Fargas, E. Paddilla, J. M. Manterola, and L. Matas.** 1998. Comparison of the Binax *Legionella* Urinary Antigen Enzyme Immunoassay (EIA) with the Biotest *Legionella* Urin EIA for detection of *Legionella* antigen in both concentrated and nonconcentrated urine samples. *J. Clin. Microbiol.* **36:**2718–2722.

4. **Dournon, E. W., F. Bibb, P. Rjagopalan, N. Desplaces, and R. M. McKinney.** 1988. Monoclonal antibody reactivity as a virulence marker for *Legionella pneumophila* serogroup 1 strains. *J. Infect. Dis.* **157:**496–501.

5. **Helbig, J. H., J. B. Kurtz, M. Castellani-Pastoris, C. Pelaz, and P. C. Lück.** 1997. Antigenic lipopolysaccharide components of *Legionella pneumophila* recognized by monoclonal antibodies: possibilities and limitations for division of the species into serogroups. *J. Clin. Microbiol.* **35:**2841–2845.

6. **Helbig, J. H., P. C. Lück, Y. A. Knirel, W. Witzleb, and U. Zähringer.** 1995. Molecular characterization of a virulence-associated epitope on the lipopolysaccharide of *Legionella pneumophila* serogroup 1. *Epidemiol. Infect.* **115:**71–78.

7. **Joly, J. R., R. M. McKinney, O. J. Tobin, W. F. Bibb, I. D. Watkins, and D. Ramsay.** 1986. Development of a standardized subgrouping scheme for *Legionella pneumophila* serogroup 1 using monoclonal antibodies. *J. Clin. Microbiol.* **23:**768–771.

8. **Joseph, C. A., J. M. Watson, T. G. Harrison, and C. L. R. Bartlett.** 1994. Nosocomial Legionnaires' disease in England and Wales, 1980-1992. *Epidemiol. Infect.* **112:**329–345.

9. **Kazandjian, D., R. Chiew, and G. L. Gilbert.** 1997. Rapid diagnosis of *Legionella pneumophila* serogroup 1 infections with the Binax enzyme immunoassay urinary antigen test. *J. Clin. Microbiol.* **35:**954–956.

10. **Plouffe, J. F, T. M. Mile, R. F. Breiman, B. A. Hackmann, S. J. Salstrom, B. J. Marston, B. S. Fields, and The Community-Based Pneumonia Incidence Study Group.** 1995. Reevaluation of the definition of Legionnaires' disease: use of the urinary antigen assay. *Clin. Infect. Dis.* **20:**1286–1291.

11. **Ruf, B., D. Schürmann, I. Horbach, F. J. Fehrenbach, and H. D. Pohle.** 1990. Prevalence and diagnosis of Legionella pneumonia: a 3-year prospective study with emphasis on application of urinary antigen detection. *J. Infect. Dis.* **162:**1341–1348.

# COMPARISON OF NON-SEROGROUP 1 DETECTION BY BIOTEST AND BINAX *LEGIONELLA* URINARY ANTIGEN ENZYME IMMUNOASSAYS

*J. Horn*

# 38

Infection due to *Legionella* species presents as either Pontiac fever or as pneumonia, Legionnaires' disease. Since the mortality rate from untreated Legionnaires' disease may range from 10 to 50% (2, 9, 10), rapid diagnosis and effective antibiotic treatment are essential. A radioimmunoassay (RIA) for the detection of *Legionella* urinary antigen was developed soon after the identification of *Legionella* as the source of Legionnaires' disease (6). The reported sensitivity of the Binax RIA was 56% for all cases in a study of community-acquired pneumonia, 80% for culture-positive *Legionella pneumophila* serogroup 1, and 38% for patients with seroconversion and negative cultures (7).

The Binax enzyme immunoassay (EIA) and RIA both showed a certain cross-reactivity with non-serogroup 1 *L. pneumophila*, as is to be expected when using polyclonal rabbit antibodies for the antigen detection. The Biotest EIA is the former urinary antigen EIA from the Robert Koch Institute in Berlin developed by Fehrenbach for extended cross-reactivity with non-serogroup 1 *L. pneumophila*. It was demonstrated by 14 World Health Organiza-

tion collaborating *Legionella* centers to have a sensitivity of 86% for all cases of *Legionella* and 94.6% in cases of *Legionella* serogroup 1 (5). The reactivity of culture-confirmed cases was higher than of culture-negative cases confirmed by serology as previously shown (H.-H Sonneborn, M. Backes, A. Hartlaub, J. Horn, D. Jürgens, and F. Fehrenbach, *Clin. Microbiol. Infect.* **3**(Suppl. 2):13, abstr. P1268, 1997). The evaluation of spiked water samples with the Biotest EIA demonstrated cross-reactivity with all *L. pneumophila* serogroups as well as other species (Table 1) (J. Horn and M. Backes, *EWGLI 1999*, 14th Meeting, 27–29 June 1999, Dresden, abstr. 37, 1999; J. Horn and M. Backes, *4th Int. Conf. Hosp. Infect. Soc.*, 13–17 Sept. 1998, Edinburgh, abstr. P.9.5.8, 1998). Benson (1) demonstrated that only 10 of 45 non-serogroup 1 urine samples previously positive in the broad-spectrum enzyme-linked immunosorbent assay described by Tang (11) were positive with the Binax EIA (22%), whereas 13 of 42 of these samples were positive with the Biotest EIA (31%); when using a lower cut-off, 20 (48%) were positive with Biotest EIA. We evaluated 28 non-serogroup 1 samples from different countries provided by users of the test to demonstrate reactivity of the two urinary antigen tests with these urines (Table 2).

*J. Horn*  Research & Development, Biotest AG, 63303 Dreieich, Germany.

*Legionella*, Edited by Reinhard Marre et al.
© 2002 ASM Press, Washington, D.C.

**TABLE 1**  Titration of *Legionella*-spiked water samples with Biotest urinary antigen EIA

| Sample | Positive endtiter | No. of *Legionella*/ml of water that endtiter corresponds to |
|---|---|---|
| *L. pneumophila* serogroup 1 | 1:1,200 | 7.5 |
| *L. pneumophila* serogroup 2 | 1:10 | $3.8 \times 10^2$ |
| *L. pneumophila* serogroup 3 | 1:4 | $1.8 \times 10^3$ |
| *L. pneumophila* serogroup 4 | 1:2 | $9.0 \times 10^3$ |
| *L. pneumophila* serogroup 5 | 1:1,200 | 9.2 |
| *L. pneumophila* serogroup 6 | 1:20 | $1.0 \times 10^3$ |
| *L. pneumophila* serogroup 7 | 1:2 | $4.8 \times 10^3$ |
| *L. pneumophila* serogroup 8 | 1:20 | $6.0 \times 10^2$ |
| *L. pneumophila* serogroup 9 | 1:2 | $3.3 \times 10^3$ |
| *L. pneumophila* serogroup 10 | 1:4 | $1.4 \times 10^3$ |
| *L. pneumophila* serogroup 12 | 1:1 | $4.8 \times 10^3$ |
| *L. pneumophila* serogroup 13 | 1:2 | $3.6 \times 10^3$ |
| *L. pneumophila* serogroup 14 | 1:40 | $4.0 \times 10^2$ |
| *L. bozemanii* | 1:4 | $2.0 \times 10^3$ |
| *L. dumoffi* | 1:8 | $1.2 \times 10^3$ |
| *L. hackeliae* | 1:4 | $1.6 \times 10^3$ |
| *L. jordanis* | 1:8 | $2.0 \times 10^3$ |
| *L. longbeachae* | 1:160 | 54.0 |
| *L. micdadei* | 1:8 | $9.3 \times 10^2$ |
| *L. sainthelensi* | 1:1 | $5.5 \times 10^3$ |

## COMPARISON OF BIOTEST AND BINAX EIA WITH PATIENT URINE SAMPLES

Binax EIA and Biotest EIA kits were used according to the test kit instructions. Binax provides a single cut-off with a ratio of ≥3.0 being positive. Biotest uses two cut-offs with a grey zone, mean of negative controls +0.200 optical density being positive, mean of negative controls +0.100 optical density (lower cut-off) being positive only if the sample is repeatedly reactive in this range. This eliminates possible washing procedure errors with low positive results since these are usually nonrepeatable in two subsequent tests.

Specificity with both Biotest cut-off values was extensively evaluated with 176 potentially cross-reactive samples (urines with high bacterial counts from urinary tract infections) and 300 negatives through testing by the manufacturer, as well as with 123 potentially cross-reactives out of the European Working Group on *Legionella* Infections study (5). A lower cut-off without extensive specificity studies has been reported for Binax (4). Samples were nonconcentrated urines from patients with *Legionella* non-serogroup 1 infections (Table 2), as confirmed by culture, serology, or direct fluorescent antibody test.

Concentration of urines was performed by boiling the urines for 5 minutes followed by a 25-fold concentration in a Urifil-10 Concentrator (Millipore Corp., Bedford, Mass.) as previously described (3). Samples were tested immediately in both tests, since reports have shown that some samples may become negative after long-term storage (8). *Legionella*-spiked water samples were concentrated by filtration. Subsequently the filters were ultrasonicated in a minimal amount of water with a Branson 250 ultrasonifier as previously reported (Horn and Backes, *EWGLI 1999*, abstr. 37, 1999; Horn and Backes, 4th ICHIS, abstr. P.9.5.8, 1998). After sonification, a turbid solution should result, indicating disintegration of the *Legionella*. This increases sensitivity considerably to less than 10 organisms/ml for serogroups 1 and 5. Further refinement of the ultrasonification resulted in

**TABLE 2** Results for Biotest EIA and Binax EIA with urines from *Legionella* non-serogroup 1 infections

| No. of samples | Organism | No. of samples positive/no. negative | | | |
|---|---|---|---|---|---|
| | | Biotest | Biotest concentrated | Binax | Binax concentrated |
| 4 | *L. pneumophila* serogroup 3 | 2/2 | 3/1 | 1/3 | 2/2 |
| 2 | *L. pneumophila* serogroup 4 | 1/1 | 2/0 | 1/1 | 1/1 |
| 1 | *L. pneumophila* serogroup 5 | 1/0 | 1/0 | 0/1 | 0/1 |
| 7 | *L. pneumophila* serogroup 6 | 5/2 | 6/1 | 3/4 | 4/3 |
| 2 | *L. pneumophila* serogroup 7 | 1/1 | 1/1 | 1/1 | 1/1 |
| 2 | *L. pneumophila* serogroup 8 | 1/1 | 1/1 | 0/2 | 1/1 |
| 1 | *L. pneumophila* serogroup 10 | 1/0 | 1/1 | 0/1 | 1/1 |
| 1 | *L. pneumophila* serogroup 12 | 1/0 | 1/0 | 1/0 | 1/0 |
| 2 | *L. longbeachae* | 1/1 | 1/1 | 0/2 | 0/2 |
| 2 | *L. hackeliae* | 1/1 | 1/1 | 1/1 | 1/1 |
| 1 | *L. jordanis* | 1/0 | 1/0 | 0/1 | 0/1 |
| 2 | *L. bozemanii* | 1/1 | 1/1 | 0/1 | 0/1 |
| 1 | *L. micdadei* | 0/1 | 0/1 | 0/1 | 0/1 |
| 28 | Total | 17/11 | 20/8 | 8/20 | 12/16 |
| | Sensitivity (%) | 60.7 | 71.4 | 28.6 | 42.9 |

about 10 organisms/liter for *L. pneumophila* serogroup 1.

Of a group of 28 non-serogroup 1 *Legionella* urines, including five non-*L. pneumophila* species and 8 serogroups other than serogroup 1 of *L. pneumophila*, the Biotest EIA detected 17 samples with a sensitivity of 60% and the Binax EIA 8 samples with a sensitivity of 30%. After concentration of the urines, the number of positives increased to 20 samples (70%) with the Biotest EIA and 12 samples (40%) with the Binax EIA (Table 2).

The Biotest EIA therefore demonstrates a considerably broader cross-reactivity with urines from non-serogroup 1 *L. pneumophila* infections than the Binax EIA. The Biotest EIA was able to detect four of eight samples from five different non-*L. pneumophila* *Legionella* species, whereas the Binax EIA detected only one of these eight samples. The examination of the spiked water samples showed that the Biotest EIA is able to react positively with a wide range of *L. pneumophila* serogroups and even other *Legionella* species.

The detection limit of the different *Legionella*, however, was not identical. This is likely to cause different sensitivities in a clinical setting. Since the production of excess lipopolysaccharide antigen is not identical in all species and during infection, differences in detecting *Legionella* in spiked water samples may not correspond to differences in detecting antigen of different *Legionella* species in clinical samples. However, the fact that *L. pneumophila* serogroup 1 is detected with high sensitivity in spiked water samples is in accordance with its excellent sensitivity in patients with *L. pneumophila* serogroup 1 infections. The potential for improving *Legionella* antigen detection with a broadly cross-reactive EIA is clearly demonstrated by the multicenter study of Harrison (5). Certainly more potential exists by fully exploiting the advantages of polyclonal antibodies from rabbits, broadly cross-reactive with *Legionella* species in the Biotest EIA, in continuing efforts to further improve reactivity with *Legionella* species other than *L. pneumophila*.

## REFERENCES

1. **Benson, R. F., W. T. Tang, and B. S. Fields.** 2000. Evaluation of the Binax and Biotest urinary antigen kits for detection of Legionnaires' disease due to multiple serogroups and species of Legionella. *J. Clin. Microbiol.* **38:**2763–2765.

2. **Brown, P. D., and S. A. Lerner.** 1998. Community acquired pneumonia. *Lancet* **352:** 1295–1302.

3. **Dominguez, J. A., N. Gali, P. Pedroso, A. Fargas, E. Padilla, J. M. Manterola, and L.**

**Matas.** 1998. Comparison of the Binax Legionella urinary antigen enzyme immunoassay (EIA) with the Biotest Legionella urine antigen EIA for detection of Legionella antigen in both concentrated and non-concentrated urine samples. *J. Clin. Microbiol.* **36:**2718–2722.

4. **Hackmann, B. A., J. F. Plouffe, R. F. Benson, B. S. Fields, and R. F. Breiman.** 1996. Comparison of Binax Legionella EIA kit with Binax RIA urinary antigen kit for detection of *Legionella pneumophila* serogroup 1 antigen. *J. Clin. Microbiol.* **34:**1579–1580.

5. **Harrison, T., S. Uldum, S. Alexion-Daniel, J. Bangsborg, S. Bernander, V. Drasar, J. Eheune, J. Helbig, D. Lindsay, I. Lochman, T. Marques, F. de Ory, J. Tartakovskii, G. Wewalka, and F. Fehrenbach.** 1998. A multicenter evaluation of the Biotest Legionella urinary antigen EIA. *Clin. Microbiol. Infect.* **4:**359–365.

6. **Kohler, R. B., S. E. Zimmermann, E. Wilson, S. D. Allen, P. H. Edelstein, I. J. Wheat, and A. White.** 1981. Rapid radioimmunoassay diagnosis of Legionnaires' disease; detection and partial characterization of urinary antigen. *Ann. Intern. Med.* **94:**601–605.

7. **Plouffe, J. F., M. File, R. F. Breiman, B. A. Hackmann, S. J. Salstrom, B. J. Marston, and B. S. Fields.** 1995. Reevaluation of the definition of Legionnaires' disease: use of the urinary antigen assay. *Clin. Infect. Dis.* **20:**1286–1291.

8. **Rigby, E. W., J. F. Plouffe, B. A. Hackmann, D. S. Hill, R. F. Benson, and R. F. Breiman.** 1997. Stability of Legionella urinary antigens over time. *Diagn. Microbiol. Infect. Dis.* **28:**1–3.

9. **Slack, M. P. E.** 1999. Legionella ssp., p. 8.20.11–8.20.13. *In* D. Armstrong and I. Cohen (ed.), *Infectious Diseases.* Harcourt Publishers Ltd., London, United Kingdom.

10. **Stout, J. E., and V. L. Yu.** 1997. Legionellosis. *N. Engl. J. Med.* **337:**682–387.

11. **Tang, P., and C. Krishnan.** 1993. Legionella antigenuria: six-year study of broad-spectrum enzyme-linked immunosorbent assay as a routine diagnostic test, p. 12–13. *In* J. M. Barbaree, R. F. Breiman, and A. P. Dufour (ed.), *Legionella: Current Status and Emerging Perspectives.* American Society for Microbiology, Washington, D.C.

# EVALUATION OF A RAPID IMMUNOCHROMATOGRAPHIC ASSAY FOR DETECTION OF *LEGIONELLA PNEUMOPHILA* IN URINE

*Norman Moore and Deborah Gentile*

# 39

An estimated 25,000 (5) to 100,000 (3) cases of legionellosis occur in the United States annually. However, one study suggests that only 3% of nonoutbreak cases are properly diagnosed (6). With mortality rates reported as high as 25 to 40% (5), a rapid and accurate diagnosis is essential to proper patient care.

Current methodologies for the diagnosis of legionellosis are time-consuming and labor-intensive, which dissuades many doctors from ordering the tests. Culturing *Legionella* on buffered charcoal-yeast extract plates may require 3 to 10 days. Moreover, in a 1989 study, only 32% of laboratories were able to correctly diagnose *Legionella* (2). Serology may be used as a retrospective diagnosis, requiring a fourfold rise in titer between acute and convalescent sera. Results may take as long as 2 to 6 weeks to obtain, while some patients never seroconvert (1). The direct fluorescent assay is also available but it is a labor-intensive test with sensitivity varying from 25 to 75% (1). Also, one of the presenting signs of patients with Legionnaires' disease is the relative lack of productive sputum (7).

Antigen can be found in the urine in as little as 1 to 3 days after the onset of symptoms (4). Commercial antibody-based enzyme tests in enzyme immunoassay format are currently available for urinary antigen. However, these tests require 90 to 180 min to perform, and since the test is not ordered often by caregivers, the samples are usually sent out or batched for analysis, which can take several days. Having a rapid and simple test available that requires only a noninvasive urine sample should allow for more appropriate and specific antibiotic therapy to be initiated in a timely manner.

To make the urinary rapid diagnostic, antibody was raised to the carbohydrate portion of *Legionella* serogroup 1. The antibody was immobilized on nitrocellulose and conjugated to colloidal gold particles to produce an immunochromatographic test (ICT). To run the assay, a swab was dipped into the urine sample and inserted into the device. Two drops of a reagent were added and the device was closed. Results were read in 15 min.

To evaluate the test, a retrospective study was performed in which 300 frozen archive urine samples were thawed and evaluated using the ICT device. Results were compared with culture diagnosis. One hundred of these urine samples were from patients positive for

*Norman Moore and Deborah Gentile*     Binax, 217 Read Street, Portland, ME 04103.

*Legionella*, Edited by Reinhard Marre et al.
© 2002 ASM Press, Washington, D.C.

*Legionella pneumophila* serogroup 1. The other 200 urine samples were evaluated to identify the specificity of the test in a proper patient population. Out of this patient population, 85 patients had non-legionellosis pneumonias, 84 had urinary tract infections, 15 had mycobacterial infections, 5 had empyema, 11 had other pulmonary conditions, and 1 had an unknown pneumonia. The sensitivity, specificity, and accuracy of the test were all reported at 95%, as seen in Table 1.

A prospective study was then performed in which 93 urine samples were collected from symptomatic patients reporting to the hospital with lower respiratory symptoms or sepsis. The purpose of this study was to evaluate the test with fresh urine samples. These patients were evaluated by culture and the ICT. In these samples, the specificity of the test was 100%. No samples were positive either by culture or ICT for *L. pneumophila*.

To ensure that the test was easy to use, a reproducibility study was performed. Three testing sites were set up with two reproducibility panels that included negative, low-positive, moderate-positive, and high-positive specimens. Two technicians at each site ran 15 controls per day on three separate days. Specimens were also evaluated with and without boric acid as a preservative. Out of these samples, 269 of 270 samples were identified correctly. The sole discrepancy was a negative that was reported as a positive. Boric acid was shown to have no effect on the test outcome.

Previous methodologies for the diagnosis of Legionnaires' disease were so time-consuming and labor-intensive that many doctors were dissuaded from ordering a test since the results would usually be too late to change the treatment pattern. As such, cases of legionellosis have always been drastically underdiagnosed. The NOW ICT test, because of its simplicity, ease of use, and accuracy, has been shown to be an effective tool in the diagnosis of Legionnaires' disease. A retrospective study provided data with a high degree of sensitivity and specificity, while the prospective study showed high specificity (no conclusions could be drawn about sensitivity). Since the test can be performed rapidly with accurate results, the test is leading to more patients being properly diagnosed and treated accordingly.

**TABLE 1** Results by culture and ICT diagnosis[a]

| ICT diagnosis | Culture diagnosis | |
| --- | --- | --- |
| | Positive result | Negative result |
| Positive result | 95 (A) | 10 (B) |
| Negative result | 5 (C) | 190 (D) |

[a] Sensitivity, specificity, and accuracy were calculated as indicated below. Values in parentheses indicate the confidence intervals.

Sensitivity = 95% (88.7–98.4%)  $A \div (A + C)$
Specificity = 95% (91.0–97.6%)  $D \div (D + B)$
Accuracy = 95% (91.9–97.2%)  $(A + D \div (A + B + C + D)$

## REFERENCES

1. **Edelstein, P. H., R. D. Meyer, and S. M. Finegold.** 1980. Laboratory diagnosis of Legionnaires' disease. *Am. Rev. Respir. Dis.* **121:**317–327.
2. **Edelstein, P. H.** 1993. Legionnaires' disease. *Clin. Infect. Dis.* **16:**741–747.
3. **Horwitz, M. A., B. J. Marston, C. V. Broome, and R. F. Breiman.** 1993. Prospects for vaccine development, p. 296–297. *In* J. M. Barbaree, R. F. Breiman, and A. P. Dufour (ed.), *Legionella: Current Status and Emerging Perspectives.* American Society for Microbiology, Washington, D.C.
4. **Kohler, R. B., W. C. Winn, Jr., and L. J. Wheat.** 1984. Onset and duration of urinary antigen excretion in Legionnaires' Disease. *J. Clin. Microbiol.* **20:**605–607.
5. **Marston, B. J., H. B. Lipman, R. F. Breiman.** 1994. Surveillance for Legionnaires' Disease: risk factors for morbidity and mortality. *Arch. Intern. Med.* **154:**2417–2422.
6. **Marston, B. J., J. F. Plouffe, R. F. Breiman, T. M. File, R. F. Benson, M. Moyenuddin, W. L. Thacker, K. H. Wong, S. Skelton, B. Hackman, S. J. Salstrom, J. M. Barbaree, and The Community-Based Pneumonia Incidence Study Group.** 1993. Preliminary findings of a community-based pneumonia incidence study, p. 36–37. *In* J. M. Barbaree, R. F. Breiman, and A. P. Dufour (ed.), *Legionella: Current Status and Emerging Perspectives.* American Society for Microbiology, Washington, D.C.
7. **Stout, J. E., V. L. Yu.** 1997. Legionellosis. *N. Engl. J. Med.* **337:**682–687.

# PCR AS A ROUTINE METHOD FOR DIAGNOSIS OF LEGIONNAIRES' DISEASE

*Søren A. Uldum and Kåre Mølbak*

# 40

We have used PCR for detection of *Legionella* DNA in respiratory samples as a routine diagnostic method for approximately 5½ years (1995 to September 2000). The aim of this study was to evaluate the performance of the method with respect to sensitivity, specificity, and predictive value of a positive test result with the help of the results obtained by the other *Legionella* diagnostic methods used in the routine laboratory.

## DATA

The calculations are based on data extracted from a database containing all results obtained by each of the routine methods in the period. No clinical or other data such as type of specimen or the timing of sample collection in relation to onset of illness were included in the evaluation. Laboratory results for the other diagnostic methods were included if samples were collected within a period of 90 days relative to the sample for PCR.

## LEGIONELLA PCR

The method is a multiplex PCR with two sets of primers, one set detecting a fragment of the macrophage infectivity potentiator (*mip*) gene of *Legionella pneumophila* (sequences from the Perkin Elmer Cetus EnviroAmp Legionella Amplification kit), the other detecting the 16S RNA gene of *Legionella* spp. (2). An internal amplification control was included in each tube for detection of inhibition and suboptimal amplification conditions. The amplification control was constructed on the basis of amplification of phage lambda DNA (position 13,663 to 14,280). The primers for construction of the amplification control included the sequence of each of the 16S rDNA primers added to the 5' ends of the corresponding lambda primers. The amplification control thus contained the binding sites of the 16S rDNA primers, was purified by gel electrophoresis, and was added to the mastermix at a concentration producing a distinct amplicon in negative controls without increasing the level of detection for the positive controls (1). The amplicons of the *Legionella* PCR were analyzed by gel electrophoresis (Fig. 1).

## CULTURE

Standard culture techniques for clinical samples were used.

*Søren A. Uldum* Department of Respiratory Infections, Meningitis and STIs, Statens Serum Institut, DK-2300 Copenhagen S, Denmark. *Kåre Mølbak* Department of Epidemiology Research, Statens Serum Institut, DK-2300 Copenhagen S, Denmark.

*Legionella*, Edited by Reinhard Marre et al.
© 2002 ASM Press, Washington, D.C.

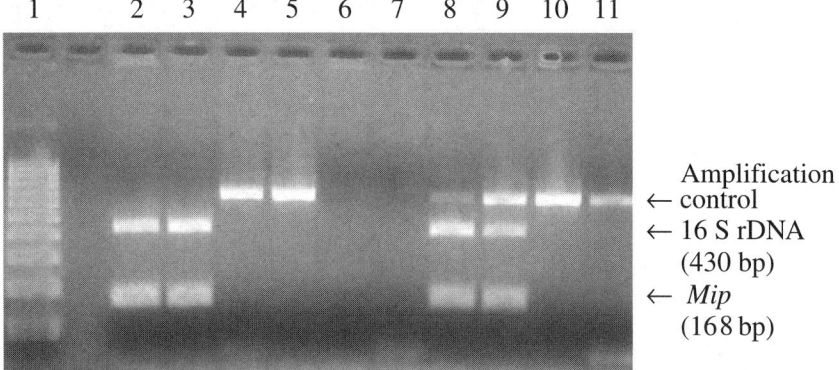

**FIGURE 1**  Gel electrophoresis of *Legionella* PCR amplicons. Lanes: 1, size marker; 2 and 3, positive samples; 4 and 5, negative samples; 6 and 7, inhibitory samples; 8 and 9, positive controls; 10 and 11, negative controls.

## *LEGIONELLA* URINARY ANTIGEN ENZYME IMMUNOASSAY

We used two different assays: from 1995 to 1999 we used an inhouse assay and from 1999 we used the Biotest *Legionella* Urin Antigen EIA (Biotest, Dreieichen, Germany). For both assays, the test results were calculated from a standard curve and expressed as arbitrary units (aU) per milliliter. For both assays, values of ≥10 aU/ml were considered diagnostic of a current or recent *Legionella* infection, values ≥5 aU/ml, but <10 aU/ml were considered equivocal, and values <5 aU/ml were considered negative.

## *LEGIONELLA* IMMUNOFLUORESCENCE ANTIBODY TEST

Heat-killed bacteria of *L. pneumophila* serogroup 1 to 6, *Legionella micdadei* and *Legionella bozemanii* were used as antigens. A fourfold or greater rise in antibody titer to a titer of ≥128 (seroconversion) to any of the antigens was considered as evidence of a recent *Legionella* infection. Single or standing titers of ≥256 to any of the antigens were considered as presumptive of a recent or past infection.

## DEFINITIONS

**Patients with *Legionella* infection:** Patients with positive culture for legionellae or seroconversion for any of the used antigens or positive urinary antigen test (≥10 aU/ml).

**Patients without *Legionella* infection:** Patients with negative culture for legionellae or no seroconversion or negative or equivocal urinary antigen results (<10 aU/ml). This group also includes patients with positive antibody titers (≥256) and patients with no tests (culture, urinary antigen, and serology) performed.

***Legionella* PCR sensitivity:** Number of patients with *Legionella* infection with positive PCR/number of patients with *Legionella* infection × 100%.

***Legionella* PCR specificity:** Number of patients without *Legionella* infection with negative PCR/number of patients without *Legionella* infection × 100%.

**Predictive value of a positive *Legionella* PCR (PVpos.):** Number of patients with *Legionella* infection with positive PCR/number of patients with positive PCR × 100%.

Patients with samples positive for the 16S RNA *Legionella* gene only were omitted from this study (<10 patients). From 1995 to September 2000 we investigated 5,402 respiratory tract specimens (predominantly from the lower respiratory tract) from 4,420 patients by *Legionella* PCR. Samples from the 4,420 patients were inhibitory in 43 (1%) patients, neg-

**TABLE 1** Distribution of the 4,420 patients with samples examined by *Legionella* PCR on positive and negative results

| PCR result | No. with *Legionella* infection | No. "without" *Legionella* infection | Total no. |
|---|---|---|---|
| Positive | 204 | 43 | 247 |
| Negative | 39 | 4,134 | 4,173 |
| Total | 243 | 4,177 | 4,420 |

ative in 4,130 (93.4%) patients, and positive in 247 (5.6%) patients. Of the 247 patients with positive results by *Legionella* PCR, the diagnosis could be confirmed for 204 by one of, or by combinations of, the other diagnostic methods: Samples from 131 patients were positive by culture; samples from 131 patients were positive by urinary antigen test ($\geq 10$ aU); and samples from 69 patients were positive by serology (seroconversion). Of the 43 patients with false-positive PCR results, three had equivocal results in *Legionella* urinary antigen test and four had a positive antibody titer of $\geq 256$. For 13 patients, no urinary antigen or antibody test was performed. Two patients had negative serology and no urinary antigen test performed; and 22 had negative results in the urinary antigen test of which 13 also had negative serology. For 39 patients with *Legionella* PCR-negative samples (false negative), samples were positive by culture (three patients) or by urinary antigen test or/and serology. The distributions of the 4,420 patients with samples examined by *Legionella* PCR on positive and negative results according to the definitions of patients with and without *Legionella* infection are shown in Table 1. In Table 2, the specificity, sensitivity, and predictive value of a positive test result (PVpos.) is calculated from the figures given in Table 1.

## CONCLUSIONS

The performance of *Legionella* PCR as a routine diagnostic method for respiratory infections caused by *L. pneumophila* was acceptable, although not all PCR-positive cases could be verified by the other diagnostic methods. The sensitivity of *Legionella* PCR is probably higher than any other single method. An important feature of the *Legionella* PCR is that the method detects all serogroups and subgroups of *L. pneumophila* equally well. The urinary antigen assays have low sensitivities for non-*L. pneumophila* serogroup 1 Pontiac subgroups and serogroups (chapter 37), which causes more than 50% of all culture-proven cases in Denmark (chapter 36). PCR is a very important method for the early diagnosis of infections caused by these serogroups that particularly are seen in nosocomial cases.

**TABLE 2** Calculation of the sensitivity, specificity, and predictive value of a positive test result (PVpos.) for *Legionella* PCR from the figures given in Table 1

| *Legionella* PCR | Calculation |
|---|---|
| Sensitivity . . . . . . . . . . . . . | 204/243 × 100% = 84% |
| Specificity . . . . . . . . . . . . . | 4134/4177 × 100% = 99% |
| PVpos. . . . . . . . . . . . . . . . . | 204/247 × 100% = 82.6% |

## REFERENCES
1. **Povlsen, K., J. S. Jensen, and I. Lind.** 1998. Detection of Ureaplasma urealyticum by PCR and biovar determination by liquid hybridization. *J. Clin. Microbiol.* **36:**3211–3216.
2. **Yamamoto, H., Y. Hashimoto, and T. Ezaki.** 1993. Comparison of detection methods for Legionella species in environmental water by colony isolation, fluorescent antibody staining, and polymerase chain reaction. *Microbiol. Immunol.* **37:** 617–622.

# DETECTION OF *LEGIONELLA*-SPECIFIC DNA IN SERUM

*Diane S. J. Lindsay, William Abraham,*
*Giles Edwards, and R. W. A. Girdwood*

# 41

## LABORATORY DIAGNOSIS OF LEGIONELLOSIS

In the United Kingdom the vast majority of cases of legionellosis are caused by *Legionella pneumophila* serogroup 1 (C. A. Joseph and E. Slaymaker, 14th Meeting Eur. Working Group *Legionella* Infections, Dresden, 1999). In Scotland, we occasionally identify patients with a serological response to other *Legionella* serogroups and species. The current methods of laboratory diagnosis of legionellosis include urinary antigen detection, serology, and culture. Urinary antigen is excreted in the acute stages of disease and can persist for weeks after onset. The Biotest urinary antigen enzyme-linked immunosorbent assay detects *Legionella* spp., predominately *L. pneumophila* serogroup 1, but has been shown to detect *L. pneumophila* serogroup 1-14 and *Legionella bozemanii* (1). Serological diagnosis of *Legionella* infection has been validated only for *L. pneumophila* serogroup 1 (12). Therefore, serological evidence of infection with other serogroups or species is difficult to interpret without concurrent laboratory or clinical evidence. The isolation of *Legionella* is diagnostically definitive (European Working Group on *Legionella* Infections) but is dependent on the quality and availability of specimens. PCR has been shown to detect DNA in respiratory secretions (4), serum (5), and urine (9). The 5S RNA gene of the *Legionellaceae* was sequenced by Mahbubani et al. (6). This gene is present in all the *Legionellaceae* and its detection in serum can provide rapid supplementary evidence of infection due to unusual species and serogroups where current tests are limited. This study investigates the presence of *Legionella*-specific DNA in patient serum using a 5S RNA PCR. In all cases, the DNA extraction was monitored by a control PCR, which amplified part of the β-globin gene, and the specificity of the PCR was verified by a combination of Southern blotting with a 50-oligomer *Legionella*-specific probe and *Taq*I restriction digestion of the PCR products.

## PCR

DNA was extracted from 200 $\mu$l of serum with Biogene nucleospin blood columns per the manufacturer's instructions (Clontech, United Kingdom). *L. pneumophila* serogroup 1 was heat shocked, and the supernatant was

*Diane S. J. Lindsay, William Abraham, Giles Edwards, and R. W. A. Girdwood* Scottish Legionella Reference Laboratory, Department of Microbiology, The North Glasgow University NHS Trust, Stobhill Hospital, Glasgow, G21 3UW, Scotland, United Kingdom.

*Legionella*, Edited by Reinhard Marre et al.
© 2002 ASM Press, Washington, D.C.

used as a positive control in the 5S RNA PCR at a concentration of 100 pg. The DNA was amplified in a control PCR to determine the efficiency of the DNA-extraction procedure. The $\beta$-globin gene was amplified using two 20-oligomer primers (CAACTTCATC-CACGTTCACC and GAAGAGCCAAGG-ACAGGTAC) in a PCR mixture containing 10 mM Tris-HCl (pH 8.3), 50 mM KCl, 2 mM $MgCl_2$, 0.4 mM deoxynucleoside triphosphates, and 1.25 U of *Taq* polymerase. The PCR consisted of an initial denaturation step at 95°C for 5 min and 35 cycles of 95°C for 30 s, 58°C for 45 s, and 72°C for 30 s. The $\beta$-globin gene product was 140 bp. The presence of the $\beta$-globin gene was an indication that the DNA extraction was successful and there were no major inhibitors present in the DNA sample. Only $\beta$-globin PCR-positive samples were tested in the 5S RNA PCR. The patient serum DNA was added to a standard PCR reaction mixture containing 20 mM Tris-HCl (pH 8.3), 100 mM KCl, 2.5 mM $MgCl_2$, 500 ng of each primer ACTATAGCGATTTGGAACCA and GCGATGACCTACTTTCGCAT, 0.25 mM deoxynucleoside triphosphates, and 1.25 U of *Taq* polymerase. The tubes were subjected to 35 cycles of 95°C for 30 s, 55°C for 1 min, and 72°C for 30 s (Hybaid omnigene thermocycler). All PCR products were analyzed by horizontal gel electrophoresis in a 1.5% agarose gel with a 100-bp ladder and run at 60 V for 1 h in 1× Tris-borate-EDTA pH 8.

## SOUTHERN BLOTTING

DNA in the agarose gel was transferred to nylon by capillary action and probed at 68°C for 2 h with 1 ng/ml of 5S RNA *Legionella*-specific digoxigenin-labelled probe CTCGAACTCAGAAGTCAAACATTTC-CGCGCCAATGATAGTGTGAGGCTTC. The nylon was washed and blocked, and an anti-digoxigenin alkaline phosphatase system (Hoffmann Le Roche) was employed to detect any probe hybridization. The color substrate was nitroblue tetrazolium-5-bromo-

4-chloro-3-indolylphosphate. The primers and probe were both produced by Perkin El-mer.

## *Taq*I DIGESTION

*Taq*I digestion was performed on all 5S RNA PCR-positive samples. The PCR product was digested with *Taq*I restriction enzyme for 16 h at 65°C. The digest was electrophoresed on a 4% GTG agarose gel (FMC products) with a 10-bp DNA ladder (Gibco BRL) at 40 V for 1 h.

## ROUTINE LABORATORY METHODS

The Biotest urinary antigen enzyme-linked immunosorbent assay was performed per the manufacturer's instruction and the serology and culture tests were performed as described previously (2, 12).

## DETECTION OF *LEGIONELLA*-SPECIFIC DNA IN SERUM

A total of 122 serum samples were analyzed for the presence of the 5S RNA gene of the *Legionellaceae*. Fifty-two serum samples came from 26 patients with laboratory evidence of *Legionella* infection, of which 88.5% were 5S RNA PCR positive (Table 1). The overall sensitivity of the PCR-Southern blotting

**TABLE 1** Summary of PCR, Southern blotting, and *Taq*I restriction digestion results

| Parameter | *Legionella* serology | |
| --- | --- | --- |
| | Presumptive positive (%) | Negative |
| Total no. tested | 52 | 70 |
| 5S RNA PCR | | |
| Positive | 46 (88.5) | 5 |
| Negative | 6 | 65 |
| Southern blotting | | |
| Positive | 42 (80.7)[a] | 0 |
| Negative | 10 | 70 |
| *Taq*I digestion | | |
| Positive | 41 (78.8)[b] | 2 |
| Negative | 5 | 3 |

[a] Overall percentage sensitivity of the PCR/Southern blotting technique.
[b] Overall percentage sensitivity of the PCR/*Taq*I digestion.

**TABLE 2** Laboratory results from presumptive *Legionella* cases[a]

| Patient no. | Serology titer | Result by: | | | | | | | |
|---|---|---|---|---|---|---|---|---|---|
| | | Serology | Urinary antigen | DFA | Culture | PCR | SB | *Taq*I | C-PCR |
| 1 | <16 | − | + | − | *L.p.* Sg 1 | + | + | + | + |
| 2 | <16 | − | + | − | *L.p.* Sg 1 | + | + | + | + |
| 3 | 256 | *L. feelei* Sg 1 | n.a. | n.a. | n.a. | − | − | n.a. | + |
| | 256 | | | | | + | + | + | + |
| | 128 | | | | | − | − | n.a | + |
| | 64 | | | | | − | − | n.a | + |
| 4 | <16 | − | n.d. | n.d. | *L. longbeachae* Sg 1 | + | + | + | + |
| | <16 | − | | | | + | + | + | + |
| 5 | <16 | − | n.d. | n.d. | *L. micdadei* | + | + | − | + |
| | 512 | *L. micdadei* | | | | + | − | − | + |
| | 512 | | | | | + | + | − | + |
| | 512 | | | | | + | + | + | + |
| | 512 | | | | | + | + | − | + |
| | 512 | | | | | + | + | + | + |
| | 512 | | | | | + | + | + | + |
| | 512 | | | | | + | + | + | + |
| 6 | <16 | − | n.a. | n.d. | *L.p.* Sg 1 | + | + | − | + |
| 7 | 256 | *L. hackeliae* Sg 1 | n.a. | n.d. | − | + | + | + | + |
| | 512 | | | | | + | + | + | + |
| | 256 | | | | | + | + | + | + |
| | 512 | | | | | + | + | + | + |
| | <16 | | | | | + | + | + | + |
| 8 | 512 | *L. birminghamensis* | n.d. | n.a. | n.a. | + | − | + | + |
| | 512 | | | | | + | − | + | + |
| | 512 | | | | | + | − | + | + |
| 9 | 1024 | *L. hackeliae* Sg 2 | n.a. | n.a. | n.a. | − | − | n.a. | + |
| | 128 | | | | | + | + | + | + |
| 10 | <16 | − | n.a. | n.a. | n.a. | + | + | + | + |
| | 512 | *L. feelei* Sg 1 | | | | + | + | + | + |
| | 256 | | | | | − | − | n.a. | + |
| | 128 | | | | | − | − | n.a. | + |
| 11 | 256 | *L.p.* Sg 3 | − | n.a. | n.a. | + | + | + | + |
| | <16 | | − | | | + | + | + | + |
| 12 | 128 | *L.p.* Sg 1 | + | n.a. | n.a. | + | + | + | + |
| | 256 | | + | − | *L.p.* Sg 1 | + | + | + | + |
| 13 | 128 | *L.p.* Sg 1 | − | − | *L.p.* Sg 1 | + | + | + | + |
| 14 | 128 | *L.p.* Sg 1 | − | − | − | + | + | + | + |
| 15 | 256 | *L.p.* Sg 1 | − | n.a. | n.a. | + | + | + | + |
| 16 | 512 | *L.p.* Sg 1 | − | n.a. | n.a. | + | + | + | + |
| 17 | <16 | − | n.a. | n.a. | n.a. | + | + | + | + |
| 18 | <16 | − | + | n.a. | n.a. | + | + | + | − |
| 19 | 512 | *L.p.* Sg 1 | − | − | − | + | + | + | + |
| 20 | 256 | *L.p.* Sg 4 | n.a. | n.a. | n.a. | + | + | + | + |
| | 256 | *L.p.* Sg 4 | | | | + | + | + | + |
| 21 | <16 | − | + | − | − | + | + | + | + |
| | 16 | *L.p.* Sg 1 | + | − | − | + | + | + | + |
| 22 | <16 | − | + | n.a. | n.a. | + | + | + | + |
| | 16 | *L.p.* Sg 1 | + | | | + | + | + | + |
| 23 | 128 | *L.p.* Sg 1 | n.a. | n.a. | n.a. | + | + | + | + |
| | | *L.p.* Sg 1 | | | | | | | |
| 24 | 512 | *L.p.* Sg 1 | n.a. | n.a. | n.a. | + | + | + | + |
| 25 | 256 | *L.p.* Sg 1 | + | n.a. | n.a. | + | + | + | + |
| 26 | 256 | *L.p.* Sg 5 | n.a. | n.a. | n.a. | + | + | + | + |

[a] A list of the laboratory results from 26 presumptive *Legionella* cases is shown. The results for each patient are listed in chronological order. PCR and Southern blotting were performed on all 52 samples from 26 patients. *Taq*I restriction digestion was only performed on 5S RNA PCR-positive samples. The control β-globin PCR was positive in all serum. +, positive; −, negative; PCR, 5S RNA PCR; SB, Southern blotting; *Taq*I, *Taq*I restriction digestion; C-PCR, β-globin control PCR; n.a., not available; n.d., not detected; *L.p.* Sg 1, *L. pneumophila* serogroup 1.

technique on these presumptive *Legionella* cases was 80% (Table 1). These were verified by culture, urinary antigen, and/or serology within the criteria of a laboratory-confirmed case of legionellosis. In most of these cases, *Legionella*-specific DNA was isolated and PCR products were amplified from the patient serum. The primers for the 5S RNA PCR have been shown to amplify DNA contaminating the *Taq* polymerase (7). This is no longer a problem since the production and synthesis of *Taq* polymerase is well controlled. The 5S RNA primers can amplify other microorganisms (8). Therefore, there is a requirement to Southern blot to confirm the specificity of the PCR findings. The *Legionellla*-specific probe was checked against all known gene sequences and found to have only 20% homology with organisms other than the *Legionellaceae*. This Southern blotting technique can detect 100 fg of *Legionella*-specific DNA, whereas the limit of the 5S RNA PCR was found to be only 1 pg (results not shown). The overall sensitivity of the PCR/*Taq* restriction digestion on the presumptive positive cases was 78.8%, which reflects the shortfall in a method that can be performed only on PCR-positive samples. Murdoch et al. (9) only showed a sensitivity of 64% in patient serum and/or urine and 21% of plasma in guinea pigs using the PCR/*Taq*I method (10).

In patients with multiple samples there were variations in PCR reactivity depending on the time of sample (Table 2). In patient 10, the 5S RNA PCR was positive in the first two serum samples (the acute- and early convalescent-phase samples) but negative in the later two convalescent-phase serum samples. However, in patient 5, the presence of DNA in the patient serum remained for more than 30 days. This suggests that the prevalence of DNA is patient dependent and is probably linked to the type of organism and immune status of the individual since there is no underlying trend of PCR positivity. Patient 8 with a serological response to *Legionella birminghamensis* gave a 5S RNA PCR product in three samples but was negative after Southern blotting. The serological reaction may be a result of a cross-reaction with some unrelated organism, since there are cases of serological cross-reactions with *Escherichia coli* (12), *Campylobacter* (3), *Coxiella burnetii* (11), and *Legionella micdadei* (11).

A further 70 serum samples were tested from non-*L. pneumophila* cases. These showed no laboratory evidence of disease. Of the 70 negative serum samples that were tested, 5 were PCR positive, but subsequently Southern blotting negative, although two were still positive after *Taq*I digestion (Table 1). The discrepancies between Southern blotting and *Taq*I restriction digestion in the negative serology group suggest that Southern blotting is more specific than *Taq*I digestion. The Southern blotting has the advantage that it can be performed on all PCR reactions, but the *Taq*I digest requires a PCR product to confirm the specificity of the PCR reaction. To verify the *Taq*I digest result, the PCR product would be required to be sequenced to be certain it was *Legionella* specific.

In conclusion, a 5S RNA PCR was devised for the identification of *Legionella*-specific DNA in patient serum. The specificity of the PCR was verified by Southern blotting and *Taq*I restriction digestion. The DNA extraction and PCR were monitored by a control PCR, which amplified part of the β-globin gene. The 5S RNA PCR was sensitive and specific and should increase laboratory diagnosis of *Legionella* infection when there is a nonvalidated serological response.

## REFERENCES

1. **Dominguez, J. A., N. Gali, P. Pedroso, A. Fargas, E. Padilla, J. M. Manterola, and L. Matas.** 1998. Comparison of the Binax *Legionella* urinary antigen enzyme immunoassay (EIA) with the Biotest *Legionella* Urin antigen EIA for detection of *Legionella* antigen in both concentrated and nonconcentrated urine samples. *J. Clin. Microbiol.* **36:**2718–2722.
2. **Fallon, R. J.** 1981. Laboratory diagnosis of Legionnaires' disease. *Anal. Cell. Pathol.* **99:**1–15.
3. **Fallon, R. J., and W. H. Abraham.** 1992. Crossreactions between *Legionella* and *Campylobacter* spp. *Lancet* **340:**551–552.

4. **Jaulhac, B., M. Nowicki, N. Bornstein, O. Meunier, G. Prevost, Y. Piemont, and J. Fleurette.** 1992. Detection of *Legionella* spp. in bronchoalveolar lavage fluids by DNA amplification. *J. Clin. Microbiol.* **30:**920–924.

5. **Lindsay, D. S. J., W. H. Abraham, and R. J. Fallon.** 1994. Detection of mip gene by PCR for diagnosis of Legionnaires' disease. *J. Clin. Microbiol.* **32:**3068–3069.

6. **Mahbubani, M. H., A. K. Bej, R. Miller, L. Haff, J. DiCesare, and R. M. Atlas.** 1990. Detection of *Legionella* with polymerase chain reaction gene probe methods. *Mol. Cell. Probes* **4:** 175–187.

7. **Maiwald, M., H. J. Ditton, H. G. Sonntag, and M. von Knebel Doeberitz.** 1994. Characterization of contaminating DNA in Taq polymerase which occurs during amplification with a primer set for *Legionella* 5S ribosomal RNA. *Mol. Cell. Probes* **8:**11–14.

8. **Maiwald, M., M. Schill, C. Stockinger, J. H. Helbig, P. C. Lück, W. Witzleb, and H.-G. Sonntag.** 1995. Detection of *Legionella* DNA in human and guinea pig urine samples by the polymerase chain reaction. *Eur. J. Clin. Micro. Infect. Dis.* **14:**25–33.

9. **Murdoch, D. R., E. J. Walford, L. C. Jennings, G. J. Light, M. I. Schousboe, A. Y. Chereshsky, S. T. Chambers, and G. I. Town.** 1996. Use of the polymerase chain reaction to detect *Legionella* DNA in urine and serum samples from patients with pneumonia. *Clin. Infect. Dis.* **23:**475–480.

10. **Murdoch, D. R., L. C. Jennings, G. J. Light, and S. T. Chambers.** 1999. Detection of *Legionella* DNA in guinea pig peripheral leukocytes, urine and plasma by the polymerase chain reaction. *Eur. J. Clin. Microbiol. Infect. Dis.* **18:**445–447.

11. **Musso, D., and D. Raoult.** 1997. Serological cross-reactions between *Coxiella burnetii* and *Legionella micdadei. Clin. Diag. Lab. Immunol.* **4:**208–212.

12. **Wilkinson, H. W., D. D. Cruce, and C. V. Broome.** 1981. Validation of *Legionella pneumophila* indirect immunofluorescence assay with epidemic sera. *J. Clin. Microbiol.* **13:**139–146.

# DIRECT DETECTION OF LEGIONELLAE IN RESPIRATORY TRACT SPECIMENS BY USING FLUORESCENCE IN SITU HYBRIDIZATION

*Jinxin Hu, Ajit P. Limaye, Matthias Horn, Stefan Juretschko, Romesh Gautom, and Thomas R. Fritsche*

# 42

Since the original description of Legionnaires' disease in 1976 (6), *Legionella pneumophila* and other *Legionella* species are well recognized as causative agents of both sporadic and epidemic community-acquired pneumonia. The case mortality rate with *Legionella* infection varies from 5 to 30%, with elderly and immunocompromised patients being most susceptible (2). Because of the need to differentiate legionellosis from other causes of respiratory tract infection to initiate targeted antimicrobial therapy, diagnostic tests that are sensitive, accurate, and timely are needed. Currently, culture is considered the gold standard for detection of legionellae; however, due to the fastidious nature and slow (minimum of 48 to 72 h) growth habit of the organism, and the usual presence of contaminating bacteria in clinical samples, the sensitivity of culture is reported to vary from 50 to 80% (5). To de-

crease the time to detection of organisms and to increase sensitivity over that of culture, a variety of diagnostic methods have been developed and include the direct fluorescent-antibody assay (DFA) technique (4), DNA hybridization assays (8), commercial DNA probes complementary to 16S rRNA (3), and PCR assays (10). The published sensitivities and specificities of these assays range from 31 to 100% and 50 to 90%, respectively. The urinary antigen test has a reported sensitivity of 75 to 90% and a specificity of 100% but has the limitation of being able to only detect infection with *L. pneumophila* serogroup 1 (12).

Fluorescence in situ hybridization (FISH), using probes targeting signature regions of the 16S rRNA molecule, is a technique that has been widely applied to the study of environmental microbiology, especially in the evaluation of complex microbial consortia (1). More recently, FISH has been reported to be a valuable diagnostic tool for the rapid and specific detection of pathogenic bacteria in clinical specimens without the need for cultivation (9, 13). Here we report the application of FISH for the direct detection and identification of *Legionella* spp. and *L. pneumophila* from respiratory tract specimens of patients with pneumonia using published 16S rRNA-based probes specific

*Jinxin Hu, Ajit P. Limaye, and Thomas R. Fritsche* Department of Laboratory Medicine, University of Washington School of Medicine, Seattle, WA 98195-7110. *Matthias Horn* Lehrstuhl für Mikrobiologie, Technische Universität München, Am Hochanger 4, 85350 Freising, Germany. *Stefan Juretschko and Romesh Gautom* Public Health Laboratories, Washington State Department of Health, 1610 NE 150th Street, Shoreline, WA 98155.

*Legionella*, Edited by Reinhard Marre et al.
© 2002 ASM Press, Washington, D.C.

for the genus *Legionella* (Leg705 [5′-ATCTGACCGTCCCAGGT-3′]) (11) and for *L. pneumophila* (LegPne1 [5′-CTGGTGTTCCTTCCGATC-3′]) (7). The probes were labeled with fluorescein isothiocyanate (green signal) or the fluorochrome Cy3 (red signal) at the 5′ end (MWG Biotech, Ebersberg, Germany), and the assay was performed as described elsewhere (7).

## DETERMINATION OF PROBE SPECIFICITY

The specificity of probe LegPne1 was evaluated by Grimm et al. with five different *Legionella* spp. (*L. bozemanii*, *L. hackeliae*, *L. longbeachae*, *L. micdadei*, and *L. anisa*) and with three non-*Legionella* species (*Burkholderia cepacia*, *Escherichia coli* K-12, and *Pseudomonas aeruginosa*) (7). To further evaluate the specificity of this probe we analyzed six additional *Legionella* species, including *L. dumoffii*, *L. feeleii*, *L. maceachernii*, *L. spiritensis*, *L. rubrilucens*, and *L. jamestownensis*, and three non-*Legionella* species, including *Pseudomonas fluorescens*, *Pseudomonas alcaligenes*, and *Bacteroides fragilis*, that are known to share similar morphology and antigens with *Legionella* species. No false-positive or false-negative hybridization reactions of the probe LegPne1 occurred with these strains under the stringency conditions employed.

## FISH ASSAY SENSITIVITY

To determine the sensitivity of FISH with probe LegPne1, we spiked 1 ml of a human bronchoalvealar lavage (BAL) specimen found to be negative for bacterial pathogens with *L. pneumophila* and performed serial dilutions of $10^{-1}$, $10^{-2}$, $10^{-3}$, $10^{-4}$, and $10^{-5}$. Five microliters of each dilution were planted onto four buffered charcoal-yeast extract (BCYE) plates for culture and simultaneously spotted onto 4 wells of 10-well glass microscope slides for FISH. All plates were incubated at 35°C for 72 h for quantitative determination of the number of CFU. The organisms on the slides were hybridized with probe LegPne1 and those organisms displaying fluorescence were enumerated. The comparative results for culture and FISH are summarized in Table 1. The results suggest that FISH is in the range of 1 to 2 orders of magnitude less sensitive than culture.

## COMPARISON OF FISH WITH STANDARD DIAGNOSTIC APPROACHES

To evaluate the usefulness of FISH as a clinical diagnostic method, we analyzed 160 respiratory samples (BAL, pleural fluid, sputum, and tissue) from patients suspected of having pneumonia caused by *Legionella* spp. FISH was performed in a double-blinded fashion in parallel with conventional culture and DFA techniques. The liquid specimens were concentrated by centrifugation at 2,000 rpm for 10 min. One drop of the pellet was applied to buffered charcoal-yeast extract (BCYE) agar without antimicrobial agents and another to BCYE agar with polymyxin B, anisomycin, and vancomycin. The plates were incubated at 35°C with 5 to 10% $CO_2$ and were examined daily for up to 7 days. DFA testing was performed with a polyvalent antibody reagent (Remel, Lenexa, Kans.) according to the manufacturer's recommendations.

In situ hybridization was performed under the conditions described by Grimm et al. (7). Five microliters of the sample pellet was spotted directly onto duplicate fields of 10-well glass microscope slides and heat fixed. Probes Leg705 and LegPne1, one labeled with fluorescein and the other labeled with Cy3, were added simultaneously to each well, except for

**TABLE 1** Detection limit of *Legionella* spp. using FISH with probe LegPne1 compared with culture on BCYE agar

| Dilution | Culture (CFU) | FISH (no. of bacteria) |
|---|---|---|
| $10^{-1}$ | >1,000 | >1,000 |
| $10^{-2}$ | >1,000 | 910 |
| $10^{-3}$ | 908 | 38 |
| $10^{-4}$ | 110 | 1 |
| $10^{-5}$ | 10 | 0 |

**TABLE 2**  Comparison of culture, DFA test, and FISH in patients with legionellosis

| Case | Sample | Result by: | | | |
|------|--------|---------|-----|------------|-----------|
| | | | | FISH probe | |
| | | Culture | DFA | Leg705 | LegPne1 |
| 1 | BAL | *L. pneumophila* | − | + | + |
| 2[a] | Pleural fluid | No growth | − | + | + |
| 3 | Sputum | *L. longbeachae* | + | + | − |
| 4 | BAL | No growth | + | + | − |
| 5 | Lung biopsy | *L. micdadei* | + | + | − |
| 6 | Sputum | *L. longbeachae* | + | + | − |
| 7 | Sputum | *L. longbeachae* | + | + | − |
| 8 | BAL | *L. longbeachae* | + | + | − |
| 9 | BAL | *L. pneumophila* | + | + | + |
| 10 | BAL | *L. micdadei* | + | + | − |

[a] Urine antigen test positive for *L. pneumophila* serogroup 1.

the negative-control well, where hybridization buffer alone was added. Positive controls consisting of *L. pneumophila* were spotted on slides and processed separately to prevent the possibility of carry-over contamination. Among the 160 clinical specimens, 10 showed a positive hybridization signal with probe Leg705; a subset of 3 of these were also reactive with probe LegPne1 (Fig. 1). Results for conventional testing and for FISH are summarized in Table 2.

## CONCLUSIONS

rRNA-targeted in situ hybridization has been employed for the identification of *L. pneumophila* in pure culture and from infected protozoa (7, 11), but to our knowledge this study represents the first report on the successful application of probes Leg705 and LegPne1 for the specific detection of *Legionella* spp. and *L. pneumophila* in clinical samples. In patient 2 (Table 2), culture and DFA were negative for *Legionella* spp. The chest X ray of the patient revealed bilateral pleural effusions and the chest CT scan revealed bilateral lower lobe infiltrates suggestive of infectious pneumonia. FISH directly identified the presence of *L. pneumophila* in pleural fluid specimens and the urine antigen assay was positive, confirming infection with *L. pneumophila* serogroup 1. The fact that *L. pneumophila* was not recovered

from culture may have been due to prior use of antimicrobial agents that inhibited growth of the organisms. Patient 4 had an equivocal (with strong peripheral staining but morphology inconsistent with *Legionella*) DFA test and negative culture but was positive with probe Leg705 by FISH. While mucoid *P. aeruginosa*

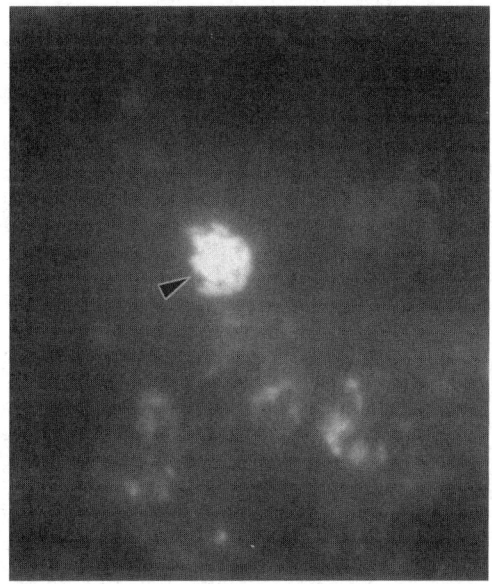

**FIGURE 1**  Microscopic examination of BAL specimen after hybridization with probe LegPne1 that is specific for *L. pnemophila*. *L. pneumophila* was seen as a cluster of intracellular bacilli (arrowhead).

grew on the BCYE plates, no hybridization signal occurred when tested with probe LegPne1. These results suggested that a non-*L. pneumophila Legionella* sp. was present, but was either nonviable due to prior antimicrobial therapy or was outgrown by the mucoid *Pseudomonas*, which displayed near-confluent growth.

From our experience, *L. pneumophila* is not the leading species producing human infection in our geographic region. Almost two-thirds of *Legionella* pneumonia cases identified were caused by either *L. longbeachae* or *L. micdadei*. Given this background, development of a series of probes specific for the predominant species may be of value for identification and epidemiologic purposes. These results further demonstrate that the direct application of FISH to clinical specimens is at least comparable to traditional methods and may offer the added advantages of enhanced specificity, rapidity (approximately 2 h are required for assay performance), and cost-effectiveness. Assay sensitivity can be determined only with the analysis of additional specimens.

## REFERENCES

1. **Amann, R. I., W. Ludwig, and K. H. Schleifer.** 1995. Phylogenetic identification and *in situ* detection of individual microbial cells without cultivation. *Microbiol. Rev.* **59:**143–169.
2. **Breiman, R. F., and J. C. Butler.** 1998. Legionnaires' disease: clinical, epidemiological, and public health perspectives. *Semin. Respir. Infect.* **13:**84–89.
3. **Doebbeling, B. N., M. J. Bale, F. P. Koontz, C. M. Helms, R. P. Wenzel, and M. A. Pfaller.** 1988. Prospective evaluation of the Gen-Probe assay for detection of legionellae in respiratory specimens. *Eur. J. Clin. Microbiol. Infect. Dis.* **7:**748–752.
4. **Edelstein, P. H., K. B. Beer, J. C. Sturge, A. J. Watson, and L. C. Goldstein.** 1985. Clinical utility of a monoclonal direct fluorescent reagent specific for *Legionella pneumophila*: comparative study with other reagents. *J. Clin. Microbiol.* **22:**419–421.
5. **Finegold, S. M.** 1988. Legionnaires' disease—still with us. *N. Engl. J. Med.* **318:**571–573.
6. **Fraser, D. W., T. R. Tsai, W. Orenstein, W. E. Parkin, H. J. Beecham, R. G. Sharrar, J. Harris, G. F. Mallison, S. M. Martin, J. E. McDade, C. C. Shepard, and P. S. Brachman.** 1977. Legionnaires' disease: description of an epidemic of pneumonia. *N. Engl. J. Med.* **297:** 1189–1197.
7. **Grimm, D., H. Merkert, W. Ludwig, K. H. Schleifer, J. Hacker, and B. C. Brand.** 1998. Specific detection of *Legionella pneumophila*: construction of a new 16S rRNA-targeted oligonucleotide probe. *Appl. Environ. Microbiol.* **64:**2686–2690.
8. **Grimont, P. A., F. Grimont, N. Desplaces, and P. Tchen.** 1985. DNA probe specific for *Legionella pneumophila*. *J. Clin. Microbiol.* **21:**431–437.
9. **Krimmer, V., H. Merkert, C. von Eiff, M. Frosch, J. Eulert, J. F. Lohr, J. Hacker, and W. Ziebuhr.** 1999. Detection of *Staphylococcus aureus* and *Staphylococcus epidermidis* in clinical samples by 16S rRNA-directed in situ hybridization. *J. Clin. Microbiol.* **37:**2667–2673.
10. **Mahbubani, M. H, A. K. Bej, R. Miller, L. Haff, J. DiCesare, and R. M. Atlas.** 1990. Detection of *Legionella* with polymerase chain reaction and gene probe methods. *Mol. Cell. Probes* **4:**175–187.
11. **Manz, W., R. Amann, R. Szewzyk, U. Szewzyk, T. A. Stenstrom, P. Hutzler, and K. H. Schleifer.** 1995. In situ identification of *Legionellaceae* using 16S rRNA-targeted oligonucleotide probes and confocal laser scanning microscopy. *Microbiology* **141:**29–39.
12. **Plouffe, J. F., T. M. File, Jr., R. F. Breiman, B. A. Hackman, S. J. Salstrom, B. J. Marston, and B. S. Fields.** 1995. Re-evaluation of the definition of Legionnaires' disease: use of the urinary antigen assay. Community Based Pneumonia Incidence Study Group. *Clin. Infect. Dis.* **20:**1286–1291.
13. **Trebesius, K., K. Panthel, S. Strobel, K. Vogt, G. Faller, T. Kirchner, M. Kist, J. Heesemann, and R. Haas.** 2000. Rapid and specific detection of *Helicobacter pylori* macrolide resistance in gastric tissue by fluorescent in situ hybridisation. *Gut* **46:**608–614.

# DETECTION AND TYPING

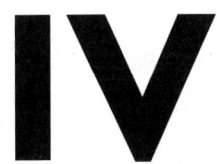

# MOLECULAR TOOLS FOR EPIDEMIOLOGICAL INVESTIGATIONS INTO *LEGIONELLA PNEUMOPHILA* INFECTIONS

*Alex van Belkum*

# 43

Approximately 2 years ago the largest outbreak of infections by *Legionella pneumophila* reported to date (3) hit the newspapers in The Netherlands (26). The source of the outbreak was traced back to a combined flower show and household exposition. Upon detailed but primarily classical epidemiological and microbiological investigations, the ultimate source was determined to be a bubble bath on display in the household exposition. In the end, 188 cases suspect to infection were traced and ultimately 133 of these individuals had really been infected. Attack rates as determined among exhibitors were three times as high as for visitors. Many people were determined to be seropositive responders to the infection. Serum antibody values matched very well with the location of the various exhibit stands and their distance to the source of infection: serum antibody levels were highest in those exhibitors close to the contaminated bubble bath. More than 30 people died as a direct result of the infection with an *L. pneumophila* serotype 1 strain. This major incident primed

the Dutch toward improvement of policies to prevent *Legionella* infections in general. During the past 2 years, the search for *L. pneumophila*, especially in water supply systems, was enormously intensified, which led to an increase in the discovery of contaminated sources. Whether this improved search-and-attack strategy has resulted in a decrease in the number of clinically manifest infections is a matter of current investigations. It is interesting to note that in the United States and the United Kingdom, additional examples of the involvement of exhibit whirlpool spas have been demonstrated recently (1, 11).

Besides regional national initiatives in various European Union member countries, the European Working Group on *Legionella* Infections (EWGLI) has been investigating *Legionella* prevalence all over Europe. This has resulted in a large database containing clinical data on more than 2,000 infections and information on, for instance, those South European holiday resorts where *Legionella* infections or at least *Legionella* presence in the water system have been noted more than once over the past years. The data gathered by EWGLI have not been made generally available, but EWGLI members do have access to the detailed descriptions in the database. The increased awareness of the Dutch public health threats

*Alex van Belkum* Department of Medical Microbiology & Infectious Diseases, Erasmus University Medical Center Rotterdam EMCR, Dr. Molewaterplein 40, 3015 GD Rotterdam, The Netherlands.

*Legionella*, Edited by Reinhard Marre et al.
© 2002 ASM Press, Washington, D.C.

posed by *L. pneumophila* initiated the discussion on whether the EWGLI data should be made publicly accessible. Suggestions put forward by the Dutch national health inspectorate to effectively do so through the Internet were not very well received by especially the South Europeans. The discussion on balancing economically detrimental effects versus the obvious health risks is still going on. One important aspect, however, has already been made clear: as long as no precise data on the dissemination of *L. pneumophila* bacteria throughout Europe have been determined accurately, the intimate association between putative sources of infections and source-related individual patients can hardly be made. This shows the need for the development of *L. pneumophila* identification networks. Only when bacterial isolates derived from patients can be adequately typed and these types can be reliably compared with, for instance, those types obtained from environmental sources that have been collated into large databases, can patients and sources possibly be directly and conveniently linked.

This chapter describes the theoretical framework within which typing networks can be established. The definitions used for identifying bacterial strains and clones will be provided, and the clinical value of typing will be illustrated as well. Current tools available for molecular typing of *L. pneumophila* will be shortly described and their reproducibility discussed. Some of the current developments in the field of bacterial genetic identification will be pinpointed, and ongoing and future developments in the field of establishing typing networks will be summarized.

## DEFINITIONS

Microbiology will always be focused on specific cultivation of the multitudes of microbial species that surround us. Viable cultures provide the microbiologist with populations of cells that can be studied in more detail and with which all sorts of laboratory-based manipulations can be performed. An important term in this respect is the bacterial isolate: a population of cells obtained in monoculture from a primary (in our medical microbiology profession, clinical) material and identified to the species level.

When additional information on the nature of a specific isolate is obtained, the isolate transforms into a strain. A strain is an isolate or a group of isolates showing traits that are distinct from those of other isolates belonging to the same species.

A reference strain is a well-characterized strain that is preserved for further study and which is frequently used as the "internal standard" during other identification studies.

Strains and references strains belong to certain types. A type is defined as a set of marker scores displayed by a strain upon application of a particular marker system (read "typing procedure").

Finally, a clone is a group of isolates or strains descending from a common (and frequently recent) ancestor as part of a direct chain of replication and transmission from host to host, environment to host, or vice versa.

In summary, typing of bacterial isolates translates these isolates into strains and possibly clones because of the designation of type information. Typing serves the purpose of defining or excluding clonal relatedness among bacterial isolates. Types can be used for the analysis or tracking of local, national, and even international bacterial dissemination.

## TECHNOLOGY

Current typing systems are very diverse in nature. The most common overall methodological distinction is the one between phenotyping and genotyping procedures. Phenotyping, which will not be discussed in detail in this chapter, is the collection of methods that define, among others, biochemical, immunological, or proteinaceous characteristics of microbial isolates (see, for instance, references 7, 16, and 18 for additional examples of phenotyping procedures). Opposite these methods are the genotyping strategies. These share the fact that they all address nucleic acid as a source of microbial polymorphism. Again, a wide variety of methods have been described, both in the past and more recently. Some of these, such as plasmid profiling or crude restriction of chromosomal DNA, have already been outdated by the newer generation of methods. Table 1 provides a concise literature review highlighting the temporal popularity of *L. pneumophila* typing methods and the changes in the frequency of usage of the various systems over the past decade. Newer methods are for instance the PCR-mediated strategies. Genes can be specifically amplified and analyzed for sequence variability on the basis of restriction site polymorphism or variable length of the PCR products. Random amplification of polymorphic DNA (RAPD) analysis and arbitrary primed PCR are methods that are essentially based on random priming of PCR primers, often using quite relaxed reaction conditions (21). This gives rise to complex mixtures of PCR fragments that can be translated into DNA fingerprints with the help of gel electrophoresis (Fig. 1). Besides direct PCR-mediated approaches, pulsed-field gel electrophoresis (PFGE) of DNA macrorestriction fragments has been introduced in the microbiology laboratory over the past 10 years. This method is electrophoresis-based and succeeds in the separation of extremely large DNA molecules of up to 5 Mb in length. Basic to the technology is that during electrophoresis, the electric field switches in direction. This results in conformational changes in the large DNA molecules on the basis of which they show size-dependent in-gel mobility. Amplification fragment length polymorphism (AFLP) analysis is another recent PCR-mediated procedure with which subsets of DNA restriction fragments can be successfully amplified. Once run on a gel, highly complex DNA fingerprints can be visualized (see Fig. 2 for a theoretical scheme and a gel picture). Currently, DNA sequence-based approaches are gaining in prevalence. This will probably result in another major shift in the usage of *L. pneumophila* typing procedures (Table 1).

Most of the methods described above generate DNA fingerprints that present as sometimes highly complex banding patterns. Interpretation and categorization of these patterns is generally complex, especially when large numbers of patterns need to be compared. Computerized methods are indispensable, but not always that user-friendly. For these and other reasons, various typing procedures that produce more robust data have been or are being developed. One of these is

**TABLE 1** Frequency of usage of various typing procedures for epidemiological analysis of *L. pneumophila* isolates: a recent historical perspective[a]

| Period | No. of times method was used | | | | | | |
|---|---|---|---|---|---|---|---|
| | Plasmic typing | REA | Ribotyping | AP PCR/RAPD | PFGE | AFLP | Sequence-based methods |
| 1990 a.e. | 10 | 4 | 0 | 0 | 0 | 0 | 0 |
| 1991–1993 | 3 | 6 | 6 | 1 | 5 | 0 | 0 |
| 1994–1996 | 2 | 2 | 4 | 9 | 15 | 0 | 0 |
| 1997–2000 | 0 | 1 | 3 | 13 | 20 | 4 | 1 |

[a] Figures indicate numbers of publications in peer-reviewed journals during the period stated in the column on the left. Data were obtained by screening the National Library of Medicine database (PubMed) at www.nlm.nih.gov/PubMed/ (December 2000 version). Both acronyms and full-spelling versions of the various terms used for the typing procedures were searched for. Some publications were included more than once due to the fact that multiple typing procedures were used simultaneously; review papers were excluded. The single hit in the sequence-based typing column involved single gene (*gyr*A) analysis; MLST data were published in the form of meeting abstracts only (not included in PubMed). REA, restriction enzyme analysis; AP PCR, arbitrarily primed polymerase chain reaction; RAPD, random amplified polymorphic DNA; PFGE, pulsed-field gel electrophoresis; AFLP, amplification fragment length polymorphism.

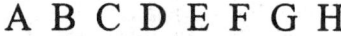
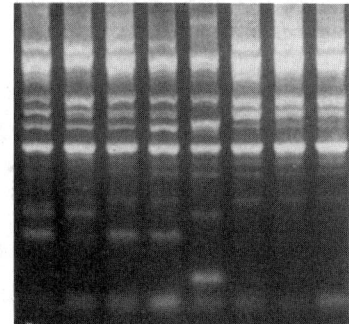

ERIC2
BG2

**FIGURE 1** RAPD analysis of *L. pneumophila* reference strains and isolates obtained during water contamination or nosocomial outbreaks of infection. A combination of two primers (ERIC2 and BG2) was applied during amplification. Lanes: A, NCTC12008-OLDA; B, NCTC11404-Bellingham; C, Hospital B, clinical isolate; D, water isolate hospital A; E through H, patient isolates obtained in hospital A. Patients F, G, and H were hospitalized simultaneously. The identity of the RAPD fingerprints suggests an ongoing outbreak of infections involving patients F, G, and H. Note, however, that not all patients who are epidemiologically linked are infected by the same strain (lane E).

the hybridization-based binary typing procedure that has already been presented for various pathogens and in different experimental formats (see later in this chapter and references 10 and 24). DNA sequencing and DNA chip technology are currently receiving much attention and it is beyond doubt that these technologies will be implemented ever more frequently in the field of epidemiological typing of microbes.

Typing methods, to be successful, should be of high quality in various aspects. Typeability should be high (preferably 100%), implying that all isolates should be amenable to data-generating analysis. The reproducibility of the method should be as high as possible and its discriminatory power should be excellent. The experimental performance should be good and the interpretation of data should be as easy as possible. The availability should be broad and the costs should be low. In the

field of legionellosis, the ideal procedure has not yet been identified, but both PFGE and AFLP are considered sufficiently adequate in all aspects listed above to make interesting candidates for the development of a novel "gold standard" *Legionella* typing forum (Table 1).

## POSITIONING *L. PNEUMOPHILA* TYPING IN CLINICAL DISEASE RESEARCH AND MANAGEMENT

An important question is whether there is an undisputed clinical need for typing of *L. pneumophila*. This can best be illustrated by highlighting a study where sources of infection and patients linked to these sources could be identified with the help of molecular typing. In a general hospital in Haarlem (The Netherlands) (1996) a man was diagnosed with *L. pneumophila* pneumonia (2). The patient contracted his pneumonia shortly after a visit to a local sauna. In the water system of the sauna, in an air-perfused foot bath in particular, a *Legionella* contamination was discovered. The isolates from patient and sauna were indiscriminate by RAPD fingerprinting. Upon retrospective analysis of all previous cases of Legionnaires' disease in the same geographic locale, five additional patients were linked to the same sauna on the basis of epidemiological data. Two of the patients succumbed to their infection and the strains isolated from the two most recently diseased individuals were still available. Typing revealed the identity of these isolates to the other two strains. Classical epidemiology suggested that heavy smoking seemed to prime individuals to infection; molecular typing definitely linked source and patients and provided direct evidence for long-term contamination and consequent infection risk due to perseverance of a single point-source of *L. pneumophila* bacteria. Upon elucidation of the transmission route, preventive measures were implemented. Improvement of the hygienic conditions in the foot bath completely eliminated *L. pneumophila* and no subsequent infections were noted.

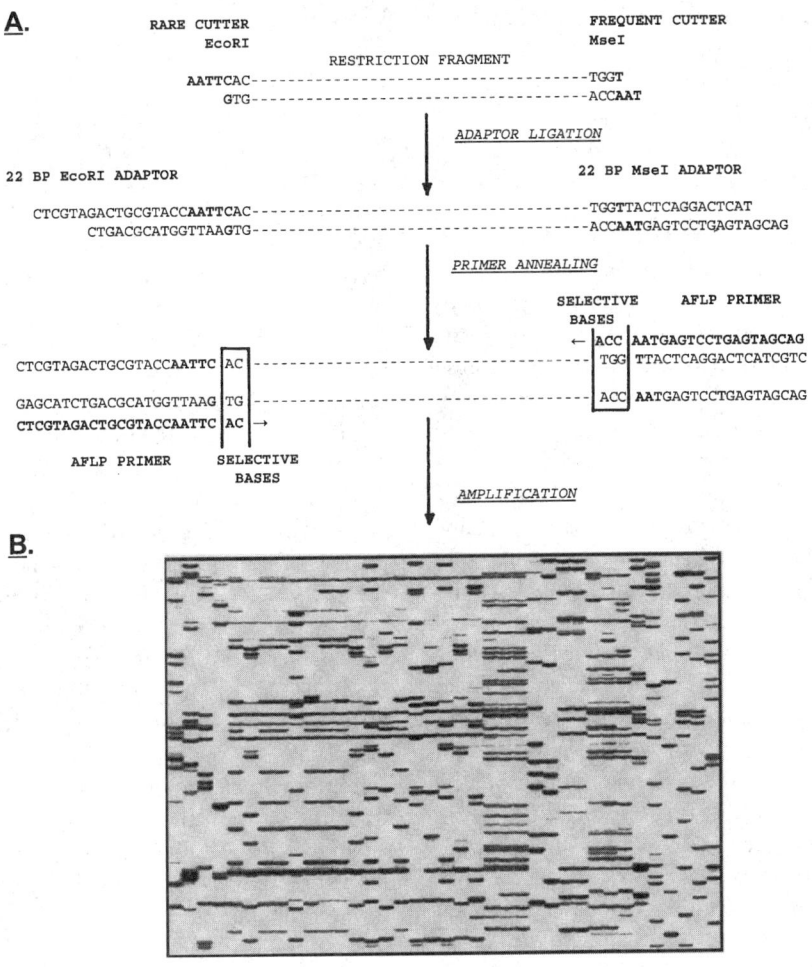

**FIGURE 2** Principle of AFLP (Keygene NV, Wageningen, The Netherlands) and example of its experimental output. Panel A delineates the various stages in the typing protocol. Initially, DNA is digested with the help of two different restriction enzymes. Specific linkers are coupled to the respective sticky ends and these linkers serve as specific anchor points for fragment amplification by PCR. Inclusion of selective bases (encoded in the neighboring region of the native restriction sites) in the primer sequences results in amplification of limited numbers of specific restriction fragments. These can be effectively separated by acryl amide gel electrophoresis and visualized by techniques for detection of haptens incorporated in primers or dNTPs used during amplification (panel B).

The example alluded to above clearly shows that molecular typing can be very helpful in the elucidation of the epidemiology of Legionnaires' disease. As such, typing can contribute to the control of epidemics and outbreaks. The study mentioned above, however, was largely retrospective in nature. To improve on timeliness, typing of clinical and environmental *L. pneumophila* isolates should be performed in a more immediate, online fashion. Although the final choice for an appropriate tool to really develop such a monitoring system has not yet been made, many studies aiming at the definition of such a system by comparative quality assessment for various methods have been described. Significant progress has been made in standardizing molecular typing of *L. pneumophila*, a field of research that will be surveyed below.

## ARE THE CURRENT TYPING PROCEDURES SUFFICIENTLY USEFUL?

To define whether the current typing procedures meet the requirements described in one of the previous sections, many studies aiming at comparative quality assessment have been described in recent literature. One of these studies described the comparison between a frequently used phenotyping test and three different DNA mediated methods (19). It appeared that serotyping suffers from limited resolution. The two systems aiming at the detection of polymorphism in ribosomal genes, ribotyping and PCR-mediated amplification of 16S-23S spacer domains, displayed intermediate resolution, whereas RAPD showed a clearly superior level of interstrain discrimination. This, however, does not unequivocally identify RAPD analysis as the method of choice, since multicenter reproducibility, for instance, was not studied. Many other comparative studies have been published over the years (6, 13, 15, 16, 18), which resulted in the selection of PFGE and AFLP as the current typing methods of choice (5). For these two latter methods, multicenter studies have revealed that AFLP may be the method most suited for the development of decentralized typing networks.

## STANDARDIZATION OF TYPING: NECESSITY OR WASTE OF ENERGY?

Typing standardization efforts were undertaken in the recent past for various species of microorganisms other than *L. pneumophila*. For instance in the case of *Staphylococcus aureus*, various multicenter typing studies have been described over the past years. Tenover et al. (17) initially compared 12 different typing procedures with respect to resolution and epidemiological coherence. This study essentially showed that if one rigorously standardizes one's favorite typing protocol, the data are generally very useful for elucidating local matters of epidemiological concern. None of the different typing procedures evaluated in this study performed in a dissatisfactory manner, although genetic typing was favorable to most authors. Two other staphylococcal studies have been described in recent literature. Both of these studies focused on a single typing strategy performed by a multitude of different research groups. Firstly, a multicenter study on RAPD analysis was performed (20). This again showed that RAPD analysis provides a method that can be very well used in a single institute: the resolving power appeared sufficient for the identification of major clonal groups of strains. However, it appeared that the nature of the RAPD fingerprints differed vastly among the datasets generated by the various participants. The conclusion was that RAPD is a high-speed method excellently suited for answering local epidemiological questions, but this method is completely unsuited for the establishment of interinstitutional or (inter)national typing networks. Secondly, PFGE was evaluated with respect to interinstitutional reproducibility (22). Although the experimental output again differed from laboratory to laboratory, this study did show successfully that several laboratories generated data that could be exchanged and put into a single, matching database. In conclusion it could be stated that standardization of typing depends on a large number of hard-to-control experimental variables. It was questioned whether banding pattern–based bacterial fingerprint analyses will be at all feasible. Currently, a project funded by the European Union (HARMONY, chaired by B. Cookson, Public Health Service Laboratories, London, United Kingdom) is investigating the feasibility of developing a trans-European PFGE network for immediate follow-up of the spread of methicillin-resistant *S. aureus*. In addition the European GENE project (Sylvain Brisse, Utrecht Medical Center, Utrecht, The Netherlands) aims at the establishment of pan-European networks for typing various pathogens using the commercially available Qualicon automated riboprinters. For both projects there is significant overlap with the PulseNet framework developed in the United States for tracking pathogenic *Escherichia coli* strains (B. Swaminathan, Centers for Disease Control and Prevention, Atlanta, Ga.).

Since the mid-1980s, many researchers have tried to develop *L. pneumophila* typing assays that adhered to a very strict and normalized experimental protocol. Efforts initially tried to capitalize on the availability of standard sets of monoclonal antibodies for *L. pneumophila* (7). However, due to the limited availability and resolving power of the antibody-mediated typing procedure, it never became widely accepted. Recently, important initiatives by EWGLI revealed the feasibility of developing typing networks using AFLP. A preliminary study revealed that AFLP may indeed be the method of choice (5), a finding that was also corroborated by epidemiological studies presented by individual research groups (8). Although the epidemiological concordance and reproducibility of AFLP appeared to be a sub-ideal 94 and 90%, respectively, AFLP was still pinpointed the procedure most likely to survive multicenter application (5). This was experimentally corroborated as well recently (4). The investigators showed that 100% reproducibility and 100% epidemiological concordance could be observed among a subset of the participants taking part in a multicenter study. It has to be emphasized, however, that overall (all participants included), the reproducibility varied between 20 and 100%, whereas the epidemiological concordance covaried between 11 and 100%. As the authors conclude: "The AFLP methodology is clearly very robust, and despite noncompliance with the standard protocol the method can still yield useful local results. However, for meaningful intercentre comparison, standardisation of the AFLP methodology requires the careful control of many experimental parameters." Apparently, the level of interlaboratory standardization obtained thus far is satisfactory albeit not (yet?) at the desired level. The question of whether genuine typing networks can be developed in the near future still is not completely answered. Finally, microbial biology is also important when considering the establishment of standard typing protocols. *L. pneumophila* has been demonstrated to possess an effective system for the exchange of DNA moieties (25) and it can survive for prolonged periods of time in biofilms (14). It is currently not known whether this and possibly other bacterial features may influence the outcome of genetic identification assays.

## CURRENT AND FUTURE ALTERNATIVES

Two major developments in the field of molecular biology have and will continue to have a clear impact on the field of bacterial epidemiology and population genetics: high-throughput nucleic acid sequencing and chip technology. DNA sequencing technology has revolutionized microbiology in general because it enabled whole genome sequencing for a variety of microorganisms. This facilitates the identification of novel target sequence motifs for epidemiological typing. Multilocus sequence typing (MLST) is one example: the sequence polymorphism detected in a number of slowly evolving genes allows for the categorization of strains on the basis of allelic diversity. Even in the absence of the complete *L. pneumophila* genome sequence (J. Russo, S. Qu, I. Morozova, M. Chien, G. Segal, R. Slotky, S. Kalachikov, E. Cayanis, B. Zhao, A. Gheorghiou, M. Glaperin, J. Chen, G. Asamani, K. Hill, H. Park, M. Feder, J. Rineer, C. Goldsberry, P. DeJong, E. Koonin, A. Rzhetsky, P. Zhang, and H. Shuman, *Abstr. Book 5th Int. Conf. Legionella*, abstr. O7, p. 6, 2000), the first examples of MLST schemes for *L. pneumophila* are now becoming available. This involves genes such as those encoding heat shock proteins, aconitase, flagellin, RecA, metalloprotease, and the major outer membrane protein (V. Gaia and R. Peduzzi, *Int. Mtg. Bacterial Epidemiol. Markers*, Noordwijkerhout, The Netherlands, abstr. S10). It is reassuring to note that this novel typing strategy shows excellent concordance with the data obtained by AFLP analysis. DNA chip technology, characterized by its extremely high-throughput probe-mediated nucleic acid identification capacity, has not yet been introduced in the field of *L. pneumophila* detection and identification. Although the technology has been used recently to map the (host) response of macrophages upon invasion by the bacteria (12), no chip-mediated typing tests are available. Since for *Mycobacterium tuberculosis* (10) and *S. aureus* (23, 24) precursors for microchip analysis have been developed, it is anticipated that also in other fields of bacterial epidemiology chip-mediated tests will be introduced shortly. These novel technologies have universal applicability, rendering them suitable for typing of other species of legionellae as well (9).

## CONCLUDING REMARKS

On the basis of the current state of affairs, it is anticipated that for the coming decade, "banding pattern-based" tests such as PFGE and AFLP will be most frequently used for the study of outbreaks of Legionnaires' disease in the individual laboratory setting. International networks will be developed on the basis of either of these or maybe even both technologies, but it is anticipated that with the progression of whole genome DNA sequencing and DNA chip technology, the gel electrophoresis-based methods will ultimately become obsolete. In the end, binary data, such as differential probe reactivity or DNA sequences, will become decisive in molecular epidemiologic studies on *L. pneumophila* and other microbial species. For the time being, centralized facilities for the establishment of typing networks are to be preferred over the decentralized approach. Future technology improvement may increase the self-sustained development of exchangeable data subdirectories in individual laboratories, but we still have to go a long way before we get there.

## ACKNOWLEDGMENTS

I gratefully acknowledge Marc Struelens (Université Libre de Bruxelles, Hopital Erasme, Bruxelles, Belgium) for introducing me to *L. pneumophila* as a clinically relevant microorganism. Nan van Leeuwen (RIVM, Bilthoven, The Netherlands), Ed Yzerman (Laboratory of Public Health, Haarlem, The Netherlands), and Jeroen den Boer (Municipal Health Service Zuid-Kennemerland, Haarlem, The Netherlands) are thanked for allowing me to participate in their past and current studies. All my colleagues from within the Department of Medical Microbiology & Infectious Diseases (University Hospital Rotterdam, The Netherlands) are thanked for continuous support and experimental expertise! The AFLP illustration has been kindly provided by Guus Simons (Keygene NV, Wageningen, The Netherlands).

## REFERENCES

1. **Benkel, D. H., E. M. McClure, D. Woolard, J. V. Rullan, G. B. Miller, S. R. Jenkins, J. H. Hershey, R. F. Benson, J. M. Pruckler, E. W. Brown, M. S. Kolczak, R. L. Hackler, B. S. Rouse, and R. F. Breiman.** 2000. Outbreak of Legionnaires' disease associated with a display whirlpool spa. *Int. J. Epidemiol.* **29:**1092–1098.
2. **Den Boer, J. W., E. Yzerman, A. van Belkum, F. Vlaspolder, and F. J. M. van Breukelen.** 1998. Legionnaire's disease and saunas. *Lancet* **351:**1056.
3. **Formica, N., G. Tallis, B. Zwolak, J. Camie, M. Beers, G. Hogg, N. Ryan, and M. Yates.** 2000. Legionnaires' Disease outbreak: Victoria's largest identified outbreak. *Commun. Dis. Intell.* **24:**199–202.
4. **Fry, N. K., J. M. Bangsborg, S. Bernarder, J. Etienne, B. Forsblom, V. Gaia, P. Hasenberger, D. Lindsay, A. Papoutsi, C. Pelaz, M. Struelens, S. A. Uldum, P. Visca, and T. G. Harrison.** 2000. Assessment of intercentre reproducibility and epidemiological concordance of *Legionella pneumophila* serogroup 1 genotyping by amplified fragment length polymorphism analysis. *Eur. J. Clin. Microbiol. Infect. Dis.* **19:**773–780.
5. **Fry, N. K., S. Alexiou-Daniel, J. M. Bangsborg, S. Bernarder, M. Castellani Pastoris, J. Etienne, B. Forsblom, V. Gaia, J. H. Helbig, D. Lindsay, P. C. Luck, C. Pelaz, S. A. Uldum, and T. G. Harrison.** 1999. A multicenter evaluation of genotypic methods for the epidemiologic typing of *Legionella pneumophila* serogroup 1: results of a pan-European study. *Clin. Microbiol. Infect.* **5:**462–477.

6. **Gomez-Lus, P., B. S. Fields, R. F. Benson, W. T. Martin, S. P. O'Connor, and C. M. Black.** 1993. Comparison of arbitrary primed polymerase chain reaction, ribotyping and monoclonal antibody analysis for subtyping *Legionella pneumophila* serogroup 1. *J. Clin. Microbiol.* **31:** 1940–1942.

7. **Joly, J. R., R. M. McKinney, J. O. Tobin, J. Bibb, I. D. Watkins, and D. Ramsay.** 1986. Development of a standardised subgrouping scheme for *Legionella pneumophila* serogroup 1 using monoclonal antibodies. *J. Clin. Microbiol.* **23:** 768–771.

8. **Jonas, D., H. G. W. Meyer, P. Matthes, D. Hartung, B. Jahn, F. D. Daschner, and B. Jansen.** 2000. Comparative evaluation of three different genotyping methods for investigation of nosocomial outbreaks of Legionnaire's Disease in hospitals. *J. Clin. Microbiol.* **38:**2284–2291.

9. **Knirsch, C. A., K. Jakob, D. Schoonmaker, J. A. Kiehlbauch, S. J. Wong, P. Delta-Latta, S. Whittier, M. Layton, and B. Scully.** 2000. An outbreak of *Legionella micdadei* pneumonia in transplant patients: evaluation, molecular epidemiology and control. *Am. J. Med.* **108:** 290–295.

10. **Kremer, K., D. van Soolingen, R. Frothingham, W. H. Haas, P. W. M. Hermans, C. Martin, P. Palittapnogarnpim, B. B. Plikaytis, L. W. Riley, M. A. Yakrus, J. M. Musser, and J. D. A. van Embden.** 1999. Comparison of methods based on different molecular epidemiological markers for typing of *Mycobacterium tuberculosis* complex strains: interlaboratory study of discriminatory power and reproducibility. *J. Clin. Microbiol.* **37:**2607–2618.

11. **McEvoy, M., N. Batchelor, G. Hamilton, A. MacDonald, M. Faiers, A. Sills, J. Lee, and T. Harrison.** 2000. A cluster of Legionnaires' disease associated with exposure to a spa pool on display. *Commun. Dis. Public Health* **3:**43–45.

12. **Nakachi, N., K. Matsunaga, T. W. Klein, H. Friedman, and Y. Yamamoto.** 2000. Differential effect of virulent versus avirulent *Legionella pneumophila* on chemokine gene expression in murine alveolar macrophages determined by cDNA expression array technique. *Infect. Immun.* **68:**6069–6072.

13. **Saunders, N. A., T. G. Harrison, T. Haththotuwa, and A. G. Taylor.** 1991. A comparison of probes for restriction fragment length polymorphism (RFLP) typing of *Legionella pneumophila* serotype 1 strains. *J. Med. Microbiol.* **35:** 152–158.

14. **Sessa, R., M. Di Pietro, M. Zamparelli, and M. Del Piano.** 2000. Biofilm formation on the surface of ceramic tiles. *New Microbiol.* **23:**407–413.

15. **Schoonmaker, D., T. Heimberger, and G. Birkhead.** 1992. Comparison of ribotyping and restriction enzyme analysis using pulsed field gel electrophoresis for distinguishing *Legionella pneumophila* isolates obtained during a nosocomial outbreak. *J. Clin. Microbiol.* **30:**1491–1498.

16. **Struelens, M. J., N. Maes, F. Rost, A. Deplano, F. Jacobs, C. Liesnard, N. Bornstein, F. Grimont, S. Lauwers, M. P. McIntyre, and E. Serruys.** 1992. Genotypic and phenotypic methods for the investigation of a nosocomial *Legionella pneumophila* outbreak and efficacy of control measures. *J. Infect. Dis.* **166:**22–30.

17. **Tenover, F. C., R. Arbeit, G. Archer, J. Biddle, S. Byrne, R. Goering, G. Hancock, G. A. Hebert, B. Hill, R. Hollis, W. J. Jarvis, B. Kreiswirth, B. Eisner, J. Maslow, L. K. MacDougal, M. Miller, M. Mulligan, and M. A. Pfaller.** 1994. Comparison of traditional and molecular methods for typing isolates of *Staphylococcus aureus*. *J. Clin. Microbiol.* **32:**407–415.

18. **Tompkins, L. S., N. J. Troup, T. Woods, W. F. Bibb, and R. M. McKinney.** 1987. Molecular epidemiology of *Legionella* species by restriction endonuclease and alloenzyme analysis. *J. Clin. Microbiol.* **25:**1875–1880.

19. **Van Belkum, A., H. Maas, H. Verbrugh, and N. van Leeuwen.** 1996. Serotyping, ribotyping, PCR-mediated ribosomal 16S-23S spacer analysis and arbitrarily primed PCR for epidemiological studies on *Legionella pneumophila*. *Res. Microbiol.* **147:**405–413.

20. **Van Belkum, A., J. Kluytmans, W. van Leeuwen, R. Bax, W. Quint, E. Peters, A. Fluit, C. Vandenbroucke-Grauls, A. van den Brule, H. Koeleman, W. Melchers, J. Meis, A. Elaichouni, M. Vaneechoutte, F. Moonens, N. Maes, M. Struelens, F. Tenover, and H. A. Verbrugh.** 1995. Multicenter evaluation of arbitrarily primed PCR for typing of *Staphylococcus aureus* strains. *J. Clin. Microbiol.* **33:**1537–1547.

21. **Van Belkum, A., M. Struelens, and W. G. V. Quint.** 1993. Typing of *Legionella pneumophila* strains by polymerase chain reaction mediated DNA fingerprinting. *J. Clin. Microbiol.* **31:**2198–2200.

22. **Van Belkum, A., W. van Leeuwen, M. E. Kaufman, B. Cookson, F. Forey, J. Etienne, R. Goering, F. Tenover, C. Steward, F. O'Brien, W. Grubb, P. Tassios, N. Legakis, N. Morvan, N. El Solh, R. de Ryck, M. Struelens, S. Salmenlinna, J. Vuopio-Varkila, M. Kooistra, A. Talens, W. Witte,**

and H. A. Verbrugh. 1998. Assessment of resolution and intercenter reproducibility of results of genotyping of *Staphylococcus aureus* by pulsed field gel electrophoresis of *Sma*I macrorestriction fragments: a multicenter study. *J. Clin. Microbiol.* **36:**1653–1659.

23. Van Leeuwen, W., H. Verbrugh, J. van der Velde, N. van Leeuwen, M. Heck, and A. van Belkum. 1999. Validation of binary typing for *Staphylococcus aureus* strains. *J. Clin. Microbiol.* **37:**664–674.

24. Van Leeuwen, W., M. Sijmons, J. Sluijs, H. A. Verbrugh, and A. van Belkum. 1996. On the nature and use of randomly amplified DNA from *Staphylococcus aureus. J. Clin. Microbiol.* **34:**2770–2777.

25. Vogel, J. P., H. L. Andrews, S. K. Wong, and R. R. Isberg. 1998. Conjugative transfer by the virulence system of *Legionella pneumophila. Science* **279:**873–876.

26. Wever, P. C., E. P. F. Yzerman, E. J. Kuiper, P. Speelman, and J. Dankert. 2000. Rapid diagnosis of Legionnaire's Disease using an immunochromatographic assay for *Legionella pneumophila* serogroup 1 antigen in urine during an outbreak in The Netherlands. *J. Clin. Microbiol.* **38:**2738–2739.

# SEQUENCE-BASED GENOTYPING SCHEME FOR *LEGIONELLA*

*Rodney M. Ratcliff, Janice A. Lanser,*
*Michael W. Heuzenroeder, and Paul A. Manning*

# 44

Sequence-based genotyping schemes have become widespread as sequencing costs reduce and suitable sequence databases are created. The digital nature of sequence, and the quantum increase in the number of measurable character states make this trend inevitable for organisms that are difficult to identify by traditional phenotypic means. The genus *Legionella* is an ideal choice: the number of species is large and the strains are relatively inert when utilizing traditional biochemical tests. Serology-based methods have been widely used, but the progressive characterization of new species has established that antigen cross-reactivity limits specificity (6). Even the promising new methods such as the quantification of cellular fatty acids and ubiquinones have similarly been proven incapable of unambiguously resolving all species, although the inclusion of monohydroxylated and dihydroxylated fatty acids has improved discrimination (5).

The gene target of choice for prokaryotes has been the 16S rRNA genes (10). The ready availability of highly conserved functionally constrained regions adjoining less conserved phylogenetically informative regions, and its universal presence in all prokaryotes, has meant that the majority of phylogenetic or genotypic studies have focused on this gene. However, these same highly conserved regions, even across several genera, and the multiplicity of gene copies may also predispose RNA genes to homologous recombination events, compromising genetic relationships inferred by such sequences (1, 9). Progressively, protein-encoding genes are being reported as targets for phylogenetic or genotypic studies. The effects of redundancy within the genetic code result in much less constrained, and hence more informative, genetic variation, especially at the third codon position. However, the homology at primer target sites is correspondingly reduced, making primer design more difficult, and often primers targeting protein-encoding genes must incorporate multiple bases at one or several sites to achieve complete consensus.

At the time this work commenced, while a number of genes from *Legionella* had been sequenced, only the 16S rRNA gene (4), and the macrophage infectivity potentiator (*mip*) gene, encoding a putative virulence factor (7), had been characterized for all species, an es-

*Rodney M. Ratcliff, Janice A. Lanser, and Michael W. Heuzenroeder* Infectious Diseases Laboratories, Institute of Medical and Veterinary Science, Adelaide, SA 5000, Australia. *Paul A. Manning* AstraZeneca R&D Boston, 35 Gatehouse Dr., Waltham, MA 02451.

*Legionella*, Edited by Reinhard Marre et al.
© 2002 ASM Press, Washington, D.C.

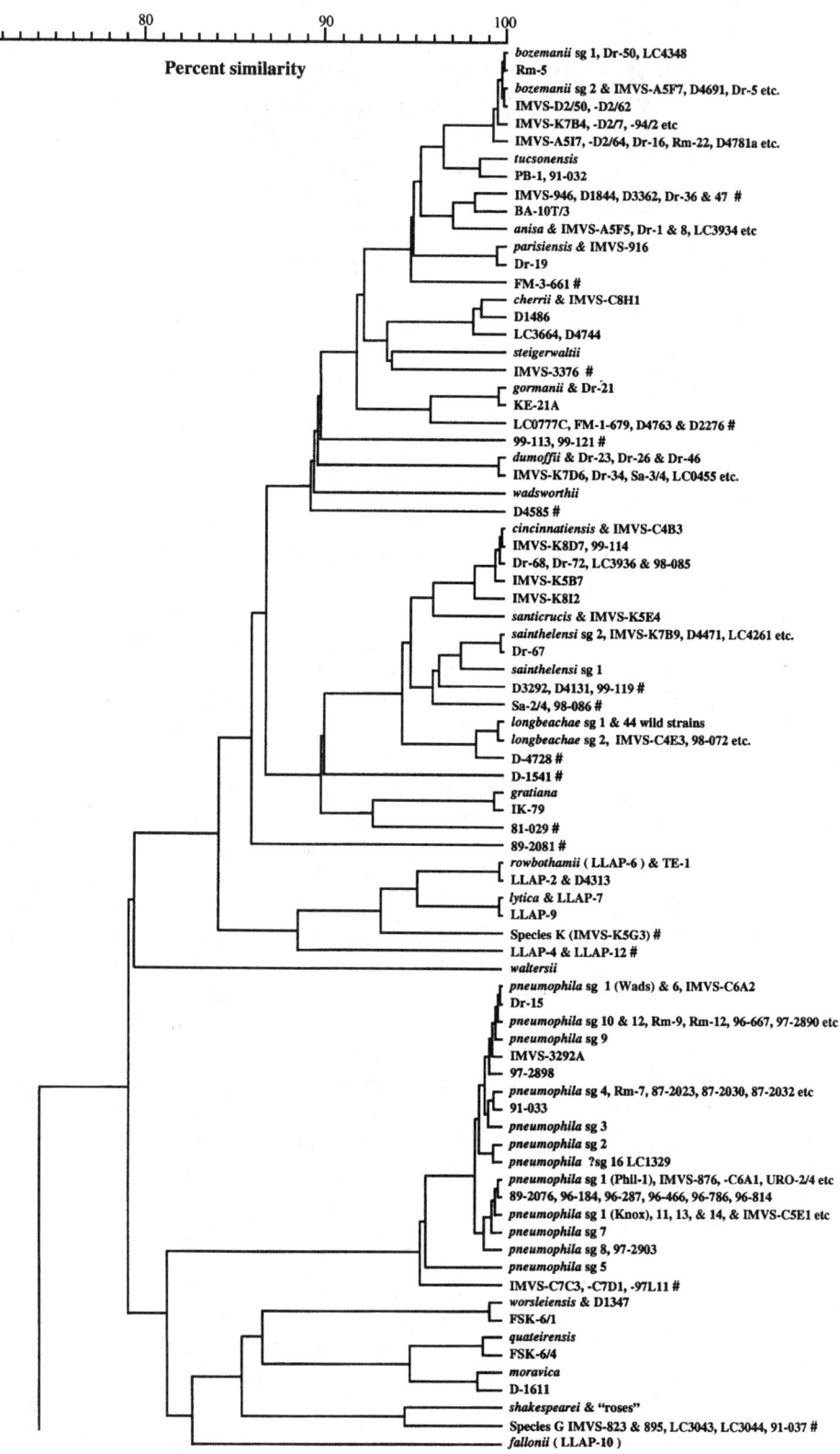

Percent similarity

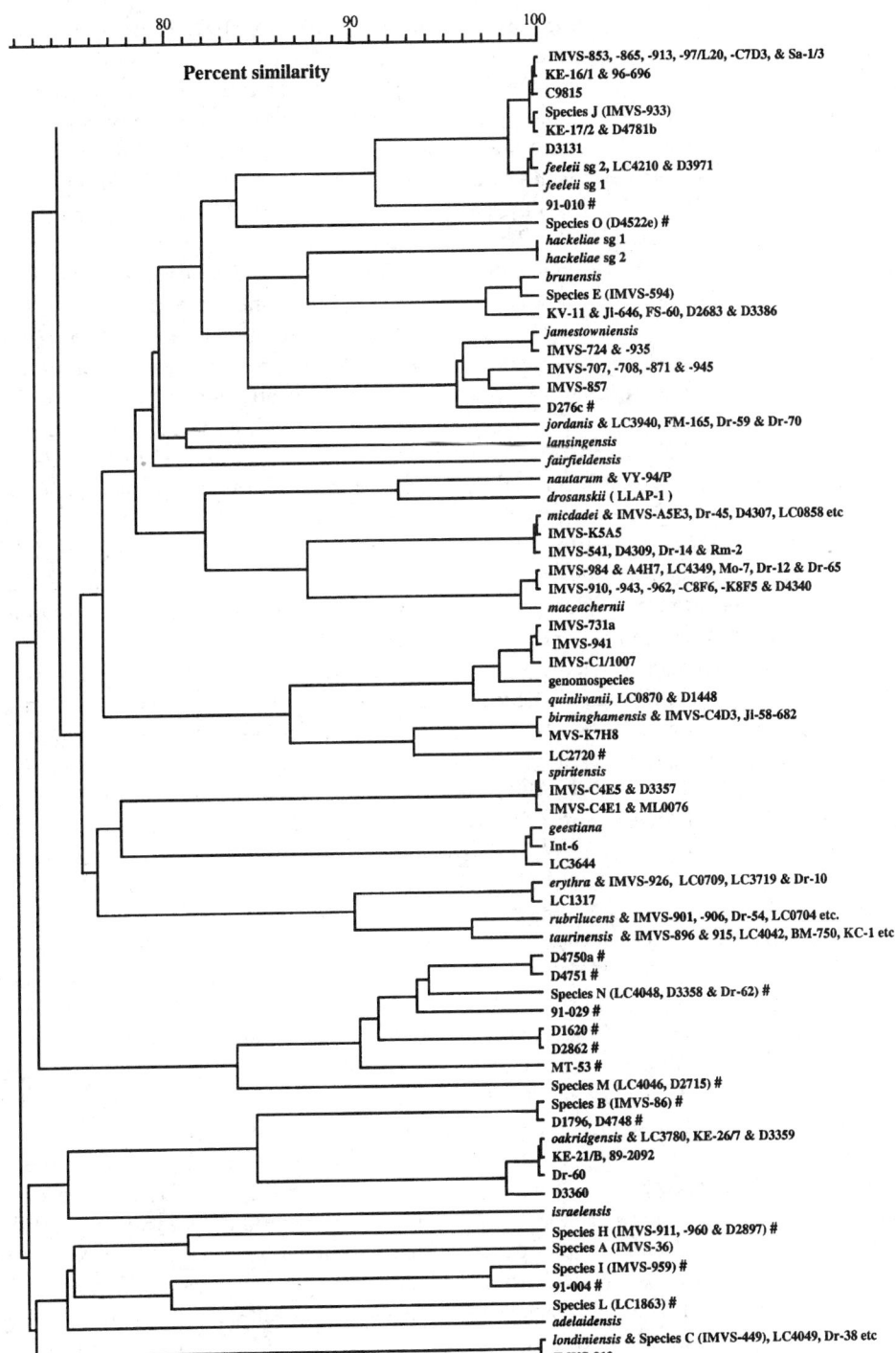

**FIGURE 1** UPGMA phylogenetic dendrogram of *mip* sequence similarities found among type and wild-type strains of *Legionella*. The vertical bar joining two isolates or clusters indicates level of similarity. Reproduced with modifications from *Journal of Clinical Microbiology* (8) with kind permission of the publishers. #, Isolates (or cluster) which represent potentially novel species.

sential requirement for a genotyping target. An analysis of the two genes revealed twice the sequence variation at a DNA level for the *mip* gene (56% of base sites) compared with that of the 16S rRNA gene (23% of base sites), with a pairwise variation between species pairs of 3 to 31% (mean 20%) and 1 to 10% (mean 6%) for the two genes, respectively (8). These statistics infer that the *mip* gene sequence is potentially three times more discriminatory than the 16S rRNA gene, and as a consequence was chosen as the target of choice.

The amplification and sequencing methods have been previously published in *Journal of Clinical Microbiology* (8). In summary (with kind permission of the publishers), a turbid suspension of a suspect culture or colony is boiled for up to 15 min to release the DNA, and an aliquot of the suspension, clarified by centrifugation, is used in a genetic amplification reaction. The forward and reverse primers, listed below, produce an amplicon of 661 to 715 bases, nearly 90% of the gene. The primer sequences are as follows:
Forward primer (Legmip-f) (27mer): 5′-GGG(AG)ATT(ACG)TTTATGAAGATGA(AG)A(CT)TGG-3′. Reverse primer (Legmip-r) (23mer): 5′-TC(AG)TT(ATCG)GG(ATG)CC(ATG)AT(ATCG)GG(ATCG)CC(ATG)CC-3′. Forward sequencing primer, which overlaps Legmip-f by seven bases (Legmip-fs) (26mer): 5′-TTTATGAAGATGA(AG)A(CT)TGGTC(AG)CTGC-3′.

Gene amplification consists of 40 cycles of 94°C for 30 s, 55°C for 60 s, and 72°C for 2 min. Products are purified using a suitable spin column or equivalent, and sequenced using dye terminator chemistry, priming the reaction with Legmip-fs, above. The sequence obtained is then compared with a library of known sequences. The Genebase computer package from Applied Maths (Kortrijk, Belgium) is very useful for the sequence analysis.

To date, the sequence database, against which a sequence from an unknown strain is tested, includes sequences from 400 type and wild-type strains encompassing some 45 characterized species, many with multiple serotypes. To ensure the scheme is robust and not affected by regional variation, strains from Europe, the United States, Australia, Japan, Singapore, Israel, and Kenya have been included, as well as several of the nonculturable *Legionella*-like Amoebic Pathogen (LLAP) strains. These sequence relationships are presented as a UPGMA phylogenetic dendrogram in Fig. 1.

All strains of *Legionella* amplify with the primers, with the exception of *L. geestiana*, a rare environmental strain; non-*Legionella* strains do not produce an amplicon of the correct size. All attempts to determine the sequence at the primer target sites for *L. geestiana* have so far failed, but a smaller 194-bp sequence fragment from the *mip* gene can be produced using an alternative forward primer Geesmip-f (5′-GTNACNGTNGANTAN-ACNGG-3′, where N represents the inclusion of all four nucleotides) with Legmip-r as the reverse primer.

The scheme unambiguously discriminates between all species. The sequence from strains for each species form a cluster of identical and near-identical sequences where the intraspecies variation is smaller than the interpecies variation with close sister species. The smallest interspecies variation of 3.6% occurs between *L. bozemanii* and *L. tucsonensis* compared with an intraspecies variation of 1 and 1.7%, respectively. Intraspecies variation greater than 3.6% does occur, e.g., in *L. pneumophila* (5.1%), *L. jamestowniensis* (4.7%), and *L. quinlivanii* (3.8%), but the interspecies variations for such species are correspondingly greater, so the strains unambiguously resolve into distinct species.

A number of multiple serogroups have been detected for some *Legionella* species. For the majority, multiple serogroups within a species share an identical sequence for the amplified *mip* gene fragment. The type strains of the two serogroups of *L. hackeliae* and *L. pneumophila* serogroups 11, 13, and 14 are examples, as are wild-type strains of *L. bozemanii* and *L. pneumophila* (especially serogroup 1). Alternatively, the current data suggest the sequence differences may be sufficient to distinguish between serogroups of *L. sainthelensi* (14 bases) and *L. longbeachae* (2 bases). The number of variant bases for the latter species is very small, but to date the sequence determined from all wild-type strains of the two serogroups of *L. longbeachae* have been identical to their corresponding type strain. In summary, this scheme is only rarely able to discriminate between different serogroups of a species.

All the LLAP strains tested by this method produce an amplicon from which the sequence could be determined, and their relationship to other LLAP strains and other *Legionella* species is informative. LLAP-7 and -9 are strains of *L. lytica*, while LLAP-1, LLAP-2 and -6, and LLAP-10 are now recognized as three new species: *L. drosanskii, L. rowbothamii*, and *L. fallonii*, respectively (2). Interestingly, two culturable wild-type strains of *L. rowbothamii* have been isolated.

In addition to the nine potentially novel species previously published (8), another 26 are now believed to exist. These are highlighted in Fig. 1. Many, and some containing multiple isolates, have been inferred because the interspecies variation with all other characterized strains is large. Others, however, are much more closely related to known species, but the uniqueness of these strains has already been suggested by DNA homology studies (R. F. Benson, personal communication). Isolates D1844 and D3362, two of five strains with identical sequence 3.9% variant from *L. anisa*, and D4728 with a sequence variation of 1.5% from *L. longbeachae*, are examples of such isolates. In total, Fig. 1 indicates 33 possible novel species, 14 of which are represented by more than one strain. None of these have an association with disease to date, in that they have only been isolated from environmental sources. If these results are confirmed by formal speciation, the *Legionella* genus may comprise nearly 80 species. Interestingly, a group of six such novel species form a clade quite distinct from all currently characterized species, and another five form a similarly distinct clade that distantly includes *L. adelaidensis*.

In conclusion, the genotyping scheme targeting the *mip* gene is currently the most tested and discriminatory of all published schemes for identifying *Legionella* strains, short of performing whole chromosome DNA hybridization studies. As with all single gene target schemes, misidentification resulting from homologous recombination events remains a theoretical possibility, although no such events have so far been detected. Parallel sequencing of a section of the zinc metallo-protease (*mspA* or *proA*) gene from wild-type strains of seven species of *Legionella* produced a classification that mirrored that from the *mip* gene (R. M. Ratcliff, unpublished data). Sequencing genes for such purposes is still in its infancy, having become affordable only relatively recently, and many suitable gene targets are yet to be elucidated. Early reports of multilocus sequence typing to type strains below the species level, as an alternative to other typing methods such as pulsed-field gel electrophoresis and amplification fragment length polymorphism, are very promising (3) but are currently significantly restricted by cost and lack of sufficiently comprehensive sequence databases from multiple gene targets and strains. As additional gene targets are reported for *Legionella*, multilocus sequence typing will become possible, which in turn will ensure that not only will homologous recombination events be detected, but the resolution of significant strain relationships at a subspecies level will be possible.

## REFERENCES

1. **Achtman, M.** A phylogenetic perspective on molecular epidemiology. *In* M. Sussman (ed.), *Molecular Medical Microbiology*, in press. Academic Press, Inc., London, England.
2. **Adeleke, A. A., B. S. Fields, R. F. Benson, M. I. Daneshvar, J. M. Pruckler, R. M. Ratcliff, T. G. Harrison, R. S. Weyant, R. J. Birtles, D. Raoult, and M. A. Halablab.** 2001. *Legionella drosanskii* sp. nov., *Legionella rowbothamii* sp. nov. and *Legionella fallonii* sp. nov: three unusual new *Legionella* species. *Int. J. Syst. Evol. Microbiol.* **51:**1151–1160.
3. **Enright, M. C., and B. G. Spratt.** 1999. Multilocus sequence typing. *Trends Microbiol.* **7:**482–487.
4. **Hookey, J. V., N. A. Saunders, N. K. Fry, R. J. Birtles, and T. G. Harrison.** 1996. Phylogeny of *Legionellaceae* base on small-subunit ribosomal DNA sequences and proposal of

*Legionella lytica* comb. nov. for *Legionella*-like amoebal pathogens. *Int. J. Syst. Bacteriol.* **46:**526–531.

5. **Jantzen, E., A. Sonesson, T. Tangen, and J. Eng.** 1993. Hydroxy-fatty acid profiles of *Legionella* species: diagnostic usefulness assessed by principal component analysis. *J. Clin. Microbiol.* **31:**1413–1419.

6. **Maiwald, M., J. H. Helbig, and P. C. Luck.** 1998. Laboratory methods for the diagnosis of *Legionella* infections. *J. Microbiol. Methods* **33:**59–79.

7. **Ratcliff, R. M., S. C. Donnellan, J. A. Lanser, P. A. Manning, and M. W. Heuzenroeder.** 1997. Interspecies sequence differences in the Mip protein from the genus *Legionella*: im-

plications for function and evolutionary relatedness. *Mol. Microbiol.* **25:**1149–1158.

8. **Ratcliff, R. M., J. A. Lanser, P. A. Manning, and M. W. Heuzenroeder.** 1998. Sequence-based classification scheme for the genus *Legionella* targeting the *mip* gene. *J. Clin. Microbiol.* **36:**1560–1567.

9. **Strätz, M., M. Mau, and K. N. Timmis.** 1996. System to study horizontal gene exchange among microorganisms without cultivation of recipients. *Mol. Microbiol.* **22:**207–215.

10. **Woese, C. R.** 1991. Reconstruction of bacterial evolution with rRNA, p. 1–24. *In* R. K. Selander, A. G. Clark, and T. S. Whittam (ed.), *Evolution at the Molecular Level*. Sinauer Associates, Sunderland, Mass.

# APPLICATION OF AMPLIFIED FRAGMENT LENGTH POLYMORPHISM ANALYSIS TO SUBTYPING OF *LEGIONELLA PNEUMOPHILA* SEROGROUP 6

*Robert F. Benson, Barry S. Fields, Andrea Benin, Heather Craddock, and Richard E. Besser*

# 45

One patient isolate and one environmental isolate of *Legionella pneumophila* serogroup 6 were obtained from an outbreak investigation associated with a whirlpool spa, in which 2 cases of Legionnaires' disease and 10 cases of Pontiac fever were diagnosed. Discriminatory subtyping methods are necessary during epidemiologic investigations to establish a link between case patients and environmental sources. Previous subtyping methods applied to *L. pneumophila* serogroup 6 include monoclonal antibodies (3, 5), arbitrarily primed polymerase chain reaction (5), ribotyping (5), pulsed-field gel electrophoresis (5), and multilocus enzyme electrophoreis (MLEE) (3). We used amplified fragment length polymorphism (AFLP) analysis to type the patient and environmental isolates. We compared the patterns obtained from our outbreak-related strains with the electrophoretic types obtained from 48 strains analyzed by MLEE. The previous analysis by MLEE had grouped the 48 unrelated strains of serogroup 6 into 11 electrophoretic types.

*Robert F. Benson, Barry S. Fields, Andrea Benin, Heather Craddock, and Richard E. Besser* Respiratory Diseases Branch, Division of Bacterial and Mycotic Diseases, National Center for Infectious Diseases, Centers for Disease Control and Prevention, Atlanta, GA 30333.

## BACTERIAL STRAINS ANALYZED

*L. pneumophila* serogroup 6 strains Chicago 2, Johannesburg 5, Albany 1, Oxford 1, SRP 39, Denver 3, Sydney 1, LD 82-683, ED 38, and Vasteras 57/1, the whirlpool and patient isolates, were selected for evaluation of the AFLP technique on the basis of previous subtyping performed by MLEE. The type strain for one of the electrophoretic types was unavailable. Strains were grown on buffered charcoal–yeast extract, and DNA was extracted using the Epicentre Technologies (Madison, Wis.) MasterPure DNA kit according to the manufacturer's instructions.

## AFLP PROCEDURE

The procedure described by Riffard et al. (4) was used for analysis of the epidemiologically related and unrelated strains in this study as follows.

### Preparation of Adapters

Adapters were constructed as previously described by Mazurek et al. (2) with oligonucleotides obtained from the BioTechnology Core Facility, Centers for Disease Control and Prevention, Atlanta, Ga. These were AX 1 (5'-PO₄– CTAGTACTGGCAGACTCT) and AX 2 (5'-GCCAGTA), as described elsewhere (2), and PS 1 (5'-GACTCGACTCG-

CATGCA) and PS2 (5′-TGCGAGT), as described by Riffard (4). The adapters were prepared by mixing 20 pmol of each complementary adapter in 1X PCR buffer (Perkin Elmer, Branchburg, N.J.) and allowing the mixture to anneal as it was cooled from 80°C to 4°C in a GeneAmp model 2400 thermocycler (Perkin Elmer, Branchburg, N.J.)

### Restriction and Adaptor Ligation

A 1μl (.2-μg) sample of DNA was digested using 40 U of XbaI and 40 U of PstI (Roche Molecular Biochemicals, Indianapolis, Ind.) in 1X sure-cut buffer H in a total volume of 12.5 μl. Reactions were prepared in 0.2-ml PCR tubes and incubated at 37°C for 90 min and then at 65°C for 20 min to inactivate the restriction enzymes.

The digested DNA (12.5 μl) was combined with 10 U of T4 DNA ligase and 1 μl each of adaptor AX and PS in a total volume of 20 μl. The reactions were incubated at 16°C for 60 min followed by heating to 65°C for 20 min to inactivate the T4 DNA ligase. The samples were redigested by adding 10 U each of XbaI and PstI directly to each tube and incubating at 37°C for 15 min.

### PCR Amplification

The digested DNA with annealed adaptors was amplified with the following primers: PS1:5′-ACGTACGCTCAGCTCAG and PXG:5′-AGAGTCTGCCAGTACTAGAG. In some experiments, the primer PXG was labeled with 6-carbo-fluorescein (FAM) for subsequent analysis using the ABI 310 (Perkin

Elmer). Each 25-μl PCR mixture contained 5.0 μl of template DNA, 0.5 μl of MgCl$_2$ (0.5 mM), 2.5 μl of PCR buffer II (Perkin Elmer), 4.0 μl of dNTP (200 μM each), 0.5 μl each of primers PS (1.0 μM/μl) and PXG (1.0 μM/μl), 0.25 μl of Taq polymerase (5 U/μl), and 11.75 μl of H$_2$O.

Amplification was performed in a GenAmp PCR system 2400 (Perkin Elmer) with an amplification profile consisting of an initial denaturation of 94°C for 5 min and then 30 cycles with denaturation at 94°C for 30 s, primer annealing at 60°C for 30 s, and extension at 72°C for 90 s.

### GEL ELECTROPHORESIS OF PCR PRODUCTS

PCR products were loaded into wells of a 3.5% Metaphor Agarose gel (FMC Bio-Products, Rockland, Maine) in 1X TBE buffer and electrophoresed at 90 V for 2 to 3 h. Bands were visualized by incorporating ethidium bromide (1 μl/100 ml agar) into the agar prior to casting the gel. DNA fragments were observed using a UV transilluminator (Fotodyne Inc., New Berlin, Wis.). The gel image is shown in Fig. 1.

### ABI PRISM 310 ANALYSIS OF PCR PRODUCTS

Fluorescence-labled PCR products were analyzed by the procedure described by Benson et al. (1) as follows: 1 μl of a 1:20 dilution of the PCR product, 0.6 μl of molecular weight standards labeled with TAMARA, and 12 μl of deionized formamide were combined. Samples were separated using an ABI Prism

**FIGURE 1** Gel electrophoresis of AFLP fragments from *L. pneumophila* serogroup 6 strains. Lanes: 1 and 15, molecular weight standards; 2, Sydney 1; 3, Albany 1; 4, LD82-683; 5, V57/1; 6, Chicago 2; 7, Denver 3; 8 and 9, SRP39; 10, ED38; 11, Johannesburg 5; 12, Oxford 1; 13, whirlpool isolate; 14, patient isolate.

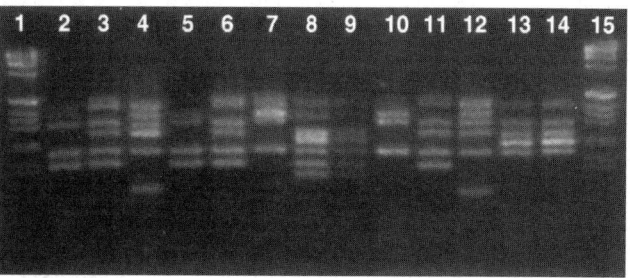

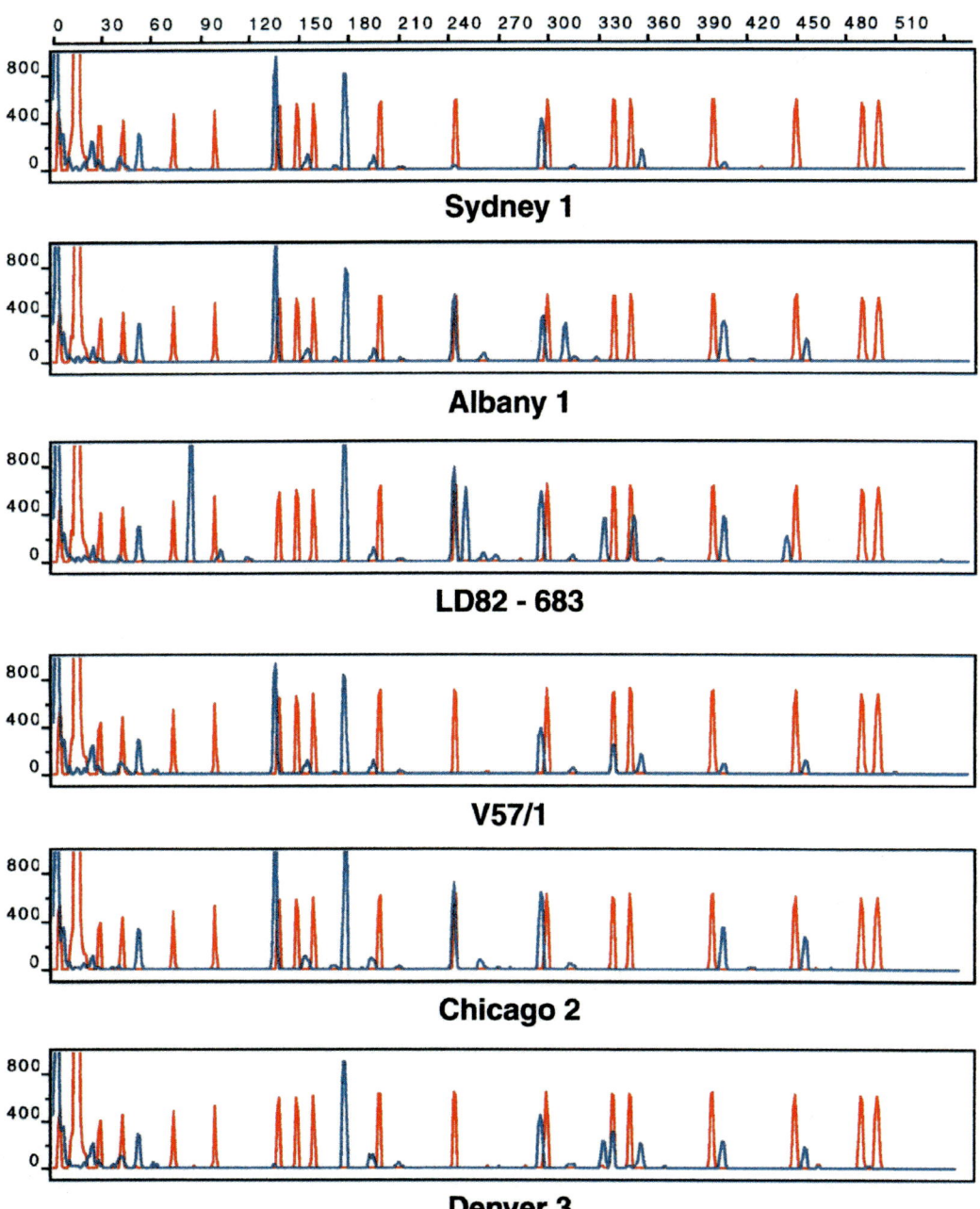

**FIGURE 2**  Electrophoretic profiles of AFLP fragments from *L. pneumophila* serogroup 6 strains separated using an ABI 310 genetic analyzer.

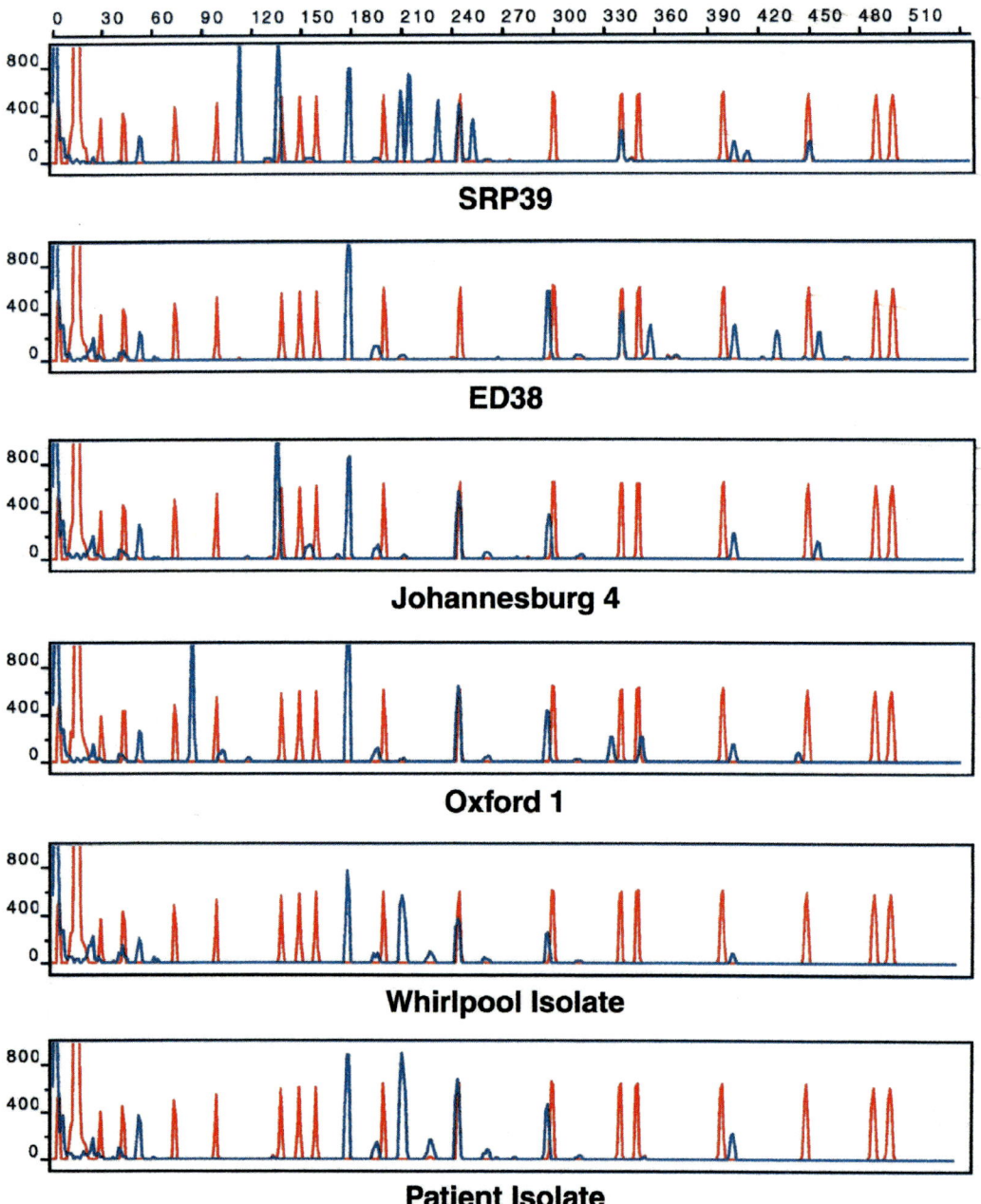

**FIGURE 3** Electrophoretic profiles of AFLP fragments from *L. pneumophila* serogroup 6 strains separated using an ABI 310 genetic analyzer.

310 genetic analyzer. The electrophoregrams for the 10 unrelated reference strains and the two outbreak-related strains are shown in Fig. 2 and 3.

## CONCLUSIONS

The fragment patterns obtained by AFLP for the environmental and patient isolate were identical and differed from the patterns obtained from 10 unrelated strains. Analysis of fragment sizes by agarose gel electrophoresis indicated that the patient and environmental strains were identical; however the 10 unique strains were divided into 7 patterns. By incorporating a fluorescent primer and separating the fragments with the ABI 310, all 10 unrelated strains could be shown to have unique patterns that were separate from the patient and environmental strains. Thus AFLP analysis yielded the same level of discrimination as MLEE. The advantages of analyzing the results with the ABI 310 over agarose gel electrophoresis are greater sensitivity and the ability to store fragment sizes in a database for comparison with other strains. An advantage of AFLP compared with pulsed-field gel electrophoresis or MLEE is that it is easier to perform and less time-consuming.

## ACKNOWLEDGMENTS

This research was supported in part by an appointment to the Emerging Infectious Diseases Fellowship Program administered by the Association of Public Health Laboratories (APHL) and funded by the Centers for Disease Control and Prevention (CDC).

## REFERENCES

1. **Benson, J. M., D. Ellingsen, M. A. Renshaw, A. G. Resler, B. L. Evatt, and W. C. Hooper.** 1999. Multiplex analysis of mutations in four genes using fluorescence scanning technology. *Thromb. Res.* **96:**57–64.
2. **Mazurek, G. H., V. Reddy, B. J. Marston, W. H. Hass, and J. T. Crawford.** 1996. DNA fingerprinting by infrequent-restriction-site amplification. *J. Clin. Microbiol.* **34:**2386–2390.
3. **McKinney, R. M., T. A. Kuffner, W. F. Bibb, C. Nokkaew, D. E. Wells, P. M. Arnow, T. C. Woods, and B. D. Plikaytis.** 1989. Antigenic and genetic variation in *Legionella pneumophila* serogroup 6. *J. Clin. Microbiol.* **27:**738–742.
4. **Riffard, S., F. Lo Presit, F. Vandenesch, F. Forey, M. Reyrolle, and J. Etienne.** 1998. Comparative analysis of infrequent-restriction-site PC and pulsed-field gel electrophoresis for epidemiological typing of *Legionella pneumophila* serogroup 1 strains. *J. Clin. Microbiol.* **36:**161–167.
5. **Visca, P., P. Goldoni, P. C. Lück, J. H. Helbig, L. Cattani, G. Giltri, S. Bramati, and M. C. Pastoris.** 1999. Multiple types of *Legionella pneumophila* serogroup 6 in a hospital heated-water system associated with sporadic infections. *J. Clin. Microbiol.* **37:**2189–2196.

# MOLECULAR TYPING OF *LEGIONELLA* STRAINS WITH PULSED-FIELD GEL ELECTROPHORESIS AND RANDOM PRIMER-AMPLIFIED POLYMORPHIC DNA IN NOSOCOMIAL LEGIONNAIRES' DISEASE

Laura Franzin, Daniela Cabodi,
Alessandro Sinicco, and Giovanni Di Perri

# 46

The nosocomial origin of legionellosis may be confirmed by strain typing, particularly by molecular typing, of isolates from the patient and the putative source. The aim of the study was to investigate the epidemiological relatedness between *Legionella* strains, isolated from a patient with Legionnaires' disease and from the hospital water supply.

Acute pneumonia occurred 5 days after discharge in a 68-year-old immunosuppressed man, hospitalized for a month. The patient was readmitted to the hospital 4 days after the onset of symptoms; the patient showed fever, cough, dyspnea and respiratory distress, confusion, and renal failure. After 2 days of therapy with ceftazidime and ciprofloxacin, the patient died. Chest radiological findings were lung opacities with alveolar-interstitial infiltrates of both lobes, prevalent on the left side. The risk factors of the patient were corticosteroid therapy, autoimmune piastrinopenia, smoking, and age >50 years.

Cultures from postmortem lung tissue were performed following Centers for Disease Control and Prevention methods (9). Colonies of *Legionella pneumophila* serogroup 1 and of *Legionella bozemanii* grew on buffered charcoal-yeast extract (BCYE), BMPA (3), and MWY (8) agar plates. The direct detection of *Legionella* by PCR using EnviroAmp (Perkin Elmer), modified for clinical samples, was positive for *Legionella* spp. and for *L. pneumophila*. Microscopic examination by Gimenez stain and by direct immunofluorescence using monoclonal antibodies (Monofluo, Diagnostic Pasteur, France) were positive.

Since a nosocomial infection was suspected, considering the incubation period of legionellosis, epidemiological and microbiological investigations for a hospital source of *Legionella* started. The methods used were previously described (4). Cold and hot water samples were collected from hospital water supply and from hot water tanks; samples were also collected from tap water (5 liters) and from the shower head (100 ml) of the patient's room from the wards where he stayed. All the samples were concentrated by filtration through cellulose acetate membrane filters (0.2-$\mu$m pore size) and resuspended in 10 ml of the same water. Aliquots (0.1 ml) of the untreated, heat-treated (50°C for 30 min), and acid-washed suspensions (1) were plated on BCYE, BMPA (3), and MWY (8). The plates were

*Laura Franzin, Daniela Cabodi, Alessandro Sinicco, and Giovanni Di Perri* Infectious Diseases Unit, University of Turin, Turin 10149, Italy.

incubated at 37°C for 15 days. The strains of *Legionella* isolated were serologically typed by slide agglutination and by immunofluorescence assay. *Legionella* colonies were isolated from all 10 hot water samples examined (20 to 45,000 CFU/liter) and from the shower head (200 CFU/ml); cold water samples were negative. Strains of *L. pneumophila* serogroups 1, 2, 3, and 6 and *Legionella* spp. were isolated.

Strains of *L. pneumophila* serogroup 1 isolated from the patient and from the hospital environment, and clinical and environmental unrelated strains were typed by pulsed-field gel electrophoresis (PFGE) and by random amplified polymorphic DNA PCR (RAPD-PCR). A standardized suspension of 72-h-old culture of *Legionella* on BCYE was mixed with an equal volume of molted 1.5% low-melting-point agarose for PFGE. The plugs were treated with digestion solution containing proteinase K (2 mg/ml) and then with restriction enzyme *Not*I and *Sfi*I (Boehringer Mannheim). The PFGE was performed on 1% agarose gel in 0.5% Tris-borate-EDTA (TBE) buffer with a contour-clamped homogenous electronic field system, CHEF-DR III (Biorad). The electrophoresis for DNAs cleaved with *Not*I and with *Sfi*I was performed following previously described methods (2, 6). Genomic fragments were stained with ethidium bromide and were photographed under UV illumination. The results were interpreted following Tenover criteria (7). For RAPD-PCR, a standardized suspension of culture was treated with 10% Chelex (5) and amplified with two primers (2 and 5, Pharmacia) using Ready-To-Go RAPD Analysis Beads (Pharmacia). The amplification products were analyzed by electrophoresis in 2% agarose gel and visualized by staining with ethidium bromide and by electrophoresis on polyacrylamide gel (CleanGel Pharmacia and silver staining) with GenePhor System (Pharmacia).

*L. pneumophila* serogroup 1 strains isolated from the patient and 11 strains isolated from hot water samples collected from different sites of the hospital water supply showed the same

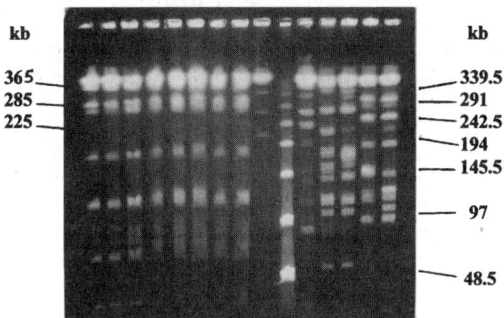

**FIGURE 1**  PFGE of *Sfi*I-cleaved genomic DNA of *L. pneumophila* serogroup 1 strains. Lanes: 1, patient's isolate; 2 through 8, environmental isolates from different sites of the hospital water supply; 11, *L. pneumophila* serogroup 1 Philadelphia 1; 12 and 13, clinical unrelated isolates; 14 and 15, environmental unrelated isolates. Lambda DNA concatamers (48.5 kb) (L, lane 10) and yeast chromosomal DNA of *Saccharomyces cerevisiae* (S, lane 9) were used as molecular size standards.

profile by PFGE with *Not*I (Fig. 1) and *Sfi*I. These strains shared identical profiles also by RAPD-PCR with the two primers used. The profiles of *L. pneumophila* serogroup 1 Philadelphia 1 type strain and of the clinical and environmental unrelated strains were different from the above strains by PFGE and by RAPD-PCR. In this study, the molecular typing results demonstrated that the strains of *L. pneumophila* serogroup 1, isolated from the patient and from the hospital hot water, were indistinguishable and thus genetically related, showing that the hospital water was the source of infection and thus confirming the nosocomial origin.

**REFERENCES**
1. **Bopp, C. A., J. W. Summer, G. K. Morris, and J. G. Wells.** 1981. Isolation of *Legionella* spp. from environmental water samples by low-pH treatment and use of a selective medium. *J. Clin. Microbiol.* **13:**714–719.
2. **Castellani Pastoris, M., L. Ciceroni, R. Lo Monaco, P. Goldoni, B. Mentore, G. Flego, L. Cattani, S. Ciarrocchi, A. Pinto, and P. Visca.** 1997. Molecular epidemiology of an out-

break of Legionnaires' disease associated with a cooling tower in Genova-Sestri Ponente, Italy. *Eur. J. Clin. Microbiol. Infect. Dis.* **16**:883–892.

3. **Edelstein, P. H.** 1981. Improved semiselective medium for isolation of *Legionella pneumophila* from contaminated clinical and environmental specimens. *J. Clin. Microbiol.* **14**:298–303.

4. **Franzin, L., M. Castellani Pastoris, P. Gioannini, and G. Villani.** 1989. Endemicity of *Legionella pneumophila* serogroup 3 in a hospital water supply. *J. Hosp. Infect.* **13**:281–288.

5. **Gomez-Lus, P., B. S. Fields, R. F. Benson, W. T. Martin, S. P. O'Connor, and C. M. Black.** 1993. Comparison of arbitrarily primed polymerase chain reaction, ribotyping, and monoclonal antibody analysis for subtyping *Legionella pneumophila* serogroup 1. *J. Clin. Microbiol.* **31**: 1940–1942.

6. **Strulens, M. J., N. Maes, F. Rost, A. Deplano, F. Jacobs, C. Liesnard, N. Bornstein,** F. Grimont, S. Lauwers, M. P. McIntyre, and E. Serruys. 1992. Genotypic and phenotypic methods for the investigation of a nosocomial *Legionella pneumophila* outbreak and efficacy of control measures. *J. Infect. Dis.* **166**:22–30.

7. **Tenover, F. C., R. D. Arbeit, R. V. Goering, P. A. Mickelsen, B. E. Murray, D. H. Persing, and B. Swaminathan.** 1995. Interpreting chromosomal DNA restriction patterns produced by pulsed-field gel electrophoresis: criteria for bacterial strain typing. *J. Clin. Microbiol.* **33**:2233–2239.

8. **Wadowsky, R. M., and R. B. Yee.** 1981. Glycine-containing selective medium for isolation of *Legionellaceae* from environmental specimens. *Appl. Environ. Microbiol.* **42**:768–772.

9. **Wilkinson, H. W.** 1987. *Hospital-Laboratory Diagnosis of Legionella Infections*. U.S. Department of Health and Human Services. Centers for Disease Control, Atlanta, Ga.

# MULTILOCUS SEQUENCE TYPING FOR CHARACTERIZATION OF *LEGIONELLA PNEUMOPHILA* SEROGROUP 1 ISOLATES

*Valeria Gaia and Raffaele Peduzzi*

# 47

*Legionella* can cause a severe form of pneumonia named Legionnaires' disease. Molecular typing of pathogenic relevant strains of *Legionella pneumophila* serogroup 1 is indispensable in determining the epidemiology of the disease. In addition to classical serotyping and subtyping using monoclonal antibodies, a variety of molecular methods have been successfully employed for epidemiological purposes including amplified fragment length polymorphism (AFLP) analysis, pulsed-field gel electrophoresis, random amplified polymorphic DNA, and many other PCR-based methods (4). These techniques are currently used because of their feasibility, rapidity, and great potential for discrimination. AFLP analysis (6) in particular is widely used in many epidemiological studies on *L. pneumophila* strains. Two recent interlaboratory studies (3, 4) have assessed the reliability of AFLP and the discrimination power for epidemiological typing of *L. pneumophila* serogroup 1 strains. While results have demonstrated that the method can be highly reproducible, intercenter reproducibility, particularly using gel analysis software, remains a problem.

The development of a unique epidemiological marker is necessary in the epidemiological investigation of the sources of contamination and infection pathways of Legionnaires' disease. Other studies have shown that during such investigations, good results are often obtained only by the application of several techniques simultaneously. Moreover, each laboratory or reference center has its own epidemiological markers and working conditions, and results obtained by different groups are not directly comparable. For this reason, further research should deal with the development of a unique universal typing method: a quick, simple, and discriminatory method that could, in the future, be applied by all microbiology laboratories to every case of Legionnaires' disease.

Multilocus sequence typing (MLST) is a sequence-based variation of multilocus enzyme electrophoresis (MLEE), where several genes are compared simultaneously at their sequence level. The advantages of MLST compared with MLEE are the detection of more variation and easy data storage, comparison, and exchange. MLST is successfully used as the "gold standard" method for typing *Neisseria meningitidis* (5), as well as *Staphylococcus*

*Valeria Gaia and Raffaele Peduzzi*   Swiss National Reference Laboratory for Legionella, Istituto Cantonale Batteriosierologico, Lugano, Switzerland.

*Legionella*, Edited by Reinhard Marre et al.
© 2002 ASM Press, Washington, D.C.

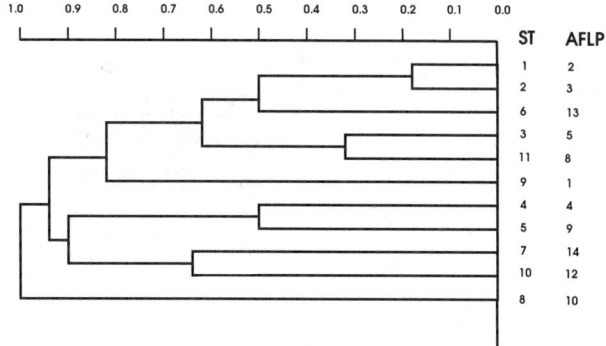

**FIGURE 1** Dendrogram of genetic relationships among 17 strains based on six gene fragments. ST and AFLP types are indicated at the right; genetic distance is indicated in the top scale.

*aureus* (2), *Streptococcus pneumoniae* (1), and many other bacterial species.

Here we report a preliminary study with genes coding for six enzymes with 17 strains of *L. pneumophila* serogroup 1, taken from the European Working Group on *Legionella* Infections (EWGLI) collection previously characterized by AFLP analysis (3, 4). Type strains corresponding to different AFLP types were included, as well as five duplicate sets (EUL19, EUL31, EUL101, EUL1, and EUL2) and two epidemiological related strains (EUL137 and EUL138). The genes chosen for MLST include some housekeeping genes (heat shock,

aconitase, *recA*) and some "virulence-associated" genes (*mompS*, flagellin, zinc metalloprotease). Nucleotide sequences of internal fragments of the following six genes were obtained: *htpB* (278-bp, 58-kDa heat shock protein, GroEL), *acn* (763 bp, aconitase), *flaA* (245 bp, flagellin), *recA* (404 bp), *proA* (480 bp, zinc metalloprotease), and *mompS* (520 bp, major outer membrane protein precursor).

Genomic DNA was isolated from single colonies with the InstaGene Purification Matrix (Bio-Rad, Hercules, Calif.). Standard PCRs were performed in a 50 $\mu$l volume with

**TABLE 1** MLST typing of 17 strains of *Legionella pneumophila* serogroup 1

| Phase 2 code no. | EUL code | AFLP type | Sequence type (ST) | | | | | | ST |
|---|---|---|---|---|---|---|---|---|---|
| | | | *htpB* | *proA* | *recA* | *acn* | *mompS* | *flaA* | |
| 3 | 19 | 2 | 1 | 2 | 1 | 1 | 1 | 1 | 1 |
| 4 | 19 | 2 | 1 | 2 | 1 | 1 | 1 | 1 | 1 |
| 6 | 79 | 3 | 1 | 2 | 1 | 1 | 1 | 2 | 2 |
| 7 | 138 | 5 | 3 | 4 | 1 | 1 | 2 | 2 | 3 |
| 8 | 137 | 5 | 3 | 4 | 1 | 1 | 2 | 2 | 3 |
| 10 | 56 | 4 | 5 | 9 | 3 | 6 | 3 | 3 | 4 |
| 11 | 31 | 9 | 1 | 5 | 3 | 3 | 3 | 3 | 5 |
| 17 | 31 | 9 | 1 | 5 | 3 | 3 | 3 | 3 | 5 |
| 19 | 101 | 13 | 1 | 6 | 1 | 1 | 4 | 4 | 6 |
| 22 | 101 | 13 | 1 | 6 | 1 | 1 | 4 | 4 | 6 |
| 33 | 77 | 14 | 1 | 1 | 4 | 4 | 6 | 5 | 7 |
| 34 | 140 | 10 | 2 | 7 | 5 | 5 | 7 | 6 | 8 |
| 38 | 40 | 1 | 4 | 8 | 6 | 1 | 8 | 8 | 9 |
| 41 | 1 | 12 | 1 | 1 | 2 | 2 | 11 | 9 | 10 |
| 47 | 1 | 12 | 1 | 1 | 2 | 2 | 11 | 9 | 10 |
| 5 | 2 | 8 | 3 | 3 | 1 | 1 | 5 | 2 | 11 |
| 50 | 2 | 8 | 3 | 3 | 1 | 1 | 5 | 2 | 11 |

1 U of *Taq* polymerase (Roche, Indianapolis, Ind.) and 10 $\mu$l of extracted DNA with the following cycling conditions: 35 cycles for 30 s at 94°C, 30 s at 50°C, and 30 s at 72°C. Amplicons were purified with columns (QIAGEN, Basle, Switzerland), cycle-sequenced with Dye Terminator Chemistry (Applied Biosystems, Foster City, Calif.), and run on an automatic sequencer ABI 310 (Applied Biosystems) following the manufacturers' instructions. Alignment of DNA data was performed with Editseq and Megalign programs included in the package DNASTAR (Lasergene, Madison, Wis.).

A sequence type (ST) is defined as the combination of alleles at a defined locus. Sequences were compared for each gene fragment, and strains with identical sequences were assigned to the same allele number. All *L. pneumophila* strains investigated in this study were typeable by using MLST. Results are represented in a dendrogram clustered from the matrix of allelic mismatches between STs (Fig. 1).

Comparison of the results obtained by MLST typing and AFLP typing are illustrated in Table 1. In general, the 17 *L. pneumophila* serogroup 1 strains could be subdivided in the same groups as with AFLP. The duplicate sets (strains with the same EUL number) always show the same ST, as do the two epidemiological related strains (EUL137 and EUL 138).

Generally, we could find more nucleotide substitutions among the virulence genes (2.5 to 4.4%) than in housekeeping genes (0.8 to 2.7%). The most variable gene is *flaA*, with 4.4% substitutions over a 240-bp total length. The largest number of different alleles was found with *mompS* (11 different alleles) matching the number of AFLP types. Strain EUL79 could be distinguished from EUL19 only by AFLP and *flaA*.

In this preliminary study, we found that the variability of the genes chosen for MLST analysis was appropriate for epidemiological typing studies on *L. pneumophila* serogroup 1 strains.

In the future we plan to validate this method for the whole panel of strains (3), and also to test other target genes, to evaluate the usefulness of MLST for *L. pneumophila* serogroup 1. MLST appears to be a promising typing technology, and by the selection of novel target genes this method has the potential of becoming the gold standard for *L. pneumophila* population studies.

## REFERENCES

1. **Enright M. C., and B. G. Spratt.** 1998. A multilocus sequence typing scheme for *Streptococcus pneumoniae*: identification of clones associated with serious invasive disease. *Microbiology* **144:**3049–3060.

2. **Enright, M. C., N. P. J. Day, C. E. Davies, S. J. Peacock, and B. G. Spratt.** 2000. Multilocus sequence typing for characterization of methicillin-resistant and methicillin-susceptible clones of *Staphylococcus aureus. J. Clin. Microbiol.* **38:**1008–1015.

3. **Fry, N. K., S. Alexiou-Daniel, J. M. Bangsborg, S. Bernander, M. Castellani-Pastoris, J. Etienne, B. Forsblom, V. Gaia, J. H. Helbig, D. Lindsay, P. C. Lück, C. Pelaz, S. A. Uldum, and T. J. Harrison.** 1999. A multicenter evaluation of genotypic methods for epidemiologic typing of *Legionella pneumophila* serogroup 1: results of a pan-European study. *Clin. Microbiol. Infect.* **5:**462–477.

4. **Fry, N. K., J. M. Bangsborg, S. Bernander, J. Etienne, B. Forsblom, V. Gaia, P. Hasenberger, D. Lindsay, A. Papoutsi, C. Pelaz, M. Streuelens, S. A. Uldum, P. Visca, and T. J. Harrison.** 2000. Assessment of intercentre reproducibility and concordance of *Legionella pneumophila* serogroup 1 genotyping by amplified fragment length polymorphism analysis. *Eur. J. Clin. Microbiol. Infect. Dis.* **19:**773–780.

5. **Maiden, M. C. J., J. A. Bygraves, E. Feil, G. Morelli, J. E. Russell, R. Urwin, Q. Zhang, J. Zhou, K. Zurth, D. A. Caugant, I. M. Feavers, M. Achtman, and B. G. Spratt.** 1998. Multilocus sequence typing: a portable approach to the identification of clones within populations of pathogenic microorganisms. *Proc. Natl. Acad. Sci. USA* **95:**3140–3145.

6. **Valsangiacomo, C., F. Baggi, V. Gaia, T. Balmelli, R. Peduzzi, and J. C. Piffaretti.** 1995. Use of amplified fragment length polymorphism in molecular typing of *Legionella pneumophila* and application to epidemiological studies. *J. Clin. Microbiol.* **33:**1716–1719.

# EVALUATION OF PCR AND RANDOM AMPLIFICATION OF POLYMORPHIC DNA FOR DETECTION AND TYPING OF *LEGIONELLA* IN ENVIRONMENTAL WATER SAMPLES

*Jafar A. A. Qasem, Ziauddin Khan, and Abu S. Mustafa*

# 48

*Legionella* is a naturally occurring aquatic bacterium found in lakes, rivers, hot springs, ponds, and moist soils (1, 7). It causes Legionnaires' disease, a respiratory illness characterized by pneumonia. The disease is predominantly acquired by inhaling mist from contaminated water sources (12, 13), and it is associated with considerable morbidity and mortality in immunocompromised hosts. Currently, more than 35 species of *Legionella* have been identified and about half of these have been associated with illness (11). Epidemiological investigations of legionellosis are complicated by the ubiquity of *Legionella* in nature (6, 9). Serological subtyping is insufficiently discriminatory when a given serogroup comprises only a few antigenically distinct subtypes, as for *Legionella pneumophila* serogroup 6 (14). Furthermore, genotypic differences have been reported in phenotypically similar organisms (2). Discriminatory molecular subtyping methods may be more informative to establish the environmental source of the illness. During the recent past, molecular diagnostic and typing methods have been employed mostly as a research tool for the detection of a wide variety of infectious agents including *Legionella* (5, 6). DNA amplification by PCR seems to be promising because it is sensitive, specific, and rapid (5, 6). In this study, we have established and evaluated PCR and random amplified polymorphic DNA (RAPD) for detection and typing of *Legionella* from environmental sources.

Water samples (2.5 liters) obtained from a water storage facility of the Mubarak Al-Kabeer Hospital, Kuwait, were filtered through 0.2-$\mu$m-pore-size Nalgene filters. A part of the filter was cultured on buffered charcoal-yeast extract agar (BCYEA-$\alpha$) with antibiotics and selective supplements. The rest of the membrane was used for DNA extraction by using standard methods (10). Swab samples were taken by twirling well inside of the wash basin taps and shower head faucets. They were streaked on a BCYEA-$\alpha$ plate with antibiotics and selective supplements. The plates were incubated at 37°C with 5% $CO_2$ and observed for up to 14 days for growth of *Legionella*. All culture-positive specimens were processed for DNA extraction by the thermic lysis method (8). PCR was per-

*Jafar A. A. Qasem* Department of Biotechnology, Kuwait Institute for Scientific Research, P.O. Box 24885, 13109 Safat, Kuwait. *Ziauddin Khan and Abu S. Mustafa* Department of Microbiology, Faculty of Medicine, Kuwait University, Kuwait, and Faculty of Medicine, Kuwait University, P.O. Box 24923, 13110 Safat, Kuwait.

*Legionella*, Edited by Reinhard Marre et al.
© 2002 ASM Press, Washington, D.C.

formed with the primer pairs L5SL9/L5SR93 and LmipL920/LmipL1548 to detect the organisms of genus *Legionella* and species *L. pneumophila* as described by Koide et al. (4). RAPD was performed according to procedures described previously (15).

A total of 263 swabs and 20 water samples were collected for 1 year. Culture of water samples did not yield *Legionella*; however, genus- and species-specific PCR could detect the presence of *Legionella* in 6 (30%) and identify *L. pneumophila* in 2 samples, respectively (Table 1). Culture of wash basin and shower head swabs yielded *Legionella* from 61 (23%) samples; all of these were positive by genus-specific PCR and 43 samples were positive by species-specific PCR for *L. pneumophila* (Table 1). Serotyping showed that all of the *L. pneumophila* isolates belonged to serotypes 1 (*n* = 8) and 3 (*n* = 35). The isolates belonging to serogroup 1 could further be divided into two groups by RAPD-PCR, i.e., one type of band pattern with isolates 25, 27, 28, 29, 32, 33, and 41 and the second type of band pattern with the isolate 24 (Fig. 1). Similarly, *L. pneumophila* isolates belonging to serogroup 3 could be divided into two distinct genotypic groups by RAPD, i.e., the first group represented by isolates 1 to 17, 19, 20, 21, 22, 23, 26, 30, 31, 34, 35, 36, 37, and 40 and the second group by isolates 18, 38, 39, and 42 (Fig. 2).

Our results confirm the previous studies that PCR is more sensitive than culture and suitable for detection of legionellae in environmental specimens to avoid overgrowth by

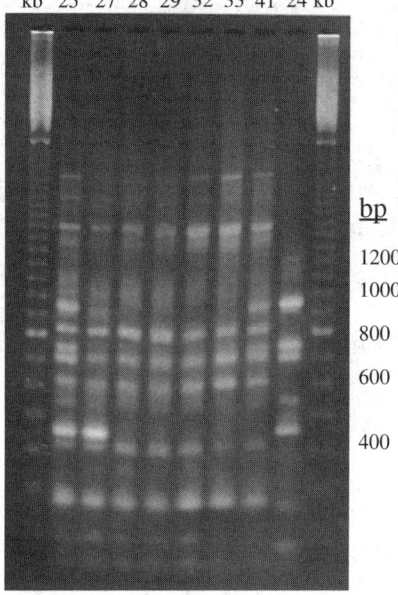

kb 25 27 28 29 32 33 41 24 kb

bp

1200
1000

800

600

400

**FIGURE 1** RAPD patterns of environmental isolates of *L. pneumophila* serogroup 1. Lanes marked 25, 27, 28, 29, 32, 33, 41, and 24 are RAPD patterns of respective *L. pneumophila* isolates. Lanes marked kb are 100-bp molecular size markers.

contaminating organisms (3). Moreover, it can identify the species *L. pneumophila* even in culture-negative specimens, which is the more relevant species for human infections. Our data also show that RAPD analysis can be a better tool to discriminate between isolates compared with serotyping. Thus, it could be more informative in epidemiological studies to determine the source of infection.

**TABLE 1** Comparison of culture, genus-specific, and species-specific PCR for detection of *Legionella* in environmental samples

| Sample type | No. tested | No. of samples positive/total no. of samples (%) | | |
| --- | --- | --- | --- | --- |
| | | Culture | *L. pneumophila*[a] | |
| | | | Genus PCR | Species PCR |
| Water | 20 | 0 | 6/20 (30) | 2/20 (10) |
| Swabs | 263 | 61/263 (23.1) | 61/263 (23.1) | 43/263 (16.3) |
| Total | 283 | 61/283 (21.5) | 67/283 (23.7) | 45/283 (16) |

[a] Genus PCR and species PCR, genus- and species-specific PCR, respectively.

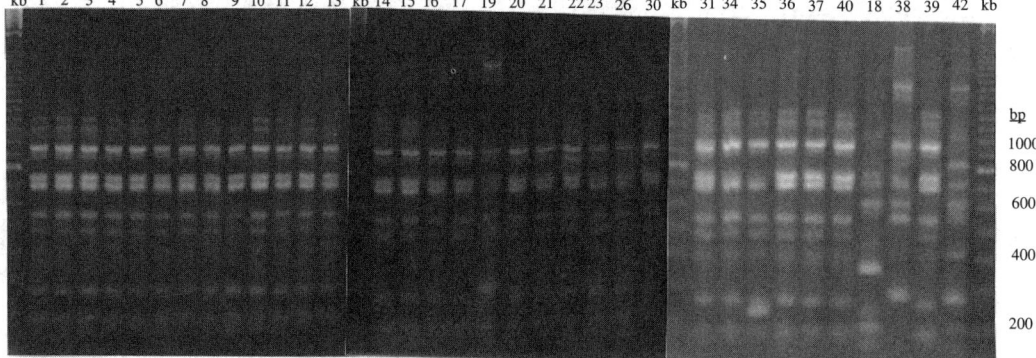

**FIGURE 2** RAPD bands of 34 environmental isolates of *L. pneumophila* belonging to serogroup 3. Lanes 1 through 42 are RAPD patterns of respective *L. pneumophila* isolates. kb, molecular weight markers (100-bp DNA ladder).

## REFRENCES

1. **Brown, A., V. L. Yu, M. H. Magnussen, G. M. Vickers, R. M. Garrity, and E. M. Elder.** 1982. Isolation of Pittsburgh pneumonia agent from a hospital shower. *Appl. Environ. Microbiol.* **43:**725–726.

2. **De Zoysa, A. S., and T. G. Harrison.** 1999. Molecular typing of *Legionella pneumophila* serogroup 1 by pulsed-field gel electrophoresis with *Sfi*I and comparison of this method with restriction fragment-length polymorphism analysis. *J. Med. Microbiol.* **48:**269–278.

3. **Ieven, M., and H. Goossens.** 1997. Relevance of nucleic acid amplification techniques for diagnosis of respiratory tract infections in the clinical laboratory. *Clin. Microbiol. Rev.* **10:**242–256.

4. **Koide, M., A. Saito, N. Kusano, and F. Higa.** 1993. Detection of *Legionella* spp. in cooling tower water by the polymerase chain reaction method. *Appl. Environ. Microbiol.* **59:**1943–1946.

5. **Lawrence, C., E. Ronco, S. Dubrou, R. Leclerco, C. Nauciel, and P. Matsiota-Bernard.** 1999. Molecular typing of *Legionella pneumophila* serogroup isolates from patients and the nosocomial environment by arbitrarily primed PCR and pulsed-field gel electrophoresis. *J. Med. Microbiol.* **48:**327–333.

6. **Maiwald, M., J. H. Helbig, and P. C. Lück.** 1998. Laboratory methods for the diagnosis of *Legionella* infections. *J. Microbiol. Methods* **33:**59–79.

7. **Muder, R. R., V. L. Yu, and A. H. Woo.** 1986. Mode of transmission of *Legionella pneumophila*. *Arch. Intern. Med.* **146:**1607–1612.

8. **Mustafa, A. S., A. Ahmed, A. T. Abal, and T. D. Chugh.** 1995. Establishment and evaluation of a multiplex polymerase chain reaction for detection of *Mycobacteria* and specific identification of *Mycobacterium tuberculosis* complex. *Tuber. Lung Dis.* **76:**336–343.

9. **Ruef, C.** 1998. Nosocomial Legionnaires' disease-strategies for prevention. *J. Microbiol. Methods* **33:**81–91.

10. **Sambrook, J., E. F. Fristch, and T. Maniatis.** 1989. *Molecular Cloning: a Laboratory Manual.* Cold Spring Harbor Laboratory, Cold Spring Harbor, N.Y.

11. **Stout, J. E., and V. L. Yu.** 1997. Legionellosis. *N. Engl. J. Med.* **337:**682–687.

12. **Stout, J., V. L. Yu, R. M. Vickers, and J. Shonnard.** 1982. Potable water supply as the hospital reservoir for Pittsburgh pneumonia agent. *Lancet* **i:**471–472.

13. **Stout, J. E., V. L. Yu, Y. C. Yee, S. Vaccarello, W. Diven, and T. C. Lee.** 1992. *Legionella pneumophila* in water supply: environmental surveillance with clinical assessment for Legionnaire disease. *Epidemiol. Infect.* **30:**537–539.

14. **Visca, P., P. Goldoni, P. C. Luck, J. H. Helbig, L. Cattani, G. Giltri, S. Bramati, and M. Castellani Pastoris.** 1999. Multiple types of *Legionella pneumophila* serogroup 6 in a hospital heated-water system associated with sporadic infections. *J. Clin. Microbiol.* **37:**2189–2196.

15. **William, J. G., A. R. Kubelik, K. J. Livak, J. A. Rafalski, and S. V. Tingey.** 1990. DNA polymorphism amplified by arbitrary primers are useful as genetic markers. *Nucleic Acids Res.* **18:**6531–6535.

# RAPID QUANTIFICATION OF *LEGIONELLA* BY PCR

Daniel Jonas and Gudrun Sahlmüller

# 49

## COUNTING OF *LEGIONELLA*

To estimate the risk of legionellosis from the plumbing systems, it is a common practice to count CFU in water samples. Interestingly, *Legionella* can survive outside of protozoa for a longer period of time and can fall—still alive—into a viable but nonculturable (VBNC) physiological state, from which it can be recovered by addition of amoebae (12). Furthermore, quantitative assays for legionellae are used in infection models to investigate virulence factors or the intracellular activity of antimicrobial agents. Because of the slow growth rate, it is advantageous to have available methods to enumerate legionellae that are faster than counting colonies after 5 to 10 days of incubation on agar plates. There already exist different approaches to numbering legionellae, e.g., by use of the bacterial cytopathic effect (5, 6), radioactive probes, chromogenic substrates of metabolic enzymes (2), or fluorescent labels, for instance, green-fluorescent-protein-expressing plasmids (9). However, these techniques lack a clear, linear correlation between CFU and the measured cytopathic effect, are less sensitive, are less versatile, or require a labeling of the bacteria before the sample is taken. This precludes counting of bacteria outside of the artificial setting of an experiment, e.g., in tap water samples.

## QUANTITATIVE PCR

The technique of quantitative competitive-template (QC)-PCR is mainly used in virology. Yet, there are also applications in microbiology for bacteria that may have low recovery rates or grow slowly (7, 11). The principle of QC-PCR is based on the simultaneous amplification of the genomic template and a recombined internal PCR standard (IS), which usually can be distinguished as the smaller template. Furthermore, the genomic template and the IS have to be amplified linearly with the same efficiencies. Therefore, if the QC-PCR results in equimolar amounts of both amplicons, the known number of competitive IS molecules added equals the unknown number of wild-type genomes. This can be inferred from the number of IS molecules. Thus QC-PCR simply works on the principle of titration of the genomic template with increasing amounts of the IS around the range of equimolarity.

*Daniel Jonas and Gudrun Sahlmüller* Institute of Environmental Medicine and Hospital Epidemiology, University Hospital Freiburg, D-79106 Freiburg, Germany.

*Legionella*, Edited by Reinhard Marre et al.

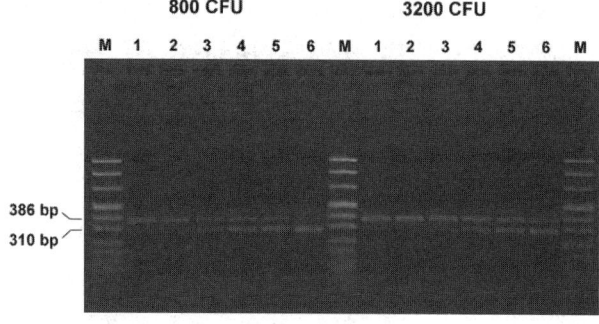

FIGURE 1 Agarose gel-electrophoresis of quantitative-competitive PCR amplification products stained with ethidium bromide and visualized under UV illumination. The two-fold dilution series of the competitive internal standard plasmid DNA ranged from 25 fg (lane 1) to 800 fg (lane 6). M, molecular size standard. Numbers of CFU are indicated above the gel.

## USE OF COMPETITIVE IS DNA

There are a large number of useful PCR targets and primers for specific detection of *Legionella* (4). To demonstrate legionellae-specific QC-PCR in principle, we chose a 16S rRNA gene-based assay, which has proven to be reliable in the routine diagnostics of clinical microbiology and has recently been proposed as one method for identification of the most common *Legionella* spp. (3, 8). A plasmid containing the competitive IS was constructed by ligation of the 386-bp PCR fragment of the 16S rRNA gene into a cloning vector. Subsequently, an internal sequence was replaced by a foreign DNA fragment, which was 76 bp smaller. After amplification of legionella DNA in the presence of the competitive IS DNA, the 310-bp IS amplicon can easily be visualized on an ethidium bromide-stained agarose gel and distinguished from the *Legionella*-specific 386-bp amplicon (Fig. 1).

Finally, to obtain equimolar amplifications of both amplicons, the amounts of the competitive IS added to the legionellae have to be increased to the same extent as the number of CFU (Fig. 1). For an equimolar amplification, around 100 fg of the competitor DNA is required in the presence of 800 CFU (Fig. 1, lane 3, left side). In the case of 3,200 CFU, 400 fg is needed (Fig. 1, lane 5, right side).

## POSSIBLE APPLICATIONS AND LIMITATIONS

QC-PCR could be evaluated as a fast and simple method for enumeration in infection models or in environmental water samples.

This approach might even detect *Legionella* genomes, which cannot be recovered on agar plates because of low plating efficiency or organisms present in a VBNC state. The method's limitation will be that it takes some hours before DNA of dead bacteria is degraded to such an extent that it can no longer be amplified efficiently (10). Therefore, a detectable decrease of genomic DNA will lag some hours behind a declining number of CFU, which are counted after 1 week of incubation. However, a multiplication of CFU should be parallel to an increased number of genomes measured by the QC-PCR. More sophisticated approaches in QC-PCR of *Legionella* have been published recently, which rely on the more expensive TaqMan or LightCycler methodologies (1; R. F. Benson, B. P. Holloway, P. Coan, T. Messmer, and B. S. Field, *Abstr. 37th Intersci. Conf. Antimicrob. Agents Chemother.*, abstr. D-66, p. 94, 1977).

## ACKNOWLEDGMENT

We thank Deborah Lawrie-Blum for assistance with the manuscript.

## REFERENCES

1. **Ballard, A. L., N. K. Fry, L. Chan, S. B. Surman, J. V. Lee, T. G. Harrison, and K. J. Towner.** 2000. Detection of *Legionella pneumophila* using a real-time PCR hybridization assay. *J. Clin. Microbiol.* **38:**4215–4218.
2. **Bej, A. K., M. H. Mahbubani, and R. M. Atlas.** 1991. Detection of viable *Legionella pneumophila* in water by polymerase chain reaction

and gene probe methods. *Appl. Environ. Microbiol.* **57:**597–600.

3. **Cloud, J. L., K. C. Carroll, P. Pixton, M. Erali, and D. R. Hillyard.** 2000. Detection of *Legionella* species in respiratory specimens using PCR with sequencing confirmation. *J. Clin. Microbiol.* **38:**1709–1712.

4. **Fry, N. K., and T. G. Harrison.** 1998. Diagnosis and epidemiology of infections caused by *Legionella* spp., p. 213–242. *In* E. N. Woodford and A. P. Johnson (ed.), *Molecular Bacteriology: Protocols and Clinical Applications.* Humana Press, Totowa, N.J.

5. **Gebran, S. J., C. A. Newton, Y. Yamamoto, T. W. Klein, and H. A. Friedman.** 1994. A rapid colorimetric assay for evaluating *Legionella pneumophila* growth in macrophages *in vitro. J. Clin. Microbiol.* **32:**127–130.

6. **Higa, F., N. Kusano, M. Tateyama, T. Shinzato, N. Arakaki, K. Kawakami, and A. Saito.** 1998. Simplified quantitative assay system for measuring activities of drugs against intracellular *Legionella pneumophila. J. Clin. Microbiol.* **36:**1392–1398.

7. **Johnsen, K., O. Enger, C. S. Jacobsen, L. Thirup, and V. Torsvik.** 1999. Quantitative selective PCR of 16S ribosomal DNA correlates well with selective agar plating in describing population dynamics of indigenous *Pseudomonas* spp. in soil hot spots. *Appl. Environ. Microbiol.* **65:** 1786–1788.

8. **Jonas, D., A. Rosenbaum, S. Weyrich, and S. Bhakdi.** 1995. Enzyme-linked immunoassay for detection of PCR-amplified DNA of legionellae in bronchoalveolar fluid. *J. Clin. Microbiol.* **33:**1247–1252.

9. **Kohler, R., A. Bubert, W. Goebel, M. Steinert, J. Hacker, and B. Bubert.** 2000 Expression and use of the green fluorescent protein as a reporter system in *Legionella pneumophila. Mol. Gen. Genet.* **262:**1060–1069.

10. **McCarty, S. C., and R. M. Atlas.** 1993. Effect of amplicon size on PCR detection of bacteria exposed to chlorine. *PCR Methods Appl.* **3:**181–185.

11. **Sidhu, H., R. P. Holmes, M. J. Allison, and A. B. Peck.** 1999. Direct quantification of the enteric bacterium *Oxalobacter formigenes* in human fecal samples by quantitative competitive-template PCR. *J. Clin. Microbiol.* **37:**1503–1509.

12. **Steinert, M., L. Emody, R. Amann, and J. Hacker.** 1997. Resuscitation of viable but nonculturable *Legionella* pneumophila Philadelphia JR32 by Acanthamoeba castellanii. *Appl. Environ. Microbiol.* **63:**2047–2053.

# MOLECULAR TYPING OF *LEGIONELLA PNEUMOPHILA* BY PULSED-FIELD GEL ELECTROPHORESIS AND AMPLIFIED FRAGMENT LENGTH POLYMORPHISM ANALYSIS

*W. J. B. Wannet, W. K. van der Zwaluw,
M. E. O. C. Heck, C. E. Elzenaar, H. M. E. Maas,
H. Brunings, J. F. P. Schellekens, A. M. C. Bergmans,
A. van der Zee, E. Thijssen, and M. F. Peeters*

# 50

*Legionella* infection (legionellosis) can vary from mild respiratory illness to acute life-threatening pneumonia. Legionellosis is acquired by inhalation or aspiration of legionellae from a contaminated environmental source, which may be established by comparing the environmental and clinical strains. When detailed epidemiologic characterization is required, standardized molecular typing methods are indispensable for the subtyping of *Legionella pneumophila* serogroups (1–4). Therefore, a comparison was made between pulsed-field gel electrophoresis (PFGE) and amplified fragment length polymorphism (AFLP) analysis for genotyping of *L. pneumophila*, using standardized protocols from the European Working Group on *Legionella* Infections (EWGLI).

*W. J. B. Wannet, W. K. van der Zwaluw, M. E. O. C. Heck, C. E. Elzenaar, H. M. E. Maas, H. Brunings, and J. F. P. Schellekens* National Institute of Public Health and the Environment (RIVM), P.O. Box 1, 3720 BA Bilthoven, The Netherlands. *A. M. C. Bergmans, A. van der Zee, E. Thijssen, and M. F. Peeters* Laboratory of Molecular Microbiology, St. Elisabeth Hospital, P.O. Box 747, 5000 AS Tilburg, The Netherlands.

## STRAINS AND METHODS

Clinical and environmental *L. pneumophila* strains used in this study were submitted to the RIVM laboratory for subtyping.

PFGE genomic fingerprinting was performed on 250 *L. pneumophila* strains using the method described by Riffard et al. (3). After cleaving the extracted DNA with *Sfi*I enzyme, banding patterns were generated by PFGE.

AFLP was performed on 400 *L. pneumophila* strains using the method of Valsangiacomo et al. (4). Genomic DNA was digested with *Pst*I restriction enzyme and specially constructed adapters were ligated to the restriction fragments in a one-step reaction. Selective amplification was carried out with a single primer, complementary to the adapters with one nucleotide extending beyond the adapters at the 3' end, in a standard PCR reaction. PCR products were separated on agarose gels and detected by staining with ethidium bromide. The banding patterns from both PFGE and AFLP were analyzed with BioNumerics software (Applied Maths, Kortrijk, Belgium). To determine the interlaboratory reproducibility, 165 *L. pneumophila* strains (obtained from the EWGLI) were AFLP subtyped by both laboratories.

**TABLE 1** Subdivision of PFGE types in AFLP types and vice versa

| PFGE type | AFLP type | AFLP type | PFGE type |
|---|---|---|---|
| A[a](2[c]) | 1[b], 2 | 12 | F, G |
| B(2) | 3, 4 | 2 | A(1), C(26) |
| C(37) | 2 (26), 5, 6 (2), 7(8) | 13 | H, I |
| D(2) | 8, 9 | | |
| E(2) | 10, 11 | | |

[a] Letters represent unique PFGE fingerprints.
[b] Numbers represent unique AFLP fingerprints.
[c] Numbers between parentheses represent number of strains.

## RESULTS

In general, AFLP yielded fingerprints that were easier to interpret than PFGE fingerprints, was less labor-intensive, was less time-consuming, and did not require expensive electrophoresis apparatus. However, with both methods we were able to divide the strains in this study into many subtypes (not shown).

As an example, among 93 unique *L. pneumophila* strains, we found 23 PFGE types and 26 AFLP types. We could further divide 5 PFGE types (approx. 20%) with AFLP and 3 AFLP types (approx. 10%) with PFGE (Table 1).

The AFLP method used by both laboratories on the 165 EWGLI strains was robust and had rather good interlaboratory concordance. Results demonstrate that the method can be highly reproducible and epidemiologically concordant, with good discrimination, yet strict adherence to the defined laboratory protocol is essential.

## CASE EXAMPLE

The RIVM laboratory received two *L. pneumophila* strains (serogroup 1 and 3) from patients suffering from severe legionellosis after a visit to a foreign hotel. We also received different *L. pneumophila* strains isolated from water samples of the same hotel. With AFLP and PFGE we were able to demonstrate that both patient strains clustered with strains isolated from the hotel (Fig. 1).

## CONCLUSIONS

- DNA fingerprint patterns derived from AFLP seem to be superior to the patterns

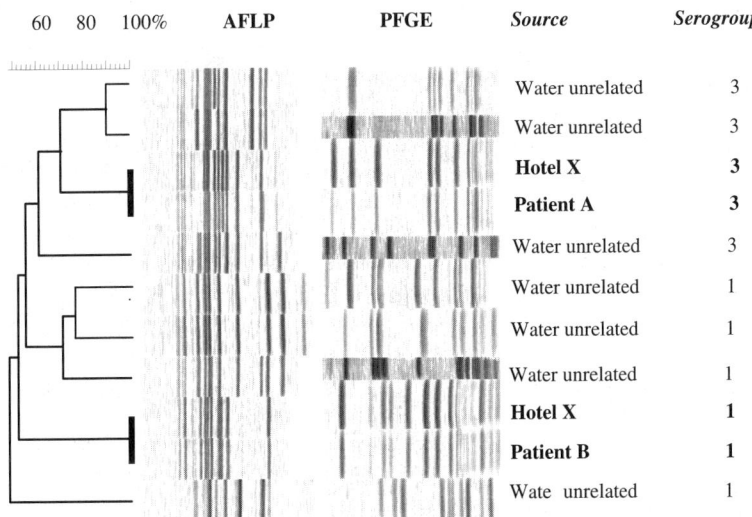

**FIGURE 1** Case example showing the application of PFGE and AFLP for the molecular subtyping of *L. pneumophila*.

derived from PFGE, in both speed and interpretability.

- AFLP and PFGE have similar discriminatory power.
- AFLP and PFGE are powerful tools for the epidemiological subtyping of *L. pneumophila*.

## FUTURE

We emphasize the importance of the standardization of data analysis and data exchange using the latest software (BioNumerics). Studies are under way to determine both the intralaboratory and interlaboratory reproducibility more extensively for further standardization of these powerful subtyping methods used by an increasing number of European countries.

## REFERENCES

1. **Fry, N. K., S. Alexiou-Daniel, J. M. Bangsborg, S. Bernander, M. Castellani Pastoris, J. Etienne, B. Forsblom, V. Gaia, J. H. Helbig, D. Lindsay, P. C. Luck, C. Pelaz, S. Uldum, and T. G. Harrison.** 1999. A multicenter evaluation of genotypic methods for the epidemiologic typing of *Legionella pneumophila* serogroup 1: results of a pan-European study. *Clin. Microbiol. Infect.* **5:** 462–477.
2. **Fry, N. K., J. M. Bangsborg, S. Bernander, J. Etienne, B. Forsblom, V. Gaia, P. Hasenberger, D. Lindsay, A. Papoutsi, C. Pelaz, M. Struelens, S. A. Uldum, P. Visca, and T. G. Harrison.** 2000. Assessment of intercentre reproducibility and epidemiological concordance of *Legionella pneumophila* serogroup 1 genotyping by amplified fragment length polymorphism analysis. *Eur. J. Clin. Microbiol. Infect. Dis.* **19:**773–780.
3. **Riffard, S., F. Lo Presti, F. Vendenesch, F. Forey, M. Reyrolle, and J. Etienne.** 1998. Comparative analysis of infrequent-restriction-site PCR and pulsed-field gel electrophoresis for epidemiological typing of *Legionella pneumophila* serogroup 1 strains. *J. Clin. Microbiol.* **36:**161–167.
4. **Valsangiacomo, C., F. Baggi, V. Gaia, T. Balmelli, R. Peduzzi, and J. C. Piffaretti.** 1995. Use of amplified fragment length polymorphism in molecular typing of *Legionella pneumophila* and application to epidemiological studies. *J. Clin. Microbiol.* **33:**1716–1719.

# THE FLUORESCENT IN SITU HYBRIDIZATION TEST IN COMPARISON WITH CULTURE FOR DETECTION OF *LEGIONELLA PNEUMOPHILA* IN WATER SAMPLES

*Bart Wullings, Remko Voogt, Harm Veenendaal,*
*and Dick van der Kooij*

# 51

The presence of *Legionella* in water installations is a potential risk to public health. *L. pneumophila* is the species most frequently isolated from water and is related to legionellosis. A semiselective agar medium (buffered charcoal-yeast extract [BCYE] agar ([3]) is used for the detection of *Legionella* in water installations. However, up to 7 days is needed before results are available. In certain situations (e.g., outbreak of legionellosis, presence of *Legionella* in an installation), time is limited and a rapid method, in which the results are available within a day, is needed. This report evaluates the fluorescent in situ hybridization (FISH) test with a specific 16S rRNA-targeted probe for detecting the presence of viable *L. pneumophila* in water. The results of this FISH test are available after 6 h (without inactivation) or 24 h (with activation). A large number of water samples, mostly from hot water systems, were tested with both test varieties and results were compared with those obtained with the culture method.

## METHODS AND MATERIALS

### Fluorescent In Situ Hybridization

FISH is a detection technique using a specific fluorescence-labeled DNA probe targeting the rRNA of the cells of the selected microorganism(s) (4, 8). Individual bacterial cells, present in concentrated water samples and biofilms, are simultaneously microscopically visualized, identified, and enumerated. A combination of a specific *L. pneumophila* probe (red excitation) and a eubacterial probe (green excitation) enables the detection of *L. pneumophila* and visualization of the total active bacterial population present in the sample. By targeting the rRNA in the cell, only metabolically active bacteria are detected. However, bacteria with a low activity and therefore a low rRNA content may remain undetected (2). Therefore, bacteria concentrated from samples were incubated on solid medium for a short time to increase their metabolic activity. This activation step makes the detection method more robust and applicable for both starved *L. pneumophila* that may be present in warm water samples and highly active cells that are observed in cooling towers.

Bacteria were concentrated from water samples (up to 250 ml) by filtration through polycarbonate membranes (with 0.2-$\mu$m

*Bart Wullings, Remko Voogt, Harm Veenendaal, and Dick van der Kooij* Kiwa Research and Consultancy, P.O. Box 1072, 3430 BB Nieuwegein, The Netherlands.

*Legionella*, Edited by Reinhard Marre et al.
© 2002 ASM Press, Washington, D.C.

pores), followed by incubation of the membranes on BCYE medium at 37°C, for 4 and 16 h, respectively. A standard FISH protocol was applied with the specific *L. pneumophila* 16S rRNA-targeted oligonucleotide probe (5) in combination with a eubacterial probe (1) for 3 h at 46°C in a hybridization solution containing 20% formamide, bovine serum albumin, and poly(U). Subsequently, filters were washed in 40 mM of NaCl buffer. A total of 100 microscopic fields were analyzed at a magnification of ×1,000 for the presence of cells giving a typical positive signal with the *L. pneumophila*-specific probe. For a 250-ml sample, the detection limit is approximately 2,000 cells/liter.

## Culture Method

The conventional culture method includes filtrating (membrane filtration with 0.2-$\mu$m pores) 500-ml samples, resuspending the cells from the membrane by vortexing in 5 ml of sterile water with glass beads, spreading 0.1 ml on BCYE medium with antibiotics, and incubating at 37°C for 5 to 7 days, respectively. The detection limit of this method is 50 CFU/liter.

## Samples

Water samples (up to 1 liter) were collected in sterile glass containers from domestic warm water systems, industrial cooling towers, and saunas. Samples were transported on ice to the laboratory and tested within 24 h with both methods.

## RESULTS AND DISCUSSION

### *Legionella* in Water Samples

*Legionella* were detected in 52 (42%) water samples, with the FISH test and/or the culture method. In 91 (73%) of 124 water samples tested, both tests gave identical results when defined as presence or absence, with 17 positive and 72 negative results (Table 1). A total of 21 (17%) water samples were positive only in FISH and negative in the culture method, and 12 were culture-positive and FISH-

**TABLE 1** Detection of *Legionella* in 124 water samples using FISH and the culture technique

| Test result | | No. (%) of samples |
| --- | --- | --- |
| FISH | Culture | |
| + | + | 19 (15) |
| − | − | 72 (58) |
| + | − | 21 (17) |
| − | + | 12 (10) |
| Total | | 124 (100) |

negative (10%). These findings are in line with results reported for PCR detection in comparison with the culture method with respectively 66 and 84% identical results obtained for both methods (7, 9). However the PCR technique gives a positive result for active as well as nonactive cells, including dead cells and remaining DNA (7). FISH detects only intact cells containing sufficient rRNA.

## Effect of Activation in FISH Test

The effect of activation of concentrated cells is demonstrated in Table 2. The direct test (no activation) resulted in *Legionella* detection in 25 of the 40 samples that gave a positive result in the FISH test. In 9 (37.5%) of the FISH-positive samples, *Legionella* was detected only after activation for 4 and/or 16 h. This demonstrates clearly the value of activation of concentrated *Legionella* cells in the FISH test. Obviously, in a significant proportion of the samples, *Legionella* cells are not active, but surviving.

**TABLE 2** Effect of activation on the result of the FISH test for detecting *L. pneumophila* in water samples

| Test procedure(s) | No. (%) of positive samples |
| --- | --- |
| No activation (direct) . . . . . . . . . . . . . . . | 7 (17.5) |
| Activation for 4 h . . . . . . . . . . . . . . . . . . | 2 (5) |
| Activation for 16 h . . . . . . . . . . . . . . . . . | 7 (17.5) |
| Activation for 4 and 16 h . . . . . . . . . . . . | 6 (15) |
| Direct and with 4 or 16 h of activation. . . . . . . . . . . . . . . . . . . . . . . . | 18 (45) |

## Quantitative Comparison

Numbers of cells detected by FISH including activation ranged from $2 \times 10^3$ to $1 \times 10^6$/liter (median: $4.6 \times 10^3$ cells/liter) and were clearly higher than the number of culturable cells, which ranged from 50 to $1 \times 10^3$ CFU/liter (median: $9.5 \times 10^2$ CFU/liter) (Fig. 1). In samples that were positive with both methods, the ratio of the number of cells detected with FISH and the colony count ranged from 0.63 to 2,500, with a median value of 56. Hence, in 50% of these samples, the number of culturable *Legionella* bacteria cells was less than 2% of the number of *L. pneumophila* cells as detected with FISH. Thus, in many samples the *Legionella* population is dominated by nonculturable cells, which contain sufficient rRNA, without or with activation, to allow detection in the FISH test. In reality the proportion of nonculturable cells may even be larger because the FISH test included only *L. pneumophila*. In a number of samples, competition with other bacteria on the agar medium may have hampered their detection with the culture method. Figure 1 shows that in two water samples, the number of culturable cells was clearly larger than the number of cells detected with FISH. In these samples, *Legionella* spp. other than *L. pneumophila* may have been present. The large difference in detection levels hampers the comparison of both tests. The high ratio between numbers detected with FISH and the number of culturable cells compensates for this difference in many samples, but not when most cells are active. Hence, improvement of the FISH test to allow detection of lower numbers of cells is needed. Interpretation of the FISH test results, in terms of hygienic significance, is even more complicated than such interpretation of colony counts. However, in several reports it has been suggested that nonculturable *Legionella* may be infectious (6).

## CONCLUSIONS

On the basis of the results reported above, the following conclusions can be drawn: (i) FISH allows detection of *L. pneumophila* in samples of water and biofilms within 24 h after sampling, but activation is needed. (ii) In many cases the numbers of cells detected with FISH are much higher than numbers detected with the culture method. (iii) Further improvement of the FISH test, e.g., a level of detection similar to the culture method, is needed.

## ACKNOWLEDGMENT

This study was conducted within the framework of the Joint Research Program of The Netherlands Water Supply Companies.

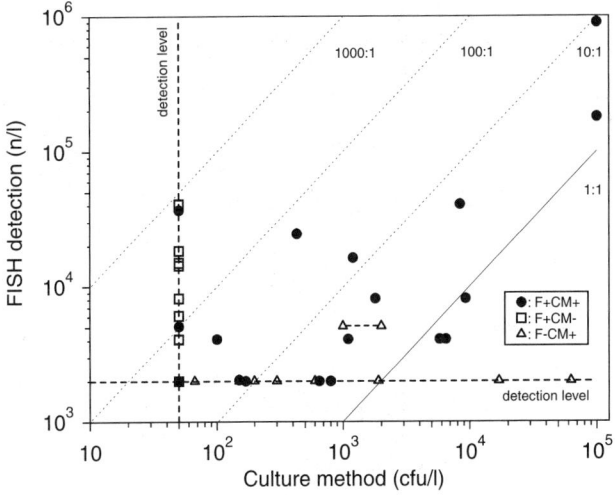

**FIGURE 1** Number of *Legionella* detected with FISH (F) compared with numbers detected with the culture method (CM). The detection limits (2,000 cells/liter in the FISH test; 50 CFU/liter for the culture method) are indicated. Also, ratios between numbers of cells detected with FISH and with the culture method are shown. Symbols on the lines, indicating the detection levels, represent samples in which the number was less than or equal to these limits.

## REFERENCES

1. **Amann, R. I., B. J. Binder, R. J. Olsen, S. W. Chrisholm, R. Devereux, and D. A. Stahl.** 1990. Combination of 16S rRNA-targeted oligonucleotide probes with flow cytometry for analyzing mixed microbial populations. *Appl. Environ. Microbiol.* **56:**1919–1925.

2. **Amann, R. I., W. Ludwig, and K.-H. Schleifer.** 1995. Phylogenetic identification and in situ detection of individual microbial cells without cultivation. *Microbiol. Rev.* **59:**143–169.

3. **Edelstein, P. H.** 1981. Improved semi-selective medium for isolation of *Legionella pneumophila* from contaminate clinical and environmental specimens. *J. Clin. Microbiol.* **14:**298–303.

4. **Giovannoni, S. J., E. F. DeLong, G. J. Olsen, and N. R. Pace.** 1988. Phylogenetic group-specific oligodeoxynucleotide probes for identification of single microbial cells. *J. Bacteriol.* **170:**720–726.

5. **Grimm, D., H. Merkert, W. Ludwig, K-H. Scheiffer, J. Hacker, and B. C. Brand.** 1998. Specific detection of *Legionella pneumophila*: construction of a new 16S rRNA-targeted oligonucleotide probe. *Appl. Environ. Microbiol.* **64:**2686–2690.

6. **Hay, J., D. V. Seal, B. Billcliffe, and J. H. Freer.** 1995. Non-culturable *Legionella pneumophila* associated with *Acanthamoeba castellanii*: detection of the bacterium using DNA amplification and hybridization. *J. Appl. Bacterial.* **78:**61–65.

7. **Maiwald, M., K. Kissel, S. Srimuang, M. von Knebel Doeberitz, and H.-G. Sonntag.** 1994. Comparison of polymerase chain reaction and conventional culture for the detection of Legionellas in hospital water samples. *J. Appl. Bacteriol.* **76:**216–225.

8. **Moter, A., and U. B. Göbel.** 2000. Fluorescence in situ hybridization (FISH) for direct visualization of microorganisms. *J. Microbial Methods* **41:**85–112.

9. **Okpara, J., M. Maiwald, M. Borneff, J. Windeler, and H.-G. Sonntag.** 1996. Evaluation of a new version of the EnvironAmp™ *Legionella* kit for the detection of *Legionellae* in water samples by the polymerase chain reaction. *Zentralbl. Hyg.* **198:**502–513.

# TYPING OF *LEGIONELLA* STRAINS ISOLATED FROM PATIENTS AND ENVIRONMENTAL SOURCES IN GERMANY, 1990-2000

*P. Christian Lück and Jürgen H. Helbig*

# 52

*Legionella* spp. are gram-negative bacteria responsible for epidemic and sporadic cases of pneumonia after inhalation of contaminated water droplets from a variety of water sources (2). Currently, at least 42 species comprise 64 serogroups of legionellae, most of which have caused disease (1). Patients with an impaired immune system or after surgery have a high risk of acquiring legionellosis (2). Here, we present the distribution of *Legionella* species, serogroups, and monoclonal subtypes of *Legionella* strains isolated in Germany and typed at the National Reference Laboratory for *Legionella*.

Strains were cultured in our institution from respiratory materials on selective buffered charcoal-yeast extract agar (BMPA-BCYE Oxoid, Wesel, Germany) or sent to our laboratory by colleagues. Environmental strains were isolated on selective buffered charcoal-yeast extract agar from water samples collected at various locations in Germany (14). For the analysis of the distribution of legionellae in the environment, we considered one strain of each species, serogroup, and

monoclonal antibody (MAb) subtype per water system.

Serological typing of *Legionella* strains was performed with a commercially available fluorescein isothiocyanate-labeled *L. pneumophila*-specific MAb (Gull Laboratories, Oberursel, Germany), with MAbs for all 15 serogroups of *L. pneumophila* (6) and with rabbit antisera against *L. micdadei, L. bozemanii* serogroups 1 and 2, *L. dumoffii, L. jordanis, L. longbeachae* serogroups 1 and 2, *L. anisa, L. wadsworthii, L. oakridgensis, L. sainthelensis, L. haeckeliae* serogroups 1 and 2, *L. maceachernii, L. israelensis, L. feelei* serogroups 1 and 2, *L. rubrilucence, L. erythra, L. santicrucis,* and *L. moravica* (9). The monoclonal subtypes were named according to the reactivity with reference strains (7).

For macrorestriction analysis, chromosomal DNAs were digested overnight with *Sfi*I, *Asc*I, and *Not*I (New England Biolabs, Schwahlbach, Germany) and separated with the CHEF III System (BioRad Laboratories, Munich, Germany) (10). For species not belonging to *L. pneumophila* we sequenced the *mip* gene to define the species (12).

In this study, all patients had a radiographically confirmed pneumonia confirmed as legionellosis by isolating a *Legionella* strain from clinical specimens. Cases were classified as nosocomial if the patient had been hospitalized

*P. Christian Lück and Jürgen H. Helbig*  Institut für Medizinische Mikrobiologie und Hygiene, TU Dresden, Fiedlerstrasse 42, D-01307 Dresden, Germany.

*Legionella*, Edited by Reinhard Marre et al.
© 2002 ASM Press, Washington, D.C.

**TABLE 1** Distribution of *Legionella* species, serogroups, and monoclonal subgroups among clinical and environmental isolates

| Species | Serogroup | Monoclonal subtype[a] | No. (%) of isolates | | | | | |
|---|---|---|---|---|---|---|---|---|
| | | | Community acquired | Travel associated | Nosocomial | Unknown | All clinical isolates | Water isolates |
| *L. pneumophila* | 1 | Philadelphia[c] | 10 | 6 | 2 | 4 | 22 | 34 |
| | 1 | Benidorm[c] | 6 | 7 | 3 | 3 | 19 | 19 |
| | 1 | Knoxville[c] | 3 | 1 | 12 | 1 | 17 | 16 |
| | 1 | France[c] | 1 | | | | 1 | 5 |
| | 1 | Allentown[c] | 1 | | | | 1 | 4 |
| | 1 | Olda | 1 | | 6 | 2 | 9 | 48 |
| | 1 | Oxford | 1 | | 1 | 1 | 3 | 21 |
| | 1 | Heysham | | | | | | 1 |
| | 1 | Camperdown | | | | | | 2 |
| | 1 | Bellingham | 5 | | 9 | 2 | 16 | 53 |
| | 1 | new[d] | | | | | | 2 |
| | 2 | | | 1 | 1 | 1 | 2 | 10 |
| | 3 | | 1 | | 1 | 3 | 3 | 46 |
| | 4 | | 1 | | 4 | 1 | 8 | 27 |
| | 5 | | 1 | | 4 | 3 | 6 | 18 |
| | 6 | | 2 | 1 | 5 | 3 | 11 | 59 |
| | 7 | | | | | | | 4 |
| | 8 | | | | | | | 9 |
| | 9 | | | | | | | 8 |
| | 10 | | 1 | | 1 | 1 | 3 | 36 |
| | 11 | | | | | | | 3 |
| | 12 | | 1 | | 1 | 1 | 3 | 10 |
| | 13 | | | | | | | 5 |
| | 14 | | | | | | | 3 |
| | 2–15[b] | | | | | 2 | 2 | 3 |
| *L. bozemanii* | 1 | | 1 | | | 2 | 2 | 3 |
| *L. longbeachae* | 1 | | 1 | | | | | 2 |
| *L. dumoffii* | | | | | 1 | | | 2 |
| *L. cincinnatensis* | | | | | 1 | | | |
| *L. haeckeliae* | 2 | | | | 1 | 1 | | |
| Other non-*L. pneumophila* | | | | | | | | 24 |
| All *L. pneumophila* | 1 | | 28 (76) | 14 (88) | 33 (61) | 13 | 88 (66) | 205 (43) |
| All *L. pneumophila* | 2–15 | | 7 (19) | 2 (12) | 17 (32) | 12 | 38 (29) | 241 (51) |
| All non-*L. pneumophila* | | | 2 (5) | | 4 (7) | 1 | 7 (5) | 31 (6) |
| All strains | | | 37 (100) | 16 (100) | 54 (100) | 26 | 133 (100) | 477 (100) |

[a] According to Joly et al. (7).
[b] Serogroup not defined because the strains did not react with serogroup-specific MAbs but only with cross-reacting MAbs (6).
[c] Reacting with MAb 3/1 (corresponding to MAb 2 of the scheme of Joly et al.) (7).
[d] Reactivity pattern did not fit with the described ones (7).

continuously for a minimum of 3 days at the time of disease onset or had been discharged from the hospital less than 10 days before the onset of symptoms (2). Furthermore, cases were defined as travel associated according to the criteria of the European Working Group on *Legionella* Infections, i.e., if the patient had a history of travel in the 10 days before the onset of illness (13). Travel was defined as staying away from home for one or more nights. Overnight stays in private accommodations were not included. Community-acquired cases were defined if both of the above-mentioned possibilities could be excluded with certainty.

All results of typing the clinical and environmental strains are summarized in Table 1. Of the 133 strains grown from clinical samples, 88 (66%) belonged to serogroup 1, 38 (29%) belonged to serogroups 2 to 15, and 7 (5%) were typed as other *Legionella* species. These data are in good agreement with results from Europe and the United States (4, 5, 11).

Only 61% of the strains isolated from nosocomial cases belonged to serogroup 1, whereas 76% of community-acquired cases were caused by strains of this serogroup. Remarkable differences were found in the frequencies of MAb 3/1 positive strains in the patient groups. MAb 3/1-positive *L. pneumophila* serogroup 1 strains accounted for only 35% among nosocomial cases, but for 58% of community-acquired cases. All but two strains isolated from travel-associated cases reacted with MAb 3/1. These two MAb 3/1-negative strains were isolated from patients with severe underlying diseases. These data confirm previous results (3, 8) and show that MAb 3/1-positive strains may be more virulent and subsequently may affect previously healthy persons.

The majority of strains isolated from environmental samples were also classified as *L. pneumophila*. Of the 477 environmental isolates serotyped, 205 (43%) were *L. pneumophila* serogroup 1, which is less than among the patient strains. A total of 241 strains (51%) belonged to other serogroups of *L. pneumophila*. The most prevalent serogroups, other than serogroup 1, were serogroup 6 (12%), serogroup 3 (10%), and serogroup 10 (8%). Thirty-one strains (6%) belonged to other species. The most frequent species were *L. bozemanii*, *L. anisa*, and *L. rubrilucence*. For determining the species, sequence analysis of the *mip* gene was a faster and more reliable method than serotyping.

In conclusion, the distribution of *Legionella* species, serogroups, and MAb subtypes among nosocomial strains reflects the distribution among environmental isolates. This is an indication that within hospitals, where patients with underlying diseases become infected, each strain might cause disease.

## ACKNOWLEDGMENTS

We thank Jutta Paasche, Sylvia Petsche, Kerstin Seeliger, Ines Wolf, and Sigrid Gäbler for technical assistance. *Legionella* strains were kindly supplied by E. Budde, Schwerin; I. Carmienke, Leipzig; E. Dinger, Wernigerode; D. Diesterweg, Eberswalde; W. Ehret, Augsburg; F. Fehrenbach, Berlin; J. Hacker, Würzburg; E. Halle, Berlin; L. Jatzwauk, Dresden; D. Jonas, Freiburg; R. Kämmerer, Lübeck; H. Kunzelmann, Chemnitz; M. Maiwald, Heidelberg; W. Matthys, Münster; R. Pfüller, Berlin; R. Marre, Ulm; D. Rimek, Heidelberg; R. Schubert, Frankfurt/M; C. Schoerner, Erlangen; B. Wiese, Göttingen; K. Zobel, Hamburg.

This study was supported by the Deutsche Forschungsgemeinschaft (Lu 485/1-2).

## REFERENCES

1. **Benson, R. F., and B. S. Fields.** 1998. Classification of the genus *Legionella*. *Semin. Respir. Infect.* **13:**90–99.
2. **Breiman, R. F., and J. C. Butler.** 1998. Legionnaires' disease: clinical, epidemiological, and public health perspectives. *Semin. Respir. Infect.* **13:**84–89.
3. **Dournon, E., W. F. Bibb, P. Rjagopalan, N. Desplaces, and R. M. McKinney.** 1988. Monoclonal antibody reactivity as a virulence marker for *Legionella pneumophila* serogroup 1 strains. *J. Infect. Dis.* **157:**496–501.
4. **European Working Group on Legionella Infections.** 1999. Legionnaires disease, Europe 1997. *Wkly. Epidemiol. Rec.* **73:**257–264.
5. **European Working Group on Legionella Infections.** 1998. Legionnaires disease, Europe 1998. *Wkly. Epidemiol. Rec.* **74:**273–280.

6. **Helbig, J. H., J. B. Kurtz, M. Castellani Pastoris, C. Pelaz, and P. C. Lück.** 1997. Antigenic lipopolysaccharide components of *Legionella pneumophila* recognized by monoclonal antibodies: possibilities and limitations for division of the species and serogroups. *J. Clin. Microbiol.* **35:**2841–2845.

7. **Joly, J. R., R. M. McKinney, J. H. Tobin, W. F. Bibb, I. D. Watkins, and D. Ramsay.** 1986. Development of a standardized subgrouping scheme for *Legionella pneumophila* serogroup 1 using monoclonal antibodies. *J. Clin. Microbiol.* **23:**768–771.

8. **Joly, J. R., Y. Y. Chen, and D. Ramsay.** 1993. Serogrouping and subtyping of *Legionella pneumophila* with monoclonal antibodies. *J. Clin. Microbiol.* **18:**1040–1046.

9. **Lück, P. C., I. Leupold, M. Hlawitschka, J. H. Helbig, I. Carmienke, L. Jatzwauk, and T. Guderitz.** 1993. Prevalence of *Legionella* species, serogroups, and monoclonal subgroups in hot water systems in south-eastern Germany. *Zentralbl. Hyg.* **193:**450–460.

10. **Lück, P. C., H. M. Wenchel, and J. H. Helbig.** 1998. Nosocomial pneumonia caused by three genetically different strains of *Legionella pneumophila* and detection of these strains in the hospital water supply. *J. Clin. Microbiol.* **36:**1160–1163.

11. **Marston, B. J., H. B. Lippman, and R. F. Breiman.** 1994. Surveillance for Legionnaires' disease. *Arch. Intern. Med.* **154:**2417–2422.

12. **Ratcliff, R. M., J. A. Lanser, P. A. Manning, and M. W. Heuzenroeder.** 1998. Sequence-based classification scheme for the genus *Legionella* targeting the *mip* gene. *J. Clin. Microbiol.* **36:**1560–1567.

13. **Slaymaker, E., C. A. Joseph, and C. L. R. Bartlett on behalf of the European Working Group on Legionella Infections.** 1999. Travel associated legionnaires' disease in Europe 1997 and 1998. *Eurosurveillance* **4:**120–124.

14. **Winn, W. C.** 1995. *Legionella*, p. 533–544. *In* P. R. Murray, E. J. Baron, M. A. Pfaller, F. C. Tenover, and R. H. Yolken (ed.), *Manual of Clinical Microbiology*, 6th ed. American Society for Microbiology, Washington, D.C.

# DEVELOPMENT OF AN INTERNATIONAL EXTERNAL QUALITY ASSURANCE SCHEME FOR ISOLATION OF *LEGIONELLA* SPECIES FROM ENVIRONMENTAL SPECIMENS

*John V. Lee, Susanne Surman,*
*Maureen Hall, and Lorraine Cuthbert*

# 53

The isolation of *Legionella* species from environmental specimens has multiple steps subject to many potential errors, which have a cumulative effect. The growth medium is relatively complex and contains heat-sensitive ingredients, and the preparation involves multiple aseptic additions after autoclaving. There may be significant variation between commercial batches of media or ingredients and even between two flasks made from the same ingredients on the same day and autoclaved together. There can be losses during concentration steps caused by legionellae remaining attached to membrane filters and centrifuge tubes. Samples require pretreatment by heat (50°C for 30 min) or acid (pH 2.2 for 5 min) and the timing must be carefully controlled to prevent loss of legionellae. The selective media and pretreatments do not suppress all background flora, and the recognition of colonies of *Legionella*, particularly non-*L. pneumophila* species, requires experience. In addition, background bacterial flora can sometimes suppress the growth of colonies of *Legionella* completely.

Competence of isolation is important for outbreak investigations, which may also cross national borders. Quantitative estimation is used increasingly to monitor control measures, and there is pressure for it to become a legal requirement in some countries. It is important that all laboratories in different countries produce equivalent reliable results. To achieve this, each laboratory needs a comprehensive quality assurance program including good internal quality control and participation in external quality assurance (EQA) schemes.

Following trials during 1991–1992, the Public Health Laboratory Service EQA scheme for the isolation of *Legionella* species from water was introduced in 1993 for laboratories in the United Kingdom and extended to overseas laboratories in 1994 with partial financial support from the European Commission. The scheme is designed to provide information on the reliability of isolation media, the concentration and selection procedure, and the identification of *Legionella* species.

Participants receive four distributions annually, each containing three 3-ml samples of simulated concentrates from water. A sample

*John. V. Lee, Susanne Surman, Maureen Hall, and Lorraine Cuthbert*  PHLS Water and Environmental Microbiology Research Unit, Public Health Laboratory, Queen's Medical Centre, University Hospital, Nottingham NG7 2UH, England.

*Legionella*, Edited by Reinhard Marre et al.
© 2002 ASM Press, Washington, D.C.

may contain one or more species of *Legionella* that have never been grown on artificial media, together with supporting natural aquatic flora; aquatic bacteria but no legionellae; a species of *Legionella* with no background organisms; or no organisms. The numbers of legionellae in the samples simulate the full range of counts that may be encountered in nature. Participants are requested to analyze the specimens on a specified date. A direct count is performed by inoculating a volume of the concentrate onto the selective medium and counting the number of colonies of *Legionella* after incubation. A further 2 ml of each sample is diluted to 1 liter to create a simulated water, which the participants are then asked to process following their routine procedures. Within 3 weeks the participants return the following information to the organizers: the direct counts, the volumes processed after concentration and inoculation onto the plates, the numbers of colonies of *Legionella* counted on each plate, the calculated number of *Legionella* organisms per liter; the identification of any *Legionella* spp., and information on the methods used to process the samples. Participants receive a preliminary report of the expected results followed by a full personalized confidential report with the participant's own results marked on bar charts of all the results.

By August 2000 the participants amounted to 148 and were distributed as follows: Austria ($n = 7$), Belgium ($n = 3$), Czech Republic ($n = 6$), Denmark ($n = 1$), England ($n = 70$), Finland ($n = 2$), France ($n = 2$), Germany ($n = 3$), Hungary ($n = 2$), Israel ($n = 1$), Italy ($n = 11$), Japan ($n = 6$), The Netherlands ($n = 1$), Northern Ireland ($n = 1$), Portugal ($n = 3$), Scotland ($n = 12$), Singapore ($n = 4$), Slovenia ($n = 1$), South Africa ($n = 1$), Spain ($n = 5$), Sweden ($n = 4$), Switzerland ($n = 1$), and Wales ($n = 1$).

In 1994, the mathematical detection limits of the methods used in the different laboratories ranged from 1 to 10,000 CFU/liter but recoveries were so low that a report of "No *Legionella* detected" could mean anything from <1 CFU/liter to <60,000 CFU/liter,

even for *L. pneumophila*. By January 2000, the mathematical detection limit range was 4 to 500 CFU/liter and for 68% of laboratories was less than or equal to 100 CFU/liter. Most laboratories now have little problem detecting *L. pneumophila*. Recoveries of *L. pneumophila* after processing have improved to range from 10 to 30% measured relative to the direct count obtained by the sending laboratory or the participant's own direct count, although some laboratories still fail completely. Recovery of non-*L. pneumophila* species remains poor (Table 1). In the organizing laboratory we use the same media as most of the participants and grow these organisms successfully. Thus, the inability of the participants to grow these organisms is almost certainly due to inadequate internal quality control failing to detect poor-quality media.

In contrast to the other *Legionella* species, detection, recovery, and identification of *L. pneumophila* is now consistently better than when the scheme started. Figures 1 and 2 display examples of the spread of results for sample C from the April 2000 distribution. These results are shown in the format in which they are included in the final reports. The early distributions to non-United Kingdom laboratories were dispatched by international mail, which was relatively cheap and convenient but often led to appreciable delays in transit. This sometimes resulted in deterioration of the material so that the numbers of legionellae recovered were lower than by the United Kingdom participants. Couriers specializing in carrying of dangerous goods now have to be used. Although much more expensive, the deliveries are now more rapid and the numbers recovered by the overseas laboratories show the same distribution as United Kingdom participants. This is illustrated in Fig. 1 and 2, where the numbers above the bars represent the numbers of non-United Kingdom laboratories included within the group represented by the bar.

The results of different distributions consistently indicate that most laboratories lose 80 to 90% of the legionellae during concentration

**TABLE 1** Proportion of laboratories detecting *Legionella* species other than *L. pneumophila*

| Month/year | Identification | Pure culture | Simulated sample CFU/liter[a] | % Laboratories detecting after: | |
|---|---|---|---|---|---|
| | | | | Direct inoculation | After processing |
| 04/93 | *L. bozemanii* | No | 1,400 | 57 | 53 |
| 07/94 | *L. birminghamensis* | Yes | 3,400 | 72 | 64 |
| 04/95 | *L. micdadei* | Yes | 16,200 | 81 | 68 |
| 10/95 | *L. bozemanii* serogroup 1 | Yes | 1,620 | 91 | 74 |
| 01/97 | *L. bozemanii* serogroup 2 | No | 680 | 70 | 58 |
| 07/97 | *L. micdadei* | Yes | 14,000 | 89 | 77 |
| 04/98 | *L. bozemanii* serogroup 2 | No | 8,600 | 46 | 42 |
| 10/98 | *L. bozemanii* serogroup 2 + *L pneumophila* | Yes | 8,400 | | 46 |
| 04/99 | *L. dumoffii* + *L. quinlavinii* | No | 9,800 (combined) | 98 | 96 |
| 01/00 | *L. jordanis* | Yes | 9,200 | 96 | 96 |
| 04/00 | *L. bozemanii* serogroup 2 | No | 4,800 | 72 | 70 |
| 07/00 | *L. anisa* | Yes | 9,200 | 90 | 85 |

[a] Based on the results obtained by the organizing laboratory.

and heat or acid treatment. Fewer laboratories now fail to isolate from all three specimens than in the earlier years, indicating that they have probably improved their media quality and/or quality control. Occasionally we distribute sterile samples. In general, false positives are not a problem, but there are always one or two laboratories that report false positives and this proportion has not changed much since 1993.

The greatest practical problem with organizing the scheme is the rules governing the

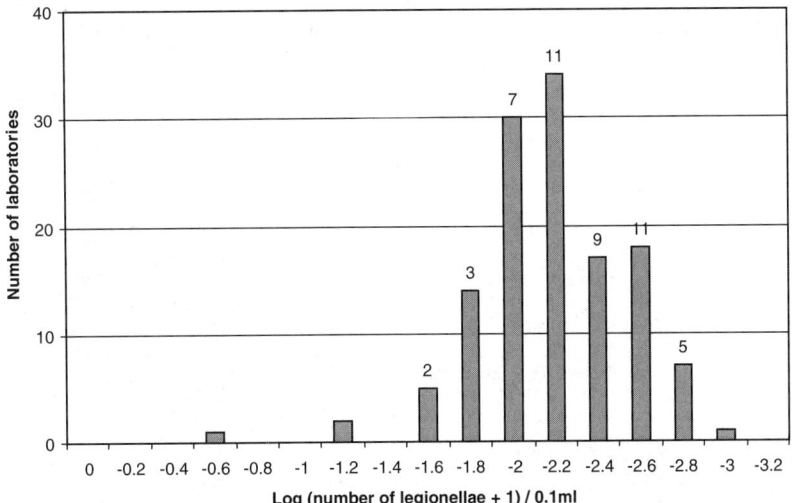

**FIGURE 1** Distribution of counts of *Legionella pneumophila* reported by participants from direct inoculation of sample C from distribution L 29, April 2000. The numbers above each bar are the number of non-United Kingdom laboratories included within the group represented by the bar.

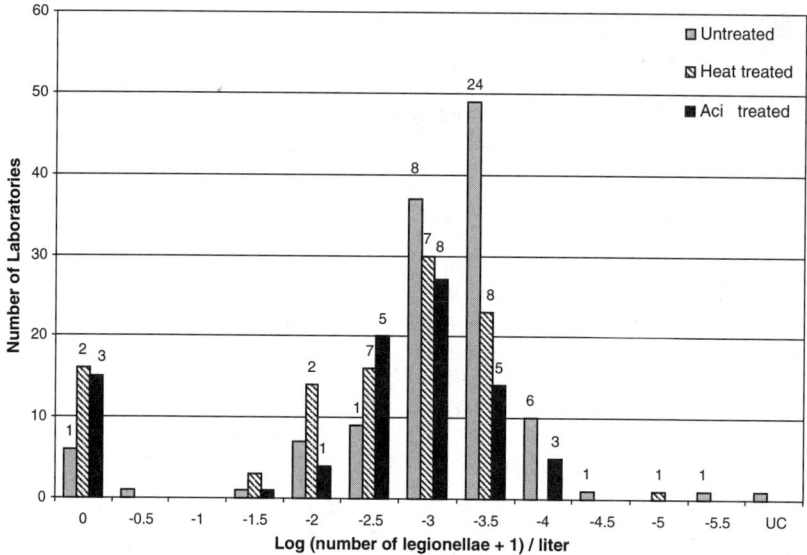

**FIGURE 2** Distribution of counts of *Legionella pneumophila* reported by participants after diluting and processing sample C from distribution L 29, April 2000. The numbers above each bar are the number of non–United Kingdom laboratories included within the group represented by the bar. UC, uncountable.

international transport of pathogens, which make it slow and expensive to transport packages. The materials we have developed are sufficiently stable over 2 or 3 weeks but not stable enough for participants to have true repeat samples. Current research is focused on developing more stable materials.

The beneficial effects of belonging to an EQA scheme have been demonstrated by the gradual improvement in the consistency of the laboratories. This in turn is leading to more reliable quantification, which is important for monitoring the effectiveness of control measures throughout the world.

# PREVALENCE OF *LEGIONELLA* IN WHIRLPOOL SPAS: CORRELATION WITH TOTAL BACTERIAL NUMBERS

*Richard D. Miller and D. Anne Koebel*

# 54

Legionnaires' disease is a bacterial pneumonia caused by *Legionella pneumophila* and related species. The disease is transmitted to humans via aerosols from building water supplies. Depending on the source, the exposure may be through indoor or outdoor routes of transmission, often leading to multiple-case outbreaks of disease. The building water sources with the highest reported risk for transmission are water cooling towers and potable water distribution systems. Heated spas (i.e., whirlpool spas, hot tubs, etc.) have been reported less commonly but still have been associated with at least 14 different outbreaks of legionellosis (1981–1996), involving 335 persons with 6 deaths. More recently, a high-profile outbreak in The Netherlands in 1999 resulted in one of the largest single outbreaks of Legionnaires' disease, with at least 188 cases and 20 deaths.

Few studies have been reported in the literature related to the prevalence of *Legionella* species in heated spas in the absence of disease. In 1983, Witherel et al. (6) examined six recreational whirlpools, isolating *L. pneumophila*

from two with no detectable chlorine, but no *Legionella* species from four whirlpools with chlorine concentrations of at least 2 mg/liter. In a larger study, Groothuis et al. (3) examined 52 whirlpools and isolated *L. pneumophila* from 11 of 28 whirlpools with free available chlorine less than 0.3 mg/liter. In contrast, no *Legionella* species were detected in 23 whirlpools with free available chlorine over 0.3 mg/liter, supporting a conclusion that this concentration of free available chlorine is sufficient to eliminate *Legionella* from whirlpools. Finally, Gonaver et al. (B. C. Gonaver, J. B. Conway, C. R. Peter, J. E. Senne, and M. A. Thompson, *Abstr. 85th Annu. Meet. Am. Soc. Microbiol. 1985*, abstr. N-27, p. 222, 1985) reported at the 1985 Annual Meeting of the American Society for Microbiology that an examination of 50 public spas in San Diego County yielded only one spa with *Legionella* species, even though 60% of the spas failed to meet California state standards for standard plate count, chlorine, or pH.

The purpose of the current study was to determine the prevalence of *Legionella* species in public whirlpool spas (in the absence of disease) by examining a large population of these spas over the past 18 years. Additionally, the presence of *Legionella* was correlated with other microbiological parameters, including

*Richard D. Miller and D. Anne Koebel* Department of Microbiology & Immunology, University of Louisville School of Medicine, Louisville, KY 40292.

the presence of another disease-causing bacterium (*Pseudomonas aeruginosa*) that may be transmitted via whirlpool spas, and the total bacterial numbers as a measure of the overall microbiology and disinfection status of the spas.

## SAMPLE DESCRIPTIONS AND MICROBIOLOGICAL METHODS

### Whirlpool Spa Samples

All samples used in this study were obtained on a volunteer basis from 1983 to 2000 from public whirlpool spas located throughout the United States, the Caribbean, and Mediterranean geographic areas. A total of 458 water samples were collected from 155 different whirlpool spas at 30 hotels and 15 cruise ships. While some spas were sampled only once during this period, most were sampled annually for as long as 10 years. A small, but unknown, percentage of the spas had additional follow-up samples taken during the year to document effectiveness of remediation procedures. One-liter (or 500-ml) samples were collected in clean containers by hotel or cruise ship personnel and shipped unrefrigerated to our laboratory for analysis via overnight (or quickest possible) express delivery. Information on the nature of the disinfection and filtration systems in use for each spa was not available, nor was the level of free available halogen or other chemical parameters of the water at the time of the sampling.

### Isolation and Quantitation of *Legionella* Species

Legionellae were isolated using a modification of the filtration, low-pH treatment, and selective media protocol as described by the Centers for Disease Control and Prevention (2). Briefly, a 500-ml sample from each spa was first filtered through a 47-mm diameter, 0.2-$\mu$m-pore-size Gelman Supor membrane filter (Gelman Sciences Inc., Ann Arbor, Mich.). The filter was then placed in a small plastic jar with 5 ml of sterile distilled water and the bacteria were removed by mild sonic vibration for 10 min in a bath-type sonicator. A 1-ml portion of the filter concentrated material was then acidified to pH 2.2 by the addition of 1 ml of 0.2 M HCl-KCl buffer. After 5 min at room temperature, the sample was neutralized by the addition of 1 ml of KOH. Portions (10:1 and 100:1) from the acid-treated sample and filter-concentrated material were spread-plated onto both buffered charcoal-yeast extract (BCYE) agar and glycine-vancomycin-polymyxin selective agar medium (both BBL Prepared Media, Becton Dickinson and Company, Cockeysville, Md.). In addition, $10^{-1}$, $10^{-2}$, $10^{-3}$, and $10^{-4}$ dilutions of the original sample were also plated on the same two media. All incubations were at 37°C. After 3 to 5 days of incubation, typical *Legionella* colonies were counted, and identification was confirmed by lack of growth on BCYE agar media without L-cysteine, as well as immunofluorescence microscopy using a monoclonal antibody reagent specific for *L. pneumophila* (Genetic Systems Corp., Redmond, Wash.). No serotyping analysis of the isolates was performed. The levels of culturable *Legionella* were expressed as CFU per milliliter of original sample.

### Total Culturable Bacteria and *Pseudomonas aeruginosa* Counts

An estimate of the "total" culturable bacteria was determined by counting all colonies on the $10^{-1}$, $10^{-2}$, $10^{-3}$, and $10^{-4}$ dilutions of the spa samples plated on the BCYE agar. The number of non-*Legionella* colonies obtained on this nonselective medium would be expected to be similar to other standard media (i.e., Trypticase soy agar, R2A, etc.) used for heterotrophic bacterial plate counts. The number of *P. aeruginosa* was determined by plating 10:1 and 100:1 portions of the original sample and the concentrated material on Cetrimide agar (Difco Laboratories, Detroit, Mich.) and incubating at 41°C. All results were expressed as CFU per milliliter of original sample.

## RESULTS

### Prevalence of *Legionella, P. aeruginosa,* and High Total Bacterial Counts

As shown in Table 1, *Legionella* was detected in 27 of 458 spa samples (5.9%). All of the isolates were further identified as the species *L. pneumophila*. The levels of *L. pneumophila* were fairly evenly distributed over a broad range of concentrations from <1/ml to 10,000/ml, with 10 of the spas in the <10/ml range, 6 spas in the 10 to 100/ml range, 7 spas in the 100 to 1,000/ml range, and 4 spas had levels of culturable *L. pneumophila* >1,000/ml. *P. aeruginosa* was also found in 50 (10.9%) of the spas (<1 to 4,000,000/ml range). Overall, 121 (26.4%) of the whirlpool spas had bacterial counts above the level (200 CFU/ml) generally accepted as satisfactory by state and local health authorities in the United States. The remaining 337 spas (73.6%) had acceptable levels of bacteria (<200/ml).

### Relationship between *Legionella, P. aeruginosa,* and Total Bacterial Counts

When the results for the 121 "dirty" spas with high bacterial counts (26.4% of the total spas) were examined in relationship to the presence or absence of *L. pneumophila* and/or *P. aeruginosa* (Table 2), it was clear that more than half (64 spas) were positive for either *Legionella* (14 spas), *P. aeruginosa* (37 spas), or both organisms (13 spas). Overall, almost one quarter (27 spas) of these spas contained *Legionella* (either alone or with *P. aeruginosa*), while 4 of every 10 of the dirty spas (41.3%) had colonization with *P. aeruginosa*. In contrast, none of the 337 spas with acceptable bacterial

**TABLE 1** Prevalence of *Legionella, P. aeruginosa,* and total bacteria in 458 whirlpool spas

| Spa category | No. (%) of spas | Range (bacteria/ml) |
| --- | --- | --- |
| *L. pneumophila* | 27 (5.9) | <1–10,000 |
| *P. aeruginosa* | 50 (10.9) | 1–4,000,000 |
| High bacteria (>200/ml) | 121 (26.4) | 300–20,000,000 |
| Acceptable bacteria | 337 (73.6) | <10–200 |

**TABLE 2** Relationship between *Legionella, P. aeruginosa,* and total bacterial counts in 458 whirlpool spas

| Spa category | No. (%) of spas |
| --- | --- |
| High bacteria only . . . . . . . . . . . . . . . . . | 57 (47.1) |
| High bacteria + *L. pneumophila* . . . . . . | 14 (11.6) |
| High bacteria + *L. pneumophila* + *P. aeruginosa* . . . . . . . . . . . . . . . . . | 13 (10.7) |
| High bacteria + *P. aeruginosa* . . . . . . . . | 37 (30.6) |
| Total spas with high bacteria (>200/ml) . . . . . . . . . . . . . . . . . . . . . | 121 (100) |
| Acceptable bacteria only . . . . . . . . . . . . | 337 (73.6) |
| Acceptable bacteria + *Legionella* . . . . . . . | 0 |
| Acceptable bacteria + *Legionella* + *P. aeruginosa* . . . . . . . . . . . . . . . . . | 0 |
| Acceptable bacteria + *P. aeruginosa* . . . . | 0 |
| Total spas with acceptable bacteria . . . . . | 337 (100) |

counts had any detectable *Legionella* or *P. aeruginosa*.

## DISCUSSION

The major finding from this study was that *Legionella* was relatively uncommon in the whirlpool spas that were examined. In fact, *Legionella* was isolated only from whirlpool spas where the total bacterial counts were unacceptable (i.e., suggesting inadequate disinfection). A similar relationship was found between *P. aeruginosa* and high total bacterial counts. On the basis of these results, it would appear that *Legionella* and *P. aeruginosa* proliferate primarily in spas where the disinfection (i.e., free halogen concentrations) and other maintenance procedures are inadequate to control the total bacterial numbers. While no measurements of free available chlorine or bromine were obtained in the current study, this overall conclusion would support the previous work of Witherel et al. (6) and Groothuis et al. (3), who failed to detect *Legionella* in spas where the chlorine concentrations were adequate.

The observation that approximately 1 of every 4 spas appeared to have inadequate disinfection for controlling the total bacterial counts should be of concern, since the conditions existing in these spas would allow for proliferation of *Legionella* and *P. aeruginosa* in the future. Because of the rapid drop in the free available halogen levels that can occur when spas are being heavily used (as in many public spas), the free halogen levels would need to be checked and adjusted frequently (or via continuous monitoring and automatic adjustment). Related to *Legionella*, the specific water chemistry guidelines for disinfection of whirlpool spas is detailed in the new ASHRAE Guideline 12-2000 entitled *Minimizing the Risk of Legionellosis Associated with Building Water Systems* (1).

This situation is somewhat different from cooling towers, where studies have shown that *Legionella* is ubiquitous (although often at low levels), and the numbers of *Legionella* are *not* correlated with the total bacterial count (4, 5). In fact, high levels (i.e., >1,000/ml) of *L. pneumophila* are often found in cooling towers when the total bacterial count is very low (4, 5). The goal for minimizing the risk of Legionnaires' disease in cooling towers is not total elimination, but rather prevention of *Legionella* growth to high levels. This is generally achieved through the use of effective biocides, often coupled with routine *Legionella* monitoring to measure their effectiveness.

In contrast, the data for whirlpool spas would suggest that the total elimination of *Legionella* is a realistic goal with tight control of free available halogen levels, particularly when combined with daily shock disinfection, regular back-flushing (or replacement) of filters, and monthly draining and scrubbing of the whirlpool surfaces. A routine monitoring of the total bacterial counts would appear to be an adequate assessment of the disinfection effectiveness, although a periodic monitoring for *Legionella* would provide more specific information about the risk for Legionnaires' disease. ASHRAE Guideline 12-2000 recognizes that "regular testing of all spas can provide an important record of safe operating conditions and may alert operators of unsafe conditions when they occur." This guideline establishes threshold values for bacteria as follows (1):

| | |
|---|---|
| Standard plate count (35°C) | 200 CFU/ml (maximum) |
| Total coliforms | 2 organisms per 100 ml (maximum) |
| Fecal coliforms | None allowable |
| *Pseudomonas aeruginosa* | None allowable |
| *Legionella* species | None allowable |

In conclusion, the current data would support a conclusion that Legionnaires' disease is a preventable illness, at least as associated with whirlpool spas. Prevention of disease would be related to tight control of free available halogen levels and other regular maintenance procedures, coupled with bacterial monitoring to assess the effectiveness of these procedures.

## ACKNOWLEDGMENT

The financial assistance of Environmental Safety Technologies, Inc. is gratefully acknowledged.

## REFERENCES

1. **American Society of Heating, Refrigerating and Air-Conditioning Engineers.** 2000. *Guideline 12-2000: Minimizing the Risk of Legionellosis Associated with Building Water Systems.* American Society of Heating, Refrigerating and Air-Conditioning Engineers, Atlanta, Ga.

2. **Barbaree, J. M., B. S. Fields, W. T. Martin, W. E. Morrill, and G. N. Sanden.** 1992. *Procedures for the Recovery of Legionella from the Environment.* Centers for Disease Control, U.S. Department of Health and Human Services, Atlanta, Ga.

3. **Groothuis, D. G., A. H. Havelaar, and H. R. Veenendaal.** 1985. A note on legionellas in whirlpool spas. *J. Appl. Bacteriol.* **58:**479–482.

4. **Miller, R. D., and K. A. Kenepp.** 1993. Risk assessments for Legionnaires disease based on routine surveillance of cooling towers for legionellae, p. 40–43. *In* J. M. Barbaree, R. F. Breiman, and A. P. Dufour (ed.), *Legionella: Current Status and Emerging Perspectives*, American Society for Microbiology, Washington, D.C.

5. **Miller, R. D., and K. A. Kenepp.** 1996. *Legionella* in cooling towers: use of *Legionella*-total bacteria ratios, p. 99–107. *In* M. Muilenberg and H. Burge (ed.), *Aerobiology.* CRC Press, Inc., Boca Raton, Fla.

6. Witherel, L. E., L. A. Orciari, K. C. Spitalny, R. A. Pelletier, W. B. Cherry, L. H. Orrison, L. F. Novick, K. M. Stone, and R. M. Vogt. 1983. Isolation of *Legionella pneumophila* from recreational whirlpool spas. *J. Environ. Health* **46:**77–80.

# PROPOSED METHOD FOR OPTIMUM RECOVERY OF *LEGIONELLA* FROM COOLING WATER IN SOUTH AFRICA

*Pauline Coubrough, Titus Modisenyane, and Bettina Genthe*

# 55

South Africa has characteristics of both the first and third world. The mining, manufacturing, building, energy, and tourist industries compare well with those of technologically developed first-world countries. However, poverty, overcrowding, and squalid conditions affect the majority of inhabitants, creating environmental factors distinctive of a third world country. Furthermore, rates of AIDS and human immunodeficiency virus-positive persons in South Africa are the highest in the world, with the numbers of the immunocompromised residents increasing daily. Therefore, accurate detection, surveillance, and control of *Legionella* in cooling water will impact positively on both human health and economic development.

## AIM

The aims of this chapter are:

- To evaluate the efficacy of international detection methods compared with an in-house-developed method for the optimum recovery of *Legionella* from cooling water.
- To determine the effect of heat and acid pretreatment procedures as well as the use of selective supplement on *Legionella* recovery.
- To investigate possible antibody cross-reactions with nonlegionellae using a polyvalent direct fluorescent antibody conjugate specific for *Legionella* species known to cause most outbreaks of legionellosis worldwide.
- To formulate guidelines to assist industry in the management and control of *Legionella* levels in cooling water.

## MATERIALS AND METHODS

The ISO 11731 (1998) (2) and the Australian Standard 3896 (1991) (3) methods were compared with the most probable number (MPN) detection method developed at the Council for Scientific and Industrial Research (1). The ISO and the Australian Standards incorporate heat and/or acid pretreatment of the water sample prior to inoculation on selective growth medium. The ISO method makes use of buffered charcoal-yeast extract (BCYE) + GVPC as the selective medium while the Australian standard utilizes the BCYE +

*Pauline Coubrough and Titus Modisenyane* Water, Environment and Forestry Technology, Council for Scientific & Industrial Research, P O Box 395, Pretoria, 0001, South Africa. *Bettina Genthe* Water, Environment and Forestry Technology, Council for Scientific & Industrial Research, P O Box 320, Stellenbosch 7599, South Africa.

*Legionella*, Edited by Reinhard Marre et al.
© 2002 ASM Press, Washington, D.C.

MWY and BCYE + BMPA selective supplements. The MPN method excludes acid and heat pretreatment but enriches water concentrates on BCYE without selective supplements.

Preliminary studies using all three methods evaluated recovery rates from sterile tap, source, and cooling water spiked with *Legionella pneumophila*. Subsequent studies determined the effect of pretreatment procedures on environmental cooling water sources only.

To determine whether heat and acid pretreatment had a negative effect on the recovery of *Legionella* or whether the negative effect was solely due to the presence of selective supplements, the MPN method was modified in this study to include pretreatment procedures. The treated and nontreated sample dilutions were, however, enriched on nonselective media and incubated at 35°C ± 1°C for 3 to 5 days. *Legionella*-like colonies were stained with the 12003-Q polyvalent conjugate (Zeus), using antibodies specific for *L. pneumophila* serogroups 1 to 6 and *Legionella micdadei*.

Smears of bacterial species, commonly found in cooling water, were examined for possible antibody cross-reactions with the conjugate.

## RESULTS

The results of the preliminary study showed that in 50 spiked tap, source, and cooling water samples, acid treatment had the most damaging effect on the recovery of *Legionella* from tap water, followed by source water and then cooling water. Heat-treated spiked cooling water gave poor *Legionella* recovery rates, followed by source water and tap water.

The main study focused on the recovery rates of *Legionella* from industrial cooling water sources. Figure 1 shows that in heat- and acid-treated environmental water concentrates, the recovery of *Legionella* was reduced by 3 to 4 logs. Acid treatment also detrimentally affected *Legionella* recovery if enriched on BCYE without selective supplements (MPN). Furthermore, fewer *Legionella* organisms were

recovered from heat-treated concentrates if enriched on BCYE + GVPC (polymyxin, vancomycin, and cycloheximide) (ISO). More *Legionella* organisms were recovered from heat-treated samples enriched on BCYE + GVPC when compared with BCYE + BMPA (cefamandole, polymyxin, and anisomycin) (Fig. 1, HT2). The lowest recovery was achieved if heat-treated samples were enriched on BCYE + MWY (glycine, polymyxin, anisomycin, and vancomycin) (Fig. 1, HT1). *Legionella* recovery was enhanced if nontreated organisms were enriched on BCYE + GVPC.

In this study the polyvalent conjugate did not cross-react with *Pseudomonas, Aeromonas, Citrobacter, Proteus, Escherichia coli, Bacillus, Serratia, Hafnia, Listeria*, and *Enterococcus* species.

## DISCUSSION

If sterile water sources were spiked with *Legionella*, heat treatment destroyed more *Legionella* organisms in water of poor quality (cooling water) while acid treatment had a greater detrimental effect on *Legionella* in water of a good quality (tap water). In the case of environmental cooling water samples, which contain impurities, other bacterial species, and biocides, the recovery of *Legionella* organisms was negatively influenced when water samples were enriched following acid and heat treatment. Acid treatment lowered recovery levels of *Legionella* organisms if plated on BCYE agar without selective supplements. However, heat-treated samples gave lower recoveries if enriched on BCYE containing selective supplements (Fig. 1). Although the results of this trial clearly show that both acid- and heat-treatment procedures had a negative impact on the recovery of *Legionella* from environmental cooling water, it is recommended that further environmental cooling water samples be evaluated to substantiate the results of the limited number of samples studied in this investigation.

The selective supplement, cycloheximide, enhanced the recovery of *Legionella* from un-

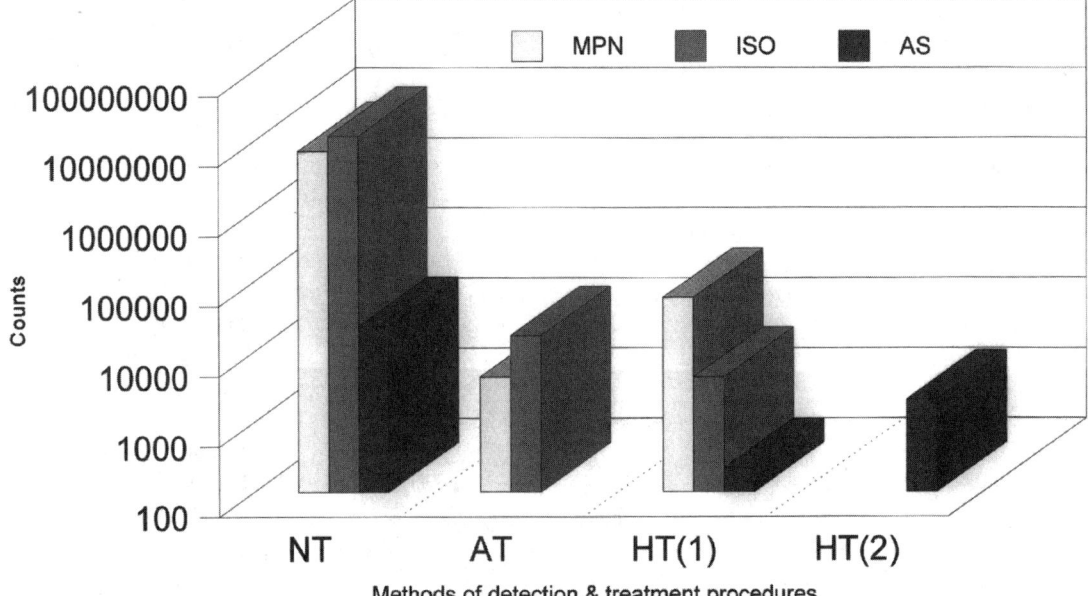

**FIGURE 1** Methods of detection and treatment procedures. Abbreviations: NT, no treatment; AT, acid treatment; HT(1), heat treatment (AS: BCYE + MWY); HT(2), heat treatment (AS: BCYE + BMPA); MPN, most probable number; ISO, international standard; AS, Australian standard.

treated water concentrates by suppressing interfering organisms (Fig. 1).

Considering the scenario where cooling water might contain low numbers of *Legionella* organisms (e.g., $10^3$/liter), utilization of recovery methods that include heat and acid pretreatment, in the light of the above findings, may lead to the recovery of nil to negligible numbers (0 to 10/liter) of *Legionella*. Furthermore, if the relative risk assessment (G. K. Morris and J. C. Feeley, *Abstr. ASHRAE Annu. Meet.*, p. 76, 1990) should be applied to cooling water containing *Legionella* levels in the high-risk category (e.g., $10^6$/liter), the use of heat and acid pretreatment would reduce the level to a category within the low-risk range (e.g., $10^3$/liter). The results would therefore provide a false picture, perceived by industry that the cooling water is well-managed and *Legionella* levels are controlled. By implication, therefore, water managers may decide to refrain from applying normal control programs to maintain low *Legionella* levels.

## CONCLUSIONS

- The MPN method is proposed as the national standard procedure for the detection of *Legionella* from cooling water in South Africa. The advantages include an optimum quantitative result of the most pathogenic species within only 3 to 5 days.
- If the ISO method is used, heat and acid pretreatment procedures need to be omitted.
- To reduce interfering bacterial growth in either the MPN or the ISO method, nontreated water sample concentrates should include a range of 10-fold dilutions with each dilution enriched on BCYE + GVPC.
- In the case of the ISO method, all representative *Legionella* colonies need to be

confirmed using blood agar, BCYE (without cysteine), latex agglutination, and/or direct fluorescent antibodies.

## REFERENCES

1. **Grabow, N. A., R. Kfir, and W. O. K. Grabow.** 1991. A most probable number method on the enumeration of *Legionella* bacteria in water. *Water Sci. Technol.* **24:**143–147.
2. **International Standards Organization.** 1998. *Report: International Standard: Water quality—Detection and Enumeration of Legionella, ISO 11731,* p. 1–16.
3. **Australian Standard.** 1991. *Report: Australian Standard: Water—Examination for Legionellae, AS 3896.*

# *LEGIONELLA* DETECTION FROM SOUTH AFRICAN COOLING WATER SYSTEMS

*Catheleen Bartie, Fanus Venter, and Louis Nel*

# 56

Large numbers of legionellae in water distribution systems present a potentially serious health risk to workers and the general public. Since the first Legionnaires' disease outbreak in 1976, numerous outbreaks have been documented and continue to occur. For example, at least three major outbreaks have been reported during the year 2000 (http://www.iol.co.za/html/frame_news.php?art_id.=qw978183300279B243; J. W. Den Boer, E. P. F. Yzerman, J. Schellekens, K. D. Lettinga, H. Boshuizen, J. Van Steenbergen, A. Bosman, S. Van der Hof, H. Van Vliet, M. F. Peeters, R. J. Van Ketel, P. Speelman, J. Kool, and M. A. Conyn-Van Spaendock, presented at the 5th Int. Conf. Legionella, Ulm, Germany, 2000; G. Tallis, J. Greig, B. Zwolak, J. Carnie, W. Hart, A. Tan, and N. Ryan, presented at the 5th Int. Conf. Legionella, Ulm, Germany, 2000), together resulting in at least 250 cases. In addition, sporadic infections are diagnosed with increasing frequency, clearly illustrating the importance of appropriate methods for *Legionella* detection.

Despite numerous new developments, culturing remains the "gold standard" for the detection of *Legionella* from environmental sources. To improve the recovery of *Legionella* by culturing, a variety of supplements and selective agents are added to culture media and are used in different combinations as preferred by different laboratories. In addition, certain treatment steps have been introduced to minimize contamination by non-legionellae during culturing procedures (2, 4, 6, 7, 9, 10, 12). However, despite these developments, no single culture method or medium has so far proven to be ideal for all sample types and environments.

Culture methods have been standardized in the United States, Britain, and Australia but such standards have not been set for South Africa. Local laboratories have thus been testing water samples using a number of methods, using a nonstandardized approach. This resulted in contradictory results regarding water quality in South Africa and a lack of confidence in local water testing, specifically for the presence of *Legionella*. Consequently, a Legionella Action Group was formed in 1995 to address this and other issues regarding *Legionella* in South Africa. The study reported here was undertaken as part of this initiative, to provide South African laboratories and in-

*Catheleen Bartie* Immunology/Microbiology Section, National Centre for Occupational Health, Johannesburg 2000 South Africa. *Fanus Venter and Louis Nel* Microbiology Department, Faculty of Biological and Agricultural Sciences, University of Pretoria, Pretoria 0002 South Africa.

*Legionella*, Edited by Reinhard Marre et al.
© 2002 ASM Press, Washington, D.C.

dustries with guidelines for the most appropriate culturing method for our environment, and with information on the prevalence of *Legionella* in our industrial waters.

Two of the internationally accepted culture methods and a locally developed adaptation of the most probable number (MPN) method, used by some laboratories in South Africa, were evaluated. The International Standard (ISO) method (5) is widely accepted as a standard and is used by some laboratories in South Africa. It is used to demonstrate the presence of confirmed legionellae in a wide range of environmental samples. The test involves sample concentration by either centrifugation or membrane filtration followed by resuspension of the concentrated organisms by vortex or sonication. The concentrates are subsequently treated with heat and acid prior to culturing on buffered charcoal-yeast extract (BCYE) agar as a nonselective medium and GVPC agar (BCYE agar supplemented with cycloheximide, glycine, polymyxin B, and vancomycin) as a selective medium. Cysteine-dependent single colonies are regarded as presumptive legionellae and confirmed by a number of methods including immunofluorescence and latex agglutination. The Australian Standard (AS) method (1) involves sample concentration and resuspension as above. The concentrates are inoculated onto BCYE agar as a nonselective medium, and onto MWY agar (BCYE agar supplemented with anisomycin, glycine, polymyxin B, vancomycin, bromocresol purple, and bromothymol blue) and BMPA agar (BCYE agar supplemented with anisomycin, cefamandole, and polymyxin B) as selective media, either as nontreated or as heat-treated portions. Acid treatment is recommended only for highly contaminated samples. Cysteine-dependent single colonies are confirmed as outlined above.

The quantitative MPN method has been adapted for enumeration of *Legionella* in water samples by South African workers (3). The method involves sample concentration by membrane filtration through 0.45-$\mu$m-pore-size cellulose filters followed by inoculation of serial dilutions of the concentrate in triplicate, using BCYE agar only. No selective media or sample pretreatment methods are incorporated into this method. After an incubation period of 3 to 7 days, representative smears of growth are stained by direct immunofluorescence (DFA) for confirmation. Cultures are recorded as positive when they contain morphologically typical *Legionella* colonies and yield a positive DFA test. MPN statistical tables are then used to calculate the number of *Legionella*-like organisms in the original sample. No further confirmatory tests are carried out.

The experimental work of this project was carried out in two stages, first by using water samples seeded with a type strain of *Legionella pneumophila* and second by using samples collected from water distribution systems. For stage one of the project, sterile and nonsterile tap water, cooling water, and makeup water samples were seeded with a type strain of *L. pneumophila* serogroup 1 (ATCC 33152). For stage two, 28 water and biofilm samples from four industries (a power station, a plastics manufacturer, a petrochemical company, and a gold mine) were tested for the presence of legionellae. These consisted of 13 cooling waters from three sources, 3 biofilms from two sources, and 12 waters from the gold mine (4 from underground processes and 8 from surface processes).

The samples were concentrated by membrane filtration through 0.45-$\mu$m-pore-size cellulose filters (these membranes are currently used by all of the laboratories in South Africa). After concentration, the membranes were aseptically removed, cut into smaller pieces, and placed into sterile containers with 10 ml of sterile distilled water for the seeded samples and 10 ml of water from the original sample for the industrial samples. These were sonicated for 10 min to dislodge the bacteria from the membranes. Using standard procedures, the sample concentrates were treated with acid (2) and/or heat (4) as indicated in the methods evaluated. Serial 10-fold dilutions were made in sterile distilled water, inoculated onto the agar media as indicated in each of the methods (reference all three), and incubated in air at 37°C. Although the screening of sample concentrates by DFA prior to culturing is not an accurate or generally accepted method for testing water for legionellae, or required by any of the methods evaluated, this step was included for the purpose of this study to indicate the possible presence of viable but nonculturable legionellae. The sample concentrates were also screened for the presence of amoebae using the method described by Page (1976) (8) prior to culturing.

Single colonies with the typical groundglass appearance of legionellae were tested for cysteine dependence by inoculating BCYE agar and nutrient agar and incubating these until growth was observed on the BCYE agar, as indicated in the ISO and AS methods. Colonies growing on BCYE agar but not on nutrient agar were regarded as cysteine-dependent and reported as presumptive legionellae. Cysteine-dependent single colonies were subsequently confirmed by DFA and/or by latex agglutination. The only DFA reagent available in South Africa is specific for *L. pneumophila* serogroups 1 to 6 and *Legionella micdadei*. The agglutination test was done using a commercially available test kit (Oxoid DR800M). The reagents supplied with the kit are specific for *L. pneumophila* serogroup 1, *L. pneumophila* serogroups 2 to 14, and *Legionella* species (including *L. longbeacheae* serogroups 1 and 2, *L. bozemanii* serogroups 1 and 2, *L. dumoffii*, *L. gormanii*, *L. jordanis*, *L. micdadei*, and *L. anisa*).

Sample concentrates that were negative by culturing, or where the presence of legionellae could not be confirmed during the first culture experiment but contained amoebae, were reincubated as described by Sanden and colleagues in 1992 (11): The concentrates were stored at 4 to 6°C until the results from the first experiment were available. After repeating the sonication step to remove aggregates that may have formed on the filter membranes during storage, the liquid was poured off into sterile, screw-capped glass containers and incubated at 37°C for 10 days. The process of

pretreatment and serial 10-fold dilution was repeated as for the first experiment. In this experiment, BCYE and GVPC agar were inoculated to represent nonselective and selective media, respectively.

For optimal recovery of legionellae from the environment, water samples have to be concentrated before culturing. Although both membrane filtration and centrifugation are widely accepted and used for this purpose, there is no consensus among workers regarding the efficiency and accuracy of either of these methods. For filtration to be effective, several factors have to be taken into account when choosing the type of filter and the pore size to use. The Centers for Disease Control and Prevention (Atlanta, Ga.) recommends the use of polycarbonate filters with a pore size of 0.2 $\mu$m, but we found it difficult to concentrate our cooling and makeup water samples through membranes with such a small pore size. We did not investigate the efficiency of different filter types and used the cellulose filters with a pore size of 0.45 $\mu$m that are commercially available and generally used for sample concentration of industrial waters in South Africa.

The data summarized in Table 1 represent a comparison of the results obtained from sterile and nonsterile seeded samples, cultured on each of the four agar media (BCYE, GVPC, BMPA, and MWY) in the absence of sample pretreatment, after acid treatment, and after heat treatment. In the absence of sample pretreatment, the recovery of confirmed *L. pneumophila* from the sterile seeded samples was high on the nonselective BCYE plates (85.9, 98.7, and 89.7% for tap, cooling, and makeup water, respectively). The use of selective media resulted in a considerable decrease in organism recovery, depending on the culture medium used. Acid treatment resulted in a further loss of organisms from the sterile samples, especially after culturing on selective agar media. The number of organisms recovered after heat treatment was negligible in all the sterile samples evaluated, regardless of the agar medium used. These results were not surpris-

**TABLE 1** Recovery of *L. pneumophila* from seeded samples: comparison of culture media and pretreatment methods[a]

| Sample | Treatment | Recovery (%) on the following culture media: | | | |
|---|---|---|---|---|---|
| | | BCYE | GVPC | BMPA | MWY |
| Sterile | | | | | |
| Tap water | N | 85.9 | 4.9 | 48.7 | — |
| | A | 76.9 | 1.4 | 44.9 | 20.0 |
| | H | <1 | <1 | <1 | <1 |
| Cooling water | N | 98.7 | 6.7 | 18.2 | 42.3 |
| | A | 8.5 | <1 | 2.3 | <1 |
| | H | <1 | <1 | <1 | — |
| Makeup water | N | 89.7 | 3.1 | 6.8 | 57.8 |
| | A | 35.9 | 1.5 | 28.2 | — |
| | H | <1 | <1 | <1 | <1 |
| Nonsterile | | | | | |
| Tap water | N | 8.1 | <1 | 4.5 | 10.1 |
| | A | <1 | <1 | <1 | <1 |
| | H | <1 | <1 | <1 | <1 |
| Cooling water | N | 38.5 | <1 | 2.6 | 1.5 |
| | A | <1 | <1 | <1 | <1 |
| | H | 12.8 | <1 | <1 | 2.6 |
| Makeup water | N | 23.1 | <1 | 14.4 | 20.5 |
| | A | 12.8 | <1 | <1 | <1 |
| | H | 9.9 | 2.2 | 4.6 | 1.2 |

[a] N, no pretreatment; A, acid treatment; H, heat treatment; —, not done.

ing given the fact that laboratory-adapted strains of *Legionella* are known to be more sensitive to adverse conditions (such as sample pretreatment) than environmental strains. The recovery rate of confirmed legionellae from the nonsterile seeded samples was considerably lower than that of the sterile samples (Table 1). In the absence of pretreatment, culturing on BCYE yielded confirmed *L. pneumophila* in only 8.1% of the tap water samples, 23.1% of the makeup water samples, and 38.5% of the cooling water samples. Pretreatment resulted in a further loss of approximately 50% of organisms in all the samples, regardless of the pretreatment method or culture medium used. The confirmation of single colonies was complicated by the presence of nonlegionellae on all the culture media.

When these results were interpreted in accordance with the ISO and AS specifications and compared with the MPN method, the following observations were made. Whereas the ISO and AS methods both provide a

means of confirming legionellae to species level, this is not possible using the MPN method. In general, the ISO and AS methods were more useful than the MPN for organism recovery from the sterile seeded samples (for example, 99.5% vs. 26.9% in the sterile cooling water samples). This may have been due to the increased specificity of the ISO and AS methods, which made it possible to perform colony counts of confirmed legionellae, a step that is excluded from the MPN method. However, for the nonsterile seeded samples the MPN method consistently yielded a higher recovery of legionellae because it does not require the confirmation of single colonies. In all the samples (sterile as well as nonsterile), the sample pretreatment steps required by the ISO and AS methods decreased the recovery of organisms significantly.

Culturing results were recorded as follows: For the ISO and AS methods, the highest dilution yielding single colonies confirmed as *Legionella* species by either DFA or agglutination or both, were recorded. For the MPN method, DFA results of representative smears for each dilution were recorded (representing presumptive legionellae). The highest dilution yielding a positive DFA test on at least one of the plates was recorded. No additional confirmation tests were carried out.

Of the 28 industrial water samples evaluated for the presence of legionellae, 26 (92.9%) were positive for *L. pneumophila* serogroups 1 to 6 and *L. micdadei* by DFA prior to culturing. Of the DFA-positive organisms, 18 (69.2%) could be confirmed with at least one of the culturing methods. Amoebae were present in 14 (87.5%) of the industrial waters and in 3 (25.0%) of the mine waters. Legionellae could be confirmed in one sample that did not contain amoebae. Small numbers of legionellae ($10^{-1}$ CFU/ml) were cultured from the two concentrates that were negative by DFA but contained amoebae.

As expected, BCYE agar was the most sensitive of the culture media evaluated, but confirmation in the absence of sample pretreatment was complicated by overgrowth of the agar plates and difficulties in distinguishing legionellae from non-legonellae (Table 2). In only 17.9% of the samples could legionellae be confirmed from this medium in the absence of sample pretreatment. A further 54.0% of BCYE plates yielded presumptive legionellae after representative smears from the plates were stained by DFA. However, these organisms could not be confirmed by cysteine dependence of latex agglutination. In the majority of cases, the only means of visualizing presumptive legionellae on this medium was by staining a representative smear of growth by DFA.

The use of selective media (GVPC, BMPA, and MWY) improved the confirmation rate of legionellae considerably (Table 2). However, the numbers recovered on these media were mostly one or two orders of magnitude lower than on BCYE agar. Although there was no statistically significant difference in the confirmation rate from GVPC, BMPA, and MWY agar (32.2, 28.6, and 25.0%, respec-

tively) in the absence of sample pretreatment, the differentiation of legionellae from non-legionellae on the basis of colony morphology was more difficult on BMPA agar than on the other two media.

The effect of sample pretreatment with acid and heat was investigated. To determine the effect of sample pretreatment on the recovery rates, all of the samples were subjected to both treatment methods. When compared with acid treatment or no treatment at all, heat treatment was shown to yield the highest number of confirmed positive samples in all cases (Table 2). Generally, the presumptive positive numbers were comparatively lower, but the percentage confirmation of these presumptive isolates was consistently high (average, 75.0%). In comparison, agar plates were also easier to read due to the lower number of viable and culturable organisms in the samples after heat treatment. Compared with no treatment, acid treatment usually allowed less growth on all media, but with higher confirmation rates of the cultured organisms. However, the total number of confirmed *Legionella* isolates was similar (Table 2).

The comparison of the three methods with regard to their relative ability to detect legionellae from the sample types and industries we evaluated indicated considerable differences in the results we obtained (Table 3). In general, the sensitivity of the ISO, AS, and MPN methods were similar (Table 2). However, in 66.7% of the samples collected from the underground processes of the mine, legionellae were detected only by using the ISO method. All of the presumptive legionellae and three samples that were negative when using the MPN method could be identified to species level using the ISO method. The AS method was not useful for any of the samples but the sensitivity of the test improved considerably and the results compared favorably with the MPN and ISO methods when appropriate sample dilutions were made (designated ASM method).

The prevalence of legionellae in samples from a plastics manufacturer, a power station,

**TABLE 2** Comparison of culture media and pretreatment methods for *Legionella* detection from environmental samples

| Culture medium | Result[a] | Recovery (%) after following pretreatment method: | | |
|---|---|---|---|---|
| | | None | Acid | Heat |
| BCYE | Presumptive | 71.4 | 64.3 | 53.6 |
| | Confirmed | 17.9 | 25.0 | 32.2 |
| | Pure growth | 0. | 9.2 | 0 |
| BMPA | Presumptive | 67.9 | 35.7 | 35.7 |
| | Confirmed | 25.0 | 17.9 | 25.0 |
| | Pure growth | 0 | 0 | 0 |
| GVPC | Presumptive | 64.3 | 57.1 | 53.6 |
| | Confirmed | 32.2 | 35.7 | 42.9 |
| | Pure growth | 0 | 0 | 22.3 |
| MWY | Presumptive | 53.6 | 57.1 | 39.3 |
| | Confirmed | 28.6 | 46.4 | 35.7 |
| | Pure growth | 0 | 0 | 23.6 |

[a] Total positive, percentage positive samples (presumptive and confirmed); Confirmed, percentage of total positive samples that were confirmed by either DFA or latex agglutination; Pure growth, percentage of confirmed positive samples that yielded pure cultures.

a petrochemical company, and a gold mine was investigated. A comparison of the culture methods, evaluated with regard to their relative ability to detect legionellae in the samples evaluated, is shown in Table 3. Legionellae were cultured from an average of 82% of the samples tested (range, 0 to 100%, depending on the detection method used). Of these, 93% were positive with at least one of the methods and 21% with all the methods (not shown). In 54% of the samples, legionellae were present in numbers equal to or greater than $10^{-3}$

CFU/ml. The majority of positive samples contained *L. pneumophila* serogroup 1 and serogroups 2 to 14, often in combination. Only one sample contained legionellae other than *L. pneumophila*, as confirmed by latex agglutination, but this organism was not identified to species level.

The effect of reincubating *Legionella* presumptive but unconfirmed samples that contained amoebae was investigated. Our results indicated that 50% of these samples yielded confirmed legionellae after 10 days of incu-

**TABLE 3** Comparison of *Legionella* prevalence by different culturing methods

| Source | n | Positive samples (%)[a] | | | |
|---|---|---|---|---|---|
| | | MPN | ISO | AS | ASM |
| Industrial water and biofilm | | | | | |
| Plastics manufacturer | 5 | 100 | 100 | 60 | 100 |
| Power station | 6 | 83 | 100 | 50 | 100 |
| Petrochemical company | 5 | 60 | 40 | 20 | 40 |
| Average | 16 | 81 | 80 | 43 | 80 |
| Mine water | | | | | |
| Underground | 4 | 25 | 100 | 0 | 0 |
| Surface | 8 | 75 | 88 | 38 | 63 |
| Average | 12 | 50 | 94 | 19 | 32 |
| Average of all samples | 28 | 69 | 86 | 34 | 61 |

[a] MPN, most probable number method; ISO, international standard method; AS, Australian standard method; ASM, Australian standard method with modifications (incorporating sample dilutions up to $10^{-5}$).

bating sample concentrates and replating onto BCYE agar. This confirmed previous findings by Sanden and colleagues (11), who reported that incubation of environmental samples with autochthonous amoebae markedly improved the sensitivity of culture techniques for legionellae. This experiment also confirmed that nonculturable legionellae remain viable and may in fact increase in numbers, to culturable levels, during periods of nutrient starvation, when they are found intracellularly within amoebae and protozoa.

In conclusion, the results from this study provided us with useful information regarding the prevalence of legionellae in South African industrial water distribution systems. It was the first step toward the development of a standard detection method specific to South African conditions and the sample types evaluated. We propose a selective approach for complex (nonpotable) samples and prefer the use of heat treatment followed by culturing on BCYE as a nonselective agar medium and MWY as a selective agar medium. To improve the sensitivity of culturing, the combination of this method with culturing on the same media in the absence of sample pretreatment (the MPN approach) is suggested. Reincubation of sample concentrates with autochthonous amoebae may improve the sensitivity further and may allow detection of viable but nonculturable legionellae or legionella-like amoebal pathogens (LLAPs), a group of organisms not previously studied in our country.

## REFERENCES

1. **Australian Standard.** 1991. *Waters–Examination for Legionellae.* AS 3896–1991.
2. **Bopp, C. A., J. W. Sumner, G. K. Morris, and J. G. Wells.** 1981. Isolation of Legionella spp. from environmental water samples by low-pH treatment and use of a selective medium. *J. Clin. Microbiol.* **13:**714–719.
3. **Grabow, N. A., R. Kfir, and W. O. K. Grabow.** 1991. A most probable number method for the enumeration of Legionella bacteria in water. *Water Sci. Tech.* **24:**143–147.
4. **Groothuis, D. G., and H. R. Veenendal.** 1983. Heat treatment as an aid for the isolation of *Legionella pneumophila* from clinical and environmental samples. *Zentralbl. Bakteriol. Mikrobiol. Hyg. [A]* **255:**39–43.
5. **International Organization for Standardization.** 1996. *Water Quality–Detection and Enumeration of Legionella.* International Standard ISO/DIS 11731. *International Organization for Standardization.*
6. **Jousimes-Somer, H. R., S. Waarala, and M. L. Väisänen.** 1993. Recovery of Legionella species from water samples by four different methods, p. 200–201. *In* J. M. Barbaree, R. F. Breiman, and A. P. Dufour (ed.), *Legionella: Current Status and Emerging Perspectives.* American Society for Microbiology, Washington, D.C.
7. **Kusnetsov, J. M., H. R. Jousimies-Somer, A. I. Nevalainen, and P. J. Martikainen.** 1994. Isolation of Legionella from water samples using various culture methods. *J. Appl. Bacteriol.* **76:**155–162.
8. **Page, F. C.** 1976. *An Illustrated Key to Freshwater and Soil Amoebae with Notes on Cultivation and Ecology. Scientific Publication no. 34.* Freshwater Biological Association, Cambridge, United Kingdom.
9. **Reinthaler, F. F., J. Sattler, K. Schaffler-Dulling, B. Weinmayr, and E. Marth.** 1993. Comparative study of procedures for isolation and cultivation of *Legionella pneumophila* from tap water in hospitals. *J. Clin. Microbiol.* **31:**1213–1216.
10. **Roberts, K. P., C. M. August, and J. D. Nelson, Jr.** 1987. Relative sensitivities of environmental legionellae to selective isolation procedures. *Appl. Environ. Microbiol.* **53:**2704–2707.
11. **Sanden, G. N., W. E. Morrill, B. S. Fields, R. F. Breiman, and J. M. Barbaree.** 1992. Incubation of water samples containing amoebae improves detection of legionellae by the culture method. *Appl. Environ. Microbiol.* **58:**2001–2004.
12. **Wilkinson, I. J., N. Sangster, R. M. Ratcliff, P. A. Mugg, D. E. Davos, and J. A. Lanser.** 1990. Problems associated with identification of Legionella species from the environment and isolation of six possible new species. *Appl. Environ. Microbiol.* **56:**796–802.

# COOLING TOWERS AND LEGIONELLOSIS: A LARGE URBAN AREA EXPERIENCE

S. Dubrou, L. Guillotin, S. Cabon, B. Van Gastel,
O. Challemel, D. Carlier, C. Lawrence, B. Decludt,
J. Etienne, and F. Squinazi

# 57

Since the first recognized outbreak of Legionnaires' disease occurred in 1976, numerous epidemics have been traced to cooling towers and evaporative condensers in Anglo-Saxon countries (3, 4). In France, the risk of legionellosis associated with cooling systems had been underestimated for a long time because until 1998, no community outbreak had been related to these devices. The health risk was not taken into account and no risk assessment was developed to manage the cooling systems. However, recommendations for prevention of legionellosis were provided in governmental guidelines published in 1997. The maintenance of cooling towers and control of *Legionella* were not mandated by law. Only compressors associated with cooling systems were submitted for regulation as detrimental devices for the environment. They are surveyed by the Technical Service of Paris Police Authority (STIIIC), which is in charge of the industrial pollution prevention and control in the Paris area and enforces the national environmental protection regulation. In 2000, 300 facilities with 600 to 900 cooling towers located in Paris (105 km$^2$) were known by STIIIC.

We are describing a Parisian experience, including two outbreaks, which should lead companies to improve the health aspects of managing cooling towers. To inform facilities managers of the *Legionella* risk linked to cooling devices, investigations were conducted by the Hygiene Laboratory of Paris in 70 facilities located in the Paris area from 1995 until 1999. They were serving air-conditioning systems of office buildings (65%), industrial installations (25%), or hospitals and hotels (10%). A total of 70 water specimens were collected from the basin in 68 cooling towers and two evaporative condensers that were all in operation. Sixty-six percent of the devices were sampled from May to October.

## LABORATORY INVESTIGATION

*Legionella* and *Legionella pneumophila* were determined in accordance with the French standard procedure XP T 90-431 (1). Briefly, the method consists of filtration of a 1-liter sam-

*S. Dubrou, O. Challemel, D. Carlier, C. Lawrence, and F. Squinazi* Hygiene Laboratory of Paris, 75013 Paris, France. *L. Guillotin and B. Van Gastel* District Health Service of Paris, 75017 Paris, France. *S. Cabon* Technical Service of Paris Police Authority, 75004 Paris, France. *B. Decludt* National Institute for Public Health Surveillance Health Survey, 94415 Saint-Maurice, France. *J. Etienne* National Reference Centre for *Legionella*, Faculté de Médecine R. Laennec, 69372 Lyon Cedex 08, France.

*Legionella*, Edited by Reinhard Marre et al.
© 2002 ASM Press, Washington, D.C.

ple through a 0.4-$\mu$m-pore-size polycarbonate membrane, decontamination by heat or acid, inoculation onto a GVPC medium, and incubation at 37°C for 10 days. A combined heat and acid decontamination procedure was added to eliminate competing bacteria, often heavily present in such samples (7). The detection level was $10^2$ CFU/liter.

## OCCURRENCE OF *LEGIONELLA* IN COOLING SYSTEMS IN THE PARIS AREA

Among the 70 devices, legionellae were detected with counts between $10^2$ and $>10^5$ CFU/liter in 75% of the samples (Fig. 1); 25% of the samples gave levels of legionellae $\geq 10^5$ CFU/liter. *L. pneumophila* was identified in all positive samples except two. The mean water temperatures were found to be 24°C in both positive (16 to 36°C) and negative specimens (18 to 31°C). Water treatment consisted of preventing scale, corrosion, and biofouling to maintain efficient thermal performance. Unfortunately it was not properly planned and controlled in most of the facilities. The water characteristics were not recovered or available, so the correlation between the presence of *Legionella* and maintenance was not possible. The location and accessibility of the devices were often critical points. Information concerning the risk of disease was insufficient.

## A FIRST OUTBREAK IN 1998

In June 1998, 20 *Legionella* cases were identified in people who had been in Paris. Eleven were French citizens and nine were European tourists. They were 29 to 77 years old and 19 were male. They had all become ill between 6 June and 14 July and four patients died (20%). The infection was diagnosed either by isolation of *Legionella pneumophila* serogroup 1 (6 cases), urinary antigen detection (11 cases), or serology (3 cases). A case control study found no common residential exposure but showed an increased level of risk associated with a delimited area (Fig. 2). The identification of the cooling towers located in this area was difficult. Fortunately the compressors of some devices were registered by STIIIC. In the suspected area, 39 facilities were identified and submitted to a questionnaire related to management. Seven facilities were selected from the cooling towers that started up in May or presented high *Legionella* counts or were located near streets where three elderly patients lived and used to walk. The environmental investigation conducted from 29 July to 5 August showed that six of seven facilities had cooling towers positive for *Legionella* and five were positive for *L. pneumophila* (Table 1).

The six patients' isolates presented an indistinguishable pulsed-field gel electrophoresis (PFGE) profile (8) that matched strains isolated from water in cooling tower 1 at high count. This profile is different from the profile of the "Paris" strain, frequently isolated in the Paris area (5). The epidemiological and microbiological studies suggest that one of the cooling towers located in the delimited area was the likely source of the outbreak (2).

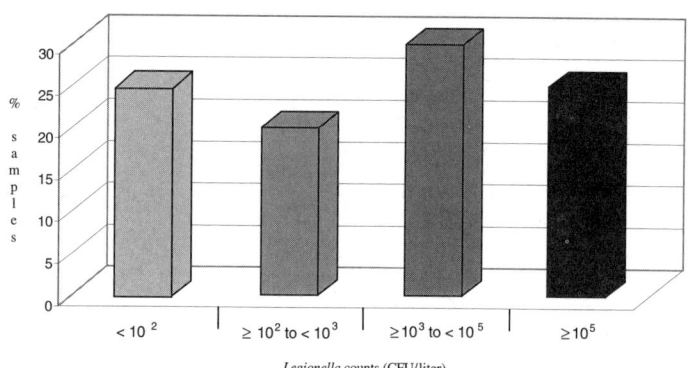

**FIGURE 1** Distribution of *Legionella* counts in cooling systems.

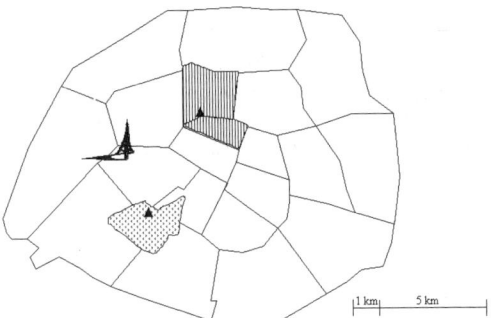

**FIGURE 2** Areas associated with two outbreaks of Legionnaires' disease linked to cooling towers in Paris. First outbreak in June 1998 ▥, 20 cases, 39 facilities with cooling systems, 3.2 km²; ▲, incriminated cooling tower. Second outbreak in August 1999 ▦, 8 cases, 20 facilities with cooling systems, 1.5 km²; ▲, incriminated cooling tower.

## A SECOND OUTBREAK IN 1999

In August 1999, a second outbreak was reported in another district of Paris. Among the eight cases, seven lived or worked in the area and one was a European tourist. They were 42 to 78 years old and seven were male. A 42-year-old worker died. The disease was diagnosed by urinary antigen detection (six cases) and isolation of *L. pneumophila* serogroup 1 (two cases). The interview of the patients showed an outdoor exposure in a living, walking, or working area corresponding to a surface of 1.5 km² (Fig. 2). The intervention was quickly defined by the District Health Service of Paris since the list of cooling systems located in the delimited area was immediately availa-

ble from STIIIC. Among 20 facilities, 6 were selected and the cooling towers were sampled for *Legionella* from 8 to 13 September. Three of six devices were contaminated with *L. pneumophila* and two were positive for *L. pneumophila* serogroup 1 (Table 1).

The two patient isolates had indistinguishable fingerprints using pulsed-field gel electrophoresis and arbitrarily primed PCR (6) to strains isolated from water of cooling tower C. The profiles obtained with both methods were different from those of the "Paris" strain and the epidemic strain of 1998. In this case, the legionellae level was found to be moderate at the sampling period. Again the epidemiological and microbiological data suggest an exposure to one cooling tower located in an urban area.

## PRACTICAL CONSEQUENCES

A working group was managed by the District Health Service of Paris in 1999 to produce technical prescriptions for the control and prevention of *Legionella* in cooling towers. A regulation was published under the supervision of the Ministry of Environment to be applied in France.

The requirements concern:

- Location: The new systems should be sited away from ventilation air intakes and open windows.
- Maintenance: The entire system has to be kept clean during the period of use and should be drained, cleaned, and disinfected

**TABLE 1** *Legionella* recovered from cooling towers examined during two outbreaks in Paris[a]

| First outbreak in 1998 | | Second outbreak in 1999 | |
|---|---|---|---|
| Cooling tower | *Legionella* culture (CFU/liter) | Cooling tower | *Legionella* culture (CFU/liter) |
| 1 | $10^6$/Lp1 | A | $3 \times 10^6$/Lp ≠ 1 |
| 2 | $5 \times 10^4$/Lp1 | B | $10^6$/Lp1 |
| 3 | $3 \times 10^4$/Lp1 | C | $5 \times 10^4$/Lp1 |
| 4 | $5 \times 10^5$/*Legionella* sp. | E | $3 \times 10^2$/*Legionella* sp. |
| 5 | $3 \times 10^2$/Lp ≠ 1 | F | $<10^2$ |
| 6 | $6 \times 10^2$/Lp ≠ 1 | G | $<10^2$ |
| 7 | $<10^2$ | | |

[a]Lp1, *L. pneumophila* serogroup 1; Lp ≠ 1, *L. pneumophila* non-serogroup 1.

before being started up, at least once a year. The disinfectants have to be effective against *Legionella*.

- Water treatment: The water treatment has to be defined by an experienced and competent company.
- Records: Records include descriptions of the system, identification of those responsible, dates of maintenance and disinfection procedures, and results of water quality including legionellae counts.

STIIIC may assess and control the effectiveness of the maintenance and treatment programs. There is no scientific evidence for a maximal acceptable safety concentration of legionellae in cooling towers. However, a review of the literature concerning legionellosis associated with cooling towers (9), the occurrence of legionellae in Parisian cooling towers, and the high counts obtained in the outbreak of 1998 suggest the need to implement the following corrective measures:

- $\geq 10^3$ to $<10^5$ CFU/liter: apply procedures to reduce the level to under $10^3$ CFU/liter.
- $\geq 10^5$ CFU/liter: shut off, clean, and disinfect.

## REFERENCES

1. **Anonymous.** 1993. Norme XP T 90-431. Essais des eaux. Recherche et dénombrement des *Legionella* et *Legionella pneumophila*. Méthode générale par ensemencement direct et filtration sur membrane. Association Française de Normalisation, Paris, France.
2. **Decludt, B., L. Guillotin, B. Van Gastel, S. Dubrou, S. Jarraud, A. Perrocheau, D. Carlier, M. Reyrolle, L. Capek, M. Ledrans, and J. Etienne.** 1999. Epidemic cluster of Legionnaires' disease Paris, June 1998. *Eurosurveillance* **4:** 115–118.
3. **Fiore, A. E., J. P. Nuorti, O. S. Levine, A. Marx, A. C. Weltman, S. Yeager, R. F. Benson, J. Pruckler, P. H. Edelstein, P. Greer, S. R. Zaki, B. S. Fields, and J. C. Butler.** 1998. Epidemic legionnaires' disease two decades later: old sources, new diagnostic methods. *Clin. Infect. Dis.* **26:**426–433.
4. **Keller, D. W., R. Hajjeh, A. DeMaria, Jr., B. S. Fields, J. M. Pruckler., R. S. Benson, P. A. Kludt, S. M. Lett, L. A. Mermel, C. Giorgio, and R. F. Breiman.** 1996. Community outbreak of legionnaires' disease: an investigation confirming the potential for cooling towers to transmit *Legionella* species. *Clin. Infect. Dis.* **22:** 257–261.
5. **Lawrence, C., M. Reyrolle, S. Dubrou, F. Forey, B. Decludt, C. Goulveste, P. Matsiota-Bernard, J. Etienne, and C. Nauciel.** 1999. Single clonal origin of high proportion of *Legionella pneumophila* serogroup 1 isolates from patients and the environment in the area of Paris over a 10-year period. *J. Clin. Microbiol.* **37:**2652–2655.
6. **Lawrence, C., E. Ronco, S. Dubrou, R. Leclercq, C. Nauciel, and P. Matsiota-Bernard.** 1999. Molecular typing of *Legionella pneumophila* serogroup 1 isolates from patients and the nosocomial environment by arbitrarily primed PCR and pulsed-field gel electrophoresis. *J. Med. Microbiol.* **48:**327–333.
7. **Nahapetian, K., and F. Squinazi.** 1987. Modalités d'isolement des *Legionella* sp. dans les eaux et les boues résiduaires, p. 165–168. *In Colloque Legionella des 6 et 7 mai 1987*. Collection Fondation Marcel, Mérieux, France.
8. **Riffard, S., F. Lo Presti, F. Vandenessch, F. Forey, M. Reyrolle, and J. Etienne.** 1998. Comparative analysis of infrequent–restriction-site PCR and pulsed-field gel electrophoresis for epidemiological typing of *Legionella pneumophila* serogroup 1 strains. *J. Clin. Microbiol.* **36:**161–167.
9. **Shelton, B. G., W. D. Flanders, and G. K. Morris.** 1994. Legionnaires' disease outbreaks and cooling towers with amplified *Legionella* concentrations. *Curr. Microbiol.* **28:**359–363.

# OCCURRENCE OF *LEGIONELLA* IN WATER FROM DENTAL UNITS AND ESTIMATION OF ANTIBIOTIC RESISTANCE OF ISOLATED STRAINS

*Bożena Krogulska, Renata Matuszewska,*
*Hanna Stypulkowska-Misiurewicz, and Katarzyna Pancer*

# 58

Water delivered to dental units can be contaminated with microorganisms. A number of different microorganisms have been found to contaminate dental unit water supplies; these include coliforms, nonhemolytic streptococci, enterococci, and opportunistic respiratory pathogens such as *Legionella* spp. (7, 11). *Legionella* species is an important cause of sporadic and epidemic pneumonia in developed countries. The principal route of transmission is probably the inhalation of aerosol contaminated with legionellae. The most common sources of such aerosol are water-cooling towers, air-conditioning systems, water faucets, shower heads, whirlpools, etc. (1, 12). Aerosol generated by the water-cooling component of dental handpieces (or air-water syringes) has recently been investigated as a source of infection with *Legionella pneumophila*.

The aim of this study was to estimate *Legionella* contamination of dental-unit waters and antimicrobial susceptibility of isolated strains.

*Bożena Krogulska and Renata Matuszewska* Department of Environmental Hygiene, National Institute of Hygiene, Chocimska Street 24, 00-791 Warsaw, Poland. *Hanna Stypulkowska-Misiurewicz and Katarzyna Pancer* Department of Bacteriology, National Institute of Hygiene, Chocimska Street 24, 00-791 Warsaw, Poland.

The membrane filtration method and growth on a buffered charcoal-yeast extract medium with GVPC selective supplement (glycine, vancomycin, polymyxin B, and cycloheximide) was used. The water samples were filtered through 0.45-$\mu$m-pore-size nitrocellulose Millipore filters. The filters with bacteria were treated with acid buffer (pH 2.2) for 10 min and then neutralized with Ringer's solution (1:40) or, after filtration, transferred to a container with Ringer's solution and incubated in a water bath at 50°C for 30 min. After the pretreatment the filters were plated on a buffered charcoal-yeast extract medium with GVPC supplement. At the same time the water samples (0.2 ml) were plated directly on the recommended medium. The plates were incubated at 35°C for up to 7 days, and colonies typical of *Legionella* spp. were counted. Colonies of presumptive *Legionella* were white-grey-blue and smooth, and had the characteristic ground-glass appearance. They were confirmed on a medium without cysteine, and they were identified by the Legionella Latex Test (Oxoid). The test consists of specific rabbit antibody grouped in three test reagents: one for *L. pneumophila* serogroup 1, the second for *L. pneumophila* serogroups 2 to 14, and the third for the following nine species and serotypes: *L. longbeachae* sero-

*Legionella*, Edited by Reinhard Marre et al.
© 2002 ASM Press, Washington, D.C.

groups 1 and 2, *L. bozemanii* serogroups 1 and 2, *L. dumoffii, L. gormanii, L. jordanis, L. micdadei,* and *L. anisa.*

A total of 66 water samples were collected from different dental clinics in Warsaw. All dental equipment was used at least 10 years. The old dental units were not regularly disinfected. Samples included tap water from elastic pipe of high-speed drills, air-water syringes, and containers for distilled water. *Legionella* spp. were detected in 24.2% of the dental-unit water samples (Fig. 1). The smallest volume of *Legionella* detected was 0.2 ml. Concentrations of *Legionella* in examined samples ranged from $1.0 \times 10^3$ CFU to $5.0 \times 10^3$ CFU per 1,000 ml (7 samples), from $1.1 \times 10^4$ CFU to $4.4 \times 10^4$ CFU per 1,000 ml (7 samples), and from $4.2 \times 10^5$ CFU to $7.2 \times 10^5$ CFU per 1,000 ml (2 samples). Among 103 isolated strains, 13 strains were identified as *L. pneumophila* serogroup 1, 64 strains as *L. pneumophila* serogroups 2 to 14, 9 strains as other species of *Legionella*, and 17 strains were undetermined.

For the estimation of antibiotic resistance, four groups of antibiotics were used: (i) inhibitors of synthesis of cell walls ($\beta$-lactam antibiotics), (ii) inhibitors of synthesis of proteins (tetracyclines, macrolides, aminoglycosides),

(iii) inhibitors of synthesis of nucleic acids (quinolones, rifampin), and (iv) inhibitors of synthesis of cell membranes (polymyxin). The filter paper disks (Bio Merieux) were used in the diffusion method. To control the disks, 24-h culture strains of *Staphylococcus aureus* ATCC 25923 and *Escherichia coli* ATCC 25 922 were used. In these studies, the following strains were selected: ATCC 33152 *L. pneumophila* serogroup 1, 7 strains typed *L. pneumophila* serogroup 1, and 24 strains typed *L. pneumophila* serogroups 2 to 14. The strains were typed on the basis of the *Legionella* Latex Test (Oxoid). The concentration of bacteria suspension used was $10^8$ CFU/ml. Within 10 to 15 min after the inoculation, disks with antimicrobial agents were distributed on the surface medium. The plates were incubated at 37°C. The results were shown in millimeters of the zone of growth inhibition. The results were read after 24 h for control strains and after 72 h for other strains.

The isolated strains from the dental units did not differ significantly from the type strain Philadelphia (3, 5). All strains tested revealed no naturally occurring in vitro resistance against $\beta$-lactam antibiotics. *L. pneumophila* is sensitive to a number of antibiotics; however, in vitro susceptibility studies do not always correlate with clinical efficacy because *Legionella* is an intracellular pathogen (5, 8, 9).

Dental-unit water is a potential source of exposure to *Legionella* species, especially since dental instruments form aerosols. Conditions affecting the survival of these organisms in aerosols are therefore of primary importance, especially relative humidity (2). Quality of dental-unit water is of considerable importance since patients and dental staff are regularly exposed to water and aerosol generated from the dental unit (6, 10, 13). Bacterial load in dental-unit water can be kept at the same recommended guidelines for drinking water (10). Water for use with drills in oral surgery should be held in sterile containers and pass down freshly sterilized tubes to sterilized handpieces (4). Appropriate procedures to decontaminate handpieces, including auto-

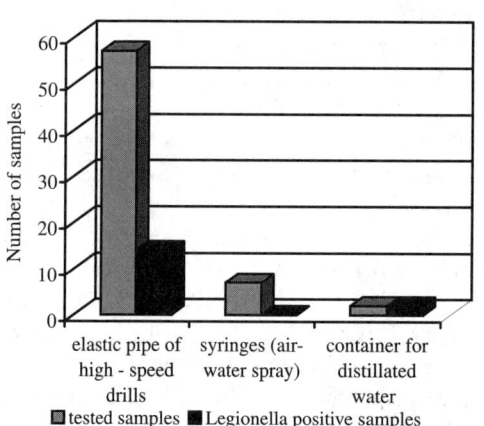

**FIGURE 1** *Legionella* spp. in water samples from dental units.

claving and handpiece replacement between patients, have been developed and implemented in dental practices. Access to the water lines to enable regular flushing with powerful disinfectant would also be desirable (10, 14).

## REFERENCES

1. **Atlas, R. M., J. F. Williams, and M. K. Huntington.** 1995. Legionella contamination of dental-unit waters. *Appl. Environ. Microbiol.* **61:**1208–1213.
2. **Berendt, R. F.** 1980. Survival of Legionella pneumophila in aerosol: effect of relative humidity. *J. Infect. Dis.* **141:**689.
3. **Holt, J. G. (ed.).** 1984. *Bergey's Manual of Systematic Bacteriology*, p. 279–288. Williams and Wilkins, Baltimore, Md.
4. **Kellett, M., and W. P. Holbrook.** 1980. Bacterial contamination of dental handpieces. *J. Dent.* **8:**249–253.
5. **Klein, C. A., and B. A. Cuhna.** 1998. Treatment of Legionnaires' disease. *Sem. Resp. Infect.* **13:**140–146.
6. **Lück, P. C., B. Lau, S. Seidel, and U. Postl.** 1992. Legionellen in Dentalenheiten— ein hygienisches Risiko? *Dtsch. Zahn-Mund.—Kieferheilkd.* **80:**341–346.
7. **Martin, M. V.** 1987. The significance of the bacterial contamination of dental unit water systems. *Br. Dent. J.* **163:**152–154.
8. **Moffie, B. G., and R. P. Mouton.** 1988. Sensitivity and resistance of Legionella pneumophila to some antibiotics and combinations of antibiotics. *J. Antmicrob. Chemother.* **22:**457–462.
9. **Nowicki, M., J. C. Paucod, N. Bornstein, H. Meugnier, P. Isoard, and J. Fleurette.** 1988. Comparative efficacy of five antibiotics on experimental airborne legionellosis in guinea pigs. *J. Antimicrob. Chemother.* **22:**513–519.
10. **Pankhurst, C. L., N. W. Johnson, and R. G. Woods.** 1998. Microbial contamination of dental unit waterlines: the scientific argument. *Int. Dent. J.* **48:**359–368.
11. **Pankhurst, C. L., and J. N. Philpott-Howard.** 1993. The microbiological quality of water in dental chair units. *J. Hosp. Infect.* **23:**167–174.
12. **Pankhurst, C. L., J. N. Philpott-Howard, J. H. Hewitt, and M. W. Casewell.** 1990. The efficacy of chlorination and filtration in the control and eradication of Legionella from dental chair water systems. *J. Hosp. Infect.* **16:**9–18.
13. **Reinthaler, F. F., F. Mascher, and D. Stunzner.** 1988. Serological examination for antibodies against Legionella species in dental personnel. *J. Dent. Res.* **67:**942–943.
14. **Scheid, R. C., C. K. Kim, J. S. Bright, M. S. Whitely, and S. Rose.** 1982. Reduction of microbes in handpieces by flushing before use. *J. Am. Dent. Assoc.* **105:**658–660.

# OCCURRENCE OF *LEGIONELLA* IN DANISH HOT WATER SYSTEMS

*Nina Pringler, Poul Brydov, and Søren A. Uldum*

# 59

In Denmark more than 50% of known cases of Legionnaires' disease are community acquired with no known association with traveling (S. A. Uldum and J. H. Helbig, 5th Int. Conf. *Legionella*, 2000). To assess the role of hot water systems in private homes and institutions as possible sources for infection, a pilot study was performed from October 1999 to May 2000.

## SYSTEMS AND SAMPLING

A total of 46 hot water systems in large buildings situated in or around Copenhagen were included in the study. Twenty-four systems were in public buildings in one municipality. The systems were visited by dk-Teknik Energy & Environment and described regarding type, size, age, and water consumption. Temperatures were recorded or measured at the hot water tanks, for the return water to tank, and at the sampling points.

The systems included 13 blocks of flats, 14 schools, seven nursing homes, eight sport centers, two industries, and two other institutions. Their ages ranged from 1 to 85 years. Most (31 of 46) had one hot water tank. Five systems had 2 to 3 tanks in series, of which one was used for preheating at lower temperatures (35 to 45°C). Two systems were heated by heat exchangers without tanks. Four systems had mixing tanks at 36 to 38°C. Most systems (41 of 46) used piping of galvanized iron. Most of the inspected systems did not appear to follow the recommended water temperatures of 60°C in hot water tanks and 50°C at all taps.

One sample of hot water (the first 1 liter) was taken at a selected tap situated at a distance from the boiler room for each system.

## ANALYSIS FOR VIABLE COUNTS

The water samples were analyzed at The National Centre for Hospital Hygiene, Statens Serum Institut, within 2 days of sampling. The method of analysis was a modification of ISO 11731 (1), consisting of direct plating (0.5 ml), as well as plating (0.1 ml) after concentration by filtration 0.2 $\mu$ ($\times$100), and further concentration ($\times$10) by centrifugation (8,000 $\times$ $g$ for 10 min). Two selective media were used in parallel: MWY (SSI Diagnostika) and

*Nina Pringler* The National Centre for Hospital Hygiene, Statens Serum Institut, DK 2300 Copenhagen S, Denmark. *Poul Brydov* dk-Teknik Energy & Environment, DK 2860 Søborg, Denmark. *Søren A. Uldum* Mycoplasma Laboratory, Department of Respiratory Infections, Meningitis and STIs, Statens Serum Institut, DK 2300 Copenhagen S, Denmark.

*Legionella*, Edited by Reinhard Marre et al.
© 2002 ASM Press, Washington, D.C.

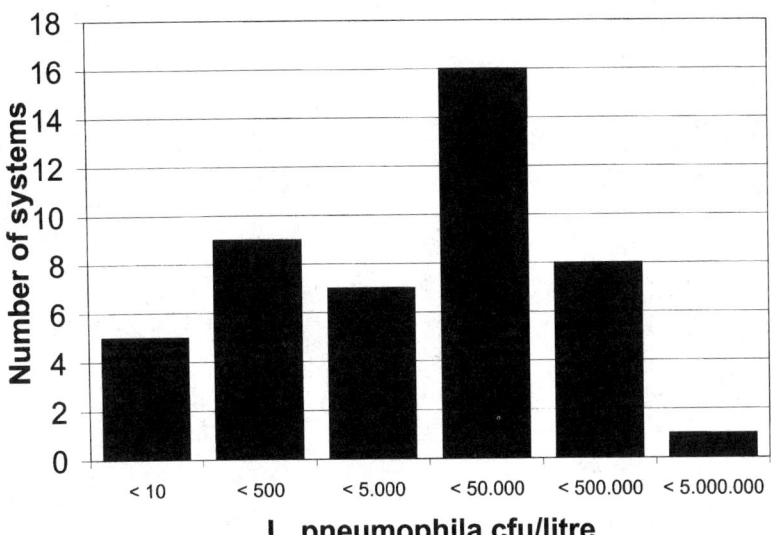

**FIGURE 1** *Legionella* viable counts in hot water samples.

GVPC (glycine, vancomycin, polymyxin B, and cycloheximide) agar (Oxoid GmbH). When necessary, an acid treatment (pH 2.2 for 5 min) and heat treatment (50°C for 30 min) were performed on the concentrated samples. All inoculated plates were incubated in parallel at 36 and 42°C for 3 to 5 and 7 to 8 days. The results were recorded as the highest number of confirmed *Legionella* (CFU/liter).

## SEROGROUP DETERMINATION

From each water sample, at least five colonies were selected. They were tested at Mycoplasma Laboratory, Statens Serum Institut by *Legionella* Latex Test (Oxoid Ltd). Two to five colonies from each water sample were further tested by monoclonal antibodies (Dresden MAb panel) that distinguish between 15 serogroups of *L. pneumophila*. All isolates determined to be *L. pneumophila* serogroup 1 were further characterized by an Enzyme Immuno Assay, distinguishing between MAb 3/1-reactive isolates (Pontiac group) and MAb 3/1-negative isolates (non-Pontiac group).

## RESULTS OF VIABLE COUNTS

*Legionella* was cultured from 41 of 46 water systems. Viable counts for the positive samples ranged from $10^1$ CFU/liter to $\geq 4.9 \times 10^6$ CFU/liter with a median of $6 \times 10^3$ CFU/liter. In nine systems the viable counts were $>5 \times 10^4$ CFU/liter (Fig. 1). Similar results were obtained for MWY and GVPC.

Relatively high counts ($8 \times 10^3$ CFU/liter to $1.8 \times 10^5$ CFU/liter) were found for three of the four systems with low-temperature mixing tanks; but for the fourth system, the viable counts were $10^2$ to $10^3$ CFU/liter. Of the five systems with two or three tanks in series, four had relatively high counts ($6 \times 10^3$ CFU/liter to $\geq 4.9 \times 10^6$ CFU/liter) and the fifth result was $1.4 \times 10^3$ CFU/liter. Low counts (one system with $10^3$ CFU/liter and four systems with $\leq 10^2$ CFU/liter) were found in five systems with copper piping (3 systems) or stainless-steel piping (2 systems) compared with systems with iron piping (41 systems).

## SEROGROUPS FROM WATER SAMPLES

Isolates from the water samples were identified as *L. pneumophila* serogroups 1, 3, 4, 6, 10, and 15 and some untypeable strains. Other *Legionella* species were identified in one sample (Fig. 2).

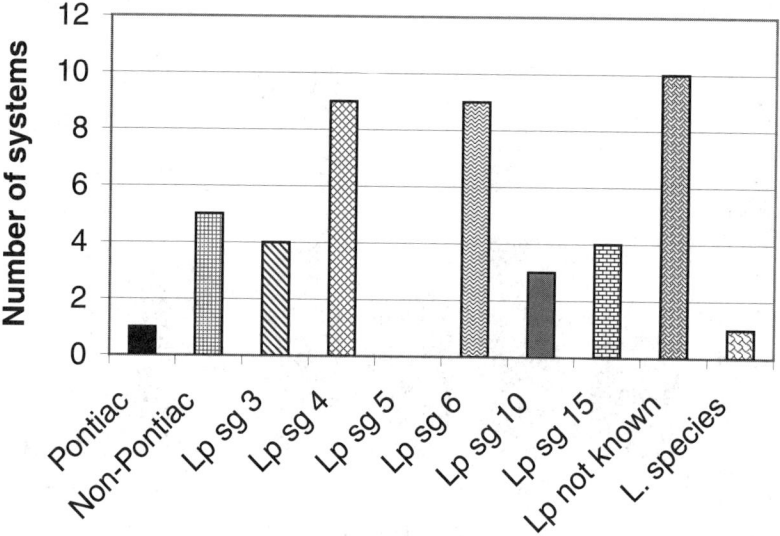

**FIGURE 2** *Legionella* species and serogroups found in 38 hot water systems. Bars indicate the number of systems containing each serogroup.

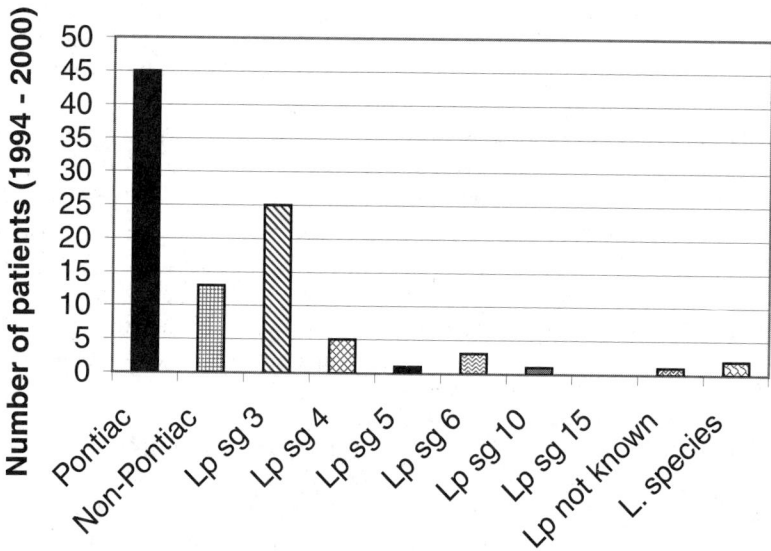

**FIGURE 3** *Legionella* species and serogroups isolated from community–acquired Legionnaires' disease cases in Denmark (Uldum and Helbig, 5th Int. Conf. *Legionella*).

## COMPARISON WITH SEROGROUPS FROM COMMUNITY-ACQUIRED LEGIONNAIRES' DISEASE

Isolates of five of the six serogroups of *L. pneumophila* identified as causing community-acquired Legionnaires' disease in Denmark (serogroups 1, 3, 4, 5, 6, and 10) (Uldum and Helbig, 5th Int. Conf. *Legionella*) (Fig. 3) were isolated from the water samples. From 1994 to 2000, serogroup 1 subgroup Pontiac accounted for the majority of infections (47%), but it was isolated from only one water system in this study. The higher proportion of cases for serogroup 1 subgroup Pontiac is probably due to the higher virulence of these strains.

Some of the serogroups isolated with comparatively high frequency from the water samples (serogroups 4, 6, 10, and 15) have only infrequently been associated with community-acquired Legionnaires' disease in Denmark. Several isolates from the water samples (from 10 water systems) were not typeable by the methods applied, in contrast to the clinical isolates, of which all except one had been typeable (Uldum and Helbig, 5th Int. Conf. *Legionella*).

## CONCLUDING REMARKS

*Legionella* was common in the tested hot water systems, often with relatively high viable counts. Five of the six serogroups of *L. pneumophila* identified as causing community-acquired Legionnaires' disease in Denmark were isolated from the water samples. The results of this pilot study are in accordance with the possibility that domestic hot water systems in private homes and institutions may be the sources of some of the community-acquired cases in Denmark.

## ACKNOWLEDGMENTS

The study was partly funded by a grant from the Danish Environmental Protection Agency, and Hvidovre Kommune (municipality) initiated and financed their part of the study.

## REFERENCE

1. **International Organization for Standardization (ISO).** 1998. *Water Quality—Detection and Enumeration of Legionella.* ISO 117311998(E). International Organization for Standardization, Geneva, Switzerland.

# ANALYSIS OF *LEGIONELLA PNEUMOPHILA* SEROGROUP 1 ISOLATES IN JAPAN BY USING PULSED-FIELD GEL ELECTROPHORESIS AND MONOCLONAL ANTIBODIES

*Junko Amemura-Maekawa, Fumiaki Kura, Haruo Watanabe, Fumio Gondaira, and Jun-ichi Sugiyama*

## 60

*Legionella pneumophila* serogroup 1 is the serogroup of *Legionella* species most frequently isolated from infected patients in Japan and all over the world. Further subgrouping of serogroup 1 is needed to determine the clonal relatedness between isolates of patients and environmental sources. The recent findings suggest that one of the most discriminative epidemiological methods is pulsed-field gel electrophoresis (PFGE) (1, 5, 6). To develop the method of epidemiological surveillance, PFGE and monoclonal antibodies were used for the analysis of 27 clinical and 20 environmental *L. pneumophila* serogroup 1 isolates in Japan.

We reported five anti-*L. pneumophila* serogroup 1 monoclonal antibodies that were specific for serogroup 1 but showed different reactivities, previously (3). We prepared monoclonal antibody-sensitized latex and performed the latex agglutination test on slide plate as described by Sugiyama et al. (7). The hypothetical antigenic factors recognized by the five kinds of antibodies were designated A, B, C, D, and E. In this study, the clinical isolates were divided into eight antigenic formulas, A, AB, ABC, ABCD, AC, AE, BC, and BCDE, and the environmental isolates were divided into six formulas, ABC, BCD, BCDE, CD, CE, and E (Fig. 1). A total of 47 isolates were divided into 12 formulas. The distributions of the hypothetical antigenic factors varied from clinical isolates to environmental isolates: the percentage of isolates with the hypothetical antigenic factor A was 78% of clinical isolates, but only 10% of environmental ones. In environmental isolates, a difference in distribution of the hypothetical antigenic factors was observed between isolates derived from cooling towers and isolates derived from hot springs. For example, 82% of isolates from cooling towers showed the BCDE type, but no isolates from hot springs showed BCDE type. Furthermore, 50% of isolates from hot springs indicated E type, but only 9% of isolates from cooling towers indicated E type.

On the other hand, PFGE using *Sfi*I DNA fragments was performed as follows. Preparation of PFGE plugs was performed as described previously (4). The DNA was digested with 20 U of restriction enzyme *Sfi*I (New England Biolabs, Boston, Mass.) at 50°C.

*Junko Amemura-Maekawa, Fumiaki Kura, and Haruo Watanabe* Department of Bacteriology, National Institute of Infectious Diseases, Tokyo 162-8640, Japan. *Fumio Gondaira and Jun-ichi Sugiyama* Denka Seiken Co., Ltd., Gosen-shi, Niigata 959-1836, Japan.

*Legionella*, Edited by Reinhard Marre et al.
© 2002 ASM Press, Washington, D.C.

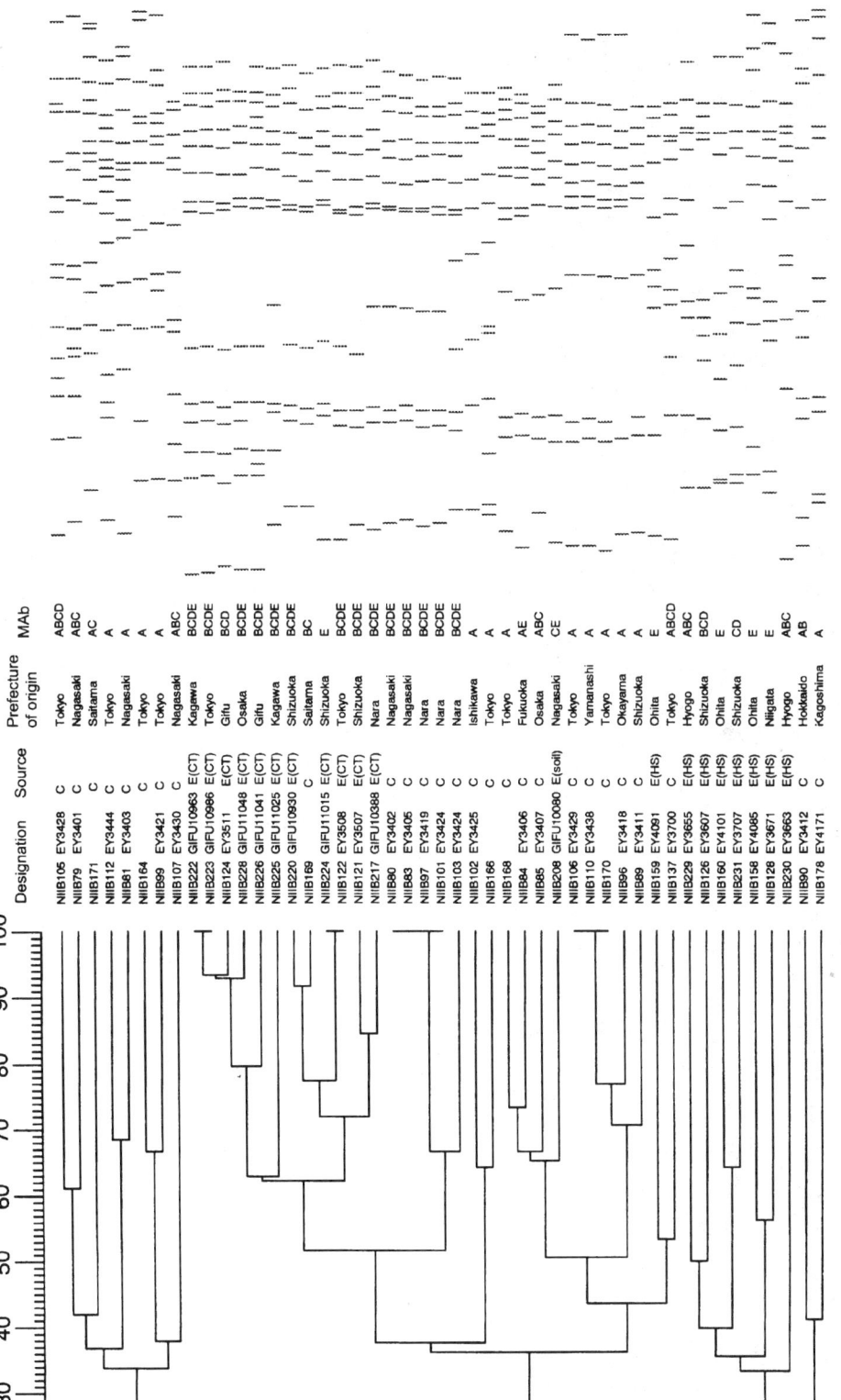

**FIGURE 1** Cluster dendrogram of Japanese *L. pneumophila* serogroup 1 isolates generated from *Sfi*I restriction fragments separated by PFGE and analyzed with the program Molecular Analyst (Bio-Rad). Designations of strains were indicated along with original ones by providers. Source is as follows: E, environmental; HS, hot spring; CT, cooling tower; C, clinical.

PFGE was performed with 1% agarose gel and 0.5X Tris-borate-EDTA running buffer by using CHEF DRII (Bio-Rad Laboratories, Richmond, Calif.). The initial switching time of 5 s was increased linearly to a final switching time of 50 s over 21 h at 6 V/cm at 14°C. The 47 unrelated isolates were discriminated into 41 PFGE types giving an index of discrimination (2) of 0.99. A dendrogram of the PFGE patterns, based on the unweighted pair group method with averages, was constructed with Molecular Analyst (Bio-Rad). The dendrogram contained two major clusters, one cluster consisting of isolates derived from both cooling towers and a few clinical isolates without antigenic factor A, and the other cluster consisting of isolates derived from hot springs. Most of the clinical isolates with factor A did not belong to these clusters (Fig. 1).

There was a close correlation between monoclonal antibody subtyping and PFGE analysis. The result by the two analyses suggested that the clinical isolates, the isolates from cooling towers, and the isolates from hot springs in Japan formed the distinctive genetical or antigenic clusters.

## ACKNOWLEDGMENTS

We are grateful to E. Yabuuchi, H. Yamamoto, and K. Yamaguchi for providing *Legionella* strains.

## REFERENCES

1. **De Zoysa, A. S., and T. G. Harrison.** 1999. Molecular typing of *Legionella pneumophila* serogroup 1 by pulsed-field gel electrophoresis with *Sfi*I and comparison of this method with restriction fragment-length polymorphism analysis. *J. Med. Microbiol.* **48:**269–278.
2. **Hunter, P. R., and M. A. Gaston.** 1988. Numerical index of the discriminatory ability of typing systems: an application of Simpson's index of diversity. *J. Clin. Microbiol.* **26:**2465–2466.
3. **Gondaira, F., and J. Sugiyama.** 1996. Subserogrouping of 49 *Legionella pneumophila* serogroup 1 strains with monoclonal antibodies by slide latex agglutination method and its usefulness for epidemiologic study. *Kansenshogaku Zasshi.* **70:**673–680.
4. **Izumiya, H., J. Terajima, A. Wada, Y. Inagaki, K.-I. Itoh, K. Tamura, and H. Watanabe.** 1997. Molecular typing of enterohemorrhagic *Escherichia coli* O157:H7 isolates in Japan by using pulsed-field gel electrophoresis. *J. Clin. Microbiol.* **35:**1675–1680.
5. **Pruckler, J. M., L. A. Mermel, R. F. Benson, C. Giorgio, P. K. Cassiday, R. F. Breiman, C. G. Whitney, and B. S. Fields.** 1995. Comparison of *Legionella pneumophila* isolates by arbitrarily primed PCR and pulsed-field gel electrophoresis: analysis from seven epidemic investigations. *J. Clin. Microbiol.* **33:**2872–2875.
6. **Schoonmaker, D., T. Heimberger, and G. Birkhead.** 1992. Comparison of ribotyping and restriction enzyme analysis using pulsed-field gel electrophoresis for distinguishing *Legionella pneumophila* isolates obtained during a nosocomial outbreak. *J. Clin. Microbiol.* **30:**1491–1498.
7. **Sugiyama, J., F. Gondaira, J. Matsuda, M. Saga, and Y. Terada.** 1987. New method for serological typing of *Vibrio cholerae* O: 1 using a monoclonal antibody-sensitized latex agglutination test. *Microbiol. Immunol.* **31:**387–391.

# RELATIONSHIP BETWEEN COLONIZATION OF BUILDING WATER SYSTEMS BY *LEGIONELLA PNEUMOPHILA* AND ENVIRONMENTAL FACTORS

*Zuhal Zeybek and Ayşın Çotuk*

# 61

*Legionella* species are widespread in aquatic environments. *Legionella pneumophila* is a pathogenic bacteria and is responsible for Legionnaires' disease. Man-made water systems are contaminated by legionellae through the municipal water supply (6, 14).

*L. pneumophila* is generally found in hot water systems and biofilms that are present in water supply systems and multiplies there within protozoan cells. Bacterial transmission to humans occurs through droplets generated from cooling towers, shower heads, and other man-made devices that generate aerosols. However, the relationship between Legionnaires' disease and contaminated water systems is still under discussion. The ecology of *Legionella* species is not clearly understood either (8, 10).

Since there are few documents (2, 7, 11) related to *L. pneumophila* in building water systems in our country, we have investigated the prevalence of *L. pneumophila* in the water supply systems of 139 hotels in Istanbul. We also examined the influences of both the natural microbial population and other environmental factors on the growth of *L. pneumophila*.

Water samples for *L. pneumophila* analysis were taken from four locations in each hotel water supply from December 1995 to June 1998:

**1.** Cold water tank drainage
**2.** Hot water tank drainage
**3.** Bathroom faucets farthest from the hot water tank
**4.** Bathroom shower heads farthest from the hot water tank

A 3000-ml water sample was collected in a sterile plastic container that contained sodium thiosulfate to neutralize any residual chlorine, after a liter preflush of water (4, 9).

The temperature and free chlorine content of water samples were also measured. In addition to the *Legionella* analysis, total viable bacterium count was determined by plate count agar. A total of 0.1 ml of water sample was inoculated to three agar plates and incubated at 22°C ± 0.5°C for 48 ± 3 h. At the end of this period, the grown colonies were counted (1).

Samples were transported immediately to the laboratory and concentrated by filtration through 0.2-μm-pore-size polyamide filters. The filtrate was resuspended for 2 min in sterile distilled water. The suspension was divided into three portions: the first one was placed in

*Zuhal Zeybek and Ayşın Çotuk* Department of Biology, Faculty of Science, University of Istanbul, Istanbul, Turkey.

*Legionella*, Edited by Reinhard Marre et al.
© 2002 ASM Press, Washington, D.C.

**TABLE 1** Relationship between the materials in hotel water systems and the isolation of *L. pneumophila*

| Material of water system | No. (%) of *L. pneumophila*-positive buildings |
|---|---|
| Iron | 27 (47.3) |
| Plastic | 0 (0) |
| Iron and plastic | 13 (22.8) |
| Iron and steel | 2 (3.5) |
| Iron and faience | 1 (1.7) |
| Iron and aluminium | 1 (1.7) |
| Iron and copper | 2 (3.5) |
| Iron and concrete | 2 (3.5) |
| Copper | 0 (0) |
| Sheet iron | 0 (0) |
| Steel | 1 (1.7) |
| Concrete and steel | 0 (0) |
| Unknown | 8 (14.0) |
| Total | 57 (99.7) |

a 50°C water bath for 30 min; the second one was acidified in HCl-KCl solution for 15 min; and the third one was not treated. All specimens were spread plated onto a selective differential agar medium containing buffered charcoal-yeast extract agar enriched with glycine, vancomycin, polymyxin B, and cycloheximide (4, 5, 6, 9, 12).

Each inoculated plate was incubated at 37°C for 10 to 14 days in a humidified environment. Colonies consistent with *Legionella* morphology were Gram stained and inoculated on Trypticase soy agar. Gram-negative rods that could not grow in Trypticase soy agar were tested serologically with a *Legionella* latex test kit (Oxoid) (3). The number of colonies was counted to determine the concentration of *Legionella* bacteria per liter of sample. The relationship between *L. pneumophila* and total viable bacteria counts (22°C) was performed by linear regression (13).

A cultural analysis of water systems of 139 hotels showed that 57 of the hotels (41%) were contaminated by *L. pneumophila*. The concentrations ranged from 6 to $2 \times 10^4$ CFU/liter.

The results also showed that the concentration of *L. pneumophila* is high in the summer. On the other hand, in general, the lowest concentration was observed in the cold water tank drainage, whereas the highest concentration was observed in bathroom shower heads farthest from the hot water tank.

*L. pneumophila*-positive results were obtained in 124 of 554 water samples. The number of positive samples isolated from the cold water tank drainage, the hot water tank drain-

**TABLE 2** Free chlorine and *L. pneumophila* content of hot water samples

| Free chlorine (ppm) | No. of samples examined | No. (%) of *L. pneumophila*-positive samples | *L. pneumophila* (CFU/liter) | |
|---|---|---|---|---|
| | | | Minimum | Maximum |
| 0 | 139 | 35 (94.5) | 72 | 20,000 |
| 0.10 | 6 | 1 (2.7) | | 20,000 |
| 0.15 | 4 | 1 (2.7) | 38 | |
| 0.20 | 2 | 0 (0) | | |
| 0.30 | 1 | 0 (0) | | |
| 0.50 | 1 | 0 (0) | | |
| 0.70 | 2 | 0 (0) | | |
| 0.80 | 1 | 0 (0) | | |
| 1 | 1 | 0 (0) | | |
| 2 | 1 | 0 (0) | | |
| 2.5 | 1 | 0 (0) | | |
| 3.5 | 2 | 0 (0) | | |
| Total | 162 | 37 (99.9) | | |

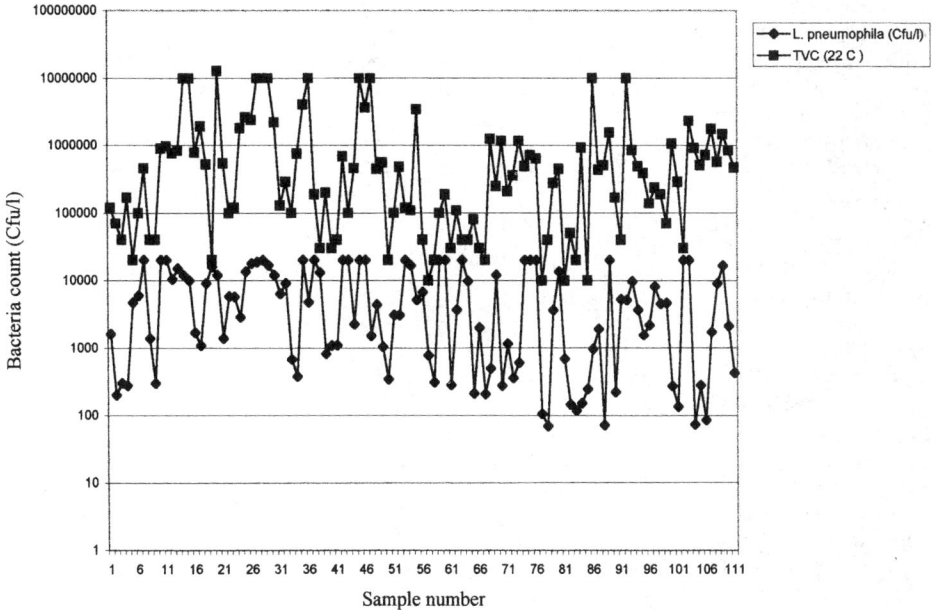

**FIGURE 1**    *L. pneumophila* and total viable bacterium count (22°C) that are isolated from the same regions.

age, the bathroom faucets farthest from the hot water tank, and the bathroom shower heads farthest from the hot water tank were 14, 25, 40, and 45, respectively. *L. pneumophila* serogroup 1 was isolated from 29 (23.3%) water samples, whereas *L. pneumophila* serogroups 2 to 14 were isolated from 95 (76.6%) water samples. The mean water temperature varied from 15 to 62°C in cold and hot water samples. It was found that the effective growth temperature of *L. pneumophila* ranged from 28°C to 41°C.

Table 1 shows the relationship between the material used in water systems of hotels and the isolation of *L. pneumophila*; there was not a significant relationship between the material and the presence of *L. pneumophila*, except iron.

Free chlorine and *L. pneumophila* content of hot water samples examined were tabulated in Table 2. These results indicated that 95% of hot water samples had *L. pneumophila*-positive culture in absence of free chlorine.

The relationship between *L. pneumophila* and total viable bacteria count was shown in

Fig. 1. There seems to be no significant relationship between *L. pneumophila* growth and total viable bacteria ($P > 0.05$).

An epidemiologic case has been notified in one of hotels surveyed in which *L. pneumophila* serogroup 1 was isolated.

In this study, we found that 41% of samples in hotel water systems were *Legionella*-positive. This percentage was 46% in Spain.

## REFERENCES

1. **American Public Health Association.** 1971. *Standard Methods for the Examination of Water and Waste Water. Bacteriological Examination of Water to Determine Its Sanitary Quality*, 13th ed. APHA, Washington, D.C.
2. **Baskin, H., O. Önal, and H. Kiratli,** 1998. A modification in *Legionella pneumophila* isolation from environmental water samples. *Turk. Microbiol. Cem. Derg.* **28:**7–10.
3. **Bridson, E. Y.** 1990. *Oxoid Manual*, 6th ed.
4. **British Standard.** 1998. *Water Quality*: Part 4: microbiological methods, detection and enumeration of Legionella. BS 6068-4.12:1998; ISO 11731:1998.
5. **DeLuca, G., S. Stampi, L. Lezzi, and F. Zannetti.** 1999. Effect of heat and acid decon-

tamination treatments on the recovery of *Legionella pneumophila* from drinking water using two selective media. *New Microbiol.* **22**:203–208.

6. **Dennis, P. J. L.** 1988. Isolation of *Legionellae* from environmental specimens, p. 31–57. *In* T. G. Harrison and A. G. Taylor (ed.), *A Laboratory Manual for Legionella.* John Wiley & Sons, Ltd., New York, N.Y.

7. **Ergin, Ç., A. N. Yalçin, A. Pinar, Ç. B. Çetin, H. Turgut, and G. Yayli.** 1998. Investigation of *Legionella* species in thermal water sources of Pamukkale Region by culture and polymerase chain reaction. *Bull. Microbiol.* **32:** 227–232.

8. **Fields, B. S.** 1993. *Legionella* and protozoa: interaction of a pathogen and its natural host, p. 129–236. *In* J. M. Barbaree, R. F. Breiman, and A. P. Dufour (ed.), *Legionella: Current Status and Emerging Perspectives.* American Society for Microbiology, Washington, D.C.

9. **Fields, B. S.** 1997. *Legionella* and Legionnaires' disease, p. 666–675. *In* C. J. Hurst, G. R. Knudsen, M. J. McInerney, L. D. Stetzenbach, and M. V. Walter (ed.), *Manual of Environmental Microbiology.* American Society for Microbiology, Washington, D.C.

10. **Kwaik, Y. A., L. Y. Gao, B. J. Stone, C. Venkataraman, and O. S. Harb.** 1998. Invasion of protozoa by *Legionella pneumophila* and its role in bacterial ecology and pathogenesis. *Appl. Environ. Microbiol.* **64:**3127–3133.

11. **Perente, S., A. Yağci, and G. Söyletir.** 1999. The prevalence of *Legionella pneumophila* in lower respiratory tract infections and hospital water samples. *Turk. Infect. Derg.* **13:**477–481.

12. **Reinthaler, F. F., J. Sattler, K. Schaffler-Dullnig, B. Weinmayr, and E. Marth.** 1993. Comparative study of procedures for isolation and cultivation of *Legionella pneumophila* from tap water in hospitals. *J. Clin. Microbiol.* **31:**1213–1216.

13. **Şenocak, M.** 1998. *Biyoistatistik* İ. Ü. Cerrahpaşa Tıp Fakültesi, Dilek Ofset Matbaacılık, Istanbul.

14. **Winn, W. C.** 1995. *Legionella*, p. 533–544. *In* P. R. Murray, E. J. Baron, F. C. Pfaller, and F. C. Tenover (ed.), *Manual of Clinical Microbiology*, 6th ed. American Society for Microbiology, Washington, D.C.

# EPIDEMIOLOGY

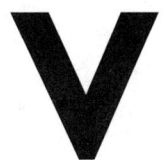

# SURVEILLANCE OF LEGIONNAIRES' DISEASE IN EUROPE

*Carol Joseph on behalf of the European
Working Group for Legionella Infections*

# 62

Identification of the organism responsible for Legionnaires' disease was first associated with an outbreak in 1976 in Philadelphia, Pa., where 189 cases and 29 deaths occurred among American Legion veterans who had attended a hotel-based convention (2). Subsequent reanalysis of sera from patients associated with earlier outbreaks of pneumonia of unknown etiology in the United States and Europe showed the organism to be the same as that implicated in the Philadelphia outbreak (14). Legionnaires' disease has since been shown to be an uncommon form of pneumonia. Estimates suggest that it accounts for less than 5% of all pneumonia cases requiring hospital admission (8), with mortality ranging from 10 to 50% depending on the individual patient's immune status and susceptibility (11). However, it has also been shown that legionella infection is hugely underdiagnosed and underreported in most countries and therefore represents a much greater burden of illness and mortality than reflected in the reported incidence data (7, 13).

Effective international cooperation in the control of communicable disease is dependent on the sharing of scientific knowledge and a willingness of national authorities to coordinate action. International surveillance of travel associated Legionnaires' disease began in 1987, following the establishment of the European Working Group for *Legionella* Infections (EWGLI) in 1986 (1). Administrative support for the surveillance scheme originally came from the World Health Organization but since 1993, funding has been obtained from the European Commission (Directorate General V, Health and Consumer Protection). The scheme is currently managed by the Public Health Laboratory Service Communicable Disease Surveillance Centre in London (12). The number of European collaborating countries has increased from 23 in 1993 to 31 in 2000. Information about EWGLI and its roles and functions can be found on the EWGLI website (www.ewgli.org).

The surveillance scheme's public health role in Europe is one of early identification of cases and clusters of travel-associated Legionnaires' disease and the rapid exchange of information on these cases so that immediate investigations and control measures can be implemented and further cases prevented. EWGLI also provides expert epidemiological, microbiological, and environmental health advice to clinical and public health officials, tour

*Carol Joseph* PHLS Communicable Disease Surveillance Centre, 61 Colindale Avenue, London NW9 5EQ, England.

*Legionella*, Edited by Reinhard Marre et al.
© 2002 ASM Press, Washington, D.C.

operators, national and international government departments, and other relevant groups such as hoteliers and members of the public. All collaborating countries in the surveillance scheme adhere to the common protocol and set of case definitions. These include a clinical and microbiological case definition for confirmed and presumptive cases of Legionnaires' disease, a definition of what counts as a travel case (one or more nights away from home in the 10 days before onset), what constitutes a cluster (two or more cases who stayed at or visited the same accommodation site and developed Legionnaires' disease within the same 6-month period), or a linked case (two or more cases who stayed at or visited the same accommodation site but developed Legionnaires' disease more than 6 months apart from each other).

EWGLI participants have held an annual scientific meeting since 1986. Prior to 1993, these meetings included a session in which individual collaborators were invited to report back on the total annual data set of Legionnaires' disease cases for their country, i.e., the community and nosocomial cases as well as the travel-associated cases. Since 1993, this annual data from the member countries of EWGLI has been obtained through completion of a set of standardized reporting forms and aggregated into an overall European data set for publication (3–6). Information is collected on total cases by population denominator, sex, number of deaths, risk group, species, and serogroup and serotype, as well as by method of diagnosis for all cases in each participating country. Details of outbreaks by type and source are also requested.

This chapter mainly presents data from 1999, which was provided by 28 of the 31 countries that currently participate in the European scheme. It also compares trends and incidence of cases in Europe from 1993.

## REPORTED INCIDENCE FROM 28 COUNTRIES

The number of cases reported in 1999 was the highest yet, with 2,136 cases of Legionnaires' disease in European residents, almost 1,000 more than were reported in 1994 (Tables 1 and 2). Absolute total number of cases per year have depended on whether large outbreaks have been reported, although the underlying trend has been upward. Sixteen countries reported more cases in 1999 than in 1998, seven reported fewer cases, and one reported the same number as in 1998. Four countries reported no cases at all. Two countries each reported more than 300 cases (France and Spain), while Italy and The Netherlands each reported more than 200 cases. A total of 193 deaths were reported in 1999—an overall case fatality rate of 9% (range, 3 to 25%) compared with 13.1% in 1998 and 10% in 1997. In 1999, 65% of the cases were male, 28% were female, and 7% were of unknown sex.

## RATE OF INFECTION PER MILLION POPULATION

Since 1993, the overall rate of infection per million residents has ranged from 3.35 to 4.46. In 1999, a population base of 398 million was used to calculate the overall European rate of infection of 5.4 cases per million population. In five countries, area rather than national statistics were used to calculate rates (Croatia, Germany, Greece, Portugal, and Russia). Belgium's infection rate was the highest at 19.5 per million population, followed by Denmark at 16.98, and The Netherlands at 16.75 per million population. Both Belgium and The Netherlands' high rates of infection were accounted for by large community outbreaks (9, 10). Denmark has consistently had a higher rate of infection than other countries, which is possibly associated with the fact that it is a small country that carries out high levels of testing for legionella in patients with pneumonia, and also has a centralized reference laboratory for diagnosing and reporting cases.

## CATEGORY OF CASES

Contributing countries report their cases according to whether they are associated with community-, hospital-, or travel-acquired infection. In 1999, 32% of the overall cases were reported as community acquired, 9% were hospital acquired, and 21% were associated

**TABLE 1**  Legionnaires' disease in Europe: cases and rate per million population from 28 countries (1999)

| Country | All reported cases (n) | Population (millions) | Rate per million |
|---|---|---|---|
| Austria | 41 | 8 | 5.13 |
| Belgium | 195 | 10 | 19.50 |
| Croatia (area) | 9 | 1.5 | 6.00 |
| Czech Republic | 23 | 10.5 | 2.19 |
| Denmark | 90 | 5.3 | 16.98 |
| England and Wales | 195 | 52.4 | 3.72 |
| Estonia | 0 | 1.4 | 0.00 |
| Finland | 9 | 5.1 | 1.76 |
| France | 445 | 58.5 | 7.60 |
| Germany (area) | 56 | 40 | 1.40 |
| Greece (area) | 12 | 1.2 | 10.00 |
| Ireland | 2 | 3.64 | 0.55 |
| Italy | 229 | 56.5 | 4.05 |
| Latvia | 0 | 2.4 | 0.00 |
| Lithuania | 0 | 3.7 | 0.00 |
| Malta | 3 | 0.38 | 7.90 |
| The Netherlands | 264 | 15.7 | 16.75 |
| Northern Ireland | 5 | 1.69 | 2.94 |
| Norway | 10 | 4.4 | 2.27 |
| Poland | 0 | 38 | 0.00 |
| Portugal (area) | 2 | 2 | 1.00 |
| Russia (Moscow) | 16 | 10 | 1.60 |
| Scotland | 35 | 5.1 | 6.81 |
| Slovak Republic | 1 | 5 | 0.20 |
| Slovenia | 25 | 1.98 | 12.62 |
| Spain | 306 | 39.42 | 7.76 |
| Sweden | 86 | 8.86 | 9.71 |
| Switzerland | 77 | 7.1 | 10.75 |
| Total[a] | 2136 | 397.72 | 5.38 |

[a] Confirmed cases = 1516 (71%), presumptive cases = 509 (24%), status unknown = 111 (5%).

with travel either in their own country or abroad. The proportion with unknown category of risk was higher in 1999 at 38% compared with 32% the previous year (Table 3).

Thirty-two outbreaks or clusters were detected in 1999 by 12 individual European countries and involved 359 cases (17%). Seven outbreaks were linked to hospitals and twelve to the community. Thirteen clusters were travel-associated, compared with twenty-nine clusters detected by the EWGLI international database for the same period, the difference relating to the surveillance scheme's detection of single cases in more than one country of residence that were associated with the same travel accommodation. The hospital outbreaks

**TABLE 2**  Legionnaires' disease in Europe: reported cases (1993–1999)

| Year | No. of cases | No. of countries contributing data | Population (millions) | Rate per million |
|---|---|---|---|---|
| 1993 | 1,242 | 19 | 300 | 4.14 |
| 1994 | 1,161 | 20 | 346 | 3.35 |
| 1995 | 1,255 | 24 | 339 | 3.70 |
| 1996 | 1,563 | 24 | 350 | 4.46 |
| 1997 | 1,360 | 24 | 351 | 3.87 |
| 1998 | 1,442 | 28 | 333 | 4.33 |
| 1999 | 2,136 | 28 | 398 | 5.38 |

**TABLE 3** Legionnaires' disease in Europe: category of cases (1994–1999)

| | No. of cases | | | | | |
|---|---|---|---|---|---|---|
| | 1994 | 1995 | 1996 | 1997 | 1998 | 1999 |
| Community | 186 | 270 | 617 | 387 | 478 | 679 |
| Nosocomial | 151 | 157 | 105 | 219 | 181 | 195 |
| Travel abroad | 157 | 170 | 215 | 263 | 245 | 288 |
| Travel home | 33 | 24 | 31 | 34 | 52 | 151 |
| Not known | 634 | 634 | 595 | 457 | 486 | 823 |
| Total | 1,161 | 1,255 | 1,563 | 1,360 | 1,442 | 2,136 |

occurred in the Czech Republic, Denmark, Germany, Italy, and Spain and the community outbreaks in Belgium, Denmark, England, France, Italy, The Netherlands, Slovenia, and Spain. One outbreak in Belgium (10) and one in The Netherlands (9), both linked to trade shows, collectively gave rise to almost 300 additional cases of Legionnaires' disease. At both trade fairs, whirlpool spas were on display and people became infected by breathing in the contaminated aerosols after walking past them. In December 1999, a meeting of experts was convened by the European Commission to review these whirlpool spa outbreaks. The objectives of the meeting were to advise the Commission on the need for European recommendations and guidelines for the control and prevention of future whirlpool spa outbreaks and to produce specific recommendations that could be addressed by the Commission.

In 1999, five travel-associated clusters occurred in the same country as the country of residence of the cases—in Belgium, England, Italy, Sweden, and Wales. The largest outbreak was reported from Sweden and involved 20 cases among their own residents who became infected after exposure to a hotel whirlpool. Two travel-associated clusters were each linked to travel in Croatia and France and one each to Portugal, Thailand, Turkey, and Spain.

## OUTBREAKS BY SOURCE OF INFECTION

Twelve of the thirty-two outbreaks in 1999 were due to hot or cold water systems. Six of these occurred in hospitals, three in the community, and three were associated with travel. Contaminated cooling towers were responsible for only one outbreak in a community setting in France. The whirlpool spa outbreaks were linked to whirlpools that were on display at two large trade shows and three other sites, mainly in hotels. Fourteen outbreaks were of unknown source.

## TRAVEL-ASSOCIATED INFECTION

Altogether, 18 countries reported 439 travel-associated cases, 142 more cases than in 1998. A total of 151 cases were linked to travel in the same country as the country of residence and 288 to travel abroad. England, France, The Netherlands, and Sweden reported a total of 269 cases, 61% of all the cases by country of residence. France, Italy, and Spain were associated with 51% of the cases by country of infection.

Travel within Europe accounted for 86% of the travel cases; the remainder were associated with the Americas, the Caribbean, the Far East, and the Middle East. The highest number of cases was associated with travel in France (86 cases), followed by Spain (77 cases), Italy (62 cases), Greece (22 cases), Sweden (22 cases), and Turkey (20 cases). However, in 121 (42%) of these cases, infection was related to travel within the same country of residence. Twelve cases involved travel in more than one European country before onset of illness and six involved travel in more than one country outside Europe. Using United Kingdom international passenger survey statistics, the rate of legionella infection per million visitors from the United Kingdom to France, Spain, Italy, Greece, and Turkey was calculated from 1999. Fourteen cases of Legionnaires' disease were reported in United Kingdom travellers returning from France—a rate of 1.2 per million United Kingdom visitors to France. Rates for Spain, Italy, and Greece were 2.1, 3.0, and 3.0 per million United Kingdom visitors, respectively, while for Turkey they were four times higher at 12 per million visitors for the United Kingdom.

## INVESTIGATION OF TRAVEL-ASSOCIATED OUTBREAKS

Although the number of travel-associated clusters detected in 1999 by both individual countries and the EWGLI surveillance scheme has increased compared with the previous year, a smaller number of cases were associated with the individual clusters in 1999. This may be accounted for by the rapid response of public health officials in the countries concerned and by the continued collaborations with tour operators to implement timely control measures and prevent further cases. Improved awareness of the dangers of legionella in water systems and effective control and prevention maintenance policies in a large number of hotels used by specific tour operators in European resorts are contributing to a decline of cases among tourists staying at these hotels.

## METHODS OF DIAGNOSIS

A total of 359 cases (17%) in 1999 were diagnosed by culture of the organism, 959 (45%) by urinary antigen detection, and 284 (13%) by seroconversion. Single high antibody titers were reported for 393 cases (18.4%) (Table 4). The remaining cases were diagnosed by respiratory antigen detection or PCR or the method was unknown. Compared with 1998, cases detected by urinary antigen detection have increased by 12%, whereas the number detected by isolation has fallen by 4.6% and by serology has fallen by 11%.

*L. pneumophila* serogroup 1 infection accounted for 1,379 (65%) of the total cases,

54% of which were diagnosed by urinary antigen. *L. pneumophila* with a different serogroup or with a serogroup not determined accounted for 647 (30%) of the reports last year. A total of 107 (17%) of these cases were diagnosed by isolation and 31% by urinary antigen detection. A total of 111 (5%) of the reports were of other legionella species or species not known, the same proportion as in 1998.

Of the 359 isolates reported, 64% were due to *L. pneumophila* serogroup 1 infection, 59 were *L. pneumophila* but serogroup unknown, and 48 were serogroups 2 to 14. Three isolates were diagnosed as *L. micdadei*, five as *L. bozemanii*, two as *L. longbeachae*, and one each as *L. dumoffii* and *L. cincinnatiensis*. For 12 isolates the *Legionella* species was not given (Table 5).

## CONCLUSIONS

The large increase in cases reported in 1999 compared with all previous years is associated with two very big community outbreaks and improved detection of cases in countries that have recently introduced enhanced national surveillance schemes. Surveillance at the international level cannot function effectively without well-developed national surveillance schemes that contribute their data in an informative and timely way. EWGLI is assisting this process through its sharing of information on cases, outbreaks, sources of infection, and continued developments in epidemiological, microbiological, and environmental aspects of legionella infection. A recent Delphi exercise to establish a list of priority diseases for European collaborative projects showed that Legionnaires' disease was ranked fourth of 35 diseases under consideration (15) in recognition of the importance of shared action at the international level for protection of European citizens at home and abroad. Two large outbreaks linked to whirlpool spas have highlighted the need for national and international guidance on their use in areas where substantial populations may be exposed to risk, for improved maintenance of these facilities, and

**TABLE 4**  Legionnaires' disease in Europe: cases by main method of diagnosis (1999)

| Main method of diagnosis | *L. pneumophila* serogroup 1 | *L. pneumophila* other serogroup or serogroup not determined | Other *Legionella* cases | All *Legionella* cases |
|---|---|---|---|---|
| Isolation | 230[a] | 107 | 23[a] | 359 |
| Antigen detection | | | | |
| Urinary | 744 | 203 | 12 | 959 |
| Respiratory | 18 | 15 | 1 | 34 |
| Serology | | | | |
| Seroconversion | 112 | 133 | 39 | 284 |
| Single high titer | 227 | 145 | 21 | 393 |
| PCR | 4 | 19 | 4 | 27 |
| Other | 0 | 3 | 5 | 8 |
| Not known | 44 | 22 | 6 | 72 |
| Total (each case counted only once) | 1,379 | 647 | 111 | 2,136[a] |

[a] One case culture positive for *L. pneumophila* serogroup 1 and *L. micdadei*.

**TABLE 5**  Legionnaires' disease by species and serogroup in Europe (1999)

| *Legionella* species or serogroup | No. of isolates |
|---|---|
| *Legionella* species | |
| *L. pneumophila* | 337[a] |
| *L. micdadei* | 3[a] |
| *L. bozemanii* | 4 |
| *L. dumoffii* | 1 |
| *L. longbeachae* | 2 |
| *L. cincinnatiensis* | 1 |
| Species unknown | 12 |
| Total | 359 |
| *L. pneumophila* serogroup | |
| sg1 | 230 |
| sg2 | 2 |
| sg3 | 16 |
| sg4 | 10 |
| sg5 | 5 |
| sg6 | 8 |
| sg8 | 4 |
| sg10 | 2 |
| sg14 | 1 |
| Not known | 59 |
| Total | 337 |

[a] One case positive for *L. pneumophila* serogroup 1 and *L. micedadei*.

for rapid control and prevention measures to be implemented when outbreaks are detected.

The big rise in the use of the urinary antigen detection test has led to more timely reporting, a consequence of which has been the earlier detection of outbreaks and the rapid implementation of control measures and prevention of further cases. However, use of this method has also resulted in fewer cases diagnosed by culture of the organism. Thus the advantages of the urinary antigen detection test in benefiting patient outcome through early appropriate antibiotic therapy are also associated with the disadvantages, which limit the power of microbiological investigations to identify sources of infection if no human isolates are available for comparison of environmental and clinical strains of legionella. Whenever possible, clinicians should try to obtain clinical specimens for culture from patients with suspected Legionnaires' disease in order to contribute to outbreak investigations and to improve our understanding of the epidemiology and microbiology of the infection.

## ACKNOWLEDGMENTS

The coordinating center in London would like to thank all the collaborators for contributing their data for use in this annual assessment of the impact of Legionnaires' disease in Europe. EWGLI has provided the impetus and the framework in which to collect the wider European national data set and also the opportunity to demonstrate the important epidemiological and microbiological trends for legionella infections within Europe.

The data in this chapter are reprinted from the *Weekly Epidemiological Record of the World Health Organization*, Geneva (6), with permission of the publisher.

## REFERENCES

1. **Anonymous.** 1990. Epidemiology, prevention and control of legionellosis. Memorandum from a WHO meeting. *Bull. W. H. O.* **68:**155–164.
2. **Anonymous.** 1997. Respiratory Infection-Pennsylvania (1st published 1976). *Morb. Mortal. Wkly. Rep.* **46:**49–56.
3. **Anonymous.** 1997. Legionnaires' disease in Europe, 1996. *Wkly. Epidemiol. Rec.* **72:**253–257.
4. **Anonymous.** 1998. Legionnaires' disease in Europe, 1997. *Wkly. Epidemiol. Rec.* **73:**257–261.
5. **Anonymous.** 1999. Legionnaires' disease in Europe, 1998. *Wkly. Epidemiol. Rec.* **74:**273–280.
6. **Anonymous.** 2000. Legionnaires' disease in Europe, 1999. *Wkly. Epidemiol. Rec.* **75:**347–352.
7. **Bohte, R., R. van Furth, and P. J. van den Broek.** 1995. Aetiology of community-acquired pneumonia: a prospective study among adults requiring admission to hospital. *Thorax* **50:**543–547.
8. **British Thoracic Society.** 1987. Community-acquired pneumonia in adults in British hospitals in 1982–1983: A BTS/PHLS survey of aetiology, mortality, prognostic factors and outcome. *Q. J. Med.* **62:**195–220.
9. **Conyn van Spaendonck, M.** 1999. Onderzoek van de epidemie van legionellose 1999. *Infect. Bull.* **10:**157–158.
10. **De Schriver, K., E. Van Bouwel, L. Mortelmans, P. Van Rossom, T. De Beukelaer, C. Vael, K. Dirven, H. Goosens, M. Leven, and O. Ronveaux.** 2000. An outbreak of legionnaires' disease among visitors to a fair in Belgium in 1999. *Eurosurveillance* **5:**115–119.
11. **Hubbard, R. B., R. M. Mathur, and J. T. Macfarlane.** 1993. Severe community-acquired legionella pneumonia: treatment, complications and outcome. *Q. J. Med.* **86:**327–332.
12. **Hutchinson, E. J., C. A. Joseph, and C. L. R. Bartlett on behalf of the European Working Group for Legionella Infections.** 1996. EWGLI: a European surveillance scheme for travel associated legionnaires' disease. *Eurosurveillance* **1:**37–39.
13. **Marston, B. J., H. B. Lipman, and R. F. Breiman.** 1994. Surveillance for Legionnaires' Disease. Risk factors for morbidity and mortality. *Arch. Intern. Med.* **154:**2417–2422.
14. **Osterholm, M. T., T. D. Y. Chin, D. O. Osborne, H. B. Dull, A. G. Dean, D. W. Fraser, et al.** 1983. 1957 outbreak of legionnaires' disease associated with a meat packing plant. *Am. J. Epidemiol.* **117:**60–67.
15. **Weinberg, J., O. Grimaud, and L. Newton.** 1999. Establishing priorities for European collaboration in communicable disease surveillance. *Eur. J. Public Health* **9:**236–240.

# USING GEOGRAPHICAL INFORMATION SYSTEMS FOR RISK ASSESSMENT AND CONTROL OF LEGIONNAIRES' DISEASE ASSOCIATED WITH COOLING TOWERS

Richard Bentham, Malcolm Pradhan,
Paul Hakendorf, and Peter Wilmot

# 63

The recent outbreak of Legionnaires' disease at the Melbourne Aquarium has prompted widespread comment by public health officials regarding testing for *Legionella*. General opinion in the media seems to suggest that state governments should institute compulsory testing of cooling tower waters for the organism. It is implied from these opinions that this strategy would reduce risks of further outbreaks.

Published reports over the last 24 years since Legionnaires' disease was first recognized have detailed a number of risk factors. There have been very few published reports in which *Legionella* culture results from cooling towers have been equated to a quantifiable risk of infection (7, 8). Of these reports, none has been based upon multiple culture results taken from single systems over prolonged periods. As such there is a lack of a scientific support for *Legionella* culture as a risk-management tool.

Cooling tower maintenance and biocide dosage have been shown to be major contributors to risk management, and review papers have stated that with proper management, *Legionella* can be readily controlled (5). Correctly fitted and designed drift eliminators are important in minimizing the release of bacteria in aerosol from the systems. Regular cleaning regimens and inspection and review of the cooling towers and water treatment equipment are also important aspects of a control strategy (reference 9; I. L. Maclaine-Cross and M. Behnia, letter, *Med. J. Aust.***157**:144).

Operation of cooling towers and cooling water temperature have been shown to positively correlate with concentrations of *Legionella* in cooling towers. Intermittent operation has been proposed as a common factor in many cooling tower-associated outbreaks (3).

The size and surface area-to-volume ratio of the cooling water systems are also significantly associated with risk of outbreaks. It is notable that outbreaks of Legionnaires' disease have not been associated with large cooling water systems (3).

Prevailing weather conditions such as cloud cover, ultraviolet light intensity, air temperature, and relative humidity have been shown to influence the survival and dispersion of legionellae in aerosol. In many cases, wind direction has been a major factor determining

*Richard Bentham* Department of Environmental Health, Flinders University, PO Box 2100, Adelaide, South Australia 5001. *Malcolm Pradhan* Health Informatics, University of Adelaide, Adelaide, South Australia 5000. *Paul Hakendorf* Epidemiology, Flinders Medical Centre, Bedford Park, South Australia 5042. *Peter Wilmot* GISCA, Pulteney St., Adelaide, South Australia 5000.

*Legionella*, Edited by Reinhard Marre et al.
© 2002 ASM Press, Washington, D.C.

whether significant exposure to aerosol could occur (1, 6). Climatic conditions determine how far the viable bacteria may be transmitted from the cooling tower. Air temperature and humidity may also influence operation and cooling water temperature (3).

The above criteria have all been the subject of review articles (2, 5). These factors are interrelated and combine to create a risk of multiplication and dissemination of the bacterium. These factors can be identified as risks without the need for *Legionella* culture.

A further confounding factor in predicting risk has been the identification of susceptible populations. Living in proximity to a cooling tower has been demonstrated to increase risk of sporadic cases of Legionnaires' disease (4). However, the demographic identification of susceptible populations and their proximity to cooling towers has not been addressed outside the context of nosocomial infection.

An alternative approach to reducing the incidence of *Legionella* outbreaks is to improve the assessment of risk of cooling tower colonization by the organism. We have constructed a Bayesian statistical model from historical data relating to cooling tower maintenance operation, climatic conditions, and factors contributing to *Legionella* multiplication to predict the risk of dissemination of *Legionella* from a cooling tower (Fig. 1).

This statistical model has been incorporated into a geographical information system (GIS), along with demographic data regarding the proximity of susceptible populations. The GIS used data from a register of cooling towers located in the Adelaide metropolitan area, South Australia. These data combined with wind directions and plume dispersions are used to predict cooling towers with the greatest likelihood of association with a case of Legionnaires' disease. Inputting patient movement data regarding location into the model enables ranking of the most likely cooling tower associated with a given case. In an outbreak situation, the system identifies the most likely cooling tower sources of infection after each case is entered. Using the register of cooling towers, the contact details for the owner/operator and the exact location of the system can be accessed immediately. This provides a desktop investigation system capable of locating the most likely sources of outbreaks within minutes of accessing patient data. The system may be used to investigate temporal variations in both climatic conditions and

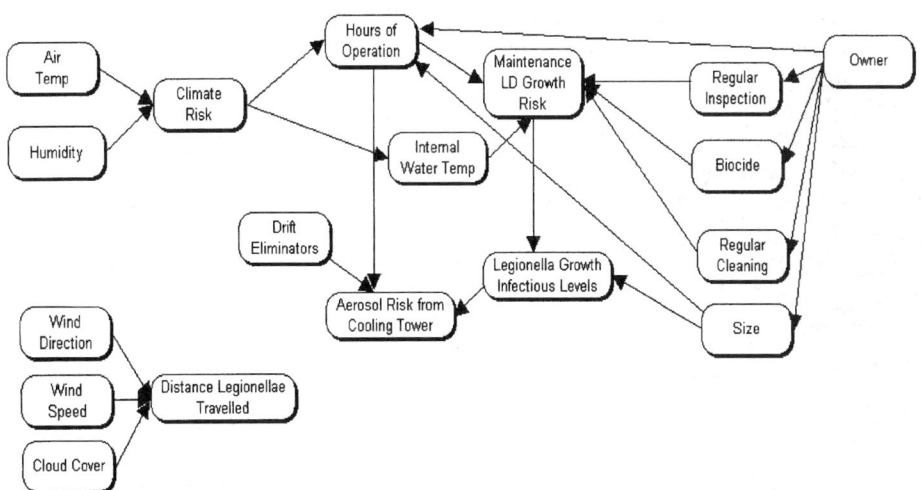

**FIGURE 1** Bayesian belief model used to establish numerical risk of dissemination of *Legionella* from cooling towers.

movements of identified cases within the incubation period.

The model could also provide a comprehensive surveillance system for cooling tower maintenance. It could be quite readily adapted to produce a web-based surveillance system Australia-wide, with access for local councils and state health departments. Routine maintenance procedures by owner/operators and water treatment personnel could be electronically reported to the system and risk assessments for each system could be made. The system provides a risk assessment on the basis of scientifically established risk factors. A cooling tower in a given location can be assessed for risk associated with Legionnaires' disease without using culture for the organism. More pertinently, the system can predict quantifiable risk on a daily basis according to climatic conditions and cooling tower specifications; it will modify risk according to system maintenance and operation characteristics.

Unreliability in *Legionella* culture is well established, and the low reliability in assessing risk from these results has probably been the reasoning behind not instituting compulsory testing. Unknowns regarding virulence within species and strains, and host immune status, further complicate culture result interpretations. We suggest that although culture may be valid as a support to a maintenance strategy, a system based on established risk factors is more functional as a surveillance, risk-assessment, and risk-management tool. The economic advantages of an interactive computer-based GIS surveillance system over routine sampling protocols and conventional outbreak investigations would be substantial.

## REFERENCES

1. **Addiss, D. G., J. P. Davis, M. LaVenture, P. J. Wand, M. A. Hutchinson, and R. M. McKinney.** 1989. Community acquired legionnaires disease associated with a cooling tower: evidence for longer distance transport of *Legionella pneumophila*. *J. Infect. Dis.* **130:**557–568.
2. **Atlas, R.M.** 1999. *Legionella*: from environmental habitats to disease pathology, detection and control. *Environ. Microbiol.* **1:**283–293.
3. **Bentham, R. H., and C. R. Broadbent.** 1993. A model for autumn outbreaks of Legionnaires' disease associated with cooling towers, linked to system operation and size. *Epidemiol. Infect.* **111:**287–295.
4. **Bhopal, R. S., R. J. Fallon, E. C. Buist, R. J. Black, and J. D. Urquhart.** 1991. Proximity of the home to a cooling tower and risk of non-outbreak Legionnaires' Disease *Br. Med. J.* **302:**378–383.
5. **Fliermans, C. B.** 1996. Ecology of *Legionella*: From data to knowledge with a little wisdom. *Microb. Ecol.* **32:**203–228.
6. **Levy, M., V. Westley-Wise, C. Blumer, M. Frommer, G. Rubin, D. Lyle, J. Brown, and G. Stewart.** 1994. Legionnaires' Disease outbreak, Fairfield 1992: public health aspects. *Aust. J. Publ. Health* **18:**137–142
7. **Miller, R. D., and K. A. Kenepp.** 1993. Risk assessments for Legionnaires disease based on routine surveillance of cooling towers for legionellae, p. 40–43. *In* J. M. Barbaree, R. F. Breiman, and A. P. Dufour (ed.), *Legionella: Current Status and Emerging Perspectives*. American Society for Microbiology, Washington, D.C.
8. **Shelton, B. G., W. D. Flanders, and G. K. Morris.** 1994. Legionnaires' disease outbreaks and cooling towers with amplified *Legionella* concentrations. *Curr. Microbiol.* **28:**359–363.
9. **Standards Australia.** 1995. *Air Handling and Water Systems of Buildings—Microbial Control*. Australia/New Zealand Standard AS/NZS 3666. Standards Australia, Sydney.

# ROUTINE SAMPLING AND TEMPORAL VARIATION OF *LEGIONELLA* CONCENTRATIONS IN COOLING TOWER WATER SYSTEMS

*Richard H. Bentham*

# 64

The routine monitoring of *Legionella* counts and total bacterial counts in cooling water systems is commonly used as a risk-assessment strategy for the potential for Legionnaires' disease outbreaks (9). To date, risk assessments have not encompassed the factors contributing to elevated counts in the systems, such as season, sporadic operation, surface area:volume ratio of the system, system size, the presence of gymnamoebae, and system water temperature (1, 2, 5, 6).

Previous studies have attempted to provide guidelines for risk assessment using samples from large numbers of cooling towers taken at a single point in time (8, 9). This chapter presents biweekly sample data from 28 small cooling towers colonized by *Legionella* over a 4-month summer period. These data were used to appraise the validity of risk assessments on the basis of routine *Legionella* sampling and to investigate the temporal variation in concentrations of *Legionella* bacteria in cooling towers.

All the cooling towers were maintained to comply with the Australian Standard AS 3666:

1989 (11), including weekly water treatment chemical dosage. The towers were all located within a 2-km radius in South Australia and received the same reticulated water supply. Samples were cultured for *Legionella* by using established methods (3, 4).

Median *Legionella* concentrations and ranges were calculated for each cooling tower. Data sets were excluded when towers had been subjected to variations in their maintenance regimes and when data sets contained <15 samples. For these 28 data sets, time series correlograms were prepared using SPSS for Windows version 6.1.3. (SPSS Inc.). From the correlograms, the sampling period after which consecutive samples were significantly correlated was determined for each cooling water system. These results were collated to identify the sampling intervals after which there was correlation between consecutive *Legionella* counts.

The median *Legionella* counts and ranges are presented in Fig. 1. Grouping the median values into categories shows that the majority of median *Legionella* counts were less than 100 CFU/ml for the summer period (Fig. 2). The median for the majority of the systems (17 of 28) was below the detection limits (4 CFU/ml). The maxima for all of the systems were greater than 100 CFU/ml, and in a significant

*Richard H. Bentham*   Department of Environmental Health, Flinders University of South Australia, PO Box 2100, Adelaide, South Australia 5001.

*Legionella*, Edited by Reinhard Marre et al.
© 2002 ASM Press, Washington, D.C.

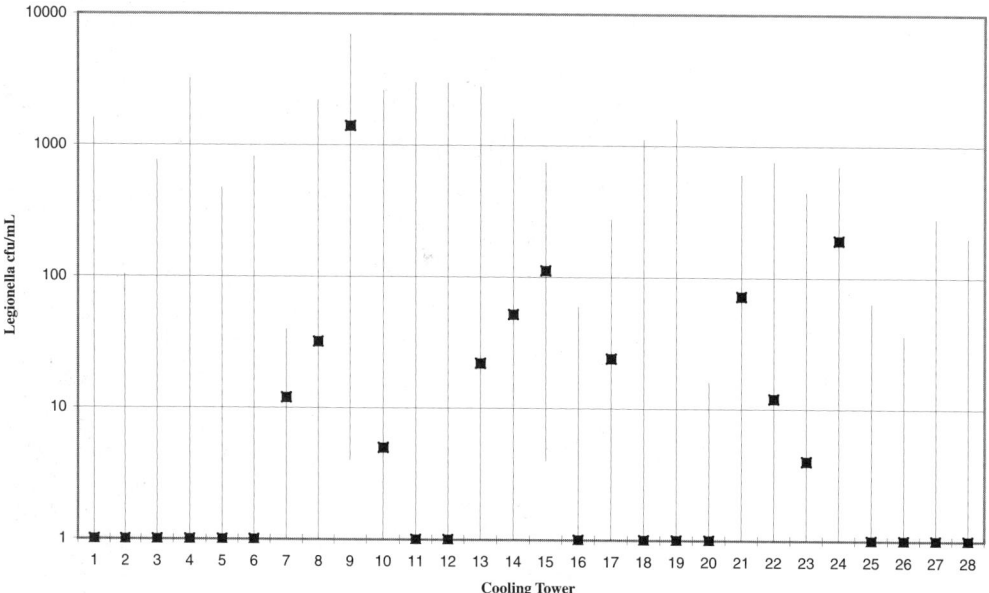

**FIGURE 1**   Median *Legionella* concentrations and ranges in cooling water systems over a 4-month summer period.

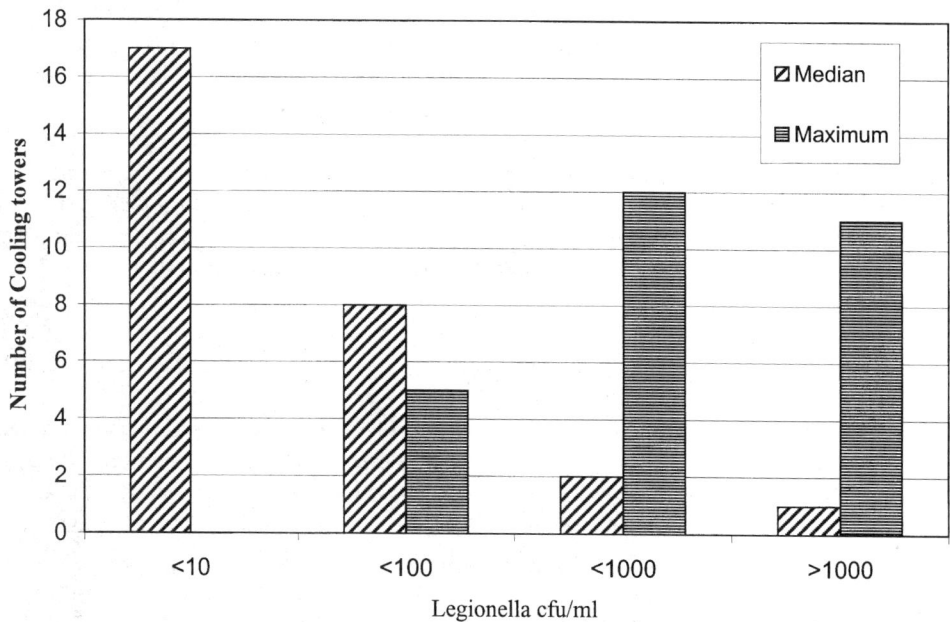

**FIGURE 2**   Number of cooling towers with median and maximum *Legionella* counts in defined ranges.

number of systems (11 of 28), they were greater than 1,000 CFU/ml.

Risk assessment based on the median *Legionella* count showed only three systems to be in the high-risk category. However, the ranges showed that during this period, 23 systems were within this category at least once at some point during the summer. Conversely, all of the systems would not have been considered a risk at some point during this same period. The correlogram results showed that in the majority (17 of 28) of cooling towers, the results of samples taken from the same cooling system less than a week apart from each other were statistically unrelated (Fig. 3). That is, before the culture result could be determined in the laboratory, it was no longer correlated to the system it came from.

After 2 weeks, 25 of 28 of the cooling tower sampling results were unrelated to the original result. Only one sample gave results that were still statistically correlated after seven samples (3½ weeks). There was no correlation

between samples taken 4 weeks apart in any of the 28 systems.

The majority (25 of 28) of cooling systems included in this study had median counts of less than 100 CFU/ml. The relatively low median concentrations and large ranges of the majority of cooling towers suggest that high concentrations of *Legionella* in cooling systems is an infrequent occurrence in these systems. This result agrees closely with a previous report that the majority of cooling systems randomly sampled had *Legionella* counts below 100 CFU/ml (10). The medians from the towers sampled in this study suggested that in most instances, single samples are likely to record a low or undetected result.

Assessment of the risk of Legionnaires' disease outbreaks based solely on counts of *Legionella* may be misleading. This study has demonstrated that *Legionella* concentrations in cooling towers are commonly in what would be accepted as low-moderate risk ranges (8, 9). In most systems, concentrations rise occa-

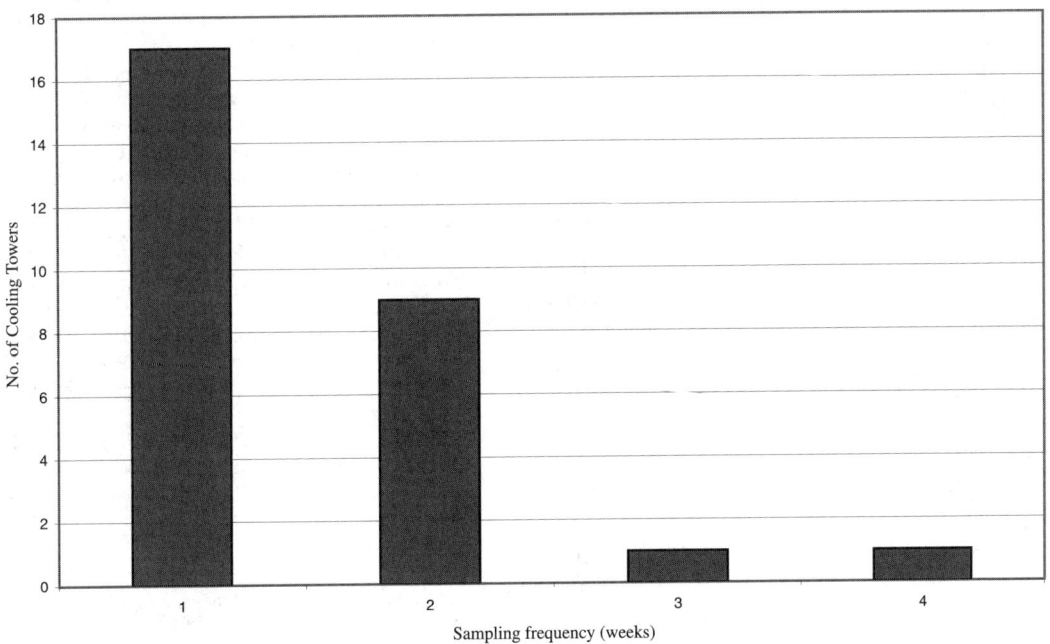

**FIGURE 3** Number of cooling towers at each sampling interval at which there was correlation between consecutive *Legionella* culture results.

sionally to high-risk ranges in response to environmental and operational influences in the system. This suggests that meaningful risk assessments using *Legionella* concentrations should be made only in the light of extended data collection and interpretation. Risk assessments based on single or limited *Legionella* test results from a tower are likely to underestimate or overestimate the risk associated with that tower. The detection of low numbers of *Legionella* in a cooling system after a single sample does not correlate to a low risk.

The time series data analyses demonstrated that in most of the systems, culture results once available gave no indication of the system status. It is highly unlikely that monthly sampling of cooling tower waters will provide data that accurately represents the microbial status of the system. Previous work related to this study has already demonstrated that *Legionella* concentrations in cooling waters are not normally distributed (1). Current action directives based on *Legionella* concentrations assume that sampling regimes are both representative and drawn from a normally distributed population; neither of these assumptions is valid.

The validity of risk assessments based on *Legionella* culture results is further compromised by factors such as the species, strain, virulence, system location, demography of the surrounding population, operating conditions, and variability in culture results between laboratories and samples (1, 7, 9, 10). *Legionella* can be readily controlled in cooling systems (7, 10). The factors contributing to successful control of the bacteria are well established, and to some extent generic, although individual systems are almost always unique in some aspect. Risk assessment of cooling towers for *Legionella* dissemination should be focused upon these established and quantifiable criteria. The role of *Legionella* culture in determining risk should be subordinate, due to the absence of a quantifiable relationship between culture results, system status, and dose response.

## REFERENCES

1. **Bentham, R. H.** 1993. Environmental factors affecting the colonization of cooling towers by *Legionella* spp. in South Australia. *Int. Biodeterior. Biodegrad.* **31:**55–63.
2. **Bhopal, R. S., and R. J. Fallon.** 1991. Seasonal variation of Legionnaires' disease in Scotland. *J. Infect.* **22:**2378–2383.
3. **Dennis, P. J.** 1988. Isolation of *Legionellae* from environmental specimens, p. 31–172. *In* T. G. Harrison and A. G. Taylor (ed.), *Laboratory Manual for Legionella.* John Wiley, London, United Kingdom.
4. **Edelstein, P. H.** 1984. *Legionnaires' Disease Laboratory Manual.* Report no. VAWMC/LD-84/1. Veterans Administration, Wadsworth Medical Centre.
5. **Fields, B. S., G. N. Sanden, J. M. Barbaree, W. E. Morrill, R. M. Wadowsky, E. H. White, and J. C. Feeley.** 1989. Intracellular multiplication of *Legionella pneumophila* in amoebae isolated from hospital hot water tanks. *Curr. Microbiol.* **18:**131–137.
6. **Fliermans, C. B., R. J. Soracco, and D. H. Pope.** 1981. Measure of *L. pneumophila* activity in situ. *Curr. Microbiol.* **6:**89–94.
7. **Fliermans, C. B.** 1996. Ecology of *Legionella*: from data to knowledge with a little wisdom. *Microb. Ecol.* **32:**203–228.
8. **Miller, R. D., and K. A. Kenepp.** 1993. Risk assessments for Legionnaires' disease based on routine surveillance of cooling towers for legionellae, p. 40–43. *In* J. M. Barbaree, R. F. Breiman, and A. P. Dufour (ed.), *Legionella: Current Status and Emerging Perspectives.* American Society for Microbiology, Washington, D.C.
9. **Shelton, B. G., G. K. Morris, and G. W. Gorman.** 1993. Reducing risks associated with *Legionella* bacteria in building water systems, p. 279–281. *In* J. M. Barbaree, R. F. Breiman, and A. P. Dufour (ed.), *Legionella: Current Status and Emerging Perspectives.* American Society for Microbiology, Washington, D.C.
10. **Shelton, B. G., W. D. Flanders, and G. K. Morris.** 1994. Legionnaires' disease outbreaks and cooling towers with amplified *Legionella* concentrations. *Curr. Microbiol.* **28:**359–363.
11. **Standards Australia.** 1989. *Air Handling and Water Systems of Buildings—Microbial Control.* Australian Standard A3666. Standards Australia, Sydney.

# PREVALENCE OF POSITIVE ANTIBODY TITERS AGAINST LEGIONELLAE IN TWO RESIDENTIAL POPULATIONS WITH DIFFERENT *LEGIONELLA* CONTAMINATIONS IN THEIR HOT WATER SYSTEMS

*Ursel Heudorf, Wolfgang Hentschel, Martin Hoffmann,*
*Christian Lück, and Ralph Schubert*

# 65

In Germany, only a few epidemiological studies on *Legionella* diseases are available, and studies on the prevalence of *Legionella* antibody response in the population are scarce (5, 7). We report on an epidemiological study on the immune responses of residents in homes with heavy and with minor *Legionella* contaminations in their hot water systems. In one of the two residential areas with a central hot water system, *Legionella* contamination of up to 1 million CFU/liter had been known for several years. Due to several redevelopment measures, *Legionella* contamination could be reduced, although it is still elevated. In the other residential area, decentralized hot water systems were installed in all houses so that no *Legionella* problem would be assumed. There were two questions to be answered in our investigation:

- Are there different prevalences of *Legionella* antibodies in the two populations with

heavy and with minor *Legionella* contamination in their hot water systems?

- Are there hints for diseases possibly caused by *Legionella*, like pneumonia, other lung diseases, or infectious fevers in the anamnesis in correlation with *Legionella* contamination in their hot water systems or with their *Legionella* antibodies?

## PARTICIPANTS AND METHODS

The inhabitants of the two housing areas were informed by leaflets on the aims of the study. Participation was voluntary, and the criteria for inclusion were age >18 years and having moved into this housing area at least 2 years ago.

In the control area, a total of 92 persons (mean age ± standard deviation, 57.5 ± 14.8 years; range, 18 to 82 years), and in the exposed housing area, 53 persons (mean age, 55.5 ± 16.4 years; range, 20 to 79 years) took part in this investigation. They were asked by questionnaire for their smoking habits, showering habits, chronic diseases such as diabetes and immune disease, and moreover for pneumonia, other lung disease (i.e., bronchitis, asthma), and infectious fever (such as Pontiac fever) during the last 8 weeks, 6 months, or 1 year.

*Ursel Heudorf, Wolfgang Hentschel, and Martin Hoffmann* Public Health Department, Braubachstr. 18-22, D-60311 Frankfurt, Germany.    *Christian Lück* National Reference Center for Legionella, Institute of Medical Microbiology and Hygiene, University Dresden, Fiedlerstr. 42, D-01307 Dresden, Germany.    *Ralph Schubert* Institut für Hygiene, University Frankfurt/M, Paul Ehrlichstr. 24, D-60596 Frankfurt, Germany.

*Legionella*, Edited by Reinhard Marre et al.
© 2002 ASM Press, Washington, D.C.

Water samples of the hot water system were taken from the flats of all of the participants and were analyzed for *Legionella pneumophila* serogroups 1 to 14 by membrane filtration and culture, and differentiation was done according to the recommendations of the German Federal Health Administration (1, 4). Serum specimens were tested for IgG antibodies by an indirect immunofluorescence test for detecting antibodies against *L. pneumophila* serogroups 1 to 14, *L. micdadei*, *L. bozemanii*, *L. dumoffii*, *L. jordanis*, and *L. longbeachae* serogroups 1 and 2 (National Reference Centre for Legionella, Dresden, Germany) (5, 6). Moreover, serum samples were tested for IgG and IgM antibodies against *L. pneumophila* serogroups 1 to 6 by enzyme-linked immunosorbent assay (ELISA) according to the manufacturer's instructions (Virion Serion GmbH, Würzburg, Germany). Urine samples were analyzed for antigen of *L. pneumophila* serogroup 1 by an immunographic method according to the criteria of the manufacturer (Binax NOW TM, Binax Diagnostics, München, Germany).

## RESULTS

Exposed and control persons did not differ in their sex, age, smoking and showering habits, and prevalence of diabetes and immune disease (Table 1). The 1-year prevalences for pneumonia, other lung disease, or infectious fever were about twice as high in the exposed versus the control persons (Table 2); differences were significant for other lung diseases (odds ratio [OR], 2.4; 95% confidence interval [95% CI], 1.04 to 5.54) and infectious fever (OR, 2.5; 95% CI, 1.25 to 5.38), but not for pneumonia (OR, 1.78; 95% CI, 0.35 to 9.15).

*Legionella* contaminations in their own hot water systems were significantly different: controls, 244 ± 1,434 CFU/liter, range of 0 to 11,700 CFU/liter; exposed, 6,049 ± 17,995 CFU/liter, range of 0 to 80,000 CFU/liter (for distribution, see Table 3). *Legionella* IgM in serum and *Legionella* antigen in urine specimens were not detectable in any partici-

pant. The prevalence of legionella IgG in serum (borderline and positive) was twice as high in the exposed versus the control persons. The differences were not significant (IgG NRC, Dresden, OR, 1.91; 95% CI, 0.74 to 4.94; IgG Virion, Würzburg, OR, 1.81; 95% CI, 0.50 to 6.58) (Table 3).

IgG antibodies of the following species were detected by immunofluorescence (numbers): *L. pneumophila* serogroups 1 to 7 (6), *L. micdadei* (6), *L. bozmanii* (5), *L. jordanis* (5), *L. dumoffii* (4), *L. longbeachae* (3).

CFU/liter in the hot water system was significantly correlated with the exposure group and with the *L. pneumophila* IgG antibodies of the participants, analyzed by ELISA or immunofluorescence method. Correlations between CFU/liter and IgG *Legionella* antibodies including other species than *L. pneumophila* failed to reach significancy; this was true for anamnestic data for pneumonia, other lung diseases, and infectious fevers.

## DISCUSSION

Prevalence of positive and/or borderline antibody titers of different *Legionella* species analyzed by immunofluorescence were 19% in the exposed and 11% in the control group, indicating former contact with *Legionella* species. Prevalence of positive and/or borderline antibody titers of *L. pneumophila* only, analyzed by ELISA (Virion), were 9% in the exposed and 6% in the control group.

Using the criterion of antibody titer of 1: 128 (immunofluorescence), 1.9% of the exposed and 1.1% of the control persons exhibited positive antibody titers against *L. pneumophila* serogroups 1 to 14, and 7.5% of the exposed and 6.5% of the control persons had positive antibody titers against *Legionella* species in total. These data may be readily compared with other epidemiological data and analyzed in the same laboratory (National Reference Center, Dresden, Germany) using identical methods. In Dresden, in 3.3% of 602 healthy inhabitants, positive IgG antibodies against *L. pneumophila* serogroups 1 to 6 were detected, and in 7%, positive antibodies

**TABLE 1** Description of study participants according to their sex, age, smoking and showering habits, and diseases such as diabetes and immune diseases[a]

| Parameter | Control group (n = 92) | | Exposed group (n = 53) | |
|---|---|---|---|---|
| | n | % | n | % |
| Sex | | | | |
| Male | 45 | 48.9 | 15 | 28.3 |
| Female | 47 | 51.1 | 38 | 71.7 |
| Age group | 91 | | 53 | |
| <40 years | 12 | 13.2 | 13 | 24.5 |
| 40–49 years | 12 | 13.2 | 4 | 7.5 |
| 50–59 years | 23 | 25.2 | 14 | 26.4 |
| 60–69 years | 22 | 24.2 | 8 | 15.2 |
| 70–79 years | 20 | 22.0 | 14 | 26.4 |
| ≥80 years | 2 | 2.2 | 0 | 0.0 |
| Nonsmoker | 82 | 89.1 | 43 | 81.1 |
| Smoker | 10 | 10.9 | 10 | 18.9 |
| <10 cigarettes/day | 2 | 2.2 | 1 | 1.9 |
| 10–<20 cigarettes/day | 2 | 2.2 | 3 | 5.7 |
| ≥20 cigarettes/day | 6 | 6.5 | 6 | 11.3 |
| Chronic diseases | | | | |
| Diabetes | 6 | 6.5 | 2 | 3.8 |
| Immune disease | 1 | 1.1 | 0 | 0 |
| Shower at home/week | | | | |
| Never | 9 | 9.8 | 7 | 13.2 |
| 1–4 | 40 | 43.4 | 24 | 45.3 |
| ≥5 | 43 | 46.8 | 22 | 41.5 |

[a] There were no significant differences in any of the parameters between the control and the exposed group.

**TABLE 2** Pneumonia, other lung disease, and infectious fever in control and exposed persons

| Parameter | Control group (n = 92) | | Exposed group (n = 53) | |
|---|---|---|---|---|
| | n | % | n | % |
| Pneumonia | | | | |
| Up to 8 weeks ago | 1 | 1.1 | 0 | 0 |
| Up to 6 months ago | 3 | 3.3 | 0 | 0 |
| Up to 1 year ago | 3 | 3.3 | 3 | 5.7 |
| Other lung disease | | | | |
| Up to 8 weeks ago | 7 | 7.6 | 8 | 15.1 |
| Up to 6 months ago | 9 | 9.8 | 9 | 17.0 |
| Up to 1 year ago | 13 | 14.1 | 15 | 28.3 |
| Infectious fever | | | | |
| Up to 8 weeks ago | 6 | 6.5 | 10 | 18.9 |
| Up to 6 months ago | 8 | 8.7 | 15 | 28.3 |
| Up to 1 year ago | 21 | 22.8 | 23 | 43.4 |

**TABLE 3** *Legionella* in home hot water systems, *Legionella* antibodies in serum, and *Legionella* antigen in urine specimen of control and exposed persons

| Parameter | Control group (n = 92) | | Exposed group (n = 53) | |
|---|---|---|---|---|
| | n | % | n | % |
| *Legionella* in hot water CFU/liter | | | | |
| 0 | 87 | 94.6 | 19 | 36.5 |
| 1–999 | 2 | 2.2 | 12 | 23.1 |
| 1,000–9,999 | 2 | 2.2 | 16 | 30.8 |
| ≥10,000 | 1 | 1.1 | 5 | 9.6 |
| IgG (National Reference Center) | | | | |
| Negative | 82 | 89.1 | 43 | 81.1 |
| Borderline (1:64) | 4 | 4.3 | 6 | 11.3 |
| Positive | 6 | 6.6 | 4 | 7.6 |
| IgG (National Reference Center), *L. pneumophila* only | | | | |
| Negative | 90 | 97.8 | 50 | 94.3 |
| Borderline (1:64) | 1 | 1.1 | 2 | 3.8 |
| Positive | 1 | 1.1 | 1 | 1.9 |
| IgG (Virion) | | | | |
| Negative | 87 | 94.6 | 48 | 90.6 |
| Borderline | 2 | 2.2 | 1 | 1.9 |
| Positive | 3 | 3.3 | 4 | 7.5 |
| IgM (Virion) | | | | |
| Negative | 92 | 100 | 53 | 100 |
| Borderline | 0 | 0 | 0 | 0 |
| Positive | 0 | 0 | 0 | 0 |
| *Legionella* antigen in urine | | | | |
| Negative | 92 | 100 | 53 | 100 |
| Positive | 0 | 0 | 0 | 0 |

against *Legionella* species were found. In Eberswalde, a small city near Berlin, the prevalences of positive antibody titers in 246 healthy inhabitants were 10.2% in the exposed group and 13.4% in the control group. In our investigation the participants exposed to heavy *Legionella* contamination in their hot water systems at home had higher antibody titers against *Legionella* than participants living in the control area. Prevalence of antibody titers (≥1:128) was not elevated in our study groups, compared with healthy persons from other regions in Germany (5). Similar results were reported from other geographical areas (2, 3, 8).

Though high *Legionella* contamination in the hot water system of the exposed area in Frankfurt had been known for up to 10 years, no cases of legionellosis had been reported from inhabitants of this area during this investigation. Anamnestic 1-year prevalence of pneumonia, other lung diseases, and infectious fevers, however, were twice as high in the exposed versus the control participants.

In summary, only one out of the six persons who stated that they suffered from pneumonia during the previous year had been treated with an antibiotic, indicating that this was the only real pneumonia. This participant—a control person—had suffered from pulmonary problems during a holiday stay abroad about 4 months before our investigation. At that time he obviously had acquired a *Legionella* pneumonia; his recent IgG antibody titer (*L. pneumophila* serogroup 1) still was 1:1024.

Only 1 out of 13 controls and 1 out of 15 exposed persons (<10%) with "other lung diseases" in their anamneses exhibited positive and borderline IgG antibodies, irrespective of the exposure to *Legionella* in their hot water system at home. In persons with infectious fever in their anamnesis, higher prevalence of IgG antibodies in the exposed versus the control group (17.3 vs. 9.5%, respectively, immunofluorescence method) was to be found, which may indicate *Legionella* causation.

In the whole group, no correlations were found between serum antibodies and anamnestic diseases. Except for the one person with obvious *Legionella* pneumonia caught during a holiday stay abroad, positive antibodies in the other persons were most likely the result of infectious fever (i.e., Pontiac fever) or asymptomatic infections (probably caused by permanent exposure to *Legionella* in their home hot water supply).

Even though no legionellosis (pneumonia) was reported in the population exposed to *Legionella* at home, we conclude that the necessity to control and to reduce *Legionella* contamination in home hot water systems is supported by our data, not only because of the higher antibody titers in the exposed vs. the nonexposed group but also because of the significant correlations of antibody titers of the participants with the *Legionella* contamination in their hot water systems.

## REFERENCES

1. **Anonymous.** 1993. Mitteilungen des Bundesgesundheitsamtes über den Nachweis von Legionellen im erwärmten Trinkwasser. *Bundesgesundheitsblatt,* p. 162.
2. **Boldur, I., M. Ergaz, G. Mor, R. Kazak, A. Pik, and D. Sompolinsky.** 1986. Exposure to Legionella in geriatric institutions. *Isr. J. Med. Sci.* **22:**728–732.
3. **Bornstein, N., D. Marmet, M. Surgot, M. Nowicki, A. Arslan, J. Esteve, and J. Fleurette.** 1989. Exposure to Legionellaceae at a hot spring spa: a prospective clinical and serological study. *Epidemiol. Infect.* **102:**31–36.
4. **Helbig, J. H., J. B. Kurtz, M. C. Pastoris, C. Pelaz, and P. C. Lück.** 1997. Antigenic lipopolysaccharide components of *Legionella pneumophila* recognized by monoclonal antibodies: possibilities and limitations for division of the species into serogroups. *J. Clin. Microbiol.* **35:**2841–2845.
5. **Lück, P. C., and J. H. Helbig.** 1993. Zur Epidemiologie der Legionellosen, p. 41–58. *In Schriftenreihe des Vereins für Wasser-, Boden- und Lufthygiene, 91.* Gustav Fischer Verlag, Stuttgart, Germany.
6. **Maiwald, M., J. H. Helbig, and P. C. Lück.** 1998. Laboratory methods for the diagnosis of Legionella infections. *J. Microb. Methods* **33:**59–79.
7. **Müller, H. E.** 1983. Antibodies against Legionellaceae in the population of West Germany and their methodical determination. *Zentralbl. Bakt. Hyg. A* **255:**84–90.
8. **Rocha, G., A. Verissimo, R. Bowker, N. Bornstein, and M. S. Da Costa.** 1995. Relationship between Legionella spp. and antibody titres at a therapeutic thermal spa in Portugal. *Epidemiol. Infect.* **155:**79–88.

# LEGIONELLOSIS IN SWEDEN

*Birgitta de Jong*

## 66

A voluntary, laboratory-based reporting system of legionellosis was initiated in Sweden in 1981 and became compulsory in January 1996. According to the Swedish Act for Communicable Diseases, clinicians have to report all diagnosed cases of legionellosis since 1 July 1989. A case is defined as a person who has a clinical diagnosis of pneumonia; preferably, the diagnosis is confirmed by a laboratory test, i.e., isolation of an organism, seroconversion (a fourfold or greater rise), or antigen detection in urine. The latter is now the most commonly used method. Reports from the clinics state where (town or country) the patient contracted the disease and other relevant epidemiological data. These reports are compiled by the Swedish Institute for Infectious Disease Control, which is responsible for the national surveillance of legionellosis in Sweden.

## EPIDEMIOLOGY OF LEGIONELLOSIS

About 50 to 100 persons are reported each year through the two different reporting systems (Table 1). The incidence rate for reported cases of legionellosis during 1995 to 1999 ranged from 0.57 to 1.15 per 100,000 inhabitants. An estimation of sources of infection indicates that about one-third of the cases had a domestic, community-acquired infection and another third contracted legionellosis during travel abroad. Each year, nosocomial cases are recorded. The age and gender of reported cases are shown in Fig. 1. Male patients accounted for 73% of all cases. During 1995 to 1999, 16% of all cases, with a known date of onset of disease, became ill during the month of September and about 10% for each month of May, June, July, and October (Fig. 2).

## OUTBREAKS OF LEGIONELLOSIS IN SWEDEN

The first recognized indigenous outbreak of legionellosis in Sweden occurred as early as 1979, when 58 persons contracted legionellosis at an indoor shopping center in a medium-sized Swedish town. The cooling tower on the roof of the shopping center was the source of the outbreak (4).

The second largest indigenous outbreak occurred in 1991. It was a nosocomial outbreak, with 29 patients infected from the showers at a hospital. Also in 1997, a nosocomial outbreak occurred in another hospital with at least 10 infected patients. This last hospital had

*Birgitta de Jong*   Department of Epidemiology, Swedish Institute for Infectious Disease Control, SE-171 82 Solna, Sweden.

**TABLE 1** Number of cases reported from the different systems and where the infection was acquired

| Year | No. of: | | | | | |
| | Clinical reports | Laboratory reports | Reported cases | Cases infected abroad | Community-acquired cases | Nosocomial cases |
| --- | --- | --- | --- | --- | --- | --- |
| 1995 | 44 | 36 | 52 | 26 | 14 | 1 |
| 1996 | 55 | 47 | 72 | 34 | 23 | 5 |
| 1997 | 87 | 67 | 104 | 30 | 31 | 17 |
| 1998 | 70 | 73 | 85 | 29 | 39 | 5 |
| 1999 | 67 | 74 | 90 | 23 | 52 | 4 |

the tap water mixed at a temperature of 40°C in the basement of the building, which was subsequently distributed to the whole building (2).

In 1999, 20 persons were reported to have acquired Pontiac fever from whirlpools at a hotel in northern Sweden. The water in the whirlpools was not automatically disinfected and no log sheets about maintenance or addition of disinfectants were available. No bacteria were isolated from the pools, but the epidemiological investigation showed that the whirlpools were the source of infection (3). Other minor nosocomial outbreaks have also occurred.

## OUTBREAKS OF LEGIONELLOSIS OUTSIDE OF SWEDEN INVOLVING SWEDISH TOURISTS

The Swedes are a travelling people, and that can explain the high number of cases of *Legionella* infection acquired abroad. The information is reported to the European Working Group for *Legionella* Infections (EWGLI) database. EWGLI runs the European surveillance scheme for travel-associated Legionnaires' disease and is funded by European Union Directorate General V. An estimated number of two million Swedes travel abroad on package tours each year.

Five persons received treatment against legionellosis at a hospital after a weekend trip to Paris in 1988. In 1990, several Nordic tourists including 13 Swedes were reported to have contracted legionellosis during a visit to Ma-

jorca. At least 20 Swedish tourists had shown symptoms of legionellosis. The disease was acquired in a newly built hotel, which had a temperature of 40 to 45°C in its hot water distribution system from which *Legionella* was isolated (1).

Several persons in a group of bridge players, who went to Kusadasi in Turkey in 1996, also contracted legionellosis. People of other nationalities were also affected in this outbreak. This hotel had had guests with Legionnaires' disease before; EWGLI had sent out reports of clusters of *Legionella* cases staying at the hotel both in 1994 and 1995.

## PREVENTING LEGIONNAIRES' DISEASE IN SWEDEN

During the last years, different channels have been used to inform landlords and their agents on how to avoid the growth of *Legionella* bacteria in the water distribution systems of their apartment buildings.

An informative brochure has been produced by the National Board of Housing, Building and Planning. It contains facts about the *Legionella* bacteria and advises on how to keep the hot water distribution system free from the bacterium. Legionnaires' disease is called an "unnecessary" disease in this brochure. The brochure is distributed free of charge to all interested persons.

In magazines for owners and managers of apartment buildings, several articles have been written about *Legionella* bacteria and Legion-

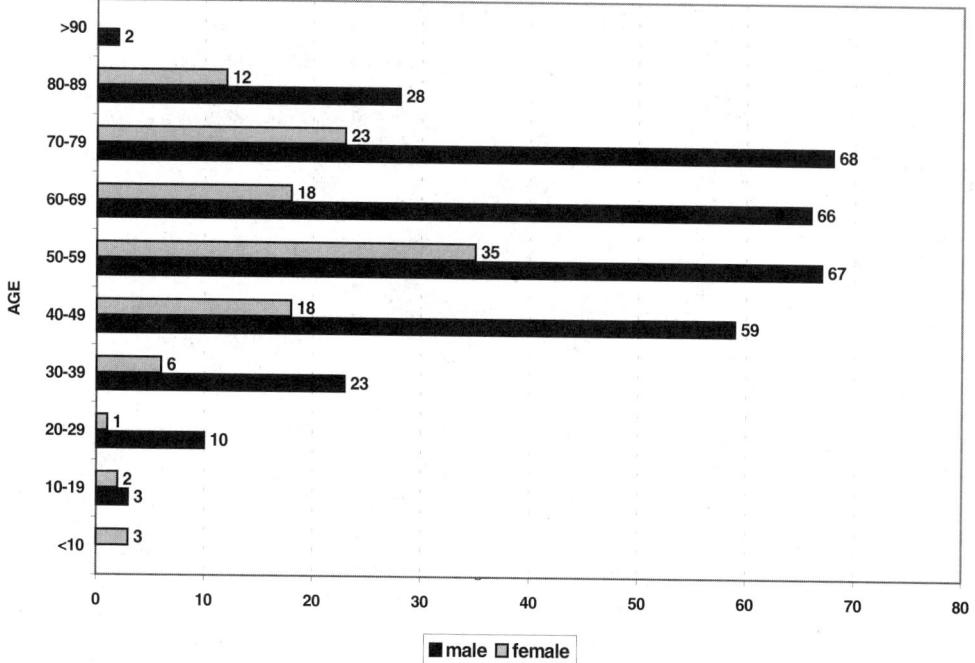

**FIGURE 1** Age and gender for reported cases of legionellosis in Sweden, 1995–1999.

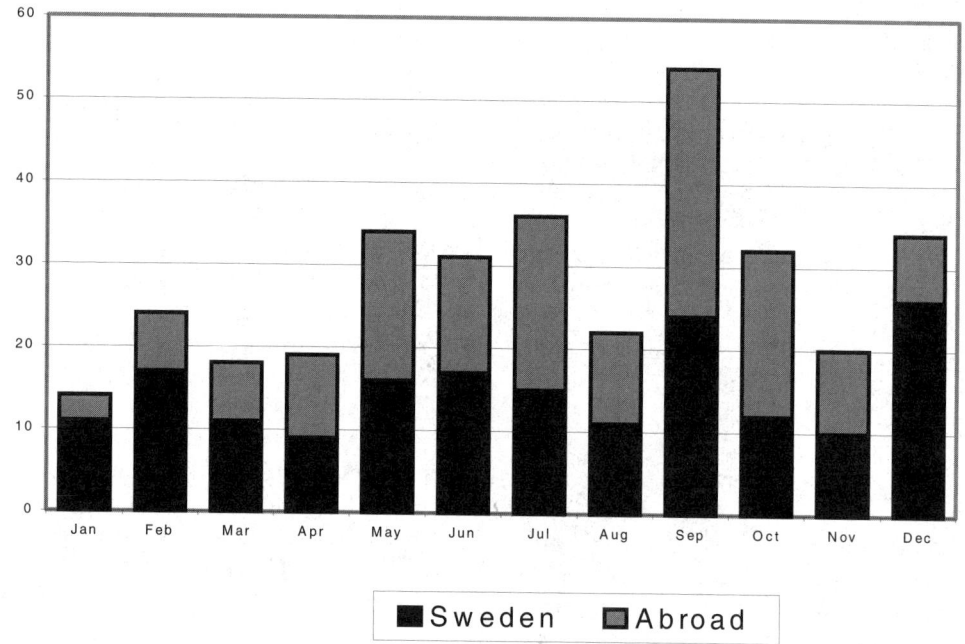

**FIGURE 2** Month of onset of disease and place of acquisition for reported cases of legionellosis in Sweden, 1995–1999.

naires' disease. These recommendations have been presented in several checklists.

## REFERENCES

1. **Anonymous.** 1990. Legionärsjukan, Mallorca. *EpidAktuellt* **6:**9–10. (In Swedish.)
2. **de Jong, B.** 1997. Ökning av anmälda fall av legionärsjuka. *Smittskydd* **12:**115–116. (In Swedish.)
3. **Götz, H. M., A. Tegnell, B. de Jong, K. A. Broholm, M. Kuusi, I. Kallings, and K. Ekdahl.** 2001. Whirlpool associated outbreak of Pontiac fever at a hotel in Northern Sweden. *Epidemiol. Infect.* **126:**241–247.
4. **Nordström, K., I. Kallings, H. Dahnsjö, and F. Clemens.** 1983. An outbreak of Legionnaires' Disease in Sweden: report of sixty-eight cases. *Scand. J. Infect. Dis.* **15:**43–55.

# RISK OF EXPOSURE IN HOSPITALS COLONIZED WITH LEGIONELLAE

*M. Spalekova and S. Bazovska*

# 67

The incidence of Legionnaires' disease in Slovakia is low (0.2/million people), though underestimated; only a few sporadic cases have been documented. The disease identification tests are not in routine use in our country. Therefore, there is no evidence of any confirmed nosocomial cases.

The present study focused on an investigation of a potable water system for *Legionella* contamination and an evaluation of the risk of possible exposure, reflecting seroreactivity or even infection of nosocomial origin in patients of the hospital, where laboratory diagnostic tests for *Legionella* infection are not performed.

The study was undertaken in two periods. During the first (1995 to 1997), epidemiological investigations included an attempt to isolate legionellae from water samples in the hospital. In the second period (1997 to 1999), an evaluation of seroreactivity in patients hospitalized for a longer period in the colonized block was performed.

The approximately 400-bed hospital that we examined consisted of nine monoblocks (designated F, A, G, P1, R, B, D, S, and P3)

supplied mostly from the central water tank (except P3). Water samples were taken from the distribution system (including swabs from shower heads, from faucets in patients' rooms, from dental syringe lines, etc.) and from hot water tanks (central and P3). The samples were cultivated with and without acid wash pretreatment on buffered charcoal-yeast extract agar (BCYE), GVPC (BCYE with glycine, vancomycin, polymyxin B, and cycloheximide), and MWY (BCYE with vancomycin, polymyxin, and anisomycin) media. Investigations of legionellae colonization of potable water in the wards and hot water storages performed from 1995 to 1997 revealed contamination in more than 30%. Completing the sampling of water from the block A and central tank in the next 2 years revealed 30.7% overall contamination with legionellae (Table 1). All of the blocks except the rehabilitation monoblock (R) were colonized; the positivity ranged from 15 to 62.5%. The most heavily colonized blocks were P1 (medical ward), S (stomatologic unit), D (pediatric ward), A (patients suffering from tuberculosis or oncological pulmonary diseases), and F (surgical ward, intensive-care unit). The mean colonization of block A was 35% in the 5-year period. The quantitative contamination of the water distribution system was $10^4$ to $10^7$ CFU/liter and

*M. Spalekova and S. Bazovska* Institute of Epidemiology, School of Medicine, Comenius University, Spitalska 24, Bratislava 811 08, Slovak Republic.

*Legionella*, Edited by Reinhard Marre et al.
© 2002 ASM Press, Washington, D.C.

**TABLE 1** *Legionella* contamination of the hospital water system, 1995 to 1999

| Blocks/tanks[a] | No. of water samples | | % Positivity |
| --- | --- | --- | --- |
| | Total | Positive | |
| F block | 124 | 31 | 25.0 |
| A block | 80 | 28 | 35.0 |
| G block | 40 | 6 | 15.0 |
| P1 block | 40 | 25 | 62.5 |
| R block | 35 | 0 | 0 |
| B block | 27 | 8 | 29.6 |
| D block | 20 | 8 | 40.0 |
| S block | 16 | 7 | 43.8 |
| P3 block | 41 | 16 | 39.0 |
| Total | 423 | 129 | 30.5 |
| Central tank | 8 | 3 | 37.5 |
| P3 tank | 2 | 1 | 50.0 |
| Total | 433 | 133 | 30.7 |

[a] All the blocks besides P3 are supplied from the central water tank. Investigation of seroreactivity of inpatients from block A was done.

was supported by the presence of legionellae in water from central and P3 tanks.

Biological, chemical, and routine microbiological analyses of water from outlets (blocks A, P3, and F) and from both hot water storages revealed that water from all sites met the standard criteria for tap water except for the presence of a very low level of free chlorine in all of them. Tested water from faucets showed a low iron content, whereas in the tank supplying the P3 block, a higher concentration of iron might have supported legionellae growth.

Identification of isolates performed by serotyping with polyclonal immune rabbit sera using microagglutination, indirect fluorescent-antibody assays, and latex agglutination tests (Oxoid) showed contamination of the drinking water system with *Legionella pneumophila* species. The most frequent isolates were *L. pneumophila* serogroup 10 (49, 6%), followed by serogroups 5 and 6 (Table 2). Block A was colonized with strains of *L. pneumophila* serogroups 10, 5, 9, and 6, and with isolates that could not be distinguished by available serotyping, identified as *L. pneumophila* serogroups 5 and 10. Contamination was supported by legionellae surviving in the central tank, pro-

moted by the nonadequate maintainance of the tank, especially in a temperature regimen (50 to 52°C) and hypochlorination.

To assess the risk of exposure to contaminated tap water for inpatients, we did a serosurvey for antibodies in patients submitted to a normal treatment regimen from block A, colonized with legionellae in 20 to 45% from 1995 to 1999 (Table 3). Paired sera from 64 inpatients, 25 to 87 years old (41 males, 23 females), were collected for 8 to 43 days (mean interval, 18.43 ± 8.6 days) and were examined in microagglutination tests using standard reference antigens for *L. pneumophila* and five *Legionella*-like organisms and homologous antigens prepared from *L. pneumophila* organisms isolated from the hospital water supply. Patients' sera presented very low reactivity with *Legionella* antigens, mostly without any antibody level changes. Sera from 15 patients (23.4%) reacted by increment of a maximum two titers (on borderline level); only six patients reacted with endemic isolates, particularly with those identified as *L. pneumophila* serogroup 5 (3 patients), *L. pneumophila* serogroup 6 (1 patient), and finally *L. pneumophila* serogroup 12 (2 patients), which originated from water from other wards. In these cases,

**TABLE 2** Serotyping of isolated legionellae from the hospital, 1995 to 1999

| L. pneumophila serogroup | No. of isolates from blocks and tanks[a] | | | Total positivity (%) |
| --- | --- | --- | --- | --- |
| | Blocks except block A, 1995–1997 | 1995–1999 | | |
| | | Block A | Tanks | |
| L.p.10 | 47 | 16 | 3 | 49.6 |
| Lp.5 | 22 | 5 | ND | 20.3 |
| L.p.5,10 | 9 | 1 | 1 | 8.3 |
| L.p.6 | 16 | 1 | ND | 12.8 |
| L.p.9 | 2 | 5 | ND | 5.3 |
| L.p.12 | 2 | ND | ND | 1.5 |
| Not determined | 3 | ND | ND | 2.2 |
| Total | 101 | 28 | 4 | 100.0 |

[a] ND, not detected.

specificity of presented low seroreactivity cannot be excluded. The other patients' sera reacted mostly with *Legionella*-like organisms.

It has not been easy to assess patients' risks in hospitals colonized with legionellae. Low seroreactivity or even absence of any confirmed or presumptive nosocomial cases are not sufficient criteria for the risk estimation. Seroreactivity of patients is influenced by many factors, including their actual immune status, age, antibiotic and immunosuppressive therapy, size of infectious dose, as well as modes and duration of aerosol exposure. Low seroreactivity of patients and therapists exposed to $10^3$ to $10^5$ CFU/liter contaminated water in thermal spas was documented (5, 9),

emphasizing the role of exposure duration followed by higher antibody titers. However, a large proportion of patients under normal treatment regimens in a *Legionella*-colonized hospital, who used only showering without any invasive procedures, did not develop the infection. Thus host susceptibility is undoubtedly a critical factor.

On the other side, the virulence of isolates and qualitative patterns of colonization are considered more important for reactivity or development of disease than the density of legionellae. Despite more than 30% contamination of the hospital water system with legionellae at $10^4$ to $10^7$ CFU/liter, only low seroreactivity of inpatients and no clinical

**TABLE 3** Seroreactivity with *Legionella* antigens in patients from block A[a]

| Year | No. of patients from whom serum samples taken | Mean age ± SD (yrs) | Mean time interval[b] ± SD (days) | Patients with elevation of 2 titers | | |
| --- | --- | --- | --- | --- | --- | --- |
| | | | | No. of patients | Reactivity with antigens[c,d] | |
| | | | | | Homologous[c] | Standard[d] |
| 1997 | 10 | 63.3 ± 13.48 | 15.3 ± 6.41 | 3 | 1 | 2 |
| 1998 | 16 | 59.8 ± 13.94 | 16.9 ± 8.86 | 5 | 0 | 5 |
| 1999 | 38 | 52.4 ± 16.97 | 19.9 ± 12.30 | 7 | 5 | 4 |
| Total | 64 | 56.0 ± 16.0 | 18.43 ± 8.6 | 15 | 6 | 12 |

[a] Block A was colonized by isolates identified as *L. pneumophila* serogroups 10, 5, 6, and 9 (and in other blocks, *L. pneumophila* serogroup 12).
[b] Time interval between first and second serum (mean ± standard deviation).
[c] Three patients reacted with isolates identified as *L. pneumophila* serogroup 5, one patient with *L. pneumophila* serogroup 6, and two patients with *L. pneumophila* serogroup 12.
[d] Five patients reacted with *L. bozemanii*, four with *L. dumoffii*, one with *L. pneumophila* serogroup 1, one with *L. pneumophila* serogroup 15, and one with *L. longbeachae*.

cases were detected. Similar inquiries of disease absence in spite of a high number of legionellae colonization sites or high degree of contamination have been reported (10). It is known that isolates from environmental sources manifest various virulence (4), but our isolates were not characterized from this point of view. The fact that there was no isolated strain of *L. pneumophila* serogroup 1, which is more than 60% responsible for legionellosis, could be explanatory, as well as the fact that isolates from this hospital belonging to other serogroups of this species are reported to be less frequently associated with the disease (1, 2, 6). Our investigations of potable water colonization in the hospitals and civil buildings of the same city revealed contamination of *L. pneumophila* non-serogroup 1 and strains of the non-Pontiac subgroup, which were isolated in 7% of samples (3).

A small group of patients suffering from pneumonia (more than 100) in the same hospital in which legionella laboratory tests are not in routine use, was investigated in order to find another explanation for the absence of nosocomial legionellosis. There was a lack of convalescent-phase sera and samples for cultivation due to insufficient cooperation with clinicians and notably missing detection by *Legionella* urinary test. This test is widely recommended for active surveillance of legionellosis in colonized hospitals (7, 8).

Despite the lack of evidence of confirmed nosocomial legionellosis in the examined hospital, the risk of exposure and the possibility of infection cannot be excluded. The implementation of more control, mainly of regimen measures, in this facility without the introduction of wider decontamination measures, and more intensive clinical surveillance of pneumonia cases with the introduction of *Legionella* laboratory tests, were recommended.

## REFERENCES

1. **Anonymous.** 1998. Legionnaires' disease in Europe, 1997. *Wkly. Epidemiol. Rec.* **73**:257–261.
2. **Anonymous.** 1999. Legionnaires' disease, Europe, 1998. *Wkly. Epidemiol. Rec.* **74**:273–277.
3. **Bazovská, S., and M. Špaleková.** 1999. Incidence of legionellae in the Bratislava region. *Hygiena.* **44**:85–90.
4. **Bollin, G. E., J. F. Plouffe, M. F. Para, and R. B. Prior.** 1985. Difference in virulence of environmental isolates of *Legionella pneumophila. J. Clin. Microbiol.* **21**:674–677.
5. **Bornstein, N., D. Marmet, M. Surgot, M. Nowicki, A. Arslan, J. Esteve, and J. Fleurette.** 1989. Exposure to legionellaceae at a hot spring spa: a prospective clinical and serological study. *Epidemiol. Infect.* **102**:31–36.
6. **Feng-Yee, C., S. L. Jacobs, S. M. Colodny, J. E. Stout, and V. L. Yu.** 1996. Nosocomial Legionnaires' disease caused by *Legionella pneumophila* serogroup 5: laboratory and epidemiologic implications. *J. Infect. Dis.* **174**:1116–1119.
7. **Kool, J. L., D. Bergmire-Sweat, J. C. Butler, E. W. Brown, D. J. Peabody, D. S. Massi, J. C. Carpenter, J. M. Pruckler, R. F. Benson, and B. S. Fields.** 1999. Hospital characteristics associated with colonization of water systems by Legionella and risk of nosocomial legionnaires' disease: a cohort study of 15 hospitals. *Infect. Control. Hosp. Epidemiol.* **20**:798–805.
8. **Lepine, L. A., B. Daniel, M. D. Jernigan, J. C. Butler, J. M. Pruckler, R. F. Benson, G. Kim, J. L. Hadler, M. L. Cartter, and B. S. Fields.** 1998. A recurrent outbreak of nosocomial legionnaires' disease detected by urinary antigen testing: evidence for long-term colonization of a hospital plumbing system. *Infect. Control Hosp. Epidemiol.* **19**:905–910.
9. **Rocha, G., A. Verissimo, R. Bowker, N. Bornstein, and M. S. Da Costa.** 1995. Relationship between *Legionella* spp. and antibody titres at a therapeutic thermal spa in Portugal. *Epidemiol. Infect.* **115**:79–88.
10. **Ruef, C.** 1998. Nosocomial Legionnaires' disease—strategies for prevention. *J. Microbiol. Methods* **33**:81–91.

# DEVELOPMENT OF SURVEILLANCE OF *LEGIONELLA* INFECTIONS IN POLAND BY SEROLOGICAL INVESTIGATION

*Hanna Stypułkowska-Misiurewicz, Katarzyna Pancer, Bożena Krogulska, and Renata Matuszewska*

# 68

Legionellosis is a new infectious disease emerging in Poland (1) although not yet registered. According to data from the European Working Group for *Legionella* Infections, 12 people returning from Poland were hospitalized with Legionnaires' disease in Sweden or Denmark from 1994 to 2000. Until recently, physicians in Poland generally were not aware of the risk for *Legionella* infections and there was a lack of diagnostic laboratory possibilities. The investigation of *Legionella* infections started in Poland in 1997, but physicians and laboratories still have problems identifying legionellosis cases. The Polish working group for *Legionella* infections was organized by the National Institute of Hygiene in Warsaw in 1997. The aim of this group was to select laboratory methods for investigating human *Legionella* infections and detecting bacterium in the environment.

The specimens from patients were examined for *Legionella* antigen in urine and for the level of antibodies to *Legionella pneumophila* serogroup 1 in patient sera (3). Methods were evaluated with control specimens.

## URINE ANTIGEN

The standard commercial BIOTEST was used for the determination of *Legionella* antigen in urine. The procedure was evaluated according to the European program of the European Working Group for *Legionella* Infections for quality of testing of *Legionella* antigen determination in urine. The 43 specimens of urine were collected from patients with pulmonary disease hospitalized all over the country. Urinary antigen has been found in only 3 of 43 received urine samples. Two cases were confirmed as legionellosis by seroconversion. From our point of view, the detection of *Legionella* antigen in urine is a rapid, easy-to-perform method. There were no problems with collecting and sending urine samples. The test is also sufficient to confirm the diagnosis of Legionnaires' disease.

## SERUM ANTIBODY LEVEL

Human serum samples of 180 patients with pneumonia and other pulmonary infectious diseases were collected and examined by microagglutination test (4). Antibody level was evaluated by reaction to antigens of *L. pneu-*

*Hanna Stypułkowska-Misiurewicz and Katarzyna Pancer* Department of Bacteriology, National Institute of Hygiene, 24, Chocimska Street, 00-791 Warsaw, Poland. *Bożena Krogulska and Renata Matuszewska* Department of Environmental Hygiene, National Institute of Hygiene, 24, Chocimska Street, 00-791 Warsaw, Poland.

*Legionella*, Edited by Reinhard Marre et al.
© 2002 ASM Press, Washington, D.C.

*mophila* serogroup 1 reference strain ATCC 33152. The level of antibodies to *L. pneumophila* serogroup 1 in patient sera was generally low, except in two cases (1%) of confirmed Legionnaires' disease (in which the titer was very high—2,048). In 5 of 180 cases (3%) the titer was raised (64) but insignificant for *Legionella* infection (Table 1). The antibodies to *L. pneumophila* serogroup 1 titer as high as 2,048 were found in only 2 of 69 sera from patients with atypical pneumonia: in one convalescent patient's serum and in serum of one nosocomial case with symptoms of pneumonia. The urine antigen of *Legionella* tests determined by the enzyme immunoassay method was also positive in both cases. Among serum samples of 25 patients with pulmonic infections due to *Mycoplasma pneumoniae*, nonspecific reactions were not observed in titer above 64. The highest titer of antibodies to *L. pneumophila* serogroup 1 antigen was 64 in 75 serum samples from patients with respiratory tract infection of unknown etiology. Among the sera of 11 patients with *Bordetella pertussis* infection (mostly children), no antibodies to *Legionella* were found in titer above 16 (Table 1). The nonspecific reactions of *L. pneumophila* serogroup 1 antigen have not been found in titer above 64 in samples of sera from patients with mycoplasma infections or with pertussis.

The most interesting results were obtained in the study of antibody level to *L. pneumophila* serogroup 1 in 503 serum samples collected from healthy hospital staff members of six hospitals in different towns. The level of antibodies to *L. pneumophila* serogroup 1 in all the sera was low with only two exceptions (titer 128) (0, 4%) (Table 2). The raised level of antibodies to *L. pneumophila* serogroup 1 (titer 64) was found in the sera of nine (2%) staff members; three of them worked in one (no. 1) hospital (Table 2). Generally the antibody level to *L. pneumophila* serogroup 1 evaluated in sera collected from staff members of six different hospitals was similar.

The risk of *Legionella* infection in the hydrotherapy ward was evaluated by determining the antibody level for *L. pneumophila* serogroup 1 (reference strain ATCC 33152) and two *L. pneumophila* serogroup 2 to 14 strains (no. 6 and no. 11) isolated from water of the unit where a Swedish patient may have been infected. The serum samples of 20 staff members of the unit were collected and examined by microagglutination test. The study was run along with the epidemiological investigation because 1 patient out of 45 became infected with *L. pneumophila* serogroup 1 and was hospitalized in Sweden. The Swedish patient was laboratory-diagnosed by I. Kallings (personal communication). The patient stayed

**TABLE 1** The antibody level to *L. pneumophila* serogroup 1 in serum samples collected from 180 patients and 523 healthy staff of hospital and spa water treatment unit

| Source of serum samples | Anti-*L. pneumophila* serogroup 1 antibody titer[a]: | | | |
|---|---|---|---|---|
| | <64 | 64 | 128 | 2,048 |
| Patients | | | | |
| Atypical pneumonia | 66 | 1 | 0 | 2 |
| Mycoplasmosis | 24 | 1 | 0 | 0 |
| Nonspecific upper respiratory tract infection | 72 | 3 | 0 | 0 |
| Pertussis | 11 | 0 | 0 | 0 |
| Healthy persons | | | | |
| Hospital staff members | 492 | 9 | 2 | 0 |
| Spa water staff members | 18 | 1 | 1 | 0 |
| Total | 683 | 15 | 3 | 2 |

[a] Determined by microagglutination test.

**TABLE 2** The comparison of antibody level to *L. pneumophila* serogroup 1 in sera collected from 503 healthy staff members of different hospitals determined by microagglutination test

| Hospital[a] | No. of persons with anti-*L. pneumophila* serogroup 1 antibody titer of: | | | |
|---|---|---|---|---|
| | <64 | 64 | 128 | 2,048 |
| I | 119 | 3 | 1 | 0 |
| II | 47 | 0 | 0 | 0 |
| III | 126 | 0 | 0 | 0 |
| IV | 29 | 0 | 0 | 0 |
| V | 27 | 1 | 1 | 0 |
| VI | 30 | 0 | 0 | 0 |
| Other | 114 | 5 | 0 | 0 |
| Total | 492 | 9 | 2 | 0 |

[a] Serum samples were taken from staff members of different hospitals for comparison.

in Poland (in the ward) from 8 to 21 September 1997; the date of onset was 20 September. Nine water samples were collected and examined in the National Institute of Hygiene by the method presented by B. Krogulska (chapter 58). The strains of *L. pneumophila* serogroups 2 to 14 were found in seven water samples collected from shower baths, whirlpools, and a hot water container. The highest number of bacteria was evaluated as $2.0 \times 10^2$ CFU/1,000 ml. No one strain of *L. pneumophila* serogroup 1 was isolated from water in the unit. The level of antibodies to *L. pneumophila* serogroup 1 as well as to *L. pneumophila* serogroups 2 to 14 strains no. 6 and no. 11 in staff members' sera was insignificant (Table 3). It was concluded that the Swedish patient had acquired the infection elsewhere, perhaps while crossing the Baltic Sea overnight on a ferry boat.

## CONCLUSIONS

Legionellosis exists in Poland and a search for cases is being conducted, but the low number of samples from patients with pulmonary diseases is proof that a period of transition in health service funding is adversely affecting the progress of the search. However, the percentage of laboratory-confirmed cases of legionellosis found in Poland among patients with respiratory tract infections is similar to that found in other countries. The percentage of patients with pneumonia having evidence of legionellosis has been reported as 1 to 30% (3, 5, 6, 7). The prospective study of community-acquired pneumonia in adults in Spain showed that legionellosis was found in 12.5% of cases (8).

The level of antibody to *L. pneumophila* serogroup 1 is low in the healthy adult population in Poland. These data are similar to those obtained by Harrison (6) and cited by Mainwald (7). The fourfold rise to 128 or higher in paired sera is significant for serological confirmation of legionellosis. However, the titer 256 or above in single serum specimens may be presumptive for *Legionella* infection (1, 7, 9), since it has not been found in any serum sample of 503 healthy staff members and the titer of 128 was found in only 0.4% of tested sera.

The risk of *L. pneumophila* infection still seems to be low for the general population in

**TABLE 3** The antibody level to *L. pneumophila* serogroup 1 ATCC 33152 and to *L. pneumophila* serogroup 2 to 14 strains isolated from spa water system in serum samples of 20 healthy spa water staff members

| Antigen obtained from the strain of *L. pneumophila* | No. of persons with anti-*L. pneumophila* antibody titer of[a]: | | | | |
|---|---|---|---|---|---|
| | 8 | 16 | 32 | 64 | 128 |
| *L. pneumophila* serogroup 1 ATCC 33152 | 9 | 6 | 3 | 2 | 0 |
| *L. pneumophila* serogroups 2 to 14 no. 6, isolated from spa water system | 14 | 3 | 3 | 0 | 0 |
| *L. pneumophila* serogroups 2 to 14 no. 11, isolated from spa water system | 2 | 6 | 3 | 1 | 0 |

[a] Serum samples were taken from healthy staff members and tested for antibodies to *Legionella* organisms found in spa water by the microagglutination test.

Poland. It might be higher for some groups, including patients in rehabilitation and transplant units, and for staff in certain institutions such as hospitals.

## ACKNOWLEDGMENT

The work was partly supported by Governmental Strategic program (SPR-1) "Safety and Protection of Human Health in Work Environment." The main coordinator was the Central Institute of Work Protection.

## REFERENCES

1. **Castellani Pastoris, M., and P. Benedetti.** 1993. *Legionella e Legionellosi.* Instituto Superiore di Sanita e dell'Assessorato alla Sanita Regione Campania, Rome, Italy.
2. **Centers for Disease Control.** 1990. Case definition for public health surveillance. *Morb. Mortal. Wkly. Rep.* **39**(RR-13):1–43.
3. **Eurosurveillance.** 1999. Special issue on legionellosis. *Eurosurveillance* **4**:111–124.
4. **Farshy, C. E., G. C. Klein, and J. C. Feeley.** 1978. A microagglutination test for detecting antibodies, p. 163–168. *In* G. L. Jones and G. A. Hebert (ed.), *"Legionnaires": the Diseases, the Bacterium and Methology.* U.S. Dept. of Health, Education, and Welfare, Atlanta, Ga.
5. **Fry, N. K., and T. G. Harrison.** 1999. Diagnosis and epidemiology of infections caused by Legionella spp., p. 213–242. *In* N. Woodford and A. P. Johnson (ed.), *Methods in Molecular Medicine.* Humana Press Inc., Totowa, N.J.
6. **Harrison, T. G., and A. G. Taylor.** 1982. A rapid microagglutination test for the diagnosis of Legionella pneumophila (serogroup 1) infection. *J. Clin. Pathol.* **35**:1028–1031.
7. **Maiwald, M., J. H. Helbig, and P. C. Lück.** 1998. Laboratory methods for the diagnosis of Legionella infections. *J. Microbiol. Methods* **33**:59–79.
8. **Sopena, N., M. Sabria, M. L. Pedro-Botet, J. M. Manterola, L. Matas, J. Dominguez, J. M. Modol, P. Tudela, V. Ausina, and M. Foz.** 1999. Prospective study of community-acquired pneumonia of bacterial etiology in adults. *Eur. J. Clin. Microbiol. Infect. Dis.* **18**:852–858.
9. **Tateda, K., H. Murakami, Y. Ishii, N. Furuya, T. Matsumoto, and K. Yamaguchi.** 1998. Evaluation of clinical usefulness of the microplate agglutination test for serological diagnosis of legionella pneumonia. *J. Med. Microbiol.* **47**:325–328.

# LEGIONELLOSIS OUTBREAK AT A COMMERCIAL FAIR IN KAPELLEN, BELGIUM, 1999: A CASE-CONTROL STUDY

*Marta Fajó Pascual, Olivier Ronveaux, Koen De Schrijver, and Frank Van Loock*

# 69

A Legionnaires' disease outbreak was detected among visitors (50,000) and workers (830) of a commercial fair being held in Kapellen from 29 October to 7 November, 1999. A total of 93 cases were identified, of whom five persons died. Exploratory interviews in connection with the early cases allowed the establishment of the epidemiological link with the Kapellen fair by 13 November. On 15 November, *Legionella pneumophila* serogroup 1 was confirmed from clinical isolates (2).

The event received huge media attention causing considerable alarm in the population. Additionally, only a few months before, another major outbreak associated with a commercial flower fair had occurred in The Netherlands (4); a whirlpool spa had been incriminated as the source of the outbreak. In Kapellen, the media immediately suspected a whirlpool spa as the source on the basis of cases detected among fair employees working

in the vicinity of the whirlpool spa stand. The whirlpool had been filled with water 1 day before the fair and heated daily for demonstration, and the water had never been replaced.

An environmental investigation and a cohort study among stand workers were initially carried out to trace the source of the outbreak. None of them had shown conclusive findings by February 2000 (2). The whirlpool spa hypothesis was biologically plausible, but other aerosol-producing devices had also been demonstrated during the fair. A case-control study was launched in February 2000 to identify the source of the outbreak.

## MATERIALS AND METHODS

### The Fair

The fair was an annual exhibition of consumable products (230 stands) hosted in a single exhibition tent (9,000 m²) with only one single entry and exit. Visitors could follow only one path, allowing each exhibitor the same opportunity to be seen. Warm air was blown into the tent through six air inlets located on both sides of the tent.

### Case Identification

Sources of information for cases were physician notifications of Legionnaires' disease and

*Marta Fajó Pascual* European Programme for Intervention Epidemiology Training (EPIET), Scientific Institute of Public Health, Rue Juliette Wytsman, 14, 1050 Brussels, Belgium. *Olivier Ronveaux and Frank Van Loock* Scientific Institute of Public Health, Rue Juliette Wytsman, 14, 1050 Brussels, Belgium. *Koen De Schrijver* Health Inspection Flemish Community, Antwerp, Coperniculaan, 1 bus 5, 2018 Antwerp, Belgium.

*Legionella*, Edited by Reinhard Marre et al.
© 2002 ASM Press, Washington, D.C.

a survey throughout Belgian hospitals and laboratories (2). All cases ($n = 93$) were persons attending the fair who developed symptoms of Legionnaires' disease within 2 weeks after their fair visit. A possible (clinical) case was defined as a patient with a radiographic diagnosis of pneumonia where no other pathogen was found. Presumptive cases were clinical cases having a single positive serological *Legionella* antibody titer (1). Confirmed cases were clinical cases with at least one of the following laboratory criteria: isolation of *Legionella*, detection of *Legionella* antigen in urine, seroconversion (a fourfold rise in serum titer), or a positive PCR along with a positive *Legionella* antibody titer in serum (1).

## Control Definition and Selection

Due to time (3 months after the outbreak) and logistical constraints, controls were selected from an available register from a nearby hospital. This register collected information about medical complaints of fair visitors who consulted the hospital, mostly to get reassured about their health status. At the hospital, they were screened for Legionnaires' disease. The control definition was a person who consulted this hospital within 2 weeks after the end of the fair, with negative X rays and/or laboratory (urinary antigen/serology) tests. Controls reporting fever and cough in the 2 weeks after the fair were excluded from the analysis to avoid misclassification of milder or undetected *Legionella* infections.

## Study Design

In February 2000, a standardized questionnaire was mailed to all persons categorized as cases (93) and as controls (350). Information was collected on personal factors such as age, sex, smoking status, visitor versus worker status, preexisting respiratory and debilitating diseases (i.e., diabetes mellitus, malignancies, etc.), and factors related to the fair visit such as the day of the visit, time spent in the fair, and visits to the aerosol-producing stands, i.e., whirlpool spa, steam iron, decorative fountain, rainproof roof demonstration, and aquarium.

## Statistical Analysis

Comparison of means with the Student's $t$ test ($\alpha = 0.05$) was used in continuous variables. Logistic regression analysis provided crude and adjusted odds ratios (OR) for discrete variables. Age, smoking, and visiting the whirlpool stand were forced into the multivariate logistic regression model. Other variables were included if they had shown in the univariate analysis a "significant" ($P \leq 0.10$) association with the disease. Variables remained in the model if the likelihood ratio test was significant ($P \leq 0.10$). Data were analyzed with the SPSS 9.0 statistical package. The analysis was repeated on confirmed cases to address the issue of potential misclassification of presumptive and possible cases. Additionally, the analysis was repeated on cases and controls who visited the fair once during the first long weekend (4 days) of the fair to account for a different risk of getting the disease related to the day of the fair visit.

## RESULTS

A total of 45 (48%) cases were confirmed, whereas 48 cases (52%) were presumptive or possible. The response rate for cases was 74.2% (69 of 93), and for controls was 46.3% (162 of 350). Eventually only 114 controls (32.6%) were eligible because the other 48 reported fever and cough within 2 weeks after the fair.

Figure 1 shows that almost every day of the fair there were persons reported ill who had visited the fair only once, with a decreasing trend in incidence over time. All cases who visited on 29 October attended the fair another day as well.

The univariate analysis indicated that cases were on average older than controls (52 versus 34 years old), were more often smokers or ex-smokers (60.8 versus 34.2%), and suffered more frequently from debilitating disease (17.4 versus 7.9%). The sex ratio (M:F) for cases was 1.1:1 and for controls it was 0.8:1 ($P = 0.2$). All cases and 95.6% of the controls completed the fair path, i.e., passed in front of all of the fair stands (Table 1).

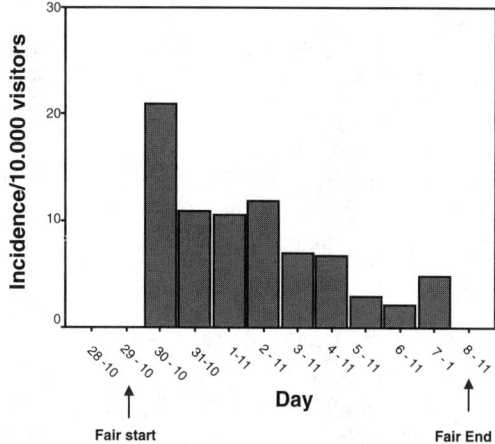

**FIGURE 1** Incidence of Legionnaires' disease by date of attendance to the Kapellen fair, Belgium, 1999. The figure includes only patients visiting the fair once ($n = 48$).

The proportion of fair employees among cases and controls was 7.2 and 11.4%, respectively ($P = 0.4$). The average time spent by cases at the fair was not significantly different from the average time spent by controls (6.2 versus 7.4 h, $P = 0.6$). Among variables measuring exposure to aerosol-producing stands, only visiting the iron steam stand was significantly associated with the disease ($OR = 2.9$, $P < 0.05$).

Variables that remained in the final logistic regression model (Table 1) were being older than 40 years ($OR_{adjusted}$, 4.5; 95% confidence interval [CI], 2.2 to 9.3), being a smoker ($OR_{adjusted}$, 2.7; 95% CI, 1.3 to 5.7) or ex-smoker ($OR_{adjusted}$, 4.5; 95% CI, 1.6 to 13.0), and having visited the steam iron stand ($OR_{adjusted}$, 3.5; 95% CI, 1.3 to 9.8).

Visiting the whirlpool stand, although not statistically significant in the univariate analysis, was forced into the model to adjust for a possible confounding effect of the variable visiting the steam iron stand. Only 24.6% of the cases (10.0% of controls) reported visiting the steam iron stand, compared with 66.7% of the cases (65.7% of controls) reporting visiting the whirlpool stand. The analysis carried out only on confirmed cases did not reveal any substantial change in the direction of the associations.

## DISCUSSION

We did not provide epidemiological evidence of an association of the disease with visiting the whirlpool stand but certain study limitations should be considered. First, controls

**TABLE 1** Univariate and multivariate logistic regression analysis and proportion of cases exposed for the Legionnaires' disease outbreak in Kapellen, Belgium, 1999

| Risk factor | % of persons exposed | Univariate[a] | | Multivariate | |
|---|---|---|---|---|---|
| | | OR | 95% CI | OR | 95% CI |
| Male | 52.2 | 1.4 | 0.8–2.6 | | |
| 41 years of age or older[a] | 55.4 | 2.5 | 1.6–3.7 | 4.5 | 2.2–9.3 |
| Smoker[a] | 39.1 | 2.4 | 1.2–4.8 | 2.7 | 1.3–5.7 |
| Ex-smoker[a] | 21.7 | 5.2 | 2.0–13.6 | 4.5 | 1.6–13.0 |
| Respiratory disease | 27.5 | 1.1 | 0.5–2.1 | | |
| Debilitating disease[a] | 17.4 | 2.5 | 1.0–6.2 | 1.6 | 0.5–4.6 |
| Visitor versus worker status | 92.8 | 1.6 | 0.7–4.8 | | |
| Visiting stand | | | | | |
| Whirlpool[b] | 66.7 | 1.0 | 0.5–2.0 | 0.8 | 0.4–1.8 |
| Steam iron[a] | 24.6 | 2.9 | 1.2–6.9 | 3.5 | 1.3–9.8 |
| Rainproof roof | 47.0 | 1.4 | 0.7–2.5 | | |
| Fountain | 32.8 | 1.1 | 0.6–2.3 | | |

[a] Variables showing a "significant" ($P \leq 0.10$) association with the disease in the univariate analysis were included in the multivariate logistic model.

[b] Variable not statistically significant in univariate analysis, forced into the model to adjust for a possible confounding effect with variable visiting steam iron stand.

were not randomly selected but rather conveniently obtained. The media had informed the population that a whirlpool spa displayed at the Kapellen fair was the most likely culprit of the outbreak. Hence, controls could have been unintentionally selected for exposure to the whirlpool, introducing a selection bias toward the null. Second, one-third of the cases did not report exposure to the whirlpool. A nondifferential exposure misclassification of cases and controls might have occurred since the investigation was launched 3 months after the outbreak. This bias effect would be again toward the null. Furthermore, just walking in the vicinity of the whirlpool stand was perhaps sufficient to get an infective dose, explaining the low proportion of cases who reported having visited the whirlpool stand. Indeed, the whole fair tour was done by nearly all study participants.

All fair days were days at risk for acquiring the disease, but the decreasing trend of the risk of infection over time is hardly compatible with the whirlpool hypothesis. Indeed, one might expect an increasing trend in incidence with increasing *Legionella* concentrations over time (water in the whirlpool was never replaced). Disinfecting of the device during the fair was reported by the whirlpool exhibitor, which could explain this finding, but this fact could not be verified. On the other hand, we found a statistical association with visiting the steam iron stand. However, the steam iron's elevated temperatures should hamper bacterial survival, providing only a weak biological plausibility. Besides, this exposure could only explain one-fourth of the cases. Nevertheless, we could hypothesize that steam iron exposure could be a proxy for exposure to the

whirlpool spa since both stands were only 15 m apart in the same corridor. Whirlpool-generated aerosols could have been pushed away by the airflow blown in the direction of the steam iron stand from the inlet behind the whirlpool.

By September 2000, results of the other investigations had not identified a definite source, and the true origin of this major outbreak may well remain unknown. In *Legionella* outbreaks, timely epidemiological investigations are crucial, particularly to guide environmental investigations (3). Routinely established communication flows between all parties involved in the control of infectious diseases will be necessary to effectively tackle future outbreaks in Belgium.

## REFERENCES

1. **Centers for Disease Control and Prevention.** 1997. Case definitions for infectious conditions under public health surveillance. *Morb. Mortal. Wkly. Rep.* **10**:10–20.
2. **De Schrijver, K., E. Bouwel, L. Mortelmans, P. Rossom, T. Beukelaer, C. Vael, K. Dirven, H. Goossens, M. Ieven, M. Fajó, and O. Ronveaux.** 2000. Infections à Legionella: épisode épidemique à une foire á Kapellen, p. 19–25. *In* F. van Loock (ed.), *Diagnostic et Surveillance des Maladies Infectieuses, 16ème Séminaire Institut Scientifique de la Santé Publique en Collaboration avec la Société Belge de Biologie Clinique.* Institut Scientific de la Santé Publique, Brussels, Belgium.
3. **Mahoney, F., C. Hoge, T. Farley, J. Barbaree, R. Breiman, R. Benson, and L. MacFarland.** 1992. Community wide outbreak of Legionnaires' disease associated with a grocery. *J. Infect. Dis.* **165**:736–739.
4. **Van Steenbergen J., F. Slijkerman, and P. Speelman.** 1999. The first 48 hours of investigation and intervention of an outbreak of legionellosis in the Netherlands. *Eurosurveillance* **4**:112–115.

# OUTBREAK OF LEGIONNAIRES' DISEASE LINKED TO A HUMIDIFIER IN A HOTEL IN WALES, UNITED KINGDOM

*Susan Hahné, Phillip Watson, Bharat Pankhania, Mark Temple, Carol Joseph, Tim Harrison, John Lee, Don Ribeiro, Robert Smith, and Roland Salmon*

# 70

Ten cases of indigenously acquired Legionnaires' disease were identified by routine laboratory surveillance in Wales, United Kingdom, over a period of 7 months. Routine investigation into itineraries during the incubation period of their disease revealed that four of these patients visited the same hotel in Cardiff. Contact with the Environmental Health Department of a neighboring area revealed a fifth Legionnaires' disease patient who had visited the same hotel during the incubation period of his disease, and a sixth patient who also visited the hotel presented himself after he learned about the outbreak in the media.

To assess the magnitude of the outbreak, active case finding was started, including checking sickness records from the hotel and an adjacent company and contacting consultants in Communicable Disease Control and Environmental Health Departments. Also, the national *Legionella* surveillance database was examined. Environmental and epidemiological investigations were carried out to determine the source of infection and, if possible, to prevent further cases.

The environmental investigations consisted of sampling water sources in and around the hotel. The hotel has an indoor swimming pool, spa, and an outdoor man-made lake with a fountain.

Epidemiological investigations started with a case-control study. Case definitions used were those of the European Working Group for Legionella Infections (http://www.phls.co.uk/International/Ewgli/ldefs2.htm); controls were taken from people who accompanied the three patients who had visited the hotel as part of a group.

A cohort study was designed with staff who worked during the weekend that two patients had visited the hotel. The hypothesis

*Susan Hahné* PHLS/CDSC in Wales/European Programme for Intervention Epidemiology Training, Abton House, Wedal Road, Cardiff CF24 4PB, United Kingdom. *Phillip Watson and Mark Temple* Bro Taf Health Authority, Temple of Peace and Health, Cathays Park, Cardiff CF1 3NW, United Kingdom. *Bharat Pankhania* Consultant in Communicable Disease Control, Wiltshire Health Authority, Southgate House, Pans Lane, Devizes, SN10 3 EQ, United Kingdom. *Carol Joseph* PHLS/CDSC, 61 Colindale Avenue, London NW9 5EQ, United Kingdom. *Tim Harrison* Respiratory and Systemic Infection Laboratory, PHLS, 61 Colindale Avenue, London NW9 5EQ, United Kingdom. *John Lee* PHLS, 61 Colindale Avenue, London NW9 5EQ, United Kingdom. *Don Ribeiro* PHLS in Wales, Department of Medical Microbiology & Public Health Laboratory, University Hospital of Wales, Heath Park, Cardiff CF4 4XW, United Kingdom. *Robert Smith and Roland Salmon* PHLS/CDSC in Wales, Abton House, Wedal Road, Cardiff CF24 4PB, United Kingdom.

*Legionella*, Edited by Reinhard Marre et al.
© 2002 ASM Press, Washington, D.C.

was that more seroconversions would have occurred among people working close to the source, so that the average titer in this group would be higher than in people not exposed to the source. In both studies, questions were asked about time spent in different places within the hotel and in its vicinity, and blood samples for *Legionella* serology were taken.

Patients (three male and three female) were between 40 and 77 years old; two of them died. Onset of illness ranged from July 1999 to February 2000 (Fig. 1).

All six patients had a lung infiltrate on chest X ray. *Legionella pneumophila* serogroup 1 was isolated from two patients at autopsy; three patients had a positive *L. pneumophila* serogroup 1 urinary antigen test (confirmed cases), and one patient had a single high titer against *L. pneumophila* serogroup 1 (probable case).

The first patient visited the hotel in July 1999, patients 2 and 3 visited in December 1999, patients 4 and 5 visited in January 2000, and patient 6 visited in February 2000. Only one stayed overnight and dined in the hotel, one used the swimming pool and spa for a week, three attended a lunch, and one attended an evening meal. Three of six patients

were active smokers; none were immunosuppressed.

Neither the case-control study nor the cohort study indicated a possible source of infection. However, as four of six patients visited the dining room of the hotel only, suspicion focused on the dining room and in particular on the buffet counter. The cold food display at the counter had an ultrasound humidifier connected to it, which generated a mist over the food. The four patients who visited the dining room were seated close to the food buffet.

The installation and maintenance of the humidifier caused concern: none of three antibacterial filters were installed; the UV lamp, which should prevent bacterial growth, was not working; the alarm that should have indicated UV failure was not working; no UV lamps were installed in the mist-delivery bars; the air inlet of the humidifier was placed underneath the enclosed food-buffet unit rather than in a clean area; the unit was placed in a difficult-to-reach position, making maintenance difficult; and the surrounding temperature of the humidifier was higher than room temperature because of adjacent bain-maries and because of an air connection to the swimming pool located on the floor below the dining room. Routine sampling for bacterial growth, which had been recommended, did not happen.

In samples from the ultrasonification unit of the humidifier taken during the outbreak investigation, *L. pneumophila* serogroup 1 was found, which was indistinguishable from the two isolates from the patients by monoclonal antibody subgrouping and amplified fragment length polymorphism analysis (2).

The humidifier was switched off on 24 February 2000. No new cases of Legionnaires' disease have subsequently been identified that could be connected to the hotel in more than 7 months. Public Health officials and local authorities were notified of the possible role of ultrasonic humidifiers in the transmission of legionellae. Furthermore, an update was made of the *Approved Code of Practice & Guid-*

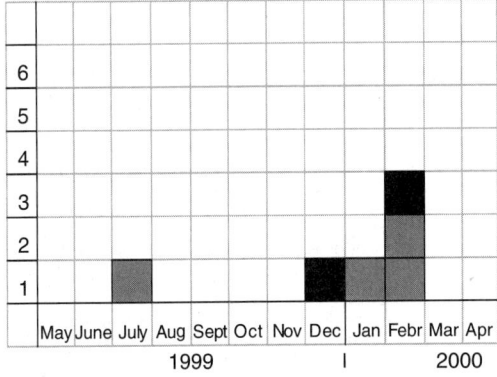

**FIGURE 1** Cases (*n* = 6) of Legionnaires' disease associated with hotel in Wales, United Kingdom, July 1999 to February 2000, by month of onset. Black boxes indicate fatal cases; gray boxes indicate nonfatal cases.

*ance L8 2000* for prevention of Legionnaires' disease (3).

This is the first time in Europe that Legionnaires' disease was associated with an ultrasonic humidifier. In the United States, a similar device had been associated with Legionnaires' disease before (1, 4).

Questions remain as to why the problem occurred intermittently and why so few people were affected. Lessons learned were shared with Public Health officials and incorporated into the revised United Kingdom guidance on the prevention of Legionnaires' disease (3). Since humidifiers are commonly used in the United Kingdom and elsewhere, improved knowledge of risks associated and improved design, installation, and maintenance may prevent further cases of Legionnaires' disease.

## REFERENCES

1. **Centers for Disease Control.** 1990. Legionnaires' disease outbreak associated with a grocery store mist machine—Louisiana, 1989. *Morb. Mortal. Wkly. Rep.* **39:**108–109.
2. **Fry, N. K., S. Alexiou-Daniel, J. M. Bangsborg, S. Bernander, M. Castellani Pastoris, J. Etienne, B. Forsblum, V. Gaia, J. H. Helbig, P. C. Lück, D. Lindsay, C. Pelaz, S. Uldum, and T. G. Harrison.** 1999. A multi-center evaluation of genotypic methods for the epidemiological typing of *Legionella pneumophila* serogroup 1: results of a pan-European study. *Clin. Microbiol. Infect.* **5:**462–477.
3. **Health and Safety Commission.** 2000. *Legionnaires' Disease—the Control of Legionella Bacteria in Water Systems. Approved Code of Practice & Guidance L8 2000.* HSE Books, Sudbury, United Kingdom.
4. **Phillips, S. J., R. H. Zeff, and D. Gervich.** 1987. Legionnaires' Disease. *Ann. Thorac. Surg.* **44:** 564.

# HOT WATER SYSTEMS WITH LOW CONCENTRATIONS OF LEGIONELLAE MAY BE A RISK ON CRUISE SHIPS

*Jaana Kusnetsov, Marjo Tiittanen, Silja Mentula, and Hannele Jousimies-Somer*

# 71

Water systems contaminated with legionellae cause outbreaks and sporadic cases of *Legionella* pneumonia. Despite improved surveillance methods in many countries, it seems that large numbers of cases are not confirmed and related water sources are left undetected. Data from 1999, collected by members of the European Working Group for *Legionella* Infections, showed that 32% of cases were reported to be community acquired, 9% were hospital acquired, 21% were travel associated, and the remaining 38% were of unknown origin (7). Legionellae are ubiquitous in water systems. In most clinical cases the source of infection can be confirmed only by using typing methods that discriminate between the patient and the environmental isolates. Strains from both the suspected water environment and the patients are unfortunately not always available.

## TRAVEL-ASSOCIATED CASES

The European surveillance scheme of travel-associated cases was introduced by members of the European Working Group for *Legionella* Infections to improve case detection of Legionnaires' disease among travellers. In 1999, the coordinator informed the Finnish collaborating laboratory of the first two unlinked cases among travelers who had visited Finland. The first patient was a 61-year-old man who fell ill with pneumonia 3 days after attending a cruise. His urinary antigen test was positive for legionellae, but no isolates were detected. The second patient was a 49-year-old man who was diagnosed with pneumonia after staying at a hotel in Helsinki. The *Legionella* pneumonia was confirmed by serology. Both patients recovered. The management of the cruise line and the hotel were informed of these cases and were given general information about legionellosis and control measures.

## ACTIVITIES ON BOARD

The cruise line management ordered a legionella investigation of all on-board water systems. In addition, the health care personnel of the company arranged a survey of recent pneumonia cases among the crew. Samples were sent for urinary antigen detection and serum antibody determination.

There were four cold water reservoirs, two hot water reservoirs, two spa pools, and one swimming pool on board. Cold water samples

*Jaana Kusnetsov and Marjo Tiittanen* Laboratory of Environmental Microbiology, National Public Health Institute (KTL), FIN-70701 Kuopio, Finland. *Silja Mentula and Hannele Jousimies-Somer* Department of Bacteriology, National Public Health Institute (KTL), FIN-00300 Helsinki, Finland.

*Legionella*, Edited by Reinhard Marre et al.
© 2002 ASM Press, Washington, D.C.

were taken from two reservoirs, a shower, and a tap. Hot water samples were taken from circulating water leaving from and returning to the reservoirs, six showers, and four taps. The shower samples were taken immediately without flushing and the tap samples after flushing until the water temperature reached the highest value. These peripheral samples represented different parts of the ship and included samples from cabins of crew members who had recently had pneumonia. All pools were also sampled.

## ANALYSES

Water samples were analyzed using legionella isolation standard method ISO 11731 (3), completed by additional concentration with centrifugation (6,000 $\times$ $g$, 10 min). The lowest detection limit of legionellae was 5 CFU/liter. Counts of viable heterotrophic bacteria were determined by incubating sample water on R2A medium (8) at 20 and 50°C. Temperatures were measured with a Fluke 51 thermometer. Chlorine concentrations were analyzed from the cold water reservoir and pool waters (1).

## HOT WATER SYSTEM CONTAMINATION

Viable legionellae were detected in four samples taken from the hot water system (Fig. 1). The legionella concentrations varied from 5 to 2,000 CFU/liter; the highest concentration was found in the tap water sample. The strains were *Legionella pneumophila* serogroup 1. The temperature of the hot water leaving the reservoirs ranged from 67 to 70°C and the returning water was 50°C. In the taps, the hot water temperature varied from 49 to 62°C. The thermophilic heterotrophic bacteria concentration was highest ($3.0 \times 10^6$ CFU/liter) in the tap water sample that contained the highest legionella counts. The mesophilic bacteria content was the highest in the legionella-positive shower sample ($5.9 \times 10^7$ CFU/liter).

The samples from cold water, spas, and the swimming pool did not contain detectable concentrations of viable legionellae. The temperature of the cold water samples varied from 12 to 17°C and the total concentration of chlorine compounds was 0.2 mg/liter in the reservoir. In pool samples, the concentration of free chlorine compounds varied from 0.4 to 0.7 mg/liter and the total concentration of chlorine compounds varied from 0.6 to 1.5 mg/liter. These temperatures and chlorine concentrations were sufficient to limit the growth of legionellae to below detectable levels.

At least one of the three crew members recently diagnosed with pneumonia had been exposed to legionellae. The shower and tap water samples from his cabin contained viable legionellae (1,000 and 5 CFU/liter, respectively). However the sera and urine samples of these crew members were all negative for legionellae.

## CONTROL PROCEDURES

Regardless of the lack of other confirmed cases and the low concentrations of legionellae detected in the distribution system, the cruise line management decided to implement preventive procedures. Initially, health personnel educated crew members about legionellae and prevention. Control measures included flushing all hot water outlets at 70°C water either daily or weekly by the crew members. The temperature of the hot water was not increased since the temperature stayed within the limits of the Finnish national guidelines on warm water temperature ($\geq$50°C) (5). This also adhered to the British guidelines on controlling the growth of legionellae in hot water systems (2). A month after the flushings began, 10 samples were taken from the three peripheral sites previously contaminated with legionellae and other sites. All sites were negative for legionellae within the detectable limits (<5 CFU/liter).

## DISCUSSION AND CONCLUSIONS

Other studies have shown that the water tanks and water systems of yachts and ships are often contaminated with legionellae (N. Temeshnikova, P. Brudny, B. Marakusha, I. Tarta-

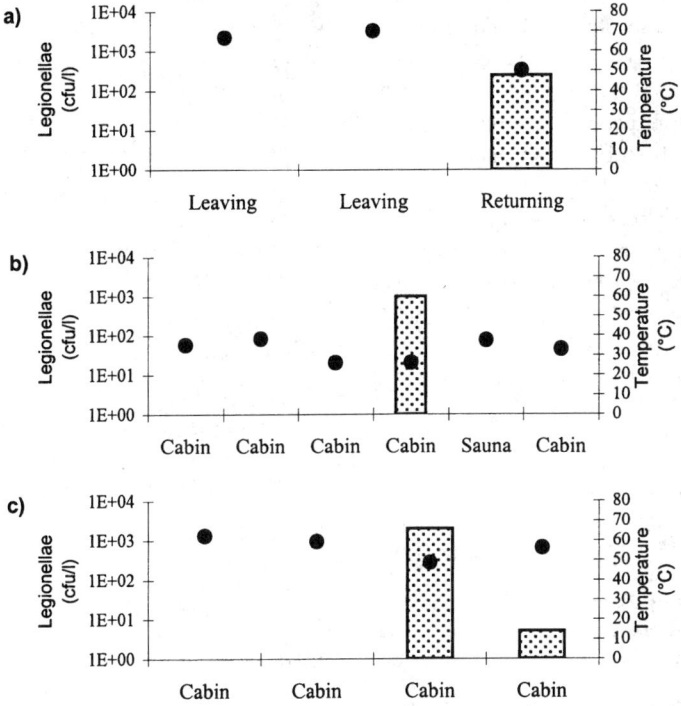

**FIGURE 1** *Legionella* concentrations (bars) and temperature (dots) in hot water samples taken from (a) circulating water, (b) shower, and (c) tap water before the control procedure.

kovskii, and S. Prosorovskii, *Proc. 11th Meet. Eur. Working Group Legionella Infect.*, Oslo, abstr., p. 71, 1996; G. Wewalka and I. Grüner, *Abstr. 9th Meet. Eur. Working Group Legionella Infect.*, abstr., p. 69–71, 1994). An unsuccessfully brominated whirlpool on a cruise ship has also been associated with an outbreak of Legionnaires' disease (4). If the *Legionella* pneumonia case of the 61-year-old man originated from the ship we studied, the most probable source was the hot water system where the recommended high water temperatures have been continuously maintained. This is addressing very high requirements for control methods of legionellae.

Further, findings of this study suggest that even low concentrations of legionellae in the water system on ships may pose a risk to health. Nowicki et al. (6) presented a theoretical infectivity level for humans of 1,000 CFU/liter, but there was no data shown relating to this concentration. The highest concentration found in this study was 2,000 CFU/liter. To suppress concentrations below 1,000 CFU/liter, in addition to high enough water temperatures, regular and frequent flushings of all the taps and showers are necessary.

The *Legionella* pneumonia case of the 61-year-old man was detected only by the urinary antigen method. Therefore, conclusive evidence of the source of this particular infection could not be confirmed. Since the incubation time for legionella infection can vary from 2 to 10 days, it is possible that the infection was contracted elsewhere, such as the patient's home. Generally absence from the home may allow bacteria to multiply in pipelines, taps, and shower heads that are not in use. Of all case detection methods, there seems to be an increasing reliance on urinary antigen at the cost of culture and serology (7). The number of cases where the source is unknown is also increasing. If these trends continue, well-focused prevention procedures will become more difficult in the future, especially following sporadic cases.

On this ship, rapid control procedures were implemented with the cooperation of the crew and the company to prevent occurrence of further cases. In the future, pneumonia cases among the crew members will be studied for the possibility of legionellosis.

## REFERENCES

1. **Finnish Standards Association.** 1987. *Determination of Available Chlorine in Water. Titrimetric method. SFS 3004.* Finnish Standards Association SFS, Helsinki, Finland.
2. **Health and Safety Executive.** 1998. The control of legionellosis in hot and cold water systems. Health and Safety Executive C130 9/98, United Kingdom.
3. **International Organization for Standardization.** 1998. Water quality–detection and enumeration of legionella. ISO 11731. International Organization for Standardization, Geneva, Switzerland.
4. **Jernigan, D., J. Hofman, M. Cetron, C. Genese, P. Nuorti, B. Fields, R. Benson, R. Carter, P. Edelstein, I. Guerrero, S. Paul, H. Lipman, and R. Breiman.** 1996. Outbreak of legionnaires' disease among cruise ship passangers exposed to a contaminated whirlpool spa. *Lancet* **347:**494–499.
5. **Ministry of Environment.** 1987. *Suomen Rakentamismääräyskokoelma D1. RT RakMK-20728.* Ministry of Environment, Helsinki, Finland.
6. **Nowicki, M., N. Bornstein, B. Jaulhac, Y. Piemont, H. Monteil, and J. Fleurette.** 1993. Rapid detection of legionellae in clinical and environmental samples by polymerase chain reaction, p. 179–181. *In* J. M. Barbaree, R. F. Breiman, and A. P. Dufour (ed.), *Legionella: Current Status and Emerging Perspectives.* American Society for Microbiology, Washington, D.C.
7. **PHLS Communicable Disease Surveillance Centre on behalf of the European Working Group for Legionella Infections.** 2000. Legionnaires' disease, Europe, 1999. *Wkly. Epidemiol. Rec.* **43:**347–352.
8. **Reasoner, D., and E. Geldreich.** 1985. A new medium for the enumeration and subculture of bacteria from potable water. *Appl. Environ. Microbiol.* **46:**1–7.

# EPIDEMIOLOGY OF *LEGIONELLA* INFECTION IN WESTERN AUSTRALIA

Tim J. J. Inglis, F. Haverkort, M. Sears,
I. Sampson, and G. Harnett

# 72

The population of Western Australia (WA) is concentrated mainly in the Perth metropolitan area and the coastal hinterland of the south-western tip of the continent. Its climate is dry and warm and is described as Mediterranean. Air-conditioning systems are therefore used extensively in public buildings and private homes during the hotter months of the year. Sporadic cases of Legionnaires' disease are diagnosed throughout the year in WA where the disease is notifiable. As in other parts of Australia, the state Health Department recommends biocide treatment of cooling towers. Maintenance of cooling towers and large-scale air-conditioning systems by engineering staff is supported by a water testing service provided by various environmental microbiology laboratories. Yet *Legionella* infection in WA has been associated with exposure to garden products such as potting mix contaminated with *Legionella longbeachae* (1, 2). Recent events in Victoria, in particular the legionellosis case cluster connected with the Melbourne oceanarium, prompted a review of

laboratory-diagnosed cases in recent years in WA.

## *LEGIONELLA* INFECTIONS IN WA

The *Legionella* urinary antigen test is not available in WA. The majority of cases of *Legionella* infection are therefore diagnosed by serological means. For purposes of laboratory-based notification, a titer of 256 is used. However, most diagnoses are made on a single titer, paired specimens being relatively uncommon. For epidemiological purposes we have used a titer of 512 or greater. Between mid-1994 and mid-2000, the vast majority of serodiagnoses were *L. longbeachae*. *Legionella pneumophila* serogroup 1 was only rarely diagnosed, and the other groups (serogroups 2 and 4) were even less common (Fig. 1). Though there were fewer culture-positive diagnoses during the same period, the same pattern was observed with *L. longbeachae* isolated significantly more often than *L. pneumophila* serogroup 1, in turn more common than other *L. pneumophila* serogroups and non-*L. pneumophila* legionellae. Nucleic acid amplification methods for diagnosis of *Legionella* infection (a *mip*-based PCR protocol) were only introduced to WA in 1998 and have led to more diagnoses of *L. pneumophila* serogroup 1 infection than *L. longbeachae* infection since then, though the

*Tim J. J. Inglis, F. Haverkort, M. Sears, I. Sampson, and G. Harnett* Division of Microbiology and Infectious Diseases, Western Australian Centre for Pathology and Medical Research, Locked Bag 2009, Nedlands, WA 6909, Australia.

*Legionella*, Edited by Reinhard Marre et al.
© 2002 ASM Press, Washington, D.C.

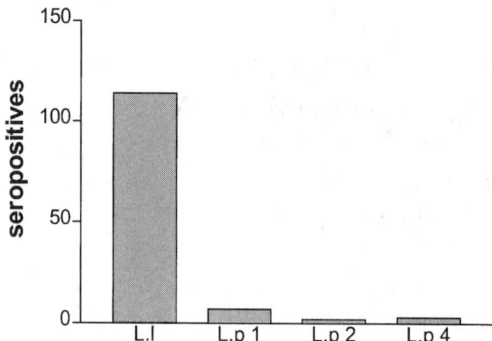

**FIGURE 1**   *Legionella* seropositives, 1994 to 2000.

*L. longbeachae* type culture strain is negative by the *mip*-PCR protocol used. It is possible that this diagnostic method underdiagnoses *L. longbeachae* infection.

## TEMPORAL DISTRIBUTION OF *LEGIONELLA* INFECTIONS IN WA

There was no evidence of temporal clustering of seropositive *Legionella* cases in WA from mid-1994 to mid-2000. Though seropositives varied in number from year to year, *L. longbeachae* seropositives remained more common than *L. pneumophila* serogroup 1 seropositives throughout the entire period. The peak months for *L. longbeachae* seropositives were October, November, December, and February, when gardening activity is at a peak (Fig. 2). January, the month when air-conditioning systems are in heaviest demand, saw a relative fall in *L. longbeachae* seropositives. By contrast, the majority of *L. pneumophila* serogroup 1

seropositives occurred during the colder months when air conditioning is not required in Perth.

## GEOGRAPHICAL DISTRIBUTION OF *LEGIONELLA* INFECTIONS IN WA

Very few patients seropositive for *L. longbeachae* lived outside the Perth metropolitan area. There was no evidence of geographical clustering of home locations of *L. longbeachae* or *L. pneumophila* serogroup 1 seropositive patients during the period studied. *L. longbeachae* seropositives were evenly distributed by postal district over the entire metropolitan area, most postal districts containing only one seropositive. The maximum was five cases per district, though these were spread evenly throughout the 6-year period.

## DEMOGRAPHIC FEATURES OF *LEGIONELLA* SEROPOSITIVE CASES

The peak age for *L. longbeachae* seropositive patients was 70 years, compared with 55 years for *L. pneumophila* serogroup 1 (Fig. 3) (Mann-Whitney U test, $P = 0.021$). For *L. longbeachae* seropositive patients there was also a sex-related difference in peak age—75 years for males and 55 years for females—though this fell short of statistical significance.

## ENVIRONMENTAL ISOLATION OF *LEGIONELLA* SPECIES IN WA

There has been no systematic survey of *Legionella* species in Western Australian environmental locations other than those required to

**FIGURE 2**   Seasonal distribution of *Legionella* seropositives, 1994 to 2000. Ll, *L. longbeachae*; Lp1, *L. pneumophila* serogroup 1.

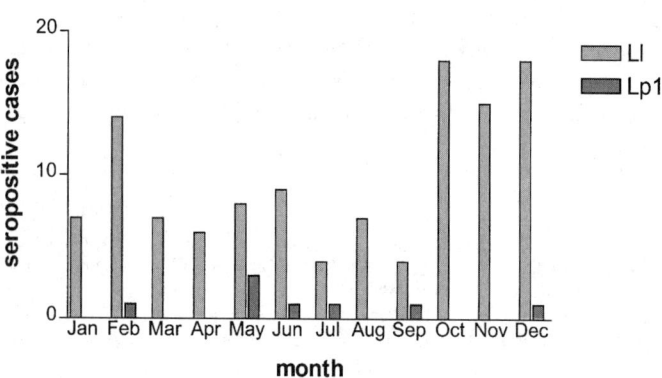

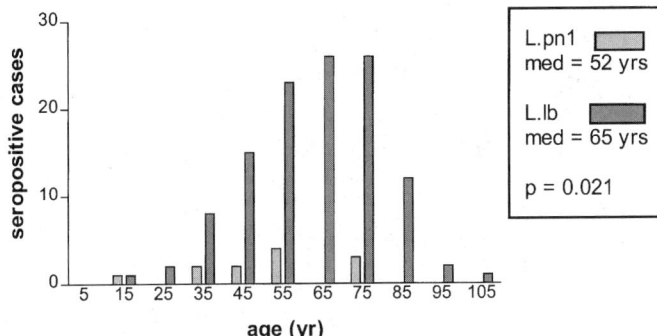

**FIGURE 3** Age distribution of *Legionella* seropositives, 1994 to 2000. L.pn1, *L. pneumophila* 1; L.lb, *L. longbeachae*; med, median.

guide the maintenance of air-conditioning and cooling systems. One representative cooling tower system on the grounds of a large public building in the Perth metropolitan area has detailed records of environmental *Legionella* testing over the last 4 years in relation to biocide and other environmental maintenance. During 1997, *L. longbeachae* was isolated from cooling tower water on three consecutive monthly samplings. From 1998 to the present this was replaced by *L. pneumophila* serogroup 1. Changes in biocide administration and thorough cleansing of the towers failed to reduce *Legionella* colony counts to recommended levels. In fact, introduction of several new biocidal agents including Stabrex 40 was associated with an increase in *Legionella* colony count by 1 to 2 × $\log_{10}$. Counts have subsequently been reduced to zero or near-zero by a combination of biocidal agents, replacement of obsolete cooling tower components, and a different biocidal regimen. Since 1997, no cases of legionellosis have been attributed to the contaminated cooling towers.

## DISCUSSION AND CONCLUSION

These data are preliminary. Nevertheless, they suggest that the epidemiology of *Legionella* infection in WA is significantly different from what has been described elsewhere. We have been unable to find any laboratory-based evidence for the occurrence of time or space clusters of legionellosis cases in WA. The serological and culture data support an environmental source widely distributed across the Perth metropolitan area and are consistent with claims that potting mix and other garden products act as the primary source. This would match with the seasonal variation and the geographical distribution. Age and sex difference may reflect differences in the populations who garden and who travel to nearby tropical destinations where air-conditioning systems are in constant use. However, further epidemiological studies are needed to confirm that *L. pneumophila* serogroup 1 infection is predominantly travel associated. Whatever the reason, *L. pneumophila* serogroup 1 infection is far less common than expected either from the experience of other Australian states or from the isolation of *L. pneumophila* serogroup 1 from WA environmental sources. In view of the predominance of *L. longbeachae* over *L. pneumophila* serogroup 1 infection in WA, it is difficult to justify the emphasis placed on controlling environmental *L. pneumophila* serogroup 1. The fact that some biocidal regimens may increase the *Legionella* count in cooling tower waters raises the possibility that biocides may in fact increase the risk of legionellosis immediately after dosing. Further studies into the epidemiology of *Legionella* infection in WA may generate useful insight into the environmental biology of this disease.

## REFERENCES

1. **Gabbay, E., W. B. de Boer, J. A. Waring, and Q. A. Summers.** 1996. *Legionella longbeachae* in Western Australia: a 12-month retrospective review. *Med. J. Aust.* **164:**704.
2. **Ross, I. S., B. J. Mee, and T. V. Riley.** 1997. *Legionella longbeachae* in Western Australian potting mix. *Med. J. Aust.* **166:**387.

# ISOLATION OF *LEGIONELLA LONGBEACHAE* AND *LEGIONELLA* SPP. FROM JAPANESE POTTING SOILS

*Michio Koide, Futoshi Higa, Noriko Arakaki, and Atsushi Saito*

# 73

*Legionella longbeachae* was first isolated in 1980 from a patient with pneumonia in Long Beach, Calif. (4). In Europe and the United States, *L. longbeachae* is rarely associated with human disease or isolated from the environment. In Australia, *L. longbeachae* serogroup 1 was first isolated from a clinical specimen in 1987, and during the following 2 years was associated with a statewide outbreak and many sporadic cases of pneumonia (3). During epidemiological investigations carried out in 1989 and 1990, *L. longbeachae* was isolated from potting mix samples and from soil surrounding potted plants collected from the homes of patients (6). These findings strongly suggest that gardening is a major risk factor in acquiring *L. longbeachae* infection.

In Japan, the first culture-proven case of legionellosis caused by *L. longbeachae* occurred in July 1996 (2). The patient was a 52-year-old male gardener, who had presented with fever, cough, and dyspnea. Despite treatment with antibiotics including erythromycin, the patient died of multiple organ failure. *L. longbeachae* serogroup 1 was isolated from his sputum. A half-year later, the potting soil manufactured by the company where the patient had worked was examined, and *Legionella bozemanii* and *Legionella spiritensis* were isolated. However, *L. longbeachae* was not isolated. This study reports a survey of ready-to-use products containing Japanese potting soils, to determine if such products are a reservoir of *L. longbeachae*.

Between January 1998 and February 1999, 32 samples were collected, consisting of 13 composted wood products, 11 potting mixes (containing composted wood products, sand, mineral fertilizer, and manure), 2 sphagnum peat moss samples, 3 peat moss-sand mixes, and 1 sample each of mineral fertilizer, manure, and hydroponic clay balls (3- to 5-mm-diameter balls used in place of sand or soil). The potting soil samples were ready-to-use products in 1.8- to 12-liter bags purchased from stores in Osaka, Hyogo, Nagasaki, and Okinawa but supplied by manufacturers from Tochigi, Tokyo, Shizuoka, Toyama, Mie, Osaka, Hyogo, and Fukuoka.

A suspension of composted wood products and potting mixes was made by mixing 50 g in 100 or 150 ml of sterile distilled water. Alternatively, a suspension of peat moss, mineral

*Michio Koide, Futoshi Higa, Noriko Arakaki, and Atsushi Saito* The First Department of Internal Medicine, Faculty of Medicine, University of the Ryukyus, 207, Uehara, Nishihara-cho, Okinawa, 903-0215, Japan.

*Legionella*, Edited by Reinhard Marre et al.
© 2002 ASM Press, Washington, D.C.

fertilizer, manure, and clay balls was made by mixing 50 g in 100 to 300 ml of sterile distilled water. The coarse particles were allowed to settle, and 1 ml of neat and 1/10, 1/100, and 1/1000 diluted suspensions were added to an equal volume of 0.2 M HCl-KCl buffer (pH 2.2), mixed, and allowed to stand for 15 min; 0.1 ml was plated on buffered charcoal-yeast extract-$\alpha$ agar containing MWY supplement (Oxoid, Hampshire, United Kingdom) and pimaricin (Sigma, St. Louis, Mo.) at a concentration of 250 mg/liter (direct method).

The original suspensions were also incubated at 33°C for 2 to 3 months (enrichment method). If amoebae were present in the sample originally, they would multiply by ingestion of soil bacteria, enabling any legionellae present to also multiply intracellularly (5). Seven cultures from which *L. longbeachae* was isolated during 2 to 3 months of amoebic enrichment were continued for 1 year. Each enrichment was subcultured onto buffered charcoal-yeast extract-$\alpha$ supplemented with MWY and pimaricin in the same way as the direct method. After incubation at 37°C for 4 days, inoculated plates were examined for *Legionella*-like colonies each day for 3 days. From each sample, 5 to 10 colonies were picked up and identified. To confirm the identity of typical colonies, the following tests were performed: biochemical identification; slide agglutination using rabbit antisera specific for *Legionella pneumophila* serogroups 1 to 15, *L. bozemanii* serogroup 1, *Legionella dumoffii*,

*Legionella gormanii*, and *Legionella micdadei* (Denkaseiken, Niigata, Japan); direct fluorescent antibody staining by using fluorescein isothiocyanate-labeled rabbit antisera specific for *L. longbeachae* serogroups 1 and 2 and *L. bozemanii* serogroups 1 and 2 (supplied by the Centers for Disease Control and Prevention, Atlanta, Ga.); and genotyping to the 25 species of *Legionella* by using a microplate DNA-DNA hybridization test kit (Kyokuto Pharm., Tokyo, Japan).

Legionellae were isolated from 11 of the 13 composted wood products samples and all 11 potting mix samples after amoebic enrichment. *L. longbeachae* was isolated from 4 and 5 samples, respectively (Table 1).

Table 2 shows the 46 strains of legionellae isolated from 22 positive samples. *L. longbeachae* was isolated from nine samples, but seven samples required enrichment before isolation was achieved. Of the nine *L. longbeachae*-positive samples, six samples were manufactured in Tokyo (three composted wood products and three potting mixes), two samples in Shizuoka (potting mixes), and one sample in Osaka (composted wood products).

Seven strains were identified as *L. longbeachae* serogroup 1 and the remaining two isolates as *L. longbeachae* serogroup 2. Interestingly, two of the samples positive for *L. longbeachae* by the direct method (both *L. longbeachae* serogroup 2) became negative within 14 weeks of incubation, in contrast to six samples from which *L. longbeachae* serogroup 1 was isolated only following enrich-

**TABLE 1** Positive rate of legionellae from 32 Japanese potting soils and gardening goods

| Kind of samples | No. of samples tested | No. of legionella-positive samples[a] | |
|---|---|---|---|
| | | Direct method | Enrichment method |
| Composted wood products | 13 | 6 (0) | 11 (4) |
| Potting mixes | 11 | 4 (2) | 11 (5) |
| Peat moss | 2 | 0 | 0 |
| Peat moss–sand mixes | 3 | 0 | 0 |
| Mineral fertilizer | 1 | 0 | 0 |
| Manure | 1 | 0 | 0 |
| Hydroponic clay balls | 1 | 0 | 0 |

[a] Values in parentheses are the number of *L. longbeachae*-positive samples.

**TABLE 2**  Species of *Legionella* isolated from 22 *Legionella*-positive samples

| *Legionella* species | No. of strains isolated | |
|---|---|---|
| | Direct method | Direct and/or enrichment method |
| *L. bozemanii* | 6 | 13 |
| *L. longbeachae* | 2 | 9 |
| *Legionella* species | 3 | 8 |
| *L. micdadei* | 1 | 7 |
| *L. oakridgensis* | 0 | 2 |
| *L cincinnatiensis* | 0 | 2 |
| *L. birminghamensis* | 1 | 1 |
| *L. gormanii* | 0 | 1 |
| *L. pneumophila* serogroup 4 | 0 | 1 |
| *L. pneumophila* serogroup 6 | 0 | 1 |
| *L. penumophila* serogroup 12 | 1 | 1 |
| Total | 14 | 46 |

**TABLE 3**  Isolation frequency of legionellae from nine samples positive for *L. longbeachae*

| Sample no. | Organism(s) isolated by[a]: | | | |
|---|---|---|---|---|
| | Direct method | Amoebic enrichment | | |
| | | 4–6 weeks | 3–4 months | 1 year |
| 1 | *L. longbeachae* serogroup 2 | *L. longbeachae* serogroup 2 | − (*Legionella* species) | ND |
| 2 | *L. longbeachae* serogroup 2 (*L. birminghamensis*) | *L. longbeachae* serogroup 2 | − | ND |
| 3 | − (*L. pneumophila*, *Legionella* species, *L. micdadei*) | − (*L. pneumophila*, *Legionella* species, *L. micdadei*) | *L. longbeachae* serogroup 1 (*L. pneumophila*, *Legionella* species) | − (*L. pneumophila*, *Legionella* species *L. micdadei*) |
| 4 | − | − (*L. bozemanii*) | *L. longbeachae* serogroup 1 (*L. bozemanii*) | *L. longbeachae* serogroup 1 (*L. bozemanii*) |
| 5 | − | *L. longbeachae* serogroup 1 (*L. bozemanii*) | *L. longbeachae* serogroup 1 (*L. bozemanii*) | *L. longbeachae* serogroup 1 (*L. bozemanii*) |
| 6 | − (*L. bozemanii*) | *L. longbeachae* serogroup 1 (*L. bozemanii*) | *L. longbeachae* serogroup 1 (*L. bozemanii*) | *L. longbeachae* serogroup 1 (*L. bozemanii*) |
| 7 | − (*L. bozemanii*) | *L. longbeachae* serogroup 1 (*L. bozemanii*) | *L. longbeachae* serogroup 1 (*L. bozemanii*) | *L. longbeachae* serogroup 1 (*L. bozemanii*) |
| 8 | − (*L. bozemanii*) | *L. longbeachae* serogroup 1 (*L. bozemanii*) | *L. longbeachae* serogroup 1 (*L. bozemanii*) | *L. longbeachae* serogroup 1 (*L. bozemanii*) |
| 9 | − (*Legionella* species) | *L. longbeachae* serogroup 1 (*Legionella* species) | *L. longbeachae* serogroup 1 (*Legionella* species) | *L. longbeachae* serogroup 1 (*Legionella* species) |

[a] ND, not done; −, negative for *L. longbeachae*; organisms in parentheses are isolated *Legionella* spp. other than *L. longbeachae*.

ment, but from which *L. longbeachae* serogroup 1 could still be isolated after incubation for 1 year (Table 3).

The most predominant species of *Legionella* obtained from potting soils was *L. bozemanii* serogroup 1, which was isolated from 13 samples (Table 2). In contrast to *L. longbeachae*, *L. bozemanii* was isolated without enrichment from six samples. In addition, *L. micdadei* and *Legionella* spp. (unclassified by the identification tests performed) were isolated from seven and eight samples each; *Legionella oakridgensis* and *Legionella cincinnatiensis* from only two samples; and *L. gormanii*, *Legionella birminghamensis*, and *L. pneumophila* serogroups 4, 6, and 12 from one sample each. Most of these species were isolated only after enrichment.

More than one *Legionella* species was isolated from all but five samples. Two species were isolated from 11 samples, and three and four species were isolated from five samples and the remaining sample, respectively.

Two peat moss samples, three peat moss-sand mixes, mineral fertilizer, manure, and the clay ball sample were negative for legionellae, similar to findings in studies that examined European peat samples (6).

In the present survey, most of the *Legionella* species isolated from Japanese potting soils have been associated with disease in humans, an important finding with respect to public health. In Japan, various types of potting soils are used for gardening, such as composted wood products, potting mixes, peat moss, and peat moss-sand mixes. Japanese potting soils contain composted wood products produced from broadleaves such as oak and Japanese oak (sometimes cryptomeria and cypress), in contrast to pines or eucalyptus in Australia. In South Australia, *L. longbeachae* was isolated from 58% of potting soils by a direct method

(all strains consisted of *L. longbeachae* serogroup 1), compared with only 8.3% (2 of 24) from Japanese potting soils by the direct method. However, the amoebic enrichment method was useful to demonstrate that legionellae are present in low numbers in most potting soils.

The first report of *L. longbeachae* in the United States in 2000 (1) consisted of three cases associated with gardening. The role of potting mixes and the mode of transmission need to be determined. The clinical relevance of the organism in potting media and its potential impact on society remain to be clarified.

## REFERENCES

1. **Duchin, J. S., J. Koehler, J. M. Kobayashi, R. M. Rakita, K. Olson, N. B. Hampson, D. N. Gilbert, J. M. Jackson, K. R. Stefonek, M. A. Kohn, J. Rosenberg, D. Vugia, and M. Marchione-Mastroianni.** 2000. Legionnaires' disease associated with potting soil—California, Oregon, and Washington, May–June 2000. *Morb. Mortal. Wkly. Rep.* **49:**777–778.
2. **Koide, M., A. Saito, M. Okazaki, B. Umeda, and R. F. Benson.** 1999. Isolation of *Legionella longbeachae* serogroup 1 from potting soils in Japan. *Clin. Infect. Dis.* **29:**943–944.
3. **Lim, I. L., N. Sangster, D. P. Reid, and J. A. Lanser.** 1989. *L. longbeachae* pneumonia: report of two cases. *Med. J. Aust.* **150:**599–601.
4. **Mckinney, R. M., R. K. Porschen, P. H. Edelstein, M. J. Bissett, P. P. Harris, S. P. Bondell, A. G. Steigerwalt, R. E. Weaver, M. E. Ein, D. S. Lindquist, R. S. Kops, and D. J. Brenner.** 1981. *Legionella longbeachae* species nova, another etiologic agent of human pneumonia. *Ann. Intern. Med.* **94:**739–743.
5. **Sanden, G. N., W. E. Morrill, B. S. Fields, R. F. Breiman, and J. M. Barbaree.** 1992. Incubation of water samples containing amoebae improves detection of *Legionellae* by the culture method. *Appl. Environ. Microbiol.* **58:**2001–2004.
6. **Steele, T. W., C. V. Moore, and N. Sangster.** 1990. Distribution of *Legionella longbeachae* serogroup 1 and other legionellae in potting soils in Australia. *Appl. Environ. Microbiol.* **56:**2984–2988.

# SPORADIC COMMUNITY-ACQUIRED LEGIONNAIRES' DISEASE AND CONTAMINATED DOMESTIC HOT WATER SUPPLIES

Michel Laverdière, Jean R. Joly, Francine Habel,
France Bernier, Guy A. Riendeau, and Emidio DeCarolis

# 74

Although *Legionella* species are a common contaminant of potable water, the epidemiological links between the source of infection and sporadic community-acquired legionellosis (CAL) is seldom established (1, 2). Domestic water supply, and particularly electric hot water systems, have been associated with *Legionella* colonization, and potential clinical implications have been suggested (1, 2, 3). In an effort to establish a link between sporadic legionellosis and hot water system colonization, patients hospitalized with documented sporadic CAL at Maisonneuve-Rosemont hospital in Montréal, Canada, were prospectively investigated.

*Michel Laverdière and Francine Habel* Department of Microbiology-Infectious Diseases, Hôpital Maisonneuve-Rosemont, 5415 Boul. L'Assomption, Montréal, Quebec H1T 2M4, Canada. *Jean R. Joly* Laboratoire de Santé Publique du Québec, 20045 Chemin Ste-Marie, Ste Anne de Bellevue, Montréal, Quebec H9X 3R5, Canada. *France Bernier* Hema-Québec, 3131 Sherbrooke E, Montréal, Quebec H1W 1B2, Canada. *Guy A. Riendeau* Services de Santé, Sécurité Santé du Publique, 75 ouest René Levesque, Montréal, Quebec H2Z 1A4, Canada. *Emidio DeCarolis* Anti-Infectives R&D, Pfizer Canada Inc., P.O. Box 800, Pointe-Claire/Dorval, Quebec H9R 4V2, Canada.

## EPIDEMIOLOGICAL SURVEILLANCE OF COMMUNITY-ACQUIRED LEGIONELLOSIS

From July 1997 through December 1999, lower respiratory tract secretions from patients admitted with symptoms of community-acquired pneumonia were cultured for *Legionella pneumophila*. The two media that were used for culture were buffered charcoal–yeast extract (BCYE) agar supplemented with ∂-ketoglutarate, and BCYE medium supplemented with cefamandole (4 mg/liter), polymyxin B (80,000 international units [IU]/liter), and anisomycin (80 mg/liter). Identifications of legionella were done according to accepted standards (6). Once a positive-culture CAL patient was identified, written informed consent was obtained to conduct an epidemiological questionnaire and to quantitatively culture for *L. pneumophila* domestic water samples from the hot water tank, sinks, showers, and tub outlets of the patient's home using BCYE and BCYE medium supplemented with glycine (3 mg/liter), polymyxin B (100,000 U/liter), and vancomycin (5 mg/liter), as previously described (1). Matching *Legionella* isolates from each patient and that patient's environment were further characterized by serotyping and by restriction endonuclease analysis (5).

*Legionella*, Edited by Reinhard Marre et al.
© 2002 ASM Press, Washington, D.C.

During our 30-month prospective surveillance period, 2,614 patients with community-acquired pneumonia were admitted at Maisonneuve-Rosemont hospital. Three culture-confirmed cases of CAL were documented. Each patient was infected with a different *L. pneumophila* serogroup (Table 1). Water samples obtained from each patient's home resulted in matching cultures in only one patient, a 62-year-old male admitted with *L. pneumophila* serogroup 1 subtype OLDA community-acquired pneumonia (patient 2). Restriction endonuclease analysis on the isolates recovered from water samples collected from this patient's hot water tank, shower head, and water faucets matched the isolate recovered from his respiratory secretions (Fig. 1). The epidemiological questionnaire revealed that the patient was a heavy smoker and an alcoholic, and that he had taken residency with his 82-year-old mother only 2 months before his first pulmonary symptoms. The mother had lived alone in this dwelling for a year and had not been sick. The patient preferred showering while the mother would mostly take baths. A few weeks before the onset of the patient's illness, plumbing work was done on the heating elements of the hot water reservoir and several water faucets in the apartment were changed.

## CONTAMINATION RATES BY *LEGIONELLA* OF DOMESTIC HOT WATER SUPPLY

To better define the population at risk in our urban population, the frequency of contamination by *Legionella* species of domestic electric hot water supply was determined at the beginning of the third year (from January to June 1999) of our prospective epidemiological surveillance of sporadic CAL. The houses selected were privately owned and located in the boundaries of the island of Montréal. Participation in the study was voluntary, and home owners were solicited through local and specialized newspapers. Houses were included in the study only if their hot water supply system was electric. In each house, a single water sample was obtained from the hot water tank. The first 500 ml of water obtained from the drainage valve of the water heater was cultured as previously described (1).

A total of 371 water samples from household electric hot water systems were cultured. The average hot water system's age was 7.2 ± 4.8 years and the average age of the houses surveyed was 48.6 ± 25.4 years. Overall, 62 of 371 (16%) hot water systems were contaminated with a *Legionella* species (Table 2). The age of the water heater and the total capacity (i.e., 182 versus 273 liters) were the only variables associated with contamination by *Legionella* species. Only 2 of 88 (2%) of the water heaters installed less than 5 years ago were contaminated compared with 24 of 94 (25%) installed ≥11 years ago. Similarly, water samples from 50 of 241 (21%) low-volume (i.e., 182 liters) water heaters compared with 11 of 114 (10%) larger-volume (i.e., 273 liters) heaters grew *Legionella*.

These findings underline the substantial contamination rates of electric hot water sys-

**TABLE 1**  Culture results for *L. pneumophila* from patients' lower respiratory tract secretions and domestic water samples from their respective residences[a]

| Sites | Culture results (concn of organism/liter) | | |
| --- | --- | --- | --- |
| | Patient 1 | Patient 2 | Patient 3 |
| Patients' LRTS | LP serogroup 8 | LP serogroup 1 | LP serogroup 5 |
| Hot water tank | LP nontypeable (1.00E + 08) | LP serogroup 1 (1.00E + 09) | Not cultured |
| Bath faucet | No growth | LP serogroup 1 (1.00E + 06) | No growth |
| Shower head | No growth | LP serogroup 1 (1.00E + 06) | No growth |
| Kitchen faucet | No growth | LP serogroup 1 (1.00E + 07) | No growth |

[a] LP, *L. pneumophila*; LRTS, lower respiratory tract secretions.

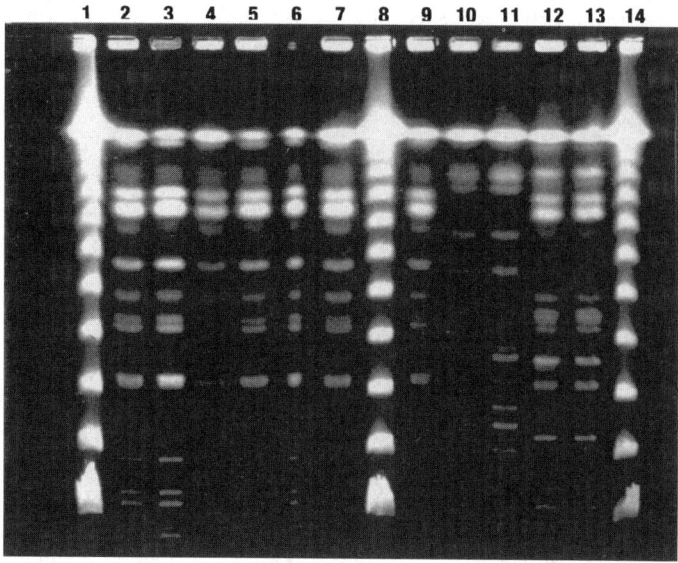

**FIGURE 1** Restriction endonuclease analysis of isolates from patient 2 and from his home water samples. Lane 1, DNA ladder; lane 2, patient's isolate: LP-1; lane 3, domestic hot water tank; lane 4, kitchen faucet; lane 5, bathroom faucet; lane 6, shower head (swab); lane 7, shower head (swab); lane 8, DNA ladder; lane 9, domestic hot water tank (1 month later); lane 10, LP-1 OLDA control no. 1 (Québec City); lane 11, LP-1 OLDA control no. 2 (Québec City no. 2); lane 12, LP-1 OLDA control no. 3 (Pittsburgh); lane 13, LP-1 OLDA control no. 4 (Pittsburgh); lane 14, DNA ladder.

tems in Montréal, and confirm results observed in other North American cities and regions (1, 2, 7). Both the location of the heating elements in electric water heater systems and the lower power of the elements in the smaller-volume systems presumably allow for a constantly relatively lower temperature in the sediment, which is adequate for the growth of *Legionella* species.

Of the 371 Montréal homes surveyed, 135 were located within the immediate territory of Maisonneuve-Rosemont hospital. Despite *Legionella* species colonization of domestic hot water systems in 34 (25%) of these 135 homes,

**TABLE 2** Distribution of *Legionella* species and serogroups isolated in water samples from 371 domestic hot water tanks

| Species and serogroups | No. (%) isolated |
| --- | --- |
| *L. pneumophila* serogroup 1 | 16 (4.3) |
| *L. pneumophila* serogroup 3 | 4 (1.1) |
| *L. pneumophila* serogroup 5 | 9 (2.4) |
| *L. pneumophila* serogroup 6 | 8 (2.2) |
| *L. pneumophila* serogroup 8 | 12 (3.2) |
| *Legionella* spp. other than *L. pneumophila* | 13 (3.5) |
| Total | 62 (16.7) |

our 30-month prospective epidemiological surveillance of more than 2,600 patients admitted at Maisonneuve-Rosemont hospital with community-acquired pneumonia showed a low incidence of severe sporadic CAL Legionnaire's disease acquired from contaminated domestic hot water supplies. Only three culture-confirmed cases of CAL were established during our 30-month prospective epidemiological surveillance study. An epidemiological link between those patients' pneumonia and their contaminated home hot water tank was established in only one patient. The first water samples from this patient's home were obtained 45 days after the patient's admission to the hospital. Additional water samples from the hot water tank taken 14 weeks after the patient's admission showed a persistence in the system of the same isolate, underlying the long-term sustained colonization of contaminated hot water systems. Debilitation by chronic alcoholism and smoking, as well as recent plumbing repair and frequent exposures to aerosols generated from the shower head, likely played predominant physiopathological roles in our patient's acquisition of Legionnaires' disease. These factors have previously been associated with higher risk for domestic acquisition of Legionnaires' disease (4, 8). Acquisition by our patient from sources outside his home is possible. However, by the time the patient moved to his mother's apartment and subsequently became ill, he was unemployed and depressed and spent most of his days at home.

The public health importance of *Legionella* colonization of domestic hot water supply systems is unknown. Large-scale epidemiological prospective studies on sporadic community-acquired legionellosis have never been done. Our study focused on severe CAL that required hospitalization and found a very low incidence linked to contaminated hot water tanks. Due to a low incidence of sporadic Legionnaires' disease, studies on the impact of *Legionella* contamination of domestic hot water supply systems might never be feasible. Individual risk factors (i.e., smoking, age, chronic lung diseases) and immunoincompetence rather than environmental factors likely represent the major contributing factors in the acquisition of severe sporadic Legionnaires' disease.

## ACKNOWLEDGMENT

We thank Johanne Ismail from the Laboratoire de Santé Publique du Québec for her technical assistance with serogrouping and molecular typing of the isolates.

## REFERENCES

1. **Alary, M., and J. R. Joly.** 1991. Risk factors for contamination of domestic hot water systems by legionellae. *Appl. Environ. Microbiol.* **57:**2360–2367.
2. **Lee, T. C., J. E. Stout, and V. L. Yu.** 1988. Factors predisposing to *Legionella pneumophila* colonization in residential water systems. *Arch. Environ. Health* **43:**59–62.
3. **Stout, J. E., V. L. Yu, P. Muraca, J. R. Joly, N. Troup, and L. S. Tompkins.** 1992. Potable water as a cause of sporadic cases of community-acquired Legionnaires' disease. *N. Engl. J. Med.* **326:**151–155.
4. **Straus, W. L., J. F. Plouffe, T. M. File, H. B. Lipman, B. H. Hackman, S. J. Salstrom, R. F. Benson, R. F. Breiman, and Ohio Legionnaires' Disease Group.** 1996. Risk factors for domestic acquisition of Legionnaires' disease. *Arch. Intern. Med.* **156:**1685–1692.
5. **Tompkins, L. S., N. J. Troup, T. Wood, W. Bibb, and R. M. McKinney.** 1986. Molecular epidemiology of Legionella species by restriction endonuclease and alloenzymes analysis. *J. Clin. Microbiol.* **25:**1875–1880.
6. **Winn, W. C.** 1999. Legionella, p. 572–585. *In* P. R. Murray, E. J. Baron, M. A. Pfaller, F. C. Tenover, and R. H. Yolken (ed.), *Manual of Clinical Microbiology*, 7th ed. American Society for Microbiology, Washington, D.C.
7. **Witherel, L. E., R. W. Duncan, K. M. Stone, L. J. Statton, L. Orclari, S. Kuppel, and D. A. Jilson.** 1988. Investigation of *Legionella pneumophila* in drinking water. *Am. Water Works Assoc. J.* **80:**87–93.
8. **Yu, V. L.** 1993. Could aspiration be the major mode of transmission for Legionella? *Am. J. Med.* **95:**13–15.

# EPIDEMIOLOGICAL TYPING OF
# *LEGIONELLA PNEUMOPHILA*
# SEROGROUP 5 STRAINS

*Björn P. Zietz, Jutta Wiese, Hartmut Dunkelberg,*
*P. Christian Lück, and Jürgen Helbig*

# 75

Following the discovery of *Legionella pneumophila* as the etiological agent of Legionnaires' disease, many different serogroups and related species of this bacterium have been detected (1). As far as is known, *L. pneumophila* serogroup 1 strains account for most cases of this acute pneumonia and have frequently been isolated from environmental samples. Despite the importance of serogroup 1, other serogroups should not be neglected. *L. pneumophila* strains identified to be serogroup 5 dominated at selected sampling sites (2). The clinical relevance of this serogroup has also been shown (2). This study aims to compare the results of two typing methods utilized for *L. pneumophila* serogroup 5 isolates. A newly developed PCR method was used to generate strain-specific DNA fingerprinting profiles. This method is compared with the results of typing the same isolates with a set of monoclonal antibodies. The test strains are isolates

cultured from water samples of different buildings in Lower Saxony, as well as strains from other parts of the world. Special interest was directed to the presence of distinct strains in hospitals and nursing homes in contrast to other isolates. This was done to evaluate the question of whether nosocomial infections can be securely differentiated from community-acquired types using the newly developed PCR analysis.

## PCR

To identify different strains of *Legionella*, we used different primers to amplify DNA fragments in crude bacterial lysates to generate banding profiles (Fig. 1). The method we used is based on a new development (6). The stored isolates were cultured on MWY agar plates at 37°C for 3 days. Next, colonies of each isolate were picked from the plates and suspended in 200 $\mu$l of 5% Chelex 100 (Biorad, Münden, Germany), vortexed for 15 s, and incubated in a heating block for 30 min at 99°C. After centrifugation at 14,500 $\times$ $g$ for 5 min, Tris-EDTA buffer (20-fold concentration) was added to the supernatant. These crude lysates were stored at $-20$°C and used in PCR reactions after adjusting them to a DNA concentration of 10 $\mu$g/ml with Tris-EDTA buffer (10 mM Tris-HCl, pH 8.0; 1 mM

*Björn P. Zietz, Jutta Wiese, and Hartmut Dunkelberg* Medical Institute of General Hygiene and Environmental Health, University of Göttingen, Windausweg 2, D-37073 Göttingen, Germany.    *P. Christian Lück and Jürgen Helbig* Institute of Medical Microbiology and Hygiene, University of Dresden, Fiedlerstraße 42, D-01307 Dresden, Germany.

*Legionella*, Edited by Reinhard Marre et al.
© 2002 ASM Press, Washington, D.C.

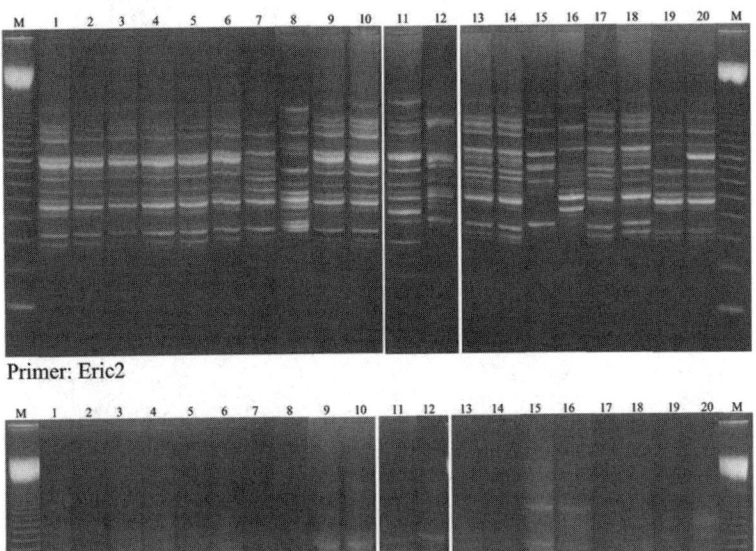

Primer: Eric2

Primer: Lpm-1 + Lpm-2

**FIGURE 1** PCR products of serogroup 5 isolates tested with primer Eric2 and a combination of Lpm-1 + Lpm-2: (lanes left to right, fit together from separate gels) molecular weight marker (M), Z 79 (lane 1), Z 132b, Z 290, WE 02 XI 1, KS E4 XII 1 (5), WL E4 XV 2, Va03335, Gö-26, Gö-215, Gö-262 (10), ATCC 33216, ATCC 33737, Denmark 6, Denmark 9, Italy 31 (15), Italy 43, Scotland 6, RingL 12A, WL 702, WL 582-4 (20), molecular weight marker (M).

EDTA, pH 8.0). DNA concentrations in the lysates were determined by UV spectroscopy (wavelength, 260 nm). PCR reactions were carried out in a final volume of 25 $\mu$l containing 5 $\mu$l of sample DNA, 2.5 $\mu$l of primer (0.01 nmol/$\mu$l), and 17.5 $\mu$l of H$_2$O. This mixture was added to Ready To Go Analysis Beads (Pharmacia Biotech Europe, Freiburg, Germany) each containing Ampli-*Taq* DNA polymerase, 0.4 mM deoxynucleotide triphosphates, 2.5 $\mu$g of bovine serum albumin, and buffer (3 mM MgCl$_2$, 30 mM KCl, 10 mM Tris [pH 8.3]). Used primers were Eric2 (5′-AAG TAA GTG ACT GGG GTG AGC G-3′, [5]) and a combination of Lpm-1 (5′-GGT GAC TGC GGC TGT TAT GG-3′)

and Lpm-2 (5′-GGC CAA TAG GTC CGC CAA CG-3′ [4]). Eric2 is an enterobacterial repetitive intergenic consensus motif. Lpm-1 and Lpm-2 are part of the macrophage infectivity potentiator (*mip*) gene of *Legionella*. The primers were synthesized and cleaned with high-pressure liquid chromatography by Biometra (Göttingen, Germany). Thermal cycling was carried out in a Crocodile III thermal cycler (Appligene Oncor, Heidelberg, Germany). Gels were stained by adding ethidium bromide to the agarose gel and bandings were visualized under UV light. Band patterns were compared visually. Isolates of a serogroup were considered to have the same PCR type when the patterns obtained with both

**TABLE 1** Results of typing serogroup 5 strains

| Designation | Source | Antigen type | PCR type with primer Eric2 | PCR type with primer Lpm-1 + Lpm-2 | PCR type, total |
|---|---|---|---|---|---|
| Z 79 | Environmental, hospital A[a] | Lp 5 Cambridge | E 1 | L 1 | I |
| Z 132b | Environmental, hospital A | Lp 5 Cambridge | E 1 | L 1 | I |
| Z 290 | Environmental, hospital A | Lp 5 Cambridge | E 1 | L 1 | I |
| WE 02 XI 1 | Environmental, hospital A | Lp 5 Cambridge | E 1 | L 1 | I |
| KS E4 XII 1 | Environmental, hospital A | Lp 5 Dallas | E 1 | L 1 | I |
| WL E4 XV 2 | Environmental, hospital A | Lp 5 Dallas | E 1 | L 1 | I |
| Va03335 | Environmental, hospital B[a] | Lp 5 Los Angeles and Lp 10[b] | E 2 | L 2 | II |
| Gö-26 | Environmental, sports hall, Göttingen | Lp 5[c] | E 3 | L 3 | III |
| Gö-215 | Environmental, hospital A | Lp 5 Cambridge | E 1 | L 1 | I |
| Gö-262 | Environmental, nursing home, Göttingen | Lp 5 Cambridge | E 1 | L 1 | I |
| ATCC 33216 | Reference strain | Lp 5 Dallas | E 4 | L 4 | IV |
| ATCC 33737 | Reference strain (= DSM 7515) | Lp 5[d] | E 5 | L 5 | V |
| Denmark 6 | Environmental, Denmark | Lp 5 Cambridge | E 6 | L 2 | VI |
| Denmark 9 | Environmental, Denmark | Lp 5 Cambridge | E 6 | L 2 | VI |
| Italy 31 | Patient, Italy | Lp 5 Dallas | E 7 | L 6 | VII |
| Italy 43 | Environmental, Italy | Lp 5 Dallas | E 8 | L 7 | VIII |
| Scotland 6 | Environmental, Scotland | Lp 5 Cambridge | E 6 | L 8 | IX |
| RingL 12A | Environmental, Great Britain | Lp 5 Cambridge | E 9 | L 2 | X |
| W 582-4 | Environmental, hospital Dresden | Lp 5 Cambridge | E 10 | L 9 | XI |
| W 702 | Environmental, Dresden | Lp 5 Cambridge | E 11 | L 10 | XII |

[a] Hospital A is located in Göttingen and hospital B in southern Lower Saxony.
[b] Strain produced positive results with MAbs for both serogroups (Dresden set).
[c] This strain gave results only with the Göttingen panel; with the Dresden panel it was not classifiable for serogroup.
[d] Antigen subtype not tested.

primers were indistinguishable. Very weak bands (not apparent on the photographs and/or not detected reproducibly) were not taken into account. In doubtful cases, the amplifications were repeated, and the patterns were compared after comigration on the same agarose gel. To guarantee reproducibility of this PCR testing, all reagents and primers were used from identical lots and solutions. Equipment was not changed during the study. Testing the method with strains other than serogroup 5 and with different lots of reagents over a longer period, no changes of banding types could be detected according to the pattern definition given above.

## TYPING WITH MONOCLONAL ANTIBODIES (MAbs)

The complete Dresden MAb panel contains 98 MAbs related to lipopolysaccharide characteristics. This panel can differentiate on the serogroup level and below. Testing of the isolates was made with these MAbs utilized in the enzyme-linked immunosorbent assay method (3).

Isolates in the Göttingen laboratory were examined by a direct fluorescent antibody technique using *L. pneumophila* serogroup 1 to 6 antibodies (rabbit) supplied by Viramed, Planegg/Steinkirchen, Germany, and *L. pneumophila* serogroup 1 to 14 MAbs (mouse) supplied by Pro-Lab Diagnostics (Mast Diagnostica, Reinfeld, Germany).

## RESULTING TYPES

In total, 20 isolates were typed that generated 12 different patterns in PCR. In some cases, both primer Eric2 and primer combination Lpm-1 + Lpm-2 were needed to differentiate between these patterns. Testing with primer Eric2 produced 11 different banding patterns, and testing with the primer combination Lpm-1 + Lpm-2 yielded 10 different banding patterns.

There were eight isolates that had PCR type I. Of these, seven isolates were water isolates from the same hospital building sampled

at different locations and on different dates. The eighth isolate with PCR type I was cultured from a water sample from a nursing home also located in Göttingen. Except for two environmental isolates from Denmark (PCR type VI), all other isolates had differing PCR types in this study.

## TYPING WITH MAbs

More than half of the isolates belong to subtype Cambridge, and subtype Dallas was less frequent (Table 1). In one case (Va03335), a strain produced positive results with MAbs for both serogroups 5 and 10. In another case (Gö-26), the strain was not classifiable for serogroup with the Dresden panel (frequency of no reaction in the Dresden MAb panel ca. 0.3%). Tested with the Göttingen direct fluorescent antibody technique panel it was classified as serogroup 5. Remarkably, PCR type I could further be differentiated in subtypes Cambridge and Dallas by MAbs (samples cultured from water from a hospital in Göttingen).

We conclude that a combination of these methods can be a useful tool for subtyping *L. pneumophila* serogroup 5 strains. The PCR fingerprinting should be done with a combination of different primers.

We plan to continue this study, especially with isolates cultured in the same outbreak from the patient and his environment to confirm the results given above.

## REFERENCES

1. **Benson, R. F., and B. S. Fields.** 1998. Classification of the genus Legionella. *Semin. Respir. Infect.* **13:**90–99.
2. **Chang, F. Y., S. L. Jacobs, S. M. Colodny, J. E. Stout, and V. L. Yu.** 1996. Nosocomial Legionnaires' disease caused by *Legionella pneumophila* serogroup 5: laboratory and epidemiologic implications. *J. Infect. Dis.* **174:**1116–1119.
3. **Helbig, J. H., J. B. Kurtz, M. C. Pastoris, C. Pelaz, and P. C. Lück.** 1997. Antigenic lipopolysaccharide components of *Legionella pneumophila* recognized by monoclonal antibodies:

possibilities and limitations for division of the species into serogroups. *J. Clin. Microbiol.* **35:**2841–2845.

4. **Jaulhac, B., M. Nowicki, N. Bornstein, O. Meunier, G. Prevost, Y. Piemont, J. Fleurette, and H. Monteil.** 1992. Detection of *Legionella* spp. in bronchoalveolar lavage fluids by DNA amplification. *J. Clin. Microbiol.* **30:**920–924.

5. **van Belkum, A., M. Struelens, and W. Quint.** 1993. Typing of *Legionella pneumophila* strains by polymerase chain reaction-mediated DNA fingerprinting. *J. Clin. Microbiol.* **31:**2198–2200.

6. **Zietz, B., J. Wiese, F. Brengelmann, and H. Dunkelberg.** 2001. Presence of *Legionellaceae* in warm water supplies and typing of strains by polymerase chain reaction. *Epidemiol. Infect.* **126:** 147–152.

# PREVENTION
# AND CONTROL

# VI

# AUSTRALIAN RISK MANAGEMENT APPROACHES TO CONTROL OF *LEGIONELLA* IN COOLING WATER SYSTEMS

*Clive Broadbent*

# 76

Cooling towers and associated systems have been refined to be highly efficient at heat rejection; they have a very important role to play in reducing the thermal pollution of the environment and in overall water management. Given appropriate conditions, these systems can act as sources of microbial growths and present a public health hazard. Table 1 summarizes the significant Australian outbreaks (February 1979 to July 2000) in which there were multiple cases attributed to a point source. Of the 21 outbreaks, 14 were traced to cooling towers/evaporative condensers.

The elevated water temperatures and large wetted surface area in cooling water systems present ideal conditions for microbial growth. To reduce contamination in cooling water systems, attention must be paid to equipment design, installation, operation, and maintenance (1, 3; website, www.health.sa.gov.au/pehs). The aim is to minimize microbial multiplication in these environments, to ensure water treatment is adequate, and to minimize the production and release of aerosols (1, 3).

Experience with cooling water systems contaminated with legionellae has led to research of the appropriate measures to control these microorganisms (2, 4). Such measures have been written into an abundance of standards and guideline documents aimed at reducing the potential for these, and other, systems to present a public health risk.

The approach taken in Australia has been to produce a prescriptive standard (6), which has been incorporated into uniform building regulations and most of the State Health acts and regulations within Australia. There are two prescriptive parts to the standard. Part 1 covers design, installation, and commissioning aspects, and part 2 covers operation and maintenance of cooling water systems and other air-handling and water systems in buildings. In regard to cooling water systems, the standard is aimed at those that are commercial-sized (cooling towers, evaporative condensers, and fluid coolers under, say, 3,000 kW of heat rejection capacity). Part 2 does not suitably address large industrial systems such as those installed at power stations and oil refineries, nor air-conditioning systems in large commercial office buildings, since there is a requirement for each system to be shut down for periodic cleaning and disinfection. In spite of this, microbiological control at such large

*Clive Broadbent*   Clive Broadbent and Associates Pty Ltd, PO Box 16, Jamison Centre 2614, Canberra, Australia.

*Legionella*, Edited by Reinhard Marre et al.
© 2002 ASM Press, Washington, D.C.

**TABLE 1** Outbreaks of Legionnaires' disease

| Source | No. of outbreaks in: | | | |
|---|---|---|---|---|
| | New South Wales | Victoria | South Australia | Other |
| Cooling towers/evaporative condensers | 6 | 6 | 1 | 1 |
| Spa pools | 1 | 1 | 2 | 1 |
| Hot water services | 0 | 1 | 0 | 0 |
| Potting mixtures | 0 | 0 | 1 | 0 |

cooling water systems (more than 3,000 kW of heat rejection capacity) is usually effective. Reported outbreaks from such sources are scant compared with those arising from smaller systems. There may be many reasons for this phenomenon but a consequence is that the typical prescriptive requirements for periodic shutdown, draining, and cleaning of smaller systems are not only impracticable and uneconomic but also unwarranted. Moreover, frequent cleaning (e.g., four times per year), while appropriate for small systems, does increase the burden on the environment, since system chemicals are drained to waste and must be replaced. It is apparent that any standard for cooling water systems needs to provide for a performance-based alternative to prescriptive approaches. To complement part 2, AS/NZS 3666 part 3 (8) was developed to provide such an option. It follows risk-management principles including hazard identification and assessment, control measures, and monitoring and corrective actions.

Table 2 sets out the risk factors that are described in part 3 of the standard as requiring assessment and control since they may contribute to source growth and dissemination of microorganisms including legionellae. The risk assessment must identify each of the risk factors and document control strategies that are effective and also appropriate to each particular site. Central to the methodology is the provision of automatically controlled water treatment to effectively minimize scale, corrosion, deposition of materials on heat-transfer surfaces, and growth of microorganisms. Performance criteria and operating control ranges

for a range of factors described in part 3 (see Table 2) need to be established and monitored for the particular installation.

Sampling for legionellae is generally not required by health authorities or by prescriptive standards such as AS/NZS 3666 part 2, but is considered to be a relevant monitoring activity in the performance-based approach described in part 3. Although the sample taken may not fully represent the microbial distribution and variety within the system, it is presently the most direct means of assessing the effectiveness of maintenance regimes on the multiplication of *Legionella* species. Such specific tests need to be complemented with other assessments such as total bacterial count (also called heterotropic colony count) and system water quality characteristics to provide reassurance that the system is well maintained and operating in a hygienic condition (e.g., that organisms such as protozoa and algae are not able to multiply).

The number of organisms required to cause infection cannot be established at this time. Indeed, infection leading to disease depends substantially on factors such as emission of protozoan vesicles or susceptibility of the person exposed. However, it is reasonable to suppose that increased risk is associated with exposure to increased concentrations of organisms (5). It is the intention of part 3 of this standard that cooling water systems operate with nondetectable concentrations of legionellae. This standard requires corrective actions to be carried out whenever a detectable concentration of *Legionella* spp. is found (10 CFU/ml is the lowest level of detection ac-

**TABLE 2** Risk factors to be assessed and controlled

| Risk area | Risk factor[a] |
|---|---|
| Opportunity for multiplication | Presence of water (especially if stagnant, e.g., deadlegs or system not in use) |
| | Concentration of legionellae (all species are considered as potential pathogens)★ |
| | Concentration of other heterotrophic bacteria★ |
| | Presence of protozoa and algae |
| | Presence of nutrients |
| | System size (surface area available for biofilm development [compared with water volume]) |
| | Presence of biofilm |
| | Characteristics of makeup water |
| | Water quality |
| | • Cleanliness★ |
| | • pH★, total alkalinity, chlorides★ |
| | • Presence of corrosion products★ |
| | • Presence of scale and fouling |
| | • Total dissolved solids/conductivity★ |
| | • Control limits out of range★ |
| | • Suspended solids (nearby construction) |
| | • Control of water treatment chemicals, bleed★ |
| | Water temperature★ |
| | Characteristics of makeup water |
| | Direct sunlight (promotes algal growth) |
| | Physical condition of system★ |
| | Microbial control program |
| | System location and environment |
| Mechanism for dissemination | Open system |
| | Aerosol generation |
| | Mode of operation |
| | • Intermittent operation |
| | • Seasonal usage |
| | Drift elimination effectiveness |
| | Aerosol dispersion |
| | System location (distance to other cooling water systems, air intakes, and passersby) |

[a] ★, Risk factor identified as a key performance indicator. Reprinted from reference 8 with permission of the publisher.

cording to AS 3896 [7], the Australian standard commonly used for enumeration of legionellae) in order to provide confidence that the system is hostile to these microorganisms. More demanding actions are required when a higher concentration is detected. Consistent total bacterial counts is a useful indicator of the hygienic condition of the cooling water system. The standard therefore sets out control strategies considered appropriate for various concentrations of heterotrophic microorganisms. Should the cooling water be drawn from a cooling pond or lake or when grey water is used, alternative control strategies should be documented and applied on the basis of case history information.

Both chemical and physical monitoring of the water-treatment program are essential for system life and performance, as well as for controlling microorganisms such as *Legionella* spp. Thus, properly implemented microbial control for disease prevention should assist in system longevity and efficiency. The water treatment needs to be well managed and more comprehensive than may suffice for those systems that are routinely cleaned and disinfected in accordance with prescriptive standards such as AS/NZS 3666 part 2. Water-management approaches may differ in detail from site to site and therefore need to be documented in a specific plan for each site.

Where the assessed risk factors (Table 2) fall outside set operating control ranges, the standard requires that remedial actions be carried out in accordance with prearranged directives to quickly bring the factors back within the specified limits. For example, high pH may be assessed as resulting in poor biocidal effectiveness; the remedial actions may be to check the chemical dosage or the concentration of salts in the system water. The standard also requires that a summary sheet of test results and actions taken be prepared monthly. The report is to include the test type, the control range, the test results, the test date, and the name of the person or organization undertaking the assessment.

Two brief case studies follow. Each involved a cooling water system for which risk factors similar to those described in Table 2 were applied.

In case study 1, an outbreak of Legionnaires' disease was associated with a hotel. *Legionella pneumophila* serogroup 1 count was 2.8 $\times$ $10^7$ CFU/ml. Control measures included:

- system decontamination
- rectification of system irregularities, e.g., absence of drift eliminators
- improved access for cleaning
- filtration of circulating water
- filtration of incoming air to plant room (construction activities at adjacent properties)
- removal of pump header piping, which was a potential deadleg
- revised biocidal regime
- water treatment automated
- monitoring plan implemented

In case study 2, several cases of Legionnaires' disease occurred at an industrial site at which there were both large process cooling towers (*L. pneumophila* serogroup 1

count, 1,000 CFU/ml) and small comfort air-conditioning towers (not sampled for legionellae). After immediate intervention measures, including decontamination of all systems, a risk-management study was carried out. Control measures included:

- extensive tower cleaning operations
- online cleaning improved by use of industrial waste cleaning trucks with vacuum hoses to clean tower basins
- installation of modern drift eliminators
- piping deadlegs eliminated
- water treatment revised and automated
- policies on personnel safety implemented
- small towers either replaced with air-cooled plant or appropriate modifications carried out
- *Legionella* management advisory committee established at site
- risk-management plan strictly enforced

At both locations, monitoring programs, including water sampling for legionellae, were implemented. No further clinical cases nor significant *Legionella* spp. detections have been experienced. These case studies are examples only of the increasing awareness of *Legionella* as an environmental pathogen that has led to control and monitoring strategies on a wide scale in Australia; sampling for legionellae may now be important as a defense under common law.

While the evidence strongly supports the view that a clean system is of fundamental importance in *Legionella* control, methods of achieving this condition may vary. One such approach is the use of risk-management techniques based on AS/NZS 3666 part 3. The approach necessarily includes microbiological monitoring, a controversial issue due to the uncertainties involved (e.g., whether the sample is representative), difficulties in interpretating results, and delays associated with laboratory culturing techniques. Nonetheless, it is believed by cooling tower owners and government regulators that sampling serves a useful management purpose when employed in conjunction with comprehensive monitoring of other system water chemical and physical characteristics. There is a need for the risk-management strategies to be further refined with use and so continue our progress in *Legionella* control in a cost-effective and environmentally sensitive manner.

## REFERENCES

1. **American Society of Heating, Refrigerating and Air-conditioning Engineers.** 2000. *Guideline 12. Minimizing the Risk of Legionellosis Associated with Building Water Systems.* American Society of Heating, Refrigerating and Air-conditioning Engineers, Atlanta, Ga.
2. **Bentham, R. H.** 1993. Environmental factors affecting the colonization of cooling towers by *Legionella* spp. in South Australia. *Int. Biodeterior. Biodegrad.* **31:**55–63.
3. **Broadbent, C.** 1996. *Guidance for the Control of Legionella.* National Environmental Health Forum Monograph, Water Series No. 1. South Australian Department of Human Services, Adelaide, Australia.
4. **Broadbent, C. R.** 1999. Control of Legionnaires' disease—an Australian perspective. *Am. Soc. Heating, Refrig. Air-cond. Eng. Trans.* **105:**595–606.
5. **Shelton, B. G., W. D. Flanders, and G. K. Morris.** 1994. Legionnaires' disease outbreaks and cooling towers with amplified *Legionella* concentrations. *Curr. Microbiol.* **28:**359–363.
6. **Standards Australia.** 1995. *Air-Handling and Water Systems of Buildings, Microbial Control. AS/NZS 3666* (parts 1 and 2). Standards Australia, Sydney, Australia.
7. **Standards Australia.** 1998. AS 3896: *Waters—Examination for Legionellae Including Legionella pneumophila.* Standards Australia, Sydney, Australia.
8. **Standards Australia.** 2000. *Air-Handling and Water Systems of Buildings, Microbial Control. AS/NZS 3666. Part 3: Performance-Based Maintenance of Cooling Water Systems.* Standards Australia, Sydney, Australia.

# AMERICAN SOCIETY OF HEATING, REFRIGERATING AND AIR-CONDITIONING ENGINEERS GUIDELINE 12-2000: MINIMIZING THE RISK OF LEGIONELLOSIS ASSOCIATED WITH BUILDING WATER SYSTEMS

*David F. Geary*

# 77

## ASHRAE

ASHRAE is an acronym for the American Society of Heating, Refrigerating and Air-Conditioning Engineers. It is an international professional society with some 50,000 members. The society is organized for the sole purpose of advancing the arts and sciences of heating, ventilation, air conditioning, and refrigeration for the public's benefit through research, writing of standards and guidelines, and continuing education and publications.

ASHRAE's annual research spending exceeds $3 million. More than 100 research projects are currently underway at a combined total cost to ASHRAE of $9 million. Results of ASHRAE research are disseminated in a number of ways. The majority of projects provide significant technical information that is used in updating the four-volume ASHRAE handbook series. Most of the remaining projects contribute to the development of standards and guidelines as well as other publications, such as design manuals.

Research projects are currently sponsored and monitored by some 54 technical committees. Research categories include indoor air quality, energy conservation, fire and safety, comfort and health, refrigeration systems, and environmentally safe materials.

## GUIDELINE 12

ASHRAE's Environmental Health Committee recognized the need for a comprehensive, nationally accepted guideline to address the public health issues surrounding Legionnaires' disease. Of course, such a guideline should also lessen legal problems and their corresponding economic impact resulting from outbreaks.

While a number of guidelines existed, none filled the requirements of the Environmental Health Committee. The Cooling Technology Institute (CTI) has a position statement, issued in 1996 (13); an emergency decontamination protocol, originally issued in 1980 (14); and a guideline issued in 2000 (12), shortly before the ASHRAE guideline. However, these all deal exclusively with cooling tower systems. ASHRAE has a position paper and a position statement, originally issued in 1981 (4) and updated in 1989 (5) and 1998 (6). These all tend to be more educational than prescriptive and do not deal with the wide range of systems deemed necessary.

*David F. Geary*  Baltimore Aircoil Company, P.O. Box 7322, Baltimore, MD 21227.

*Legionella*, Edited by Reinhard Marre et al.
© 2002 ASM Press, Washington, D.C.

Allegheny County in western Pennsylvania has a document titled *Approaches to Prevention and Control of Legionella Infection in Allegheny County Health Care Facilities* (1). However, this is limited in scope to potable water systems in health care facilities.

The Wisconsin protocol, *Control of Legionella in Cooling Towers—Summary Guidelines* (28), was issued in 1987 but was limited in scope to routine maintenance and emergency cleaning of cooling towers. The CDC has published *Recommendations for Prevention of Nosocomial Legionnaires' Disease* (11). However, this document is of limited scope dealing with nebulizers, cooling towers, and water distribution systems in hospitals. It does not fill the bill of a comprehensive guideline. Section II, chapter 7, of the *OSHA Technical Manual* (23), also does not fill the need since it deals with investigative procedures and its stated intent is to assist industrial hygienists in the assessment of work sites for potential Legionnaires' disease. The primary focus is on control and prevention of contaminated water sources, but it is limited to discussion of cooling towers and domestic water systems.

Finally, the state of Maryland has recently issued a guideline on *Legionella* in health care institutions (24). This document is limited to potable water systems and cooling towers and the focus is on acute care hospitals.

Guideline 12-2000 (3) was developed to fill a void in the United States.

## GUIDELINE PROJECT COMMITTEE (GPC)-12

Guideline 12 was drafted by ASHRAE Guideline Project Committee (GPC) 12, which was formed in 1993 and held its first meeting at the winter meeting in 1994. The committee averaged 18 to 19 voting members from January 1994 to June 1999 with approximately half of the voting members remaining active throughout the entire period.

GPC-12 was composed of members with diverse backgrounds ranging from physicians to consulting engineers and microbiologists to manufacturers. The membership was characterized as falling into one of the following categories: general interest, users, equipment suppliers, chemical suppliers, and biological testing/monitoring services. GPC-12 was a balanced committee in that no one or two categories constituted a majority.

## BACKGROUND

*Legionella* thrives when favorable conditions are encountered. Conditions that are favorable to amplification of legionellae include water temperatures of 25 to 42°C (77 to 108°F), plus the presence of scale, sediment, biofilms, and protozoa. Growth of legionellae within protozoa and/or within complex biofilms may be the primary means of proliferation. Controlling the populations of protozoa and other microorganisms may be the best means of minimizing *Legionella* (15).

Investigation of Legionnaires' disease outbreaks has suggested that, in most instances, transmission to humans has occurred when water containing the organism is aerosolized into droplets less than 5 $\mu$m in diameter, allowing inhalation into the lungs of a susceptible host.

A chain of events must occur in order for Legionnaires' disease to result. As depicted in Fig. 1 (8), the chain begins with a source of *Legionella*. This event is generally outside the scope of building engineering and management practices. However, the next three events in the chain—amplification, dissemination, and transmission—can be influenced by engineering design and maintenance practices. Subsequent events are influenced by the individual's health.

The strategy for the control of most diseases, including legionellosis, is to break the chain of transmission at as many points as possible. Guideline 12 presents information intended to allow readers to develop an understanding of the types of conditions that may allow amplification and transmission of *Legionella*. With this understanding it should be possible to define strategies to break the chain to prevent the disease.

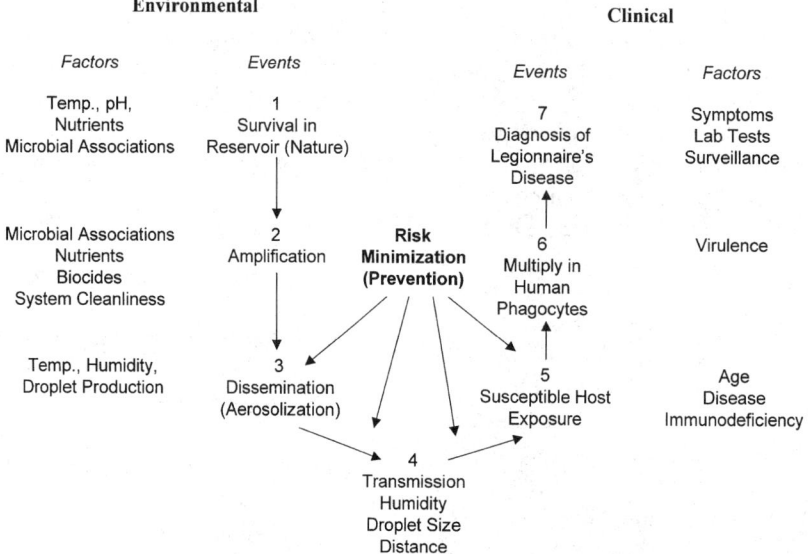

**FIGURE 1** *Legionella* transmission. © 2000, American Society of Heating, Refrigerating and Air-Conditioning Engineers, Inc., www.ashrae.org. Reprinted by permission from *Guideline 12-2000—Minimizing the Risk of Legionellosis Associated with Building Water Systems* (3).

## AMPLIFIERS

Systems that receive legionellae from a water or air source and offer conditions favorable for the amplification of the organism are referred to as amplifiers. Amplifiers that are covered by Guideline 12 include potable (hot as well as cold) and emergency water systems, cooling towers and evaporative condensers, heated spas, architectural fountains and waterfall systems, evaporative air coolers, misters, air washers, humidifiers, and metal working systems. Information is presented on operation, nutrient availability, operating temperature level, water droplet sizes, and most importantly, recommended treatment. A review of all of the amplifier systems is beyond the scope of this chapter. Rather, the discussion will be limited to potable water systems, cooling towers and evaporative condensers, and heated spas. Readers are referred to ASHRAE Guideline 12-2000 for information on amplifiers not covered here, as well as additional information on amplifiers that are covered.

## Potable Water Systems

Potable water systems include all piping from the point where the water enters the building, as well as hot water heaters, storage tanks, faucets, nozzles, and any other distribution outlets. Water delivered to these systems from most municipal water systems has been chlorinated to control the presence of microorganisms. However, legionellae are more tolerant of chlorine than many other bacteria and are presumed present, in low concentrations, in municipal water supplies (19) and thus the potable water system.

Potable cold water systems are generally below the 25°C (77°F) level required for amplification. Potable hot water temperatures typically range from 41 (105°F) to 60°C (140°F). Temperatures below 42°C (108°F) are in the amplification range for legionellae. Both dead and living microorganisms, biofilms, and debris may provide nutrient sources required for legionellae growth. Water droplets of very small size (less than 5 $\mu$m) that can be inhaled deeply into the lungs can be created by shower heads, aerators, spray nozzles, water impacting on hard surfaces, and bubbles breaking up.

Many reports link legionellae in hospital tap water to outbreaks of nosocomial (hospital-acquired) Legionnaires' disease, often with immunosuppressed patients (18). Potable hot water systems are an important potential source of legionellosis in all buildings and are of particular importance in hospitals, nursing homes, and other health care facilities (26).

The principal treatment strategy for potable water systems is control of the water temperature level. Cold water should be stored and/or delivered at temperatures below 20°C (68°F). In health care facilities including nursing homes, the hot water should be stored at or above 60°C (140°F) and where it is recirculated, the minimum return temperature should be 51°C (124°F).

Operating at these temperature levels requires that great care be taken to avoid scalding problems. One means of accomplishing this is to install preset thermostatic mixing valves. Where this is not practical, periodically increasing the temperature to at least 66°C (150°F) or chlorination followed by flushing should be considered. Systems should be inspected annually to ensure that thermostats are functioning properly. Where practical in other situations, hot water should be stored at temperatures of 49°C (120°F) or above.

Elevated holding tanks in hot or cold water systems should be inspected and cleaned annually. Lids should fit closely to exclude foreign materials.

Insulated recirculation loops should be incorporated as a design feature in high-risk applications. For all situations the pipe runs should be as short as practical. New shower systems in large buildings, hospitals, and nursing homes should be designed to permit mixing of hot and cold water near the shower head. The warm water section of pipe between the control valve and the shower head should be self-draining.

An optional treatment strategy involving copper-silver ionization is a relatively new approach to controlling Legionella in hot water distribution systems and has been used successfully in a number of hospitals (16, 20, 22). Copper and silver ions are generated electrolytically and build up in the hot water recirculating system to levels effective in eradicating Legionella, typically in the range of 0.2 to 0.8 mg of copper per liter and 0.02 to 0.08 mg of silver per liter. The optimum concentration of copper-silver ions for controlling Legionella in hot water systems is not known. Also, a specific concentration may not be universally effective due to variables in water quality and system design. It is also important to note that the efficacy of copper-silver ions, like chlorine, is adversely affected by elevated pH (25).

In high-risk applications, monthly removal of shower heads and top aerators to clean out sediment and scale and then cleaning them in a chlorine bleach solution is recommended.

Where decontamination of hot water systems is required (typically due to implication of an outbreak of legionellosis), this can be accomplished by either thermal shock treatment or by shock chlorination. See Guideline 12 for details.

Once the decontamination is complete, recolonization is likely to occur unless preventative steps are taken. Such steps could involve maintaining the recommended temperatures, using continuous supplemental chlorination, or using an alternative approach such as copper-silver ionization.

For potable water systems that were opened for repair or construction or for systems that were subjected to water pressure changes associated with construction (which may cause water to become brown and the concentration of Legionella to dramatically increase) (21), it is recommended that as a minimum the system be thoroughly flushed. High-temperature flushing or chlorination may be appropriate, and that judgment should be made on a job-specific basis.

## Cooling Towers and Evaporative Condensers

Conventional open cooling towers are evaporative heat-transfer devices in which atmospheric air mixes with and cools warm water by evaporating a portion of the water. Air movement through the tower is generally achieved by fans. Cooling towers typically use some media, referred to as "fill," to provide improved contact between the water and the cooling air.

As shown in Fig. 2, cooling towers associated with building water systems are typically used for rejecting waste heat from the chiller providing air conditioning for the building, though they could also be rejecting process heat.

Closed-circuit cooling towers and evaporative condensers are also evaporative heat-transfer devices. As evident from Fig. 3, both are similar to conventional open cooling towers, but there is one very significant difference. The process fluid (either a liquid such as water, an ethylene glycol/water mixture, oil, etc., or a condensing refrigerant) does not directly contact the cooling air. Rather, the process fluid is contained in a tubular coil assembly.

Water that is evaporated as part of the heat rejection process is replaced by make-up water, generally from the municipal water supply. Since this water is likely to contain legionellae (19), in low concentrations, it is reasonable to presume that some concentration of legionellae will be present in the cooling tower or evaporative condenser.

Cooling towers (both conventional open designs as well as closed-circuit designs) and evaporative condensers frequently, if not generally, offer conditions that are favorable to the growth of legionellae. The operating temperature is likely to be in the range of 25 to 42°C (77 to 108°F), which is favorable to amplification, although temperatures can be above 49°C (120°F) or below 21°C (70°F) depending on system heat load, ambient temperature, and system operating strategy.

Because cooling towers and evaporative condensers are highly efficient air scrubbers and also move large volumes of air, organic material and other debris can be accumulated. This material may serve as a nutrient source for legionella growth. Diverse biofilms, which can support the growth of legionellae, may be present on heat-exchanger surfaces, structural surfaces, sump surfaces, and other miscellaneous surfaces.

Cooling towers and evaporative condensers incorporate inertial stripping devices called drift eliminators to remove water droplets generated within the unit. While the effectiveness of these eliminators can vary significantly with the design (new state-of-the-art eliminators are significantly more efficient than older designs) and the condition of the eliminators, it should be assumed that some water droplets of less than 5 $\mu$m in diameter

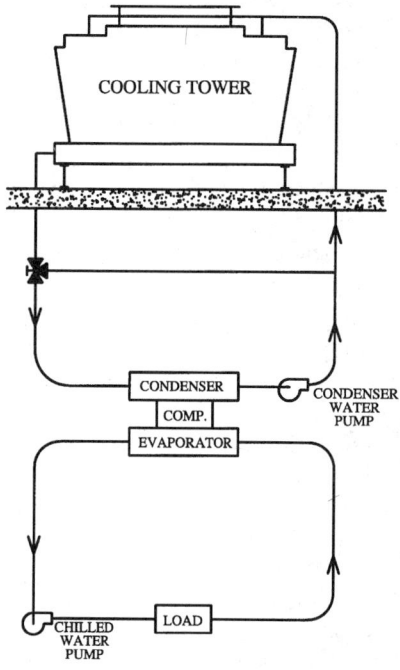

**FIGURE 2** Typical cooling tower/chiller system. © 2000, American Society of Heating, Refrigerating and Air-Conditioning Engineers, Inc., www. ashrae.org. Reprinted by permission from *Guideline 12-2000—Minimizing the Risk of Legionellosis Associated with Building Water Systems* (3).

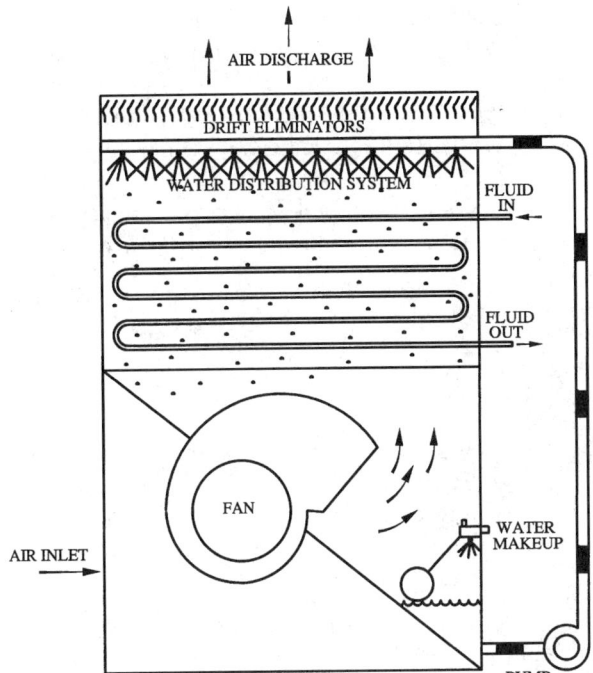

**FIGURE 3** Typical closed-circuit cooling tower or evaporative condenser. © 2000, American Society of Heating, Refrigerating and Air-Conditioning Engineers, Inc., www.ashrae.org. Reprinted by permission from *Guideline 12-2000—Minimizing the Risk of Legionellosis Associated with Building Water Systems* (3).

leave the unit. In addition, some larger droplets leaving the unit may be reduced to 5 $\mu$m or less by evaporation.

The key treatment recommendations of Guideline 12 are that the system be maintained clean and that a biocidal treatment program be employed. Further, it is recommended that a qualified water-treatment specialist be used to define and oversee the treatment program.

Maintaining a clean system reduces the nutrients available for *Legionella* growth. Regular visual inspections of the equipment should be made and the cold water basin should be cleaned when any buildup of dirt, organic matter, or other debris is visible or found through sampling. Mechanical filters or centrifugal-gravity-type separators can be useful in assisting to control such buildup. The drift eliminators should also be inspected regularly and cleaned or replaced as needed.

Operating and maintenance records should be maintained. These records should include manufacturers' operating and maintenance manuals, a description of the water-treatment program, dates of all inspections and maintenance, material safety data sheets for all chemicals used, dates of any repairs, records of the system water volume, and names of persons responsible for system startup, shut down, and operation.

A water-treatment program should be employed to minimize scale and corrosion, to control microbial growth, and to minimize the deposition of solids (organic and inorganic). Details are presented in Guideline 12.

Systems that have been inactive for more than 3 days require special attention before being returned to service (7). Specific actions vary according to whether the system was drained or not and whether a remote storage tank is used or not. See Guideline 12 for details.

Where a system is known to be contaminated and is to be decontaminated, Guideline 12 recommends that the CTI "Emergency Protocol" for decontaminating cooling towers and evaporative condensers be used (14). It is pointed out that this procedure must not be used routinely because it can be very corrosive and produces toxic fumes. Also, it is important to note that recontamination is likely if proper routine treatment is not provided.

## Heated Spas

Heated spas are small baths or pools used for recreational, hygienic, or therapeutic purposes. Whirlpool spas and hot tubs both feature recirculated water. Whirlpools and whirlpool baths are single-use systems where the water is drained after each use. Whirlpools are traditionally used for therapy, frequently for athletes, while whirlpool baths are often found in upscale hotel rooms and are gaining popularity in new houses in the United States.

Heated spas generally operate in the temperature range of 32 to 40°C, which is in the range that favors amplification. Nutrients in the form of sun lotion, body oils, and other organic materials are likely to be present. The aerosol mist that is created has 1- to 5-$\mu$m droplets and extends to a height of at least 0.5 m above the water surface. Several multiple-case outbreaks of legionellosis have been traced to spas and hot tubs (17, 27). No cases have been traced to whirlpool baths (10, 17).

The American National Standards Institute, as well as the National Spa and Pool Institute, have established chemical standards related to pool disinfection. These are generally used as the basis for most state and local regulations. They govern the operating halogen level and call for daily superchlorination. Filter maintenance includes back flushing as often as daily and cleaning or replacing filter cartridges once or twice weekly. The water should also be changed frequently, in fact, daily during continuous conditions of high use. The spa should also be physically cleaned when the water is changed.

The halogen level should be checked frequently, as often as hourly during periods of high use. Regular testing for bacteria levels may alert operators of unsafe conditions when they occur. And since the filter is likely to be the least hygienic part of the system, it is de-

sirable to inject the biocide downstream of the filter as well as into the pool.

## MONITORING FOR *LEGIONELLA*

While routine culturing of building water systems for *Legionella* is not recommended, Guideline 12 advises that it may be appropriate under the following circumstances:

- Caring for high-risk patients in health care facilities (9, 29; A. E. Fiore, J. C. Butler, T. G. Emori, and R. P. Gaynes, *35th Annu. Meet. Infect. Dis. Soc. Am.*, abstr. 332).
- Tracing the source of an outbreak.
- Evaluating the potential amplifier/transmission sources at a facility.
- Verifying the effectiveness of decontamination procedures.

Routine culturing may not be predictive of the risk of transmission for the following reasons:

- The presence of the organism cannot be equated to the risk of infection. The bacterium is frequently present in water systems without known cases of disease.
- The risk of illness is influenced by factors other than the concentration of organisms. These factors include strain virulence, susceptibility of the host, and the degree of aerosolization (i.e., water droplet sizes created).
- Test results only represent the condition at the time the sample was taken. A negative result could lead to a false sense of security because any amplifier can quickly become heavily colonized if it is neglected.
- Interpretation of the results is confounded by use of different bacteriologic methods in various laboratories, by variable culture results among different sites sampled within a water system, and by fluctuations in the concentration of *Legionella* from a single site.

If the decision is made to monitor, it should be in addition to, not in place of, sound maintenance practices and proper treatment.

## CONCLUSIONS

ASHRAE Guideline 12 presents information on several building water systems that can amplify and disseminate *Legionella*. This chapter has focused on three of these amplifiers: cooling towers, evaporative condensers, and heated spas. Specific guidance is presented to minimize the risk of legionellosis associated with these devices. Greater detail, as well as guidance on additional amplifiers, is given in Guideline 12-2000, which is available for purchase from ASHRAE and is available as a free download at www.BaltimoreAircoil.com.

## REFERENCES

1. **Allegheny County Health Department.** 1993. *Approaches to Prevention and Control of Legionella Infection in Allegheny County Health Care Facilities.* Allegheny County Health Department, Allegheny, Pa.
2. **ANSI/NSPI.** 1999. *ANSI/NSPI-2 1999 Standard for Public Spas.* ANSI/NSPI.
3. **American Society of Heating, Refrigerating and Air-Conditioning Engineers.** 2000. *ASHRAE Guideline 12-2000. Minimizing the Risk of Legionellosis Associated With Building Water Systems, 2000.* American Society of Heating, Refrigerating and Air-Conditioning Engineers, Atlanta, Ga.
4. **American Society of Heating, Refrigerating and Air-Conditioning Engineers.** 1981. *ASHRAE Legionellosis Position Paper and Statement, 1981.* American Society of Heating, Refrigerating and Air-Conditioning Engineers, Atlanta, Ga.
5. **American Society of Heating, Refrigerating and Air-Conditioning Engineers.** 1989. *ASHRAE Legionellosis Position Paper and Statement, 1989.* American Society of Heating, Refrigerating and Air-Conditioning Engineers, Atlanta, Ga.
6. **American Society of Heating, Refrigerating and Air-Conditioning Engineers.** 1998. *ASHRAE Legionellosis Position Paper and Statement, 1998.* American Society of Heating, Refrigerating and Air-Conditioning Engineers, Atlanta, Ga.
7. **American Society of Heating, Refrigerating and Air-Conditioning Engineers.** 1995. *ASHRAE TC 3.6 Letter to the Centers of Disease Control and Prevention, 1995.* American Society of Heating, Refrigerating and Air-Conditioning Engineers, Atlanta, Ga.
8. **Barbaree, J. M.** 1991. Controlling *Legionella* in cooling towers. *ASHRAE J.* **33:**38–42.
9. **Butler, J., B. S. Fields, and R. F. Breiman.** 1997. Prevention and control of legionellosis. *Infect. Dis. Clin. Pract.* **6:**458–464.
10. **Centers for Disease Control and Prevention.** 1997. Legionnaires' disease associated with a whirlpool spa display—Virginia, September-October 1996. *Morb. Mortal. Wkly. Rep.* **46:**83–86.
11. **Centers for Disease Control and Prevention.** 1996. *Recommendations for Prevention of Nosocomial Legionnaires' Disease, 1996.*
12. **Cooling Technology Institute.** 2000. *Legionellosis Guideline: Best Practices for Control of Legionella, 2000.* Cooling Technology Institute.
13. **Cooling Technology Institute.** 1996. *Cooling Technology Institute Legionellosis Position Statement, 1996.* Cooling Technology Institute.
14. **Cooling Technology Institute.** 1980. *Suggested Protocol for Emergency Cleaning of Cooling Towers and Related Equipment Suspected of Infection by Legionnaires' Disease Bacteria (L. Pneumophila), 1980.* Cooling Technology Institute.
15. **Fields, B. S.** 1993. *Legionella* and protozoa: interaction of a pathogen and its natural host, p. 129–136. *In* J. M. Barbaree, R. F. Breiman, and A. P. Dufour (ed.), *Legionella: Current Status and Emerging Perspectives.* American Society for Microbiology, Washington, D.C.
16. **Goetz, A., and V. L. Yu.** 1997. Copper-silver ionization: cautious optimism for *Legionella* disinfection and implications for environmental culturing. *Am. J. Infect. Control* **25:**449–451.
17. **Jernigan, D. B., J. Hofmann, M. S. Cetron, C. A. Genese, J. P. Nuorti, B. S. Fields, R. F. Benson, R. J. Carter, P. H. Edelstein, I. C. Guerrero, S. M. Paul, H. B. Lipman, and R. F. Breiman.** 1996. Outbreak of Legionnaires' disease among cruise ship passengers exposed to a contaminated whirlpool spa. *Lancet* **347:**494–499.
18. **Joseph, C. A., J. M. Watson, T. G. Harrison, and C. L. R. Bartlett.** 1994. Nosocomial Legionnaires' disease in England and Wales. *Epidemiol. Infect.* **112:**329–345.
19. **Kutcha, J. M., S. J. States, and A. M. McNamara.** 1983. Suceptibility of *Legionella pneumophilia* to chlorine in tap water. *Appl. Environ. Microbiol.* **46:**1134–1139.
20. **Liu, Z., J. E. Stout, M. Boldin, J. Rugh, W. F. Diven, and V. L. Yu.** 1998. Intermittent use of copper-silver ionization for *Legionella* control in water distribution systems: a potential option in buildings housing individuals at low risk for infection. *Clin. Infect. Dis.* **26:**138–140.

21. **Mermel, L. A., S. L. Josephson, C. H. Girogio, J. Dempsey, and S. Parenteau.** 1995. Association of Legionnaires' disease with construction: contamination of potable water. *Infect. Control Hosp. Epidemiol.* **16:**76–81.

22. **Metizner, S., R. C. Schwille, A. Farley, E. R. Wald, J. H. Ge, S. J. States, T. Libert, and R. M. Wadowsky.** 1997. Efficacy of thermal treatment and copper-silver ionization for controlling *Legionella pneumophila* in high volume hot water plumbing systems in hospitals. *Am. J. Infect. Control* **25:**452–457.

23. **Occupational Safety and Health Administration.** Legionnaires' Disease. *OSHA Technical Manual.* Occupational Safety and Health Administration.

24. **State of Maryland Department of Health and Mental Hygiene.** 2000. *Report of the Maryland Scientific Working Group to Study Legionella in Water Systems in Health Care Institutions, 2000.* State of Maryland Department of Health and Mental Hygiene, Baltimore, Md.

25. **Stout, J. E., and V. L. Yu.** 1997. Eradicating *Legionella* from hospital water. *JAMA* **278:**1404.

26. **Stout, J. E., V. L. Yu, P. Muraca, J. Joly, N. Troup, and L. S. Tompkins.** 1992. Potable water as the cause of sporadic cases of community-acquired Legionnaires' disease. *N. Engl. J. Med.* **326:**151–154.

27. **Thomas, D., L. Mundy, and P. Tucker.** 1993. Hot tub legionellosis: Legionnaires' disease and Pontiac fever after a point-source to *Legionella pneumophila. Arch. Intern. Med.* **153:**2597–2599.

28. **Wisconsin Division of Health.** 1987. *Control of Legionella in Cooling Towers Summary Guidelines, 1987.* Wisconsin Division of Health, Madison, Wis.

29. **Yu, V. L.** 1997. Prevention and control of *Legionella*: an idea whose time has come. *Infect. Dis. Clin. Pract.* **6:**420–421.

# STRATEGIES FOR PREVENTION AND CONTROL OF LEGIONNAIRES' DISEASE IN GERMANY

*Martin Exner, Michael H. Kramer, and Stefan Pleischl*

# 78

Measures to improve technical water systems should aim at limiting concentrations of *Legionella* spp. to levels safe for exposed persons. In Germany, several standards and regulations have been published with the objective of preventing cases and outbreaks of legionellosis; these standards and regulations need to be considered for the planning, operation, and maintenance of technical water systems.

## HOT WATER DISTRIBUTION SYSTEMS

### Background

Temperatures between 30 and 40°C provide optimal growth conditions for *Legionella*. However, *Legionella* can multiply even at temperatures >40°C and can survive temperatures close to 60°C. In the past, energy conservation measures resulted in the introduction of low-temperature hot water systems, especially in large buildings (e.g., hospitals, office buildings). Recent investigations showed that the percentage of hot water systems colonized with *Legionella* ranged from 50 to 79% (S.

Pleischl, unpublished data). To minimize the number of systems with low hot water temperatures contaminated with *Legionella*, the technical standard W 551 was established by the German Association of Gas and Water Branches (DVGW) in 1996 (3).

Following their investigation of hot water systems in large buildings, Exner et al. (7) proposed this distinction between systemic and local contamination with *Legionella*: a systemic contamination is characterized by contamination of central (e.g., hot water holding tank) and peripheral parts of the system, and a local contamination is limited to the peripheral parts, such as single shower heads or peripheral pipes. This distinction is important because remedial actions may differ for systemic and peripheral contaminations.

The following are environmental factors that generally favor the multiplication of *Legionella*:

- Inorganic deposits in heating elements, distribution beams, pipes, and fittings. These deposits have large surfaces, which can become colonized by microorganisms.
- The use of materials such as rubber or silicon (e.g., in washers, membrane expansion vessels, shower hoses), which quickly can become colonized by microorganisms generating a biofilm.

*Martin Exner, Michael Kramer, and Stefan Pleischl*  Hygiene-Institut der Universität Bonn, Sigmund-Freud-Str. 25, 53105 Bonn, Germany.

*Legionella*, Edited by Reinhard Marre et al.
© 2002 ASM Press, Washington, D.C.

• Stagnant water in parts of the installation with inadequate or absent circulation (e.g., dead ends), in which *Legionella* can reach high concentrations.

Remedial actions against contamination with *Legionella* in hot water systems, especially in large buildings, may be labor-intensive and quite expensive.

## Hygienic-Microbiologic Investigations

To effectively determine whether an installation is contaminated systemically, the combination of a site inspection with sampling, testing, and interpretation of the results is critical. These tasks should be performed by trained personnel from qualified institutions. The characterization of a system needs to be done in a structured way, allowing the identification of its special characteristics (e.g., structure of the installation, operating conditions, technical and operating parameters). This characterization, together with the testing of only a limited number of water samples, usually will enable the investigator to assess whether a given contamination is systemic or not.

Typically, samples should be taken from the following sites of a hot water system:

• Cold water (before the water heater)
• Proximal hot water and/or mixed water (after exiting the water heater)
• Returning circulating hot water (before reentering the water heater)
• Most distant outlets in the periphery of the installation system

The same sampling sites, selected during the first site inspection, are also used for subsequent testing, which may be done on a regular basis or after interventions. This practice complies with the initial screening described in the DVGW Manual W 552 (4); sampling procedures should follow the standard DIN 38402-14 (2). During the initial investigation, at least one sample has to be taken from the water heater and from the most distant peripheral point (i.e., shower or tap) of the system. On the basis of our experience, an additional sample should be taken from the returning circulating hot water because a comparison with the results from the proximal hot water samples will permit a first assessment about the nature of the contamination if *Legionella* is found. If the concentration of *Legionella* exceeds 1 CFU/ml in one of the samples, additional investigations should be performed. Sampling more sites in the periphery will enable the investigators to better identify the likely source of contamination.

### Interpretation of Results

According to the DVGW Manual W 552, remedial actions need to be taken when the concentration of *Legionella* exceeds 1 CFU/ml in at least one of the water samples. Short-term violation of this value can be tolerated without complete cessation of water use until the sanitation of the system. For a discussion of the legal aspects in Germany, see Roth 1997 (13).

Note that these recommendations are not fully applicable to hospitals. In high-risk areas, including intensive care and transplantation units, additional measures need to be taken to ensure the provision of safe water (e.g., through installation of distal water filters). Table 1 gives an overview of action levels and necessary remedial measures in hospitals, nursing homes, and other settings (5, 8).

## WATER TREATMENT INSTALLATIONS FOR SWIMMING AND HOT WHIRLPOOLS

### Background

The filters in water treatment units for swimming and hot whirlpools are the most critical areas for colonization with *Legionella*. Usually, first the filters are colonized, and a detectable contamination of the pool water occurs only after *Legionella* grows through the filter material.

### Hygienic-Microbiologic Investigations

According to DIN 19643 (1), either samples of the filtrate after flocculation (i.e., 100 ml) or pool water samples of a treatment unit for

**TABLE 1** Criteria for the interpretation of results of water testing and necessary interventions (simplified after Exner et al. [5])

| Category | Description | Microbiologic criteria | Necessary actions |
|---|---|---|---|
| I-1 | Transplantation units, units for immunosuppressed patients, intensive care units, households with immunosuppressed persons | *Legionella* must not be detectable in 1 liter | Limit water use: no processing of medical devices, no use of tap water in humidifiers (respiratory therapy and ambient air) or showering |
| I-2 | Hospitals, nursing homes, hotels, and large apartment buildings[a], facilities with showers | $\geq 10^4$ CFU/liter independent of serogroup $\leq 10^2$ KBEL/liter of highly virulent subgroups[b] | Preliminary sanitation (e.g., thermal disinfection, high-level chlorination), raising temperature to $>60°C$, and weekly monitoring |
| II | Same as category I-2 | $10^2$–$10^4$ CFU/liter for not highly virulent subgroups | Limit water use (see category I), technical sanitation (e.g., removal of boiler sediments, elimination of unused pipe segments, and control after 6 months) |
| III | Same as category I-2 | 1–$10^2$ CFU/liter | No sanitation necessary and control after 1 year |

[a]With central hot water distribution systems.
[b]e.g., *Legionella pneumophila* serogroup 1, subgroup Pontiac.

water from swimming or hot whirlpools (i.e., 1 ml) need to be tested every 2 months. Testing of the filtrate allows larger facilities with multiple pools treated by one or a few filter units to comply with the standard while minimizing the number of, and thus the cost for, the samples tested.

### Interpretation of Results
According to DIN 19643, *Legionella* must not be detectable in the tested water samples (i.e., 100 ml of filtrate or 1 ml of pool water). If this action level is exceeded, remedial actions should be taken immediately.

## EVAPORATION CONDENSERS AND COOLING TOWERS

### Background
In contrast to closed systems, which are not a direct source of contamination for the environment, mist from open or half-open cooling towers and evaporation condensers is released into the environment and can be a source of *Legionella* infection if the system is contaminated. Operating parameters such as water volume, evaporation loss, maintenance conditions, and possible biocidal treatment of the cooling water greatly influence the extent to which conditions are favorable or adverse for the multiplication of *Legionella*.

### Hygienic-Microbiologic Investigations
Water samples can be obtained directly from the cooling water reservoirs of evaporation condensers and cooling towers. Since guidelines or regulations for sampling and interpretation of results are not yet established in Germany, the VDI-Standard 6022 for air-conditioning systems in office buildings ([15]; see Air-Conditioning Systems, Hygienic-Microbiologic Investigations) could be used as a point of reference.

## AIR-CONDITIONING SYSTEMS

### Background
Only air conditioning systems with spray humidifiers, in which the water is recycled, are relevant sources for *Legionella,* but not the sys-

**TABLE 2** Objectives and reference values for *Legionella* testing in hot water systems, swimming pools and hot whirlpool waters, and air-conditioning systems according to German regulations and recommendations[a]

| Reference | Type of water | Volume needed for testing | Sampling interval | No. of samples | Action value (CFU/volume) | Actions needed if action value is exceeded | Aim and description |
|---|---|---|---|---|---|---|---|
| Exner, 1991 (6) | Hot water | 1 liter (currently 100 ml) | Annually | Determined after site inspection | ≤10/100 ml (stepwise approach) | Technical improvements, additional testing (stepwise approach) | Prevention of legionelloses Recommendations for investigation, evaluation, and technical improvement of contaminated hot water systems in large buildings |
| DVGW W 551, 1993 (3) | Hot water | | | | | | Prevention of growth of *Legionella* in drinking water heating systems and pipes |
| RKI-Richtlinie, Anl. 4.4.6 and 6.7/5.6, 1988/94 (12) | Drinking water, hot water, water from dental units | n.d. | Twice a yr/suspected nosocomial infections | n.d. | n.d. | n.d. | Hygienic standards for the water supply in hospitals Description of technical standards to minimize contaminations with *Legionella* |
| DVGW W 552, 1996 (4) | Hot water | ≥100 ml | Annually | ≥2 | 1/ml | Additional testing, technical improvements | Operation and rehabilitation of drinking water heating systems and pipes by targeted measures |
| DIN 19643-1, 1997 (1) | Pool water | 1 ml (pool water), 100 ml | Every 2 mo | 1 / 1 | 1/ml / 1/100 ml | Disinfection, filter back wash | Processing of bathing water from swimming pools Prevention of growth of *Legionella* |
| Merkblatt 64.01, 1997 (10) | Hot water in baths | 100 ml | Annually | ≥3 | 1/ml | Disinfection, additional testing | Prevention of contamination with *Legionella* in hot water heating systems of public swimming pools |
| VDI 6022, 1998 (15) | Humidifier water | 1 ml | Every 2 yr | 1 | 1/ml | Cleaning, disinfection | Hygienic requirements for air-conditioning systems (offices and conference rooms) Prevention of growth of *Legionella* |

[a] n.d. = no description.

tems with steam humidifiers, in which water is evaporated by heating to $\geq 100°C$. Presently, the latter systems are being installed in almost all newly constructed, larger air-conditioning systems.

## Hygienic–Microbiologic Investigations

According to the VDI-Standard 6022 for air-conditioning systems in office buildings (15), water samples should be obtained directly from the reservoirs for the circulated humidifier water. *Legionella* should not be detectable in 1 ml.

On the basis of our experience, concentrations of *Legionella* exceeding the guideline value of 1 CFU/ml can be reached within 1 to 2 months. Thus, regular and careful maintenance and cleaning is critical for maintaining the necessary microbiologic safety of these installations.

Table 2 gives an overview of the objectives and reference values for testing for *Legionella* in hot water systems, swimming pools and hot whirlpools, and air-conditioning systems, according to German regulations and recommendations.

## STANDARD METHODS FOR *LEGIONELLA* TESTING IN TECHNICAL WATER INSTALLATIONS

Until recently, no approved testing standard for *Legionella* had been set forth, and each microbiology laboratory could use its own testing method. The various methods used often made it difficult to compare test results among different laboratories. In May 1998, the ISO-Norm 11731 (9) was published as an international standard for *Legionella* testing, intended to facilitate the comparison of test results among different laboratories. However, the standard allows for many variations in the methods used since it is designed for testing a variety of samples with very different qualities, including samples containing sediments, mucus, or sewage. Since the standard does not ensure that the details of the method used are uniform, the test results still may not be comparable.

In Germany, most water samples tested for *Legionella* are relatively unpolluted and usually have only little sediment (e.g., drinking or recreational water, humidifier water). Thus, an alternative standard method, specifically designed for the testing of these waters, was developed and recently published (11). In 2000, this alternative method was approved by the German Environmental Protection Agency (Umweltbundesamt, UBA) for the testing of drinking and pool waters (14).

## REFERENCES

1. **Deutsches Institut für Normung.** 1997. *Treatment of the Water of Swimming-Pools and Baths-Part 1: General Requirements.* DIN 19643-1. Deutsches Institut für Normung.
2. **Deutsches Institut für Normung.** 1986. *German Standard Methods for the Examination of Water, Waste Water and Sludge; General Information (Group A); Sampling of Untreated Water and Drinking Water (A 14).* DIN 38402-14. Deutsches Institut für Normung.
3. **Deutscher Verein des Gas- und Wasserfaches e.V.** 1993. *Hot Water Systems and Pipes; Technical Improvements for the Reduction of the Growth of Legionella.* DVGW Manual W 551. Deutscher Verein des Gas- und Wasserfaches e.V.
4. **Deutscher Verein des Gas- und Wasserfaches e.V.** 1996. *Hot Water Systems and Pipes; Technical Improvements for the Reduction of the Growth of Legionella; Renovation and Operation.* DVGW Manual W 552. Deutscher Verein des Gas- und Wasserfaches e.V.
5. **Exner, M., K. D. Jung, et al.** 1990. Nosocomial Legionella-infections connnected with a systemic legionella-contamination of a hot water system and experiences of renovation. *Forum Städte-Hygiene* **41:**289–293.
6. **Exner, M.** 1991. Incidence and evaluation of *Legionella* in hospitals and other large buildings. *Forum Städte-Hygiene* **42:**178–191.
7. **Exner, M., G.-J. Tuschewitzki, et al.** 1992. Incidence and evaluation of *Legionella* in hospitals and other large buildings. *Forum Städte-Hygiene* **43:**130–140.
8. **Exner, M., and S. Pleischl.** 1996. Technical and hygienic improvements for prevention of infections with *Legionella.* Hygiene and technology in hospitals. W. Steuer. Esslingen, Bartz, W. J. **207:**151–181.

9. **ISO.** 1998. *Water Quality–Detection and Enumeration of Legionella.* ISO 11731. ISO.

10. **Federal Trade Association for Public Swimming Pools.** 1997. *Prevention of Legionella in Hot Water Systems of Bathes.* Leaflet 64.01. Federal Trade Association for Public Swimming Pools.

11. **Pleischl, S., E. Frahm, et al.** 1999. Comparison of two methods to recover *Legionella* out of water samples; results of a validation test by the DIN ad-hoc-working-group "*Legionella.*" *Bundesgesundheitsblatt* **42:**650–656.

12. **Robert-Koch-Institut.** 1994. *Guidelines for Hospital Hygiene and Infection Prevention.* Enclosures 4.4.6 and 6.7/5.6, delivery 9/12. Robert-Koch-Institut.

13. **Roth, S.** 1997. Occurence of *Legionella* in hot water systems–danger or hysteria? *ZdW Bay* **9/97:**47–52.

14. **Umweltbundesamt.** 2000. Detection of Legionella in drinking water and water of swimming pools. *Bundesgesundheitsblatt* **43:**911–915.

15. **Verein Deutscher Ingenieure.** 1998. *Hygienic Standards for Ventilation and Air-Conditioning Systems—Offices and Assembly Rooms.* VDI Guideline 6022. Verein Deutscher Ingenieure.

# LEGIONNAIRES' DISEASE IN THE UNITED STATES: OPPORTUNITIES FOR PREVENTION

*Richard E. Besser*

# 79

Much of what we know about the epidemiology and prevention of Legionnaires'disease (LD) comes from outbreak investigations and special studies. These have shed light on new and underutilized prevention strategies for both community- and hospital-acquired disease. In this chapter I will focus on three areas where our knowledge is expanding and where new prevention opportunities have emerged: surveillance for travel-related legionellosis, the use of LD diagnostic tests, and new directions in water disinfection.

## TRAVEL-RELATED LD IN THE UNITED STATES

In 1999, a 64-year-old woman was diagnosed with LD in New York after returning from a wedding in Georgia (A. Benin, K. Arnold, R. Benson, A. Fiore, P. Cook, K. Williams, E. Brown, V. Galvin, B. Fields, and R. Besser, presented at the 37th Annu. Meet. Infect. Dis. Soc. Am., 1999). Five of her extended family members in Massachusetts developed a flu-like illness shortly after returning from the same

wedding. No other wedding guests were ill, and no other guests had stayed at the same hotel as the affected family. Case finding among hotel guests identified one other case of LD and six cases of Pontiac fever. A cohort study implicated the hotel whirlpool spa as the source of the outbreak. Strains of *Legionella pneumophila* serogroup 6, identical by pulsed-field gel electrophoresis, were isolated from one patient with LD and from the whirlpool spa. The spa was disinfected and no further cases occurred.

This outbreak was identified only because it occurred in one family with only one common source of exposure. The investigation uncovered additional cases of LD and Pontiac fever that would not have otherwise been detected or reported. The investigation allowed for measures to be taken that may have prevented additional cases from occurring.

This outbreak demonstrates many of the characteristics of typical travel-related LD outbreaks that make detection very difficult: low attack rates, long incubation periods, dispersal of persons away from the source of the infection, and inadequate surveillance. Only 2 of 414 (0.5%) hotel guests developed LD. Had one of these patients not been tested for LD, it is unlikely that the outbreak would have been linked to the hotel. The incubation pe-

*Richard E. Besser* Respiratory Diseases Branch, Division of Bacterial and Mycotic Diseases, National Center for Infectious Diseases, Centers for Disease Control and Prevention, 1600 Clifton Rd., NE, Mailstop C23, Atlanta, GA 30333.

*Legionella*, Edited by Reinhard Marre et al.
© 2002 ASM Press, Washington, D.C.

riod for LD, 2 to 10 days, allows time for infected persons to disperse from the source of the infection. This makes it less likely that any one clinician would see more than one case. During the incubation period in this outbreak, the two infected persons returned to different states. Had there not been associated Pontiac fever occurring in the family of a patient with LD, this outbreak would have been missed. Finally, clinicians treating these two persons did not suspect travel-related disease and did not report back to the state in which the infection was acquired.

In the United States, surveillance for LD is unable to detect clusters of travel-associated LD. There are two national reporting systems in place at the Centers for Disease Control and Prevention (CDC): the National Electronic Telecommunications System for Surveillance, an electronic system that collects data on LD in addition to all reportable diseases; and the Legionnaires' Disease Reporting System, a paper-based system that collects detailed information on LD alone. Although the electronic system is timely, it does not collect any information on travel. The paper system, while collecting detailed information on travel as well as other risk factors for LD, is very insensitive and is used mainly for tracking major epidemiologic trends. Although we estimate that there are between 8,000 and 18,000 cases of LD each year in the United States (15), only 250 to 450 cases are reported to the paper-based system. This difference relates to many factors: failure to properly test patients presenting with symptoms consistent with LD, failure of clinicians to report cases to local and state health departments, and failure of state health departments to report to the CDC.

The true burden of travel-related legionellosis in the United States is not clear. Although 21% of cases reported to the CDC through the paper LD reporting system indicate an out-of-home stay during the incubation period (CDC, unpublished data), a case-control study of risk factors for sporadic Legionnaires' disease in Ohio found that the rate of travel was similar between patients and controls (18). Unfortunately, this study did not look in detail at travel-related activities to determine whether particular exposures when traveling or returning home were associated with LD. Further studies are needed to determine the proportion of disease attributable to travel, and to design appropriate prevention strategies.

Detection of travel-related outbreaks offers the potential for providing new prevention opportunities. The European Working Group for *Legionella* Infections conducts surveillance for travel-related LD in Europe (7). This system has been quite successful at identifying clusters of travel-associated LD. We propose to modify the existing National Electronic Telecommunications System for Surveillance by adding a supplemental page to collect information on travel and other risk factors for infection. This could then be linked to a detection algorithm that would automatically flag cases that were associated with a common hotel exposure. Eventually, this system could be used to compare isolates associated with outbreak strains by molecular subtyping. In this way, outbreaks would be identified in a timely fashion so that preventive actions could be taken. Prevention of travel-related disease will be difficult without such a system.

## DIAGNOSTIC ISSUES FOR PUBLIC HEALTH IN THE HOSPITAL AND THE COMMUNITY

To prevent LD, one must be able to recognize situations in which transmission is occurring. Several studies indicate that our ability to identify outbreaks of LD is inadequate and that the adoption of new diagnostic tests may be further eroding our capacity to identify certain types of *Legionella* infections. Prevention of health care-associated LD and community-acquired LD requires an appreciation of the shifting diagnostic landscape.

### Diagnostic Issues in the Hospital

Health care-associated legionellosis is a significant public health problem. During the

1980s, approximately 23% of cases reported to the CDC were health care-associated, and the mortality rate was almost 40% (14). Although the mortality rate in the 1990s declined significantly, nearly 20% of patients with health care-associated LD still die (CDC, unpublished data). Hospitals present an optimal situation for LD transmission: many hospitalized patients have chronic medical conditions that are risk factors for LD; to prevent scalding, water is often circulated at temperatures favoring amplification of legionellae; and plumbing systems are often complex, providing areas within pipes where water can stagnate and legionellae can multiply and avoid disinfectants.

To prevent LD in hospitals, CDC recommends a strategy based on proper maintenance of water systems, universal testing of appropriate patients, and thorough investigations in situations where disease transmission is occurring (4). Infection-control personnel should educate medical staff to heighten suspicion for health care-associated LD, especially in high-risk patients. Appropriate diagnostic testing should be available and used for evaluating patients with health care-associated pneumonia. This includes having access to a laboratory that is proficient in isolating legionellae from cultures and having on-site urine antigen testing. Serologic testing can be used to make the diagnosis, but is not helpful acutely, since a fourfold rise in antibody titer from specimens obtained 3 to 6 weeks apart is necessary to make the clinical diagnosis of LD. Direct fluorescent antibody testing can be used to make the diagnosis but can be difficult to interpret if not performed frequently. In situations where health care-associated LD is occurring, detailed epidemiologic and environmental investigations should be undertaken to identify the source of transmission so that further transmission can be prevented.

Surveillance for health care-associated LD involves appropriately testing patients and recognizing and investigating situations in which transmission is occurring. Two recent reports indicate the perils of not routinely testing

health care-associated pneumonia patients for LD. In 1998, Kool et al. published a report describing transmission over a 17-year period in an Arizona hospital (12). Seven cases of LD were diagnosed in 1996. This prompted an investigation that documented 25 confirmed LD cases since 1979. Of the persons with confirmed cases, 48% died, probably indicating some degree of ascertainment bias and the likelihood that additional cases went unrecognized. This hospital did not routinely test patients with hospital-acquired pneumonia for LD and did not conduct investigations when cases were diagnosed. After the investigations, corrective measures were taken that halted disease transmission.

In 1998, Lepine et al. reported on a cluster of health care-associated LD cases in a hospital soon after introduction of urinary antigen testing (13). There was no increase in the overall rate of health care-associated pneumonia. This hospital had experienced an outbreak of health care-associated LD 16 years earlier, and isolates from the two outbreaks were identical by molecular subtyping methods. This study suggests that persistent transmission of *Legionella* infections may have gone unrecognized over a long period of time. Not until appropriate diagnostic tests were introduced was the transmission recognized and halted.

While these two reports are useful as illustrations of the problem of underutilization of diagnostic testing, they are by no means unique. In 1999, Fiore et al. published a survey of 253 hospitals participating in a CDC-sponsored surveillance system for hospital-acquired infections (6). Of 192 responding hospitals, only 60% had in-house testing available for LD, and only 21% had established routine testing procedures that included LD for respiratory specimens from patients with health care-associated pneumonia.

To prevent health care-associated LD, transmission must be identified, investigated, and interrupted. It is clear that a major prevention opportunity exists in the United States if hospitals would make better use of existing diagnostic tools and make surveillance for LD an infection control priority. Hospitals must have policies in place so that patients with health care-associated pneumonia are appropriately tested for LD.

## Diagnostic Issues in the Community

The passive LD reporting system at the CDC captures information on diagnostic testing. During the early 1990s, use of the urine antigen tests began to increase (Fig. 1). By 1997, it was the leading diagnostic method for reported cases. Beginning in 1993, the number of cases with a positive culture began to decline. This was preceded by a decline in the number of cases diagnosed by direct fluorescent antibody and serology.

The public health implications of these changes are mixed. On the one hand, it is clearly beneficial to have available the urine antigen test, a rapid diagnostic test for LD that is sensitive and specific for *L. pneumophila* serogroup 1, the leading cause of LD in the United States. This should increase the likelihood of clinicians testing for LD since results can be available within minutes if the test is

run on-site. On the other hand, if clinicians are no longer obtaining cultures of respiratory specimens, cases of LD caused by non-*L. pneumophila* serogroup 1 strains will be missed. These strains accounted for 29% of cases reported to the CDC between 1980 and 1989 for which complete culture results were available (14). Outbreaks of health care-associated disease linked to these strains continue to occur (9), as do outbreaks of LD in the community. Recently, public health officials in the Pacific Northwest reported cases of LD in which *Legionella longbeachae* was isolated (5). These cases were temporally associated with exposure to potting soil. We attempted to review previously reported cases of *L. longbeachae* in prelude to conducting a study to assess risk factors for acquisition. In several countries these infections have been postulated as resulting from exposure to potting soils (2, 17). However, over the past 10 years, there has been a dramatic drop in *L. longbeachae* reports in the United States (Fig. 2). Although it is possible that this reflects a true drop in incidence, it more likely is due to the overall decline in the use of cultures. Whether we will lose our ability to detect rare species and serogroups of *Legionella* remains to be seen.

The shift in diagnostic approach also has implications for the ability of the public health community to respond to outbreaks of LD. Although the urine antigen tests identify cases

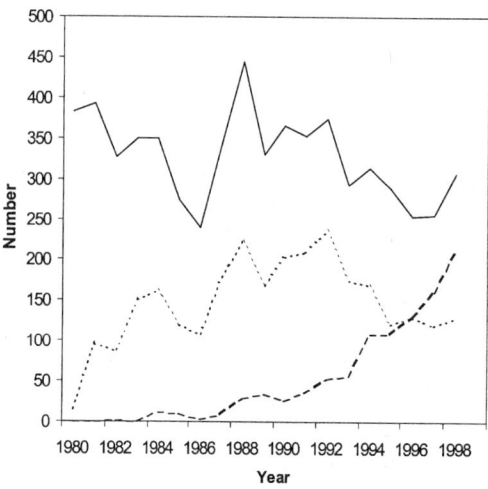

**FIGURE 1** Legionnaires' disease cases reported to Legionnaires' Disease Reporting System, by diagnostic method, United States, 1980 to 1998. Solid line, total number of cases; dotted line, cases diagnosed by culture; dashed line, cases diagnosed by urine antigen.

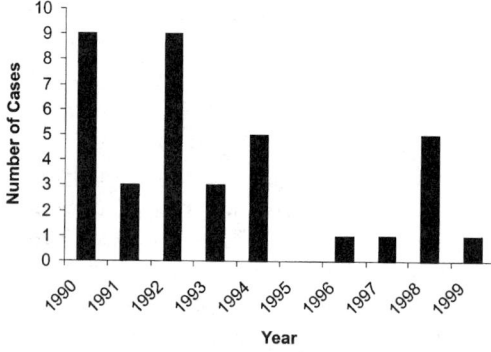

**FIGURE 2** *Legionella longbeachae* cases per year reported to Legionnaires' Disease Reporting System, United States, 1990 to 1999.

of LD, they do not provide bacterial isolates, which can be crucial during an investigation. Without a clinical isolate, it can be difficult to definitively implicate a potential source of transmission. During an investigation, multiple strains of *Legionella* often will be isolated from a variety of sources. Molecular epidemiology is used to determine whether strains from the environment are identical to patient isolates (19).

A number of guidelines are available to assist clinicians in selecting appropriate diagnostic tests for patients at risk for LD (3, 4; Maryland State Health Department, http://www.dhmh.state.md.us/html/legionella.htm). Hospitalized patients who develop pneumonia need to have respiratory specimens cultured for *Legionella*, as well as be tested for the presence of the urinary antigen. Patients with community-acquired pneumonia who are sick enough to be hospitalized and have known risk factors for LD should also be evaluated using both tests (1).

## NEW DIRECTIONS IN WATER DISINFECTION: POTENTIAL IMPACT OF MONOCHLORAMINE

During the past 5 years, epidemiologic and laboratory data have begun to accumulate that suggest that a new prevention strategy may have arrived. Studies indicate that the use of monochloramine as a biocide in municipal water systems is more effective than chlorine in preventing transmission of *Legionella* and has the potential to greatly reduce the incidence of LD. Laboratory data support this finding. During the next 5 years it will be essential that this biocide be evaluated prospectively to truly determine its impact.

Monochloramine is currently used by nearly 25% of municipalities as a residual disinfectant in their public water distribution system. It is more stable than chlorine and may provide better residual disinfection over long distribution systems (8). The U.S. Environmental Protection Agency issued regulations that require reductions in the levels of certain disinfection byproducts that have been asso-

ciated with cancer in laboratory animals (16). Monochloramine is attractive to municipal water systems since it results in reduced production of these regulated disinfection byproducts.

Epidemiologic studies support using monochloramine as part of a strategy for reducing outbreaks of LD. In 1999, Kool et al. published the results of a case-control study assessing the risk of a hospital having a health care-associated outbreak of LD based upon the type of disinfectant used by the municipality (11). Hospitals that had drinking water outbreaks of LD were matched to hospitals that had not had an LD outbreak by size, presence of a transplant program, and year of the outbreak. The authors then contacted the municipality to determine what type of disinfectant was used at the time of the outbreak. Hospitals that had had an outbreak were significantly more likely to be in municipalities that disinfected with chlorine. These results suggest that 90% of the health care-associated outbreaks associated with drinking water would not have occurred if monochloramine had been used as the residual disinfectant.

In 1999, Kool et al. published results of a cohort study of hospital risk factors for LD in San Antonio, Temple, and Austin, Texas (10). They reviewed laboratory databases for cases of LD in the preceding 3 years, collected information on water treatment and diagnostic testing, and cultured water from water tanks and patient rooms. They found that hospitals in municipalities using chlorine as the residual disinfectant were significantly more likely to have legionellae isolated from the water supply. These hospitals were also more likely to have had health care-associated cases, although this difference did not reach statistical significance.

To further assess whether municipal disinfection with monochloramine was associated with a lower occurrence of health care-associated LD, Heffelfinger et al. conducted a survey of hospital epidemiologists who were members of the Society of Healthcare Epidemiologists of America (J. Heffelfinger and C.

Whitney, Presented at the 4th Decennial Int. Conf. Nosocomial Infections, 2000). They collected information on the occurrence of outbreaks of LD, hospital characteristics including presence of a transplant unit, and type of hospital and municipal water disinfection. They found that hospitals using chlorine as the residual disinfectant were significantly more likely to have cases of health care-associated LD (odds ratio, 3.57; 95% confidence interval, 1.04 to 12.5). These data suggest that 72% of health care-associated LD cases might not have occurred if monochloramine had been used instead of free chlorine for residual disinfection.

In addition to epidemiologic studies supporting the use of monochloramine, laboratory data demonstrate increased efficacy of monochloramine compared with chlorine in eliminating biofilm-associated *Legionella*. Recently, Donlan et al. compared the effects of monochloramine and chlorine on *Hartmanella vermiformis*-associated *L. pneumophila* in a laboratory-grown potable water biofilm (R. Donlan, R. Murga, E. Brown, J. Carpenter, R. Besser, and B. Fields, presented at 5th Int. Conf. Legionellosis, 2000). While both chlorine and monochloramine were effective at eradicating planktonic *Legionella*, monochloramine was significantly more effective than chlorine at killing *Legionella* in the biofilm.

The results of these studies are encouraging and suggest a possible new approach to LD prevention for both hospitals and the wider community. It is now time for prospective large-scale intervention trials to assess the effectiveness of monochloramine in reducing colonization of water systems and in preventing community-acquired and health care-associated legionellosis. Given that many municipalities are already planning to convert from chlorine to monochloramine disinfection in response to EPA regulations, there should be many opportunities to address this important public health question.

## CONCLUSIONS

Many opportunities exist to improve the prevention of legionellosis in the United States.

Computer-based reporting systems provide a means of conducting timely surveillance for previously undetected outbreaks of travel-related LD. New rapid diagnostic tests can improve case detection, but only as long as these new methodologies do not replace bacterial cultures. Municipal disinfection with monochloramine may provide a means of reducing the incidence of both health care-associated and community-acquired LD.

## REFERENCES

1. **Bartlett, J. G., S. Dowell, L. A. Mandell, T. M. J. File, D. Musher, and M. Fine.** 2000. Practice guidelines for the management of community-acquired pneumonia in adults. *Clin. Infect. Dis.* **31:**347–382.
2. **Cameron, S., D. Roder, C. Walker, and J. Feldheim.** 1991. Epidemiological characteristics of Legionella infection in South Australia: implications for disease control. *Aust. N.Z. J. Med.* **21:** 65–70.
3. **Centers for Disease Control and Prevention.** 2000. CDC/IDSA/ASBMT guidelines for the prevention of opportunistic infections in hematopoietic stem cell transplant recipients. *Morb. Mortal. Wkly. Rep.* **49**(RR-10)**:**36–38.
4. **Centers for Disease Control and Prevention.** 1997. Guidelines for prevention of nosocomial pneumonia. *Morb. Mortal. Wkly. Rep.* **46**(RR-1)**:** 1–79.
5. **Centers for Disease Control and Prevention.** 2000. Legionnaires' disease associated with potting soil—California, Oregon, and Washington, May–June 2000. *Morb. Mortal. Wkly. Rep.* **49:** 777–778.
6. **Fiore, A. E., J. C. Butler, T. G. Emori, and R. P. Gaynes.** 1999. A survey of methods used to detect nosocomial legionellosis among participants in the National Nosocomial Infections Surveillance System. *Infect. Control Hosp. Epidemiol.* **20:**412–416.
7. **Hutchinson, E. J., C. A. Joseph, and C. L. R. Bartlett.** 1996. EWGLI: a European surveillance scheme for travel associated legionnaires' disease. *Eurosurveillance* **1:**37–39.
8. **Kirmeyer, G., G. Foust, G. Pierson, J. Simmler, and M. MeChevalier.** 1993. *Optimizing Chloramine Treatment.* American Water Works Research Foundation, Denver, Colo.
9. **Knirsch, C. A., K. Jakob, D. Schoonmaker, J. A. Kiehlbauch, S. J. Wong, P. Della-Latta, S. Whittier, M. Layton, and B. Scully.** 2000. An outbreak of *Legionella micdadei* pneumonia in

transplant patients: evaluation, molecular epidemiology, and control. *Am. J. Med.* **108**:290–295.

10. **Kool, J. L., D. Bergmire-Sweat, J. C. Butler, E. W. Brown, D. J. Peabody, D. S. Massi, J. C. Carpenter, J. M. Pruckler, R. F. Benson, and B. S. Fields.** 1999. Hospital characteristics associated with colonization of water systems by *Legionella* and risk of nosocomial legionnaires' disease: a cohort study of 15 hospitals. *Infect. Control Hosp. Epidemiol.* **20**:798–805.

11. **Kool, J. L., J. C. Carpenter, and B. S. Fields.** 1999. Effect of monochloramine disinfection of municipal drinking water on risk of nosocomial Legionnaires' disease. *Lancet* **353**:272–277.

12. **Kool, J. L., A. E. Fiore, C. M. Kioski, E. W. Brown, R. F. Benson, J. M. Pruckler, C. Glasby, J. C. Butler, G. D. Cage, J. C. Carpenter, R. M. Mandel, B. England, and R. F. Breiman.** 1998. More than 10 years of unrecognized nosocomial transmission of legionnaires' disease among transplant patients. *Infect. Control Hosp. Epidemiol.* **19**:898–904.

13. **Lepine, L. A., D. B. Jernigan, J. C. Butler, J. M. Pruckler, R. F. Benson, G. Kim, J. L. Hadler, M. L. Cartter, and B. S. Fields.** 1998. A recurrent outbreak of nosocomial legionnaires' disease detected by urinary antigen testing: evidence for long-term colonization of a hospital plumbing system. *Infect. Control Hosp. Epidemiol.* **19**:905–910.

14. **Marston, B. J., H. B. Lipman, and R. F. Breiman.** 1994. Surveillance for legionnaires' disease. Risk factors for morbidity and mortality. *Arch. Intern. Med.* **154**:2417–2422.

15. **Marston, B. J., J. F. Plouffe, T. M. File, B. A. Hackman, S. J. Salstrom, H. B. Lipman, M. S. Kolczak, and R. F. Breiman.** 1997. Incidence of community-acquired pneumonia requiring hospitalization—results of a population-based active surveillance study in Ohio. *Arch. Intern. Med.* **157**:1709–1718.

16. **Office of Water, U.S. Environmental Protection Agency.** 1999. *National Primary Drinking Water Regulations: Disinfectants and Disinfection Byproducts.* 40 CFR Parts 9, 141, and 142. U.S. Environmental Protection Agency, Washington, D.C.

17. **Okazaki, M., B. Umeda, M. Koide, and A. Saito.** 1998. [Legionella longbeachae pneumonia in a gardener]. *Jpn. J. Infect. Dis.* **72**:1076–1079. (In Japanese.)

18. **Straus, W. L., J. F. Plouffe, T. M. File, Jr., H. B. Lipman, B. H. Hackman, S. J. Salstrom, R. F. Benson, and R. F. Breiman.** 1996. Risk factors for domestic acquisition of legionnaires disease. Ohio legionnaires Disease Group. *Arch. Intern. Med.* **156**:1685–1692.

19. **Whitney, C. G., J. Hofmann, J. M. Pruckler, R. F. Benson, B. S. Fields, U. Bandyopadhyay, E. F. Donnally, C. Giorgio-Almonte, L. A. Mermel, S. Boland, B. T. Matyas, and R. F. Breiman.** 1997. The role of arbitrarily primed PCR in identifying the source of an outbreak of Legionnaires' disease. *J. Clin. Microbiol.* **35**:1800–1804.

# ELEVEN YEARS OF EXPERIENCE WITH NOVEL STRATEGIES FOR *LEGIONELLA* CONTROL IN A LARGE TEACHING HOSPITAL

*J. V. Lee, S. B. Surman, A. Kirby, and F. Seddon*

# 80

The Queen's Medical Centre (QMC) is a large teaching hospital housing approximately 1,400 beds. The center consists of four blocks. The Medical School was completed in 1976, the West Block was completed in 1978, the East Block was completed in 1981, and the South Block was completed in 1984. The water supply for the hospital is normally taken from its own borehole supply but can also be taken from the municipal supply. The cold water is hard and chlorinated to provide a residual of 0.4 mg/liter at the outlets throughout the hospital.

Cooling towers are situated on the Medical School, West Block, and East Block. Currently each of these is automatically dosed with an oxidizing biocide. The West Block and East Block towers are treated continuously with a combination of bromine and chlorine maintained at a residual equivalent to chlorine at 1 to 2 mg/liter. The Medical School towers are treated with similar levels of chlorine dioxide. All of the towers are also treated with corrosion inhibitors and have automatic control of pH and conductivity. In view of their high-risk environment, the cooling systems are monitored once a week for the aerobic heterotrophic colony count (determined at 30°C) and for legionellae. The samples are collected from sampling points installed on the return from the refrigeration condensers to the cooling towers. Legionellae are usually not detectable with our methods, which have a detection limit of 10 CFU/liter.

Each block has its own independent circulating hot water system (HWS). The West Block and Medical School have storage calorifiers (water heaters) equipped with antistratification pumps, and the water is circulated at 60 to 62°C. The East and South Blocks were originally each equipped with two HWSs heated by Angeleri-type instantaneous calorifiers. One system circulated water at 60°C and supplied kitchens and sluice rooms and the other system, the "low temperature hot water system," circulated water at 43°C and supplied water to the wash hand basins, bathrooms, and showers.

During 1988 and 1989, 12 cases of Legionnaires' disease were associated with the 43°C system in the South Block (1). This outbreak was controlled by raising the hot water tem-

*J. V. Lee and S. B. Surman* PHLS Water and Environmental Microbiology Research Unit, Public Health Laboratory, Queen's Medical Centre, University Hospital, Nottingham NG7 2UH, England. *A. Kirby and F. Seddon* Estates Department, Queen's Medical Centre, University Hospital, Nottingham NG7 2UH, England.

*Legionella*, Edited by Reinhard Marre et al.
© 2002 ASM Press, Washington, D.C.

perature in the 43°C system to 60°C and removing all unused outlets, dead legs, and blind ends. The control measures were monitored by measuring the temperature of the calorifier inlet and outlet continuously, and weekly at selected taps representative of each loop of the circulating hot water systems on each floor. In addition, the levels of *Legionella* were monitored at selected taps. Initially, monitoring of the legionellae was carried out weekly, but this was then reduced to monthly for several years and finally quarterly. The 43°C hot water system of the South Block was extensively colonized with *Legionella pneumophila* serogroup 1 that was indistinguishable by monoclonal subtyping and restriction fragment length polymorphism typing from the strains isolated from the patients. A total of 31 sites were examined for *Legionella* species, 7 or 8 per week on a 4-week rotation. From April 1989 until April 1991 there was a progressive decline in the numbers and incidence of *L. pneumophila*. This correlated with the progressive removal of unused outlets and with cutting back any unused pipes to the circulating main rather than variation in the temperature control. In April 1991, a silver/copper ionizer was installed on the return to the calorifier in the former 43°C system in the South Block. From that time, *L. pneumophila* has rarely been isolated from the circulating HWSs in the South Block.

The 43°C system in the East Block was also extensively and heavily colonized with *L. pneumophila* serogroup 1 but of a different type than the outbreak strain in the South Block. In late 1992, a silver/copper ionizer was installed in the East Block. The results of monitoring the silver concentrations and legionellae in the East Block hot water are shown in Fig. 1. Twelve samples, two per floor, were examined for *Legionella* spp. each week. These points were representative of the extremes of the circulation system on each floor and had been consistently contaminated with legionellae previously. Silver concentrations were monitored weekly at the return to the calorifier and at representative sample points on the top and bottom floors. The *Legionella* counts and silver concentrations in Fig. 1 are the means of the 12 *Legionella* counts and three silver concentrations, respectively. The counts of *Legionella* dropped as soon as the ionizer was put into operation. However, this ionizer was from a different manufacturer than that installed in the South Block, was not as well designed, and had to be subjected to a number of modifications before the silver concentrations could be consistently maintained at levels above 20 $\mu$g/liter. Adequate silver levels were achieved in late January 1993 and *L. pneumophila* remained undetectable until 5 August 1993, when it reappeared and remained in low numbers until 22 September 1993. The appearance of *L. pneumophila* was preceded by a rise in the heterotrophic colony count. One sample in August of the following year also yielded legionellae at low numbers, below 50 per liter. The colony count of the aerobic heterotrophs followed a similar pattern to that of *L. pneumophila*. Before the ionizer was installed, the mean counts at 37°C were between $10^3$ and $10^4$ CFU/ml. After the installation of the ionizer, the numbers dropped to between 10 and 100 CFU/ml for the first 8 months, after which the counts were less than 10 CFU/ml. *L. pneumophila* has continued to be undetectable or present in only low numbers to this day.

The circulation of hot water at 60°C so that it is delivered to every outlet at 50°C within 1 min of opening is the recommended strategy for the control of *Legionella* (2, 3) in the United Kingdom. However, this means that there is a risk of scalding, particularly where there is whole body immersion such as in baths or showers. To combat this risk, in 1992 the UK Department of Health published a health guidance note advising that all outlets in patient, resident, and visitor areas of health-care premises should be fitted with thermostatic mixer valves (TMVs) adjusted to deliver water at temperatures not exceeding 43°C (4). For showers and baths, the TMVs should be of a fail-safe design. At the QMC, like most other hospitals in the United Kingdom, TMVs

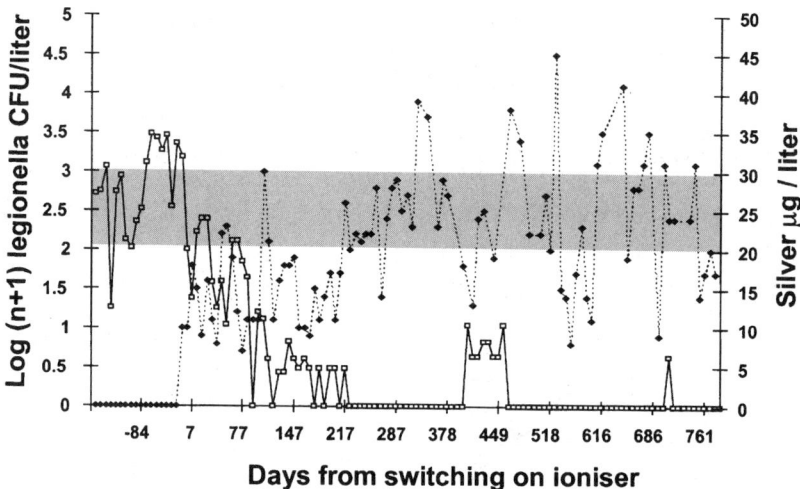

**FIGURE 1** The mean numbers of *Legionella* species (□, log CFU + 1/liter) and mean silver concentrations (♦, μg/liter) in the QMC East Block former 43°C hot water system before and following the installation of a silver/copper ionizer. The shaded area indicates the target range of silver concentrations when the study began.

have been progressively installed since 1992. Frequently, in new or refurbished installations, all outlets are protected by fail-safe TMVs.

A number of problems are associated with the installation of TMVs. They are expensive to purchase; require much maintenance, particularly if the water is hard; and the failure of the nonreturn valves fitted within them can result in cold water passing into the hot or vice versa, depending on the relative pressure differences. The dead volume in some TMVs can be more than 100 ml, and they are equipped with a variety of seals that may also be conducive to the multiplication of legionellae. In common with a number of other hospitals in the United Kingdom, following the installation of TMVs we have experienced a decline in our ability to control the colonization of hot water outlets with legionellae. Downstream of the mixer, not only is the effect of the heat removed but also the concentration of the added silver ions is diluted by the cold water. Because of its hardness, we do not treat our cold water with an ionizer. Although we have not observed significant numbers of *L. pneumophila*, we have increas-

ingly seen autofluorescent *Legionella* species, especially *L. anisa*, at outlets, particularly showers. *L. anisa* has been detected in the incoming municipal water supply but not in the raw hospital borehole supply water. *L. anisa* can occasionally be detected in low numbers in the hospital cold water but not in the circulating hot water. The circulating hot water is probably incompatible with their long-term survival because they appear to be more heat-sensitive than *L. pneumophila*, giving very poor or no recovery after heat treatment at 50°C for 30 min. The hematology ward in one of the blocks is considered to house patients particularly at risk of Legionnaires' disease. We are examining a number of strategies to improve the control of *Legionella* in this ward.

The hot water to the hematology ward is treated with copper and silver ions and the supply maintained at 60 to 62°C. Wash hand basin taps without TMVs rarely yield legionellae and when present, they are always less than $10^2$ CFU/liter. Wash hand basin taps fitted with TMVs frequently yield legionellae, often at numbers between $10^2$ and $10^3$ CFU/liter. The ward is equipped with a number of single-bedded side rooms, each with their own shower. When the patients are very ill, the showers may go unused for several weeks at a time but they are flushed at least once a week by staff. The showers frequently yield high numbers of legionellae, between $10^3$ and $10^5$ CFU/liter. Following replacement of the TMVs and shower fittings with new or disinfected replacements, the legionellae remained undetectable for only 1 to 3 weeks. Flushing the outlet daily for 5 min did not reduce the number of legionellae. At the end of March 2000, the cold water supply to the ward was equipped with a chlorine dioxide dosing system, which ensures that a chlorine dioxide residual of at least 0.5 mg/liter reaches beyond the TMV to the shower hose and head. To date, this does not appear to have significantly reduced the legionellae. We also modified two showers so that the water flowed over special ceramic beads that had been shown to have antibacterial properties in vitro, but this also had no effect, probably because the contact time was insufficient.

Until now we have not discovered a strategy that can consistently control colonization in showers downstream of the TMVs so that legionellae remain consistently undetectable for any longer than a couple of weeks at a time. It may be that legionellae can only be maintained at undetectable levels by routinely removing and disinfecting the TMVs and shower components. To enable this, the units would have to be designed for quick release so that they can be rapidly recycled.

Our experience has been that long-term control is achievable in cooling systems using oxidizing biocides. In circulating hot water systems, control can be achieved by good system design, meticulous maintenance, ensuring that the circulating temperature is close to 60°C, and ensuring that water is delivered to the outlet or TMV inlet at greater than 50°C.

These measures prevented further cases of Legionnaires' disease in the South Block but did not reduce the level of *L. pneumophila* to below the detection limit. This was achieved only by supplementing the temperature regime with a silver/copper ionizer and maintaining the silver at a concentration of 20 to 40 $\mu$g/liter.

Although legionellae may be controlled in cold water and circulating hot water systems to the point where they are not detectable, this control will only persist as long as the hot and cold water are kept separate. The introduction of TMVs is incompatible with the control of legionellae if the target is that they are not readily detectable. TMVs should be avoided in intensive-care facilities and wherever possible in areas where patients may be considered to be particularly at risk. In such areas, electrically heated instantaneous showers may be more appropriate. Despite the problems with TMVs, the incidence of nosocomial Legionnaires' disease in England and Wales has been consistently low in recent years, and this probably reflects the widespread application in the United Kingdom of the heat regime and good maintenance as advised by the Health and Safety Executive (3).

## REFERENCES

1. **Colville, A., J. Crowley, D. Dearden, R. C. B. Slack, and J. V. Lee.** 1993. Outbreak of Legionnaires' disease at University Hospital, Nottingham—epidemiology, microbiology and control. *Epidemiol. Infect.* **110:**105–116.
2. **Health and Safety Commission**. 1995. *Health and Safety Commission Approved Code of Practice L8. The Prevention and Control of Legionellosis (Including Legionnaires' Disease)*. HMSO, London, United Kingdom.
3. **Health and Safety Executive.** 1993. *Health and Safety Executive Series booklet HS(G)70. The Control of Legionellosis Including Legionnaires' Disease*, 2nd ed. HMSO, London, United Kingdom.
4. **NHS Estates.** 1992. *Health Guidance Note— ''Safe'' Hot Water and Surface Temperatures*. HMSO, London, United Kingdom.

# UV LIGHT FOR ELIMINATION
# OF LEGIONELLAE

*Tim Eckmanns, Frank Schwab, Hans Posselt,*
*Petra Gastmeier, and Henning Rüden*

# 81

Aquatic bacteria of the genus *Legionella* are causative agents of severe nosocomial pneumonia with high case-fatality rates. There are different methods for the control and eradication of legionellae in water systems. Focal modalities include UV light, instantaneous heating, and ozone. Systemic modalities include hyperchlorination, copper/silver ionization, superheat and flush sterilization, and maintaining hot water temperatures in water heaters at >60°C (140°F) (2). Total sterility is difficult to achieve with any disinfection modality (5).

The investigation took place in an internal hospital department with 375 beds (11,331 patients in 1999) with a separate copper pipe water system. The department was built in 1993. Because of calcification of the water plumbing system, we wanted to decrease the hot water temperature (1).

In this investigation we determined whether maintaining a hot water temperature in water heaters at >50°C (122°F) with an additional central flowthrough UV sterilizer (power 85 W, 5 m³/h) was as efficient as maintaining a hot water temperature in water heaters at >60°C to control legionellae in a hospital water system (4).

## THE METHOD, THE HOSPITAL WATER SYSTEM, THE SAMPLES, AND THE SAMPLE WORK UP

Since 1993, maintaining a hot water temperature in the main water tank at >60°C has minimized *Legionella* colonization. The tested method was a combination of focal modality (UV light) and systemic modality (maintaining hot water temperature in the main water tank at >50°C).

To get information about different locations of the hospital water circulation system, samples were taken in three different rooms, A, B, and C (Fig. 1) (each at a different distance from the main tank) and from the water of the main water pipe directly after the tank and the UV sterilizer (outlet D). On each occasion, we took four samples of hot water from the sink water outlets in the three rooms (sample series: from the faucet where the hot and cold water are already mixed and from a special outlet from the hot water pipe, immediately after the water reached a stable temperature). The means of the sample series are given in Table 1.

*Tim Eckmanns* Institute of Hygiene, Free University Berlin, 14059 Berlin, Germany. *Frank Schwab, Petra Gastmeier, and Henning Rüden* Institute of Hygiene, Free University Berlin, Berlin, Germany. *Hans Posselt* Clinitec Ltd. Facility Management, Berlin, Germany.

*Legionella*, Edited by Reinhard Marre et al.
© 2002 ASM Press, Washington, D.C.

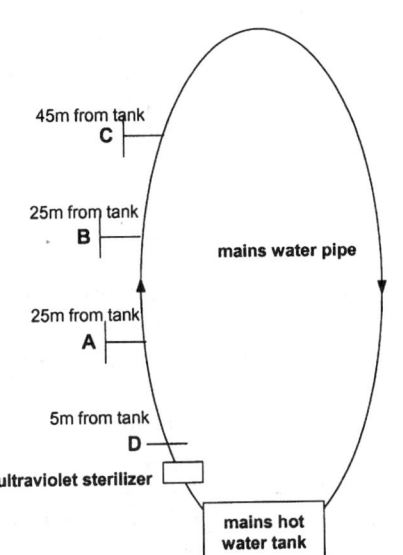

**FIGURE 1** Water system with different water outlets. The water outlets A, B, C, and D are at different distances from the main tank.

When the temperature was >60°C, samples from the four different locations (A, B, C, and D) were taken six times in 4 weeks in October. While the temperature was >50°C with the UV sterilizer installed, six samples from the four locations were taken in 5 months to get information about when the system had stabilized. All samples were taken in the winter (October through March) when *Legionella* counts might be lower (6; unpublished data).

Samples (100 ml) were concentrated by filtration (0.2-$\mu$m-pore-size polycarbonate membrane) and plated on buffered charcoal-yeast extract supplement with alpha-ketoglutarate and incubated at 36°C for 7 to 10 days (7).

## *LEGIONELLA* COUNTS AND TEMPERATURES OF THE WATER AT THE OUTLETS

In the water sinks of rooms A and B, no legionellae were found when the hot water temperature was >60°C (the corresponding water temperatures of the outlets A, B, C, and D are given in Table 1). In the room with the

**TABLE 1** Number of legionellae in samples of hot water maintained at a temperature of >60°C and hot water maintained at a temperature of >50°C with additional UV sterilization and corresponding P values

| Source[a] | No. of legionellae (CFU/ml)[b] | | | | | | | | | | | | | | P value[c] |
|---|---|---|---|---|---|---|---|---|---|---|---|---|---|---|---|
| | Water temp >60°C | | | | | | | Water temp >50°C and UV sterilization | | | | | | | |
| | 1 | 2 | 3 | 4 | 5 | 6 | Mean | 1 | 2 | 3 | 4 | 5 | 6 | Mean | |
| A | <0.3 | <0.3 | <0.3 | <0.3 | <0.3 | <0.3 | <0.3 | 2.5 | 0.3 | <0.3 | <0.3 | <0.3 | 2.8 | 0.9 | <0.005 |
| T | 61 | 59 | 59 | 49 | 56 | 57 | 57 | 50 | 50 | 50 | 49 | 50 | 44 | 49 | >0.05 |
| B | <0.3 | <0.3 | <0.3 | <0.3 | <0.3 | <0.3 | <0.3 | 1.5 | <0.3 | <0.3 | 1 | 0.5 | 3.5 | 1.2 | <0.005 |
| T | 59 | 58 | 53 | 54 | 53 | 51 | 55 | 49 | 45 | 48 | 45 | 48 | 47 | 47 | >0.05 |
| C | 6.8 | 12.5 | 2 | 2 | <0.3 | <0.3 | 3.9 | 113 | 23 | 66 | 128.3 | 4.8 | 163.3 | 83.1 | <0.001 |
| T | 57 | 55 | 54 | 45 | 44 | 43 | 50 | 47 | 44 | 48 | 45 | 46 | 38 | 45 | <0.05 |
| D | <1 | <1 | <1 | <1 | <1 | 1 | 0.2 | 1 | <1 | 1 | <1 | <1 | <1 | 0.3 | >0.05 |
| T | 62 | 62 | 62 | 60 | 59 | 58 | 61 | 52 | 51 | 51 | 50 | 51 | 51 | 51 | <0.01 |

[a] A, B, C, and D, rooms A, B, C, and D, respectively; T, tank.
[b] In rooms A, B, and C the numbers are the means of sample series of four samples; from outlet D, only one sample was taken.
[c] Student's t test (two-sample).

longest distance from the main tank (outlet C), the highest numbers of legionellae (mean of the six-sample series, 3.9 CFU/ml) and the lowest water temperatures at the outlets (mean of the six-sample series, 50°C) were found. In the main water pipe directly after the water tank (outlet D), 1 CFU/ml was in one of the six samples when the hot water temperature was at >60°C (mean of the sample series, 0.2 CFU/ml; mean of temperature at outlet, 61°C).

When the hot water temperature in the tank was at >50°C with the UV sterilizer installed in three of the six sample series of room A, no legionellae were found (mean of series, 0.9 CFU/ml; temperature, 49°C). In room B in two of the six series, no legionellae were found (mean of series, 1.2 CFU/ml; temperature, 47°C). In room C in all series legionellae were found with an overall mean count of 83.1 CFU/ml (temperature, 45°C). In outlet D in two of the six samples, legionellae were detected (mean, 0.3 CFU/ml; temperature, 51°C).

In all the rooms A, B, and C, the differences of legionellae counts between a hot water temperature in the water tank at >60°C and a temperature of >50°C with UV light were significant. The differences in temperature were significant in room C and outlet D. There was no significant difference in legionella count in the probes of location D.

## DISCUSSION AND CONCLUSIONS

The water sampled closest to the sterilizer (outlet D) has the same results with both types of water preparation in spite of different water temperatures at the outlet. That means a hot water temperature of >50°C with UV sterilization kills legionellae in the incoming water as efficiently as a water temperature of >60°C.

But the significant increase of legionellae in rooms A, B, and C, with a huge increase in room C, demonstrates that a hot water temperature of >50°C and UV sterilization provide no residual protection, not even in a

water system where in the beginning, only a small number of legionellae were detected, like in this study. The temperature of the water at the outlet is the crucial point, in spite of the UV sterilization.

Another remarkable point is that even the differences between room C, with >60°C (mean, 3.9 CFU/ml), and rooms A and B, with >50°C and UV sterilization (mean, 0.9 and 1.2 CFU/ml, respectively), are significant ($P = 0.006$) or almost significant ($P = 0.053$). That means that locations at a long distance from the main tank are at much higher risk of an increased number of legionellae. These results are not only a consequence of the water temperature at the outlets, because at the outlet of room C, the mean temperature when the maintaining hot water temperature was at >60°C was higher (50°C) than at the outlets of rooms A and B, when the maintaining water temperature was at >50°C (49 and 47°C). It is therefore important to carefully choose the location of the outlets that will be sampled to get an overview of a hospital water system.

According to these results, we do not recommend lowering the hot water temperature from >60°C to >50°C with the additional installation of a central flowthrough UV sterilizer to prevent transmission of legionellae in a hospital setting, because the lower temperature with UV sterilization provides no residual protection (3).

## REFERENCES

1. **Deutsche Industrienorm 1988-7.** 1988. Technische Regeln für Trinkwasser-Installationen; Vermeidung von Korrosionsschäden und Steinbildung; technische Regel des DVGW. Beuth, Berlin, Germany.
2. **Hospital Infection Control Practices Advisory Committee.** 1997. Guidelines for prevention of nosocomial pneumonia. *Morb. Mortal. Wkly. Rep.* **46:**1–79.
3. **Kusnetsov, J. M., P. J. Keskitalo, H. E. Ahonen, A. I. Tulkki, I. T. Miettinen, and P. J. Martikanen.** 1994. Growth of Legionella and other heterotrophic bacteria in a circulating cooling water system exposed to ultraviolet irradiation. *J. Appl. Bacteriol.* **77:**461–466.

4. **Miyamoto, M., Y. Yamaguchi, and M. Sasatsu.** 2000. Disinfectant effects of hot water, ultraviolet light, silver ions and chlorine on strains of Legionella and nontuberculous mycobacteria. *Microbios* **101:**7–13.

5. **Stout, J. E., and V. L. Yu.** 1999. Nosocomial legionella infection, p. 453–465. *In* C. G. Mayhall (ed.), *Hospital Epidemiology and Infection Control*, 2nd ed. Lippincott Williams & Wilkins, Philadelphia, Pa.

6. **Tobiansky, L., A. Drath, B. Dubery, and H. J. Koornhof.** 1986. Seasonality of Legionella isolates from environmental sources. *Isr. J. Med. Sci.* **22:**640–643.

7. **Wendt, C., K. Weist, E. Dietz, P. Schlattmann, and H. Rüden.** 1995. Field study to obtain Legionella-free water from showers and sinks of a transplantation unit by a system of water filters. *Zentbl. Hyg. Umweltmed.* **196:**515–531.

# MONOCHLORAMINE DISINFECTION OF BIOFILM-ASSOCIATED *LEGIONELLA PNEUMOPHILA* IN A POTABLE WATER MODEL SYSTEM

Rodney Donlan, Ricardo Murga, Joseph Carpenter,
Ellen Brown, Richard Besser, and Barry Fields

# 82

Microbial biofilms are ubiquitous in potable water systems and may provide a habitat for the survival of pathogenic organisms. *Legionella pneumophila* has been shown to survive in water system biofilms. Biofilm-associated microorganisms are significantly more resistant to antimicrobial agents either due to the mass transport limitations provided by the biofilm matrix or because these organisms are physiologically different from planktonic organisms (2). A recently published study provided evidence that hospitals supplied with drinking water containing free chlorine as the residual disinfectant were more likely to have a reported outbreak of Legionnaires' disease than those that used drinking water containing monochloramine as the residual disinfectant (4). Other published studies showed that monochloramine inactivated biofilm bacteria more effectively than free chlorine when compared on the basis of equal activity (5).

We undertook a study to compare free chlorine and monochloramine as disinfectants against *L. pneumophila* cells in a mixed culture bacterial biofilm. Our approach was to develop a heterotrophic-bacterial biofilm containing the amoeba *Hartmannella vermiformis* in a laboratory potable water system, then colonize these biofilms with *L. pneumophila*. The goal of this study was to determine the susceptibility of biofilm-associated *L. pneumophila* to free chlorine and monochloramine.

## MATERIALS AND METHODS

A biofilm reactor, developed in the Centers for Disease Control and Prevention (CDC) Biofilm Laboratory and containing 316L stainless-steel coupons (1.3-cm diameter), was used for all experiments (Fig. 1). Temperature was maintained at 30°C by placing the reactor in a water bath. The biofilm reactor had a lid with a vent, a sampling port for the bulk liquid, and an inlet through which fresh nutrients were added. A side arm at the 400-ml level provided overflow drainage. Mixing was provided by a digitally controlled mixing plate (Mirak Thermolyne, Fisher Scientific, Pittsburgh, Pa.) placed beneath the water bath. The medium initially used in the biofilm reactor contained 0.05 g of yeast extract, proteose peptone no. 3, Casamino Acids, and

*Rodney Donlan, Ricardo Murga, and Joseph Carpenter* Biofilm Laboratory, Division of Healthcare Quality Promotion, Centers for Disease Control and Prevention, Atlanta, GA 30333. *Ellen Brown, Richard Besser, and Barry Fields* Respiratory Diseases Branch, Division of Bacterial and Mycotic Diseases, Centers for Disease Control and Prevention, Atlanta, GA 30333.

*Legionella*, Edited by Reinhard Marre et al.
© 2002 ASM Press, Washington, D.C.

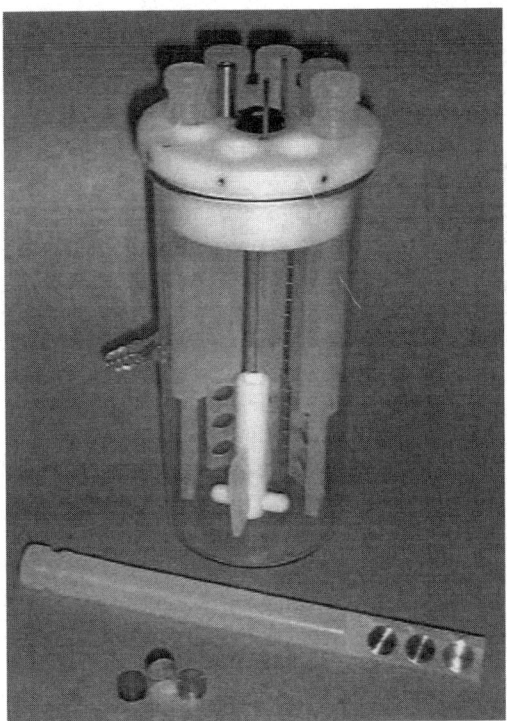

**FIGURE 1** Potable water biofilm reactor.

dextrose; 0.03 g of sodium pyruvate and dibasic potassium phosphate; and 0.005 g of magnesium phosphate per liter of filter-sterilized reverse-osmosis water. It was operated in batch mode for the first 72 h to establish the biofilms on the steel substrata. The system was then operated as an open system by continuously pumping a 1/10 dilution of the medium formulation given above at a flow rate of 1 ml/min for 24 h to dilute the medium, after which the feed to the reactors was changed to filter sterilized, dechlorinated tap water (Atlanta, Ga., municipal tap water dechlorinated using 0.1 N sodium thiosulfate) for the remaining 21 days.

Each of two reactors was inoculated with *Pseudomonas aeruginosa* (ATCC 7700), *Klebsiella pneumoniae* (CDC Strain Designation DMDS Lab No. 92-08-28a), and *Flavobacterium* spp. (CDC-65). Cultures were stored at −70°C, transferred to R2A agar plates, and resuspended in phosphate buffered water (pH 7.2) to a concentration equivalent to a 0.5 McFarland Standard. A total of 1 ml of each cell suspension ($10^8$ cells per ml) was added to each reactor. *H. vermiformis* (CDC-19) stocks were kept in axenic growth medium at 35°C without $CO_2$ and were split twice a week into T75 cell culture flasks. Flasks were tapped to dislodge *H. vermiformis* trophozoites from the growth surface, and 50 ml of the culture was transferred to individual conical tubes that were centrifuged to pellet the amoebae and then was resuspended in phosphate buffered saline. Reactors were inoculated with *H. vermiformis* to obtain a final concentration of $10^4$ cells/ml. A virulent strain of *L. pneumophila* (RI-243-GFP) was stored as a suspension in defibrinated rabbit blood in liquid nitrogen (−120°C). Four days before the isolate was needed, the mutant was cultured on buffered charcoal-yeast extract medium containing kanamycin and incubated at 36°C with 2.5% $CO_2$. After 4 days, the isolate was resuspended in sterile reverse-osmosis-treated water and diluted to the desired concentration. A total of 1 ml of this suspension was added to each reactor.

Coupons were removed from the reactor, rinsed in sterile phosphate buffered water, and placed into 250-ml beakers containing 200 ml of either 0.2-, 0.5-, or 1.5-mg/liter concentrations of either free chlorine or monochloramine for contact times of either 15, 60, or 180 min at ambient temperature. All glassware used was demand-free. Free chlorine and monochloramine residual concentrations were measured with a Hach Amperometric Digital Titrator (model 19300, Hach Co., Loveland, Colo.). Monochloramine stock solution was prepared by mixing 0.11 g of ammonium chloride with 100 ml of phosphate buffered water and then slowly adding 1 ml of 5% sodium hypochlorite and stirring for 20 min. Final concentration of this stock solution was 300 to 400 mg of total chlorine per liter. Reverse-osmosis (RO) water was used to dilute the stock solution to obtain the desired working concentration. Free chlorine was prepared by adding 20 to 25 $\mu$l of 5.25% sodium hypochlorite (commercial bleach) to 1 liter of RO water to obtain a stock solution final concentration of 1.5 mg/liter. Additional RO water was added as required to obtain the desired concentration. The pH of the monochloramine working solution was 7.5; the pH of the free chlorine solution was 7.8.

Coupons were then placed into 10 ml of a 0.12 M solution of sodium thiosulfate in phosphate buffered saline, processed to remove the attached organisms by three 30-s cycles of sonication and vortexing, homogenized for 1 min, then spread plated onto R2A medium for quantification of the base biofilm. For recovery of *H. vermiformis*, 100 μl from several dilutions were plated onto nonnutritive agar, which had been spread with viable *Escherichia coli*. Plates were read for the presence or absence of *H. vermiformis* at the dilution plated. For recovery of *L. pneumophila*, the remaining suspension was treated with a KCl-HCl solution, filtered through a 0.2-μm-pore-size filter (part no. GTTP, Millipore Corp., Bedford, Mass.), resuspended, and plated onto glycine-polymyxin B-anisomycin-vancomycin plates.

## RESULTS AND DISCUSSION

A biofilm reactor was developed to grow biofilms containing *L. pneumophila* on 24 replicate stainless-steel surfaces in potable water. The ability of this reactor to produce reproducible biofilms was validated by the fact that the standard deviations of the base biofilm densities on stainless-steel coupons ($n = 3$) ranged from 0.06 to 0.18 log CFU per coupon. Tilt and Hamilton (7) reviewed the literature to determine the range of repeatability (within laboratory precision of log reduction data during germicide testing) and found that standard deviation values ranged between 0.25 and 1.21, and that a test can be considered very good if it achieves a value of less than 0.3. Our results were well within this range.

*Legionella* levels in the biofilms exceeded $10^3$ per coupon surface on the pretreated coupons. When *Legionella*-containing biofilms were exposed to three different concentrations of free chlorine (0.2, 1.0, 1.5 mg/liter) for three different contact periods (15, 60, 180 min), this disinfectant was relatively ineffective, providing a 1.1 log reduction only at the highest dosage/contact time tested (1.5 mg/liter for 3 h) (Fig. 2). When *Legionella*-containing biofilms were exposed to the same dosages of monochloramine for identical contact periods, the treatments were significantly more effective (Fig. 3). Even though the 0.2-mg/liter treatment was ineffective for all contact times examined, the 0.5-mg/liter dosage

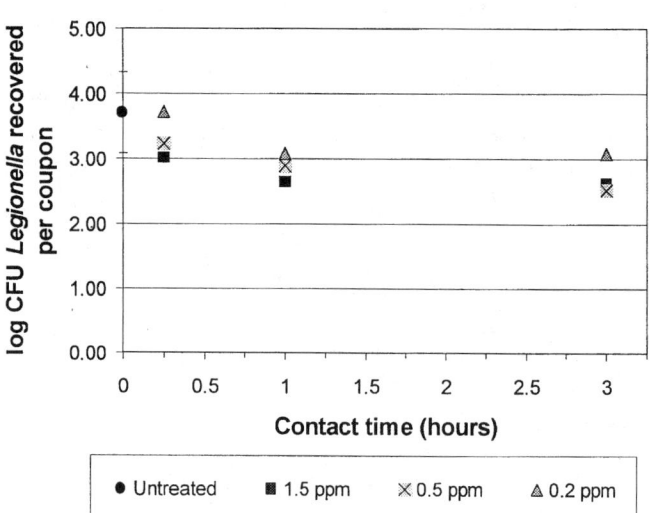

**FIGURE 2** Biofilm-associated *Legionella* disinfection with free chlorine.

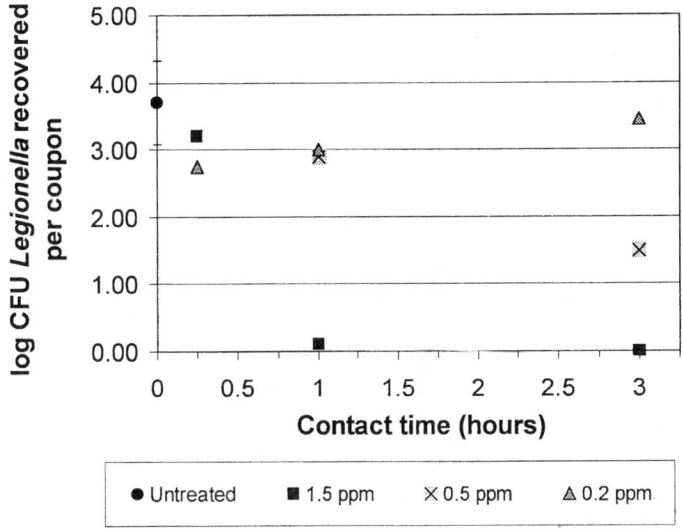

**FIGURE 3** Biofilm-associated *Legionella* disinfection with monochloramine.

reduced *Legionella* levels by 99% for the 180-min contact period. The 1.5-mg/liter concentration reduced levels by more than 99.9% for both the 60- and 180-min contact periods. A second study comparing 1.5 mg of free chlorine per liter with the same concentration of monochloramine showed that monochloramine was significantly more effective than free chlorine for a 3-h contact period. These results are shown in Fig. 4.

LeChevallier et al. (5) found that the concentration-times-time coefficient (CT) values (milligram minutes per liter to achieve a 99% reduction in viability) for hypochlorous acid (pH 7.0, 1 to 2° C) against heterotrophic plate count bacteria was 0.08. For monochloramine under the same conditions, the value was 94. They showed that three times the CT was required to inactivate biofilm–associated *Klebsiella* cells on glass slides using mono-

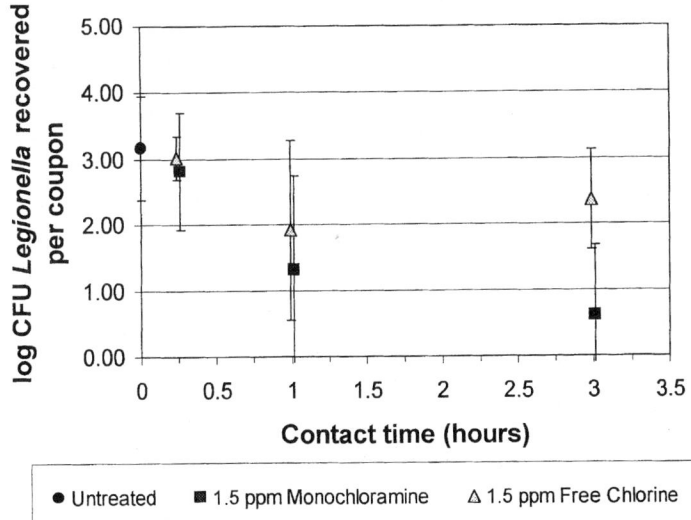

**FIGURE 4** Comparison of free chlorine and monochloramine disinfection efficacy of biofilm-associated *Legionella*. Error bars represent standard deviations ($n = 3$).

chloramine; one CT was required to inactivate 99% of heterotrophic bacteria on metal surfaces with monochloramine. Our results show that the CT value for inactivation of biofilm-associated *Legionella* was 90, which is similar to the results obtained by LeChevallier et al. for biofilm-associated heterotrophic bacteria.

In summary, we have shown that biofilm-associated *L. pneumophila* are significantly less susceptible to chlorine than are planktonic *L. pneumophila*, while susceptibility of planktonic and biofilm-associated *L. pneumophila* to monochloramine are similar. When monochloramine and free chlorine were compared under identical conditions, monochloramine was significantly more effective, indicating that monochloramine may be an effective disinfectant for the inactivation of *L. pneumophila* within potable water distribution systems. Since it is known that *L. pneumophila* is indigenous to potable water system biofilms (8), and that biofilms readily form in these systems (3), an effective control strategy could incorporate monochloramine as a disinfectant for these organisms. This has been suggested by LeChevallier et al. (6) for general biofilm control and by Cunliffe (1) specifically for *Legionella* control. Further research using open system biofilm reactors and model distribution systems is needed to determine the utility of monochloramine as a disinfectant against biofilm-associated *L. pneumophila*.

## REFERENCES

1. **Cunliffe, D. A.** 1990. Inactivation of *Legionella pneumophila* by monochloramine. *J. Appl. Bacteriol.* **68**:453–459.
2. **Donlan, R. M.** 2000. Role of biofilms in antimicrobial resistance. *Am. Soc. Artif. Intern. Organs* **46**:S47–S52.
3. **Donlan, R. M., W. O. Pipes, and T. L. Yohe.** 1994. Biofilm formation on cast iron substrata in water distribution systems. *Water Res.* **28**:1497–1503.
4. **Kool, J. L., J. C. Carpenter, and B. S. Fields.** 1999. Effect of monochloramine disinfection of municipal drinking water on risk of nosocomial Legionnaires' disease. *Lancet* **353**:272–277.
5. **LeChevallier, M. W., C. D. Cawthon, and R. G. Lee.** 1988. Inactivation of biofilm bacteria. *Appl. Environ. Microbiol.* **54**:2492–2499.
6. **LeChevallier, M. W., C. D. Lowry, and R. G. Lee.** 1990. Disinfecting biofilms in a model distribution system. *J. Am. Water Works Assoc.* **87**:99.
7. **Tilt, N., and M. A. Hamilton.** 1999. Repeatability and reproducibility of germicide tests: a literature review. *J. AOAC Int.* **82**:384–389.
8. **Wright, J. B.** 2000. *Legionella* biofilms: their implications, study, and control, p. 291–310. *In* L. V. Evans (ed.), *Biofilms: Recent Advances in Their Study and Control.* Harwood Academic Publishers, Amsterdam, The Netherlands.

# CONTROL OF *LEGIONELLA* IN DRINKING WATER SYSTEMS: IMPACT OF MONOCHLORAMINE

Jacob L. Kool

# 83

*Legionella* and *Legionella*-like organisms live as facultative intracellular parasites of amoebae in the biofilm that covers the inside of tanks and pipes in water systems. Most drinking-water disinfectants penetrate poorly into biofilm (20) and *Legionella* is further shielded by its amoebal host (13). In addition, *Legionella* often proliferates peripherally, while disinfectants often do not reach distant points in a distribution system.

Use of new diagnostic techniques and recent pneumonia-etiology studies have shown that the burden of disease due to *Legionella pneumophila* is large: *L. pneumophila* causes between 2 and 16% of all community-acquired pneumonias, which makes it the second to third most common causative organism (2). Non-*L. pneumophila* species and *Legionella*-like organisms that are not detected by routine diagnostic testing may cause significant additional morbidity (1, 21, 24).

*Legionella*-control efforts have often focused on hospitals and hotels because the outbreaks happen there. However, it should be emphasized that the great majority of Legionnaires'

disease cases are sporadic and community acquired (23). It is likely that in a large number of these sporadic cases, the disease was contracted in their homes or from other incidental sources that expose only a few persons at a time (28). A control measure that reduces *Legionella* and *Legionella*-like organism exposure in the community will therefore have great impact. Recent investigations, which will be discussed at the end of this chapter, have indicated that it is possible to prevent 90% of drinking-water-associated Legionnaires' disease (community acquired as well as nosocomial; sporadic disease as well as outbreaks) through the use of monochloramine for residual municipal water disinfection.

A selection of available *Legionella* control measures for drinking-water systems will be discussed in more detail hereunder. All of these methods have their drawbacks and none are 100% efficacious, so it may often be necessary to combine two or more. Moreover, any measure is likely to fail if it is not accompanied by a thorough analysis of the water system and correction of problems such as stagnation, cross-connections, and tepid temperatures.

## HEAT

Temporarily increasing the water temperature to above 65°C and flushing all outlets for a

*Jacob L. Kool* Bacterial Zoonoses Branch, Division of Vector-Borne Infectious Diseases, Centers for Disease Control and Prevention, P.O. Box 2087, Ft. Collins, CO 80522.

*Legionella*, Edited by Reinhard Marre et al.
© 2002 ASM Press, Washington, D.C.

few minutes (termed "superheat-and-flush") will result in a short-term reduction of *Legionella* counts. This has to be repeated regularly because the bacteria will otherwise grow back within a few weeks. In practice, this method is time-consuming, since the maximum number of outlets that can be flushed at once is limited by the capacity of the water heaters. To reduce risk of scalding, superheat-and-flush is preferably carried out at night or during weekends. The large number of staff needed for opening and closing outlets and the unusual work hours make this method expensive and impractical as a long-term solution. Superheat-and-flush was used unsuccessfully in one hospital for 13 years; *Legionella* continued to be recovered and nosocomial infection continued to occur during the entire period (27). Very few hospitals currently use this method for long-term *Legionella* control (9).

For long-term effect, the hot water temperature should be continuously maintained above 50 to 60°C in every part of the hot water system. One disadvantage of this method is the risk of scalding. Another potential problem is that an increase of the hot water temperature can lead to warming of the cold water side because of heat exchange between the two systems, resulting in an increased risk of cold water-associated *Legionella* transmission (12).

## FREE CHLORINE

Supplemental chlorination is a simple method that has been proven effective in numerous instances. It is currently the most commonly used measure for U.S. hospitals (9). Standard free chlorine levels in municipal drinking water are often inadequate to kill biofilm-associated sessile *Legionella* and *Legionella*-like organisms: chlorine does not penetrate well into biofilm (6) and it often does not reach peripheral areas or areas of stagnation within the plumbing system. Nevertheless, free chlorine can be effective if the concentration is sufficiently high in all reaches of the distribution system and after necessary changes are made to prevent stagnation (10, 18, 25). Con-

centrations below 0.5 mg/liter are often not enough (Fig. 1) (16). The Centers for Disease Control and Prevention (CDC) recommends a concentration of at least 1.0 mg of free chlorine per liter (4), but some hospitals have had to go up to 3 to 4 mg/liter. The required chlorine concentration seems to depend mostly on the success that hospital staff have with maintaining temperatures and preventing stagnation. Also, free chlorine is less effective at high pH. To achieve chlorine concentrations of >1 mg/liter, facilities will usually have to install a supplemental chlorine injector. The main drawback of high chlorine concentrations is that some hospitals have reported increased corrosion of plumbing materials, with a resulting increase in operating costs (11). This corrosion apparently does not affect every hospital and some hospitals have reported that corrosion could be controlled with addition of silicates, which would form a protective "coating" (25).

Formation of potentially carcinogenic disinfection byproducts (DBPs) has been put forward as another argument against use of free chlorine. A causal relationship between consumption of chlorinated drinking water and risk of cancer has not been confirmed. The U.S. Environmental Protection Agency did a meta-analysis in 1998 of available research on this subject. The agency concluded that among the 240 million U.S. citizens exposed to disinfected water, there may be 0 to 100 excess cases of bladder cancer per year based on toxicological data, or 0 to 9,300 based on epidemiological studies (8). To be on the safe side, authorities in many countries have put limits on the maximum concentrations of certain DBPs in drinking water. This has led many municipal water suppliers to switch from chlorine to alternative disinfectants such as monochloramine. For supplemental chlorination, however, the concern for cancer seems less relevant: any possible cancer risk will probably be negligible for short-term exposure such as for hospital patients or hotel guests.

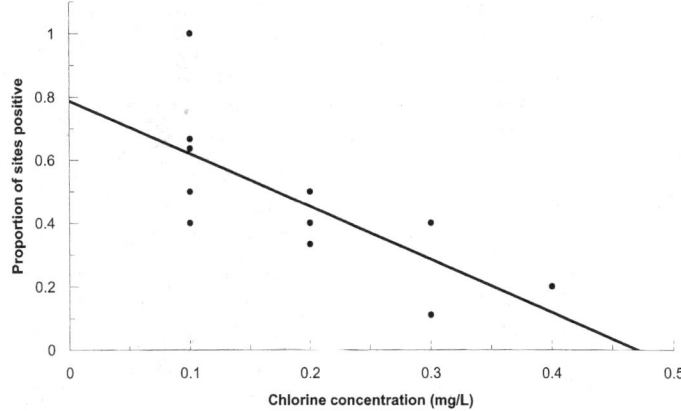

**FIGURE 1** Average free residual chlorine concentration as measured in patient room tap water and proportion of sites positive for *Legionella* in 11 San Antonio hospitals. Each dot represents one hospital; a regression line is shown. Reprinted from *Infection Control and Hospital Epidemiology* (16) with permission of the publisher.

## COPPER-SILVER IONIZATION

Experts disagree on the merits of this method. A review of the available literature gives the impression that *Legionella* counts generally decrease by about two logs after application of copper-silver ionization. Its effectiveness is sensitive to many parameters such as pH, water hardness, and dissolved solids. Furthermore, it is difficult to calibrate levels of copper and silver within the narrow range between minimum inhibitory levels and maximum allowable concentrations. Scale buildup may necessitate frequent replacing of the electrodes. For the above reasons, this is often a labor-intensive and expensive method. A hospital in Arizona was able to control *Legionella* with a combination of copper-silver and 0.5 mg of free chlorine per liter, but the entire process of installation and calibration of the copper-silver system was estimated to cost approximately $1 million (15).

The first study on the effectiveness of copper and silver against *Legionella* reported that it had an effect only in the presence of at least 0.4 mg of free chlorine per liter (19). It is possible that, in some situations, this chlorine concentration could by itself achieve the reported effect. Unfortunately, later papers on the effectiveness of copper-silver have often failed to report chlorine concentrations. In addition to positive experience with copper-silver ionization (3, 22), failures have been documented frequently (5, 9, 26, 27). A hospital in Ohio reported that a copper-silver system neither reduced the number of positive samples nor terminated transmission and the system was discontinued (5). In a hospital in Pittsburgh, a copper-silver system was installed in 1994. *Legionella* counts decreased, but the bacteria continued to be recovered from the water system and at least six nosocomial Legionnaires' disease cases occurred in the 3 years after the system was installed (27). In a 4-year study in a German university hospital, copper-silver had an effect in the first 2 years, but *Legionella* counts increased thereafter. The researchers concluded that copper-silver was ineffective in the long term, perhaps because of the development of resistance, and the use of the system was discontinued (26). Another German hospital reports in these proceedings that the use of copper-silver required intensive maintenance but that it had only limited effect on *Legionella*, concluding that copper-silver cannot be recommended for control of *Legionella* in German hospitals (see chapter 84). In a survey of U.S. hospitals participating in the National Nosocomial Infections Surveillance System, 38 reported using long-term *Legionella* control measures: 22 (58%) used supplemental chlorination compared with 9 (24%) that used copper-silver. Five hospitals reported that nosocomial infection continued to occur despite the control measures, and of these five, three used copper-silver (9). The conclusion is that copper-silver is used less frequently than chlorine and that it has a higher failure rate.

In view of the above evidence it seems that copper-silver alone does not reliably control *Legionella* and that it is less effective than, for example, free chlorine. However, copper-silver can be a useful addition to free chlorine because it allows for a reduction in the concentration of the latter (3, 15, 19), thereby reducing corrosion problems and improving taste and odor.

## OTHER METHODS

Other disinfectants such as ozone and chlorine dioxide have been tried with limited success. These disinfectants appear to have the same problem that free chlorine has: they do not penetrate biofilm. UV light stops *Legionella* growth only at the point of application; it has no effect on peripheral *Legionella* growth and therefore has very limited value for water systems.

## MONOCHLORAMINE

### General Description

Monochloramine (combined chlorine) is formed when ammonia and free chlorine are mixed in water in the correct ratio (14). It penetrates better into biofilm than free chlorine and it is better at killing biofilm bacteria such as some *Pseudomonas* spp. (20). It has been used for drinking-water disinfection since 1916 (7). Municipal drinking-water disinfection has two stages: initial disinfection at the water-treatment plant, and residual disinfection to maintain biocidal activity throughout the distribution system. Monochloramine's disinfecting action is slower than that of free chlorine, so it is less useful for initial disinfection. On the other hand, it is more stable than free chlorine, so a disinfecting residual can be maintained over long distances in a distribution system, which can reduce cost (14). It is believed to form less potentially carcinogenic disinfection by products than free chlorine (8). Another advantage is that it causes fewer taste and odor problems.

A survey in 1989 and 1990 of municipal water utilities in the United States that served populations greater than 50,000 found that 23% were using monochloramine as a residual disinfectant (14), and this percentage has undoubtedly gone up since then. It is also used in other countries, such as Canada and the United Kingdom. A typical monochloramine-using water treatment plant presently uses free chlorine or ozone for initial disinfection, and monochloramine for residual disinfection (14).

Disadvantages of monochloramine are that it is toxic to some fish and it causes a febrile reaction when the water is used for dialysis. It can be removed from water by granular activated carbon filters or it can be neutralized with agents such as ascorbic acid or thiosulphate. Although corrosion usually is not a problem associated with monochloramine, it does deteriorate some artificial rubbers.

### Evidence for the Effect of Monochloramine on *Legionella*

Recent research has shown that monochloramine may be considerably more effective against *Legionella* and *Legionella*-like organisms than free chlorine. In an investigation in Texas in 1997, we did not recover *Legionella* or *Legionella*-like organisms from the water systems of hospitals in cities that treated their water with monochloramine. These hospitals also did not detect cases of Legionnaires' disease among their patients. In contrast, 11 of 12 studied hospitals in a nearby chlorine-using municipality were found to contain *Legionella* in their water system and 5 had detected nosocomial Legionnaires' disease among their patients. The only hospital in the chlorine-using city where we did not recover *Legionella* had just experienced a nosocomial Legionnaires' disease outbreak and had already implemented control measures (16). This observation led us to do a retrospective analysis of published nosocomial outbreaks of Legionnaires' disease in the United States (17). Through literature searches we identified 32 hospitals that had experienced outbreaks re-

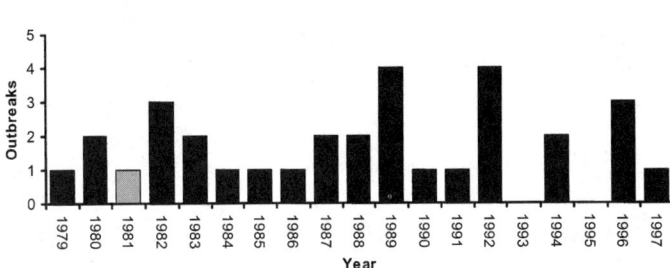

**FIGURE** 2 Potable water-associated nosocomial Legionnaires' disease outbreaks identified through literature review in the United States, by year. Solid bars represent hospitals supplied with free chlorine-containing water; the shaded bar is the hospital that was supplied with monochloramine-containing water. Reprinted from *The Lancet* (17) with permission of the publisher. © by The Lancet Ltd., 1999.

lated to their water system (Fig. 2). Forty-eight control hospitals were randomly selected and matched by hospital size and the presence of a transplant program. We then collected information on the type of water disinfection by interviewing the local water-treatment authorities. A total of 31 of the 32 case hospitals were supplied with water containing free chlorine. Only one, a hospital in Denver, was supplied with water that was disinfected with monochloramine (Fig. 3). This hospital experienced a small outbreak of three cases in 1981. At the time, it had an unusual water system configuration: large hot water storage tanks were in turn taken off-line but were

kept warm and full of water for weeks at a time before being reconnected. After the hospital corrected this problem by replacing the tanks with instantaneous heaters, no nosocomial Legionnaires' disease cases were detected in the following two decades in spite of intensive surveillance. Of the control hospitals, 12 (25%) were supplied with drinking water containing monochloramine. Interestingly, the Denver hospital with the outbreak received water with a lower monochloramine concentration (1 mg/liter) than all control hospitals (1.5 to 4.3 mg/liter; Table 1). Denver later increased the monochloramine level because the municipality had difficulty main-

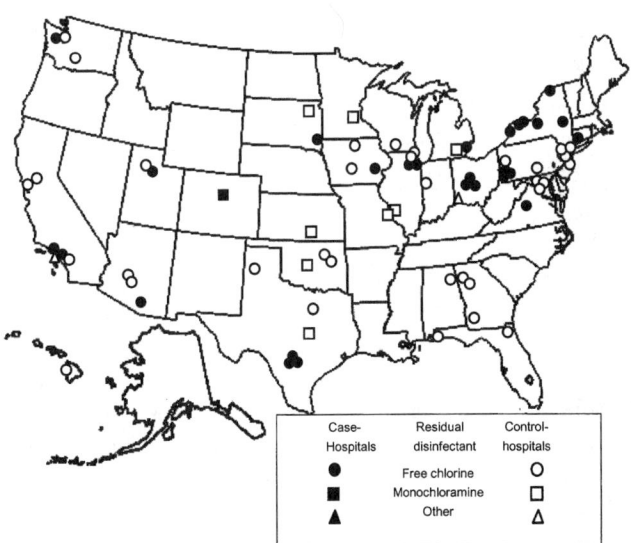

**FIGURE** 3 Geographical distribution of hospitals with reported Legionnaires' disease outbreaks associated with potable water and of randomly selected control hospitals. Some overlapping points were dispersed to improve legibility. Reprinted from *The Lancet* (17) with permission of the publisher. © by The Lancet Ltd., 1999.

**TABLE 1** Characteristics of 32 hospitals with drinking water-associated Legionnaires' disease outbreaks, 42 control hospitals, and their municipal water suppliers[a]

| Characteristic | Outbreak hospitals (n = 32) | Control hospitals (n = 48) | Adjusted OR (95% CI)[b] | P |
|---|---|---|---|---|
| Hospital characteristics | | | | |
| No. of municipal water distribution systems | 26 | 45 | | |
| No. with 200 beds or more | 31 | 46 | | |
| No. (%) with a transplant program | 23 (72%) | 35 (73%) | | 0.89[f] |
| Median year (range) | 1988.5 (1979–1997) | 1988 (1979–1997) | | |
| Residual disinfectant | | | | |
| No. using free chlorine | 31 | 36 | 10.2 (1.4–460) | 0.007 |
| No. using monochloramine | 1 | 12[c] | 1.0[d] | |
| Median free chlorine concn (range)[e] | 0.55 (0.0–1.8) | 0.6 (0.0–2.1) | | 0.34[f] |
| Median monochloramine concn (range)[e] | 1.0 (1.0–1.0) | 2.7 (1.5–4.3) | | 0.11[f] |
| Initial disinfectant | | | | |
| No. using free chlorine | 31 | 43 | 2.1 (0.16-114) | 0.46 |
| No. using monochloramine | 1 | 3 | 1.0[d] | |
| No. alternating chlorine and monochloramine | 0 | 1 | Excluded | |
| Ozone | 0 | 1 | Excluded | |
| Water source | | | | |
| Surface | 22 | 33 | | 0.91[f,g] |
| Ground | 5 | 10 | | |
| Mix of surface/ground | 5 | 5 | | |
| Median no. of persons supplied by water utility (range) | 242,500 (5,000–4,000,000) | 198,000 (3,500–9,000,000) | | 0.28[f] |
| Median pH of finished water (range) | 7.6 (7.0–10.0) | 7.8 (7.0–10.5) | | 0.82[f] |

[a] Reprinted from *The Lancet* (17) with permission of the publisher. © by The Lancet Ltd., 1999.
[b] CI, confidence interval; OR, odds ratio.
[c] Including one hospital supplied with water that contained free chlorine for 2 weeks per year.
[d] Reference category.
[e] Values are calculated for those water systems that used this disinfectant and are the water-treatment specialist's estimate of the concentration at the location of the hospital. Free chlorine concentration is in mg/liter, monochloramine concentration is expressed as mg of combined chlorine per liter.
[f] Mann-Whitney U test.
[g] Analyzing the proportion surface water as a continuous variable.

taining sufficient residual in warm summer months (15).

The data from the above case-control study gave an odds ratio of 10.2 (95% confidence interval, 1.4 to 460). In other words, the likelihood of having an outbreak of nosocomial drinking water-associated Legionnaires' disease was 10 times higher for hospitals in chlorine-using municipalities than for those in monochloramine-using cities. This result suggests that 90% of drinking-water-associated outbreaks would not have occurred if all hospitals had been supplied with monochloramine-disinfected water. Apart from the municipal residual disinfection method, no other parameters were associated with risk of outbreaks (Table 1). Because we collected data on water treatment at the time of the beginning of each Legionnaires' disease outbreak, none of the hospitals in our study were implementing control measures against *Legionella*.

The protective effect of monochloramine was confirmed in a survey of more than 300 hospitals, which found that hospitals supplied with chlorinated water were 3.6 times more likely to experience a problem with nosocomial Legionnaires' disease. This result suggested that 72% of occurrences of nosocomial transmission could have been prevented if all municipalities had used monochloramine as a residual disinfectant (J. D. Heffelfinger, S. K. Fridkin, J. L. Kool, V. Fraser, J. C. Hageman, E. R. Zell, B. Kupronis, and C. G. Whitney, 4th Decennial Int. Conf. Nosocomial Healthcare-Associated Infections, May 2000). A pilot study of monochloramine injection in the water system of one wing of a Washington, D.C., hospital showed promising results (Shelton, B. G., N. Donegan, W. D. Flanders, J. Kool, L. Pic-Aluas, and L. Witherell, Efficacy of point of use monochloramine treatment to control *Legionella* in colonized building water system. 5th International Conference on Legionella, Ulm, Germany, 2000). The municipal water supplier of that hospital later switched to monochloramine, and since then, no *Legionella* could be recovered from any of the other hospital wings (personal communication, L. Pic-Aluas, February 2001). A laboratory study on the effect of monochloramine on *Legionella* in a biofilm model is described in chapter 82. Monochloramine was more effective at killing biofilm-associated *Legionella* than free chlorine.

It is likely that the superior effect of monochloramine is mostly due to its better penetration into biofilm. This effect may be further enhanced by its higher chemical stability, enabling it to penetrate the far reaches of a distribution system and to persist longer in areas of stagnation. An interesting hypothesis is that monochloramine may also be better at killing the amoebae that serve as hosts to *Legionella* and *Legionella*-like organisms. More research is needed to elucidate the mechanisms by which monochloramine inhibits *Legionella* colonization.

## CONCLUSIONS

To this author's knowledge, monochloramine is the only disinfectant that has been shown to reduce the incidence of Legionnaires' disease when used at the municipal level. This finding is not just important for control of nosocomial infections. More than 75% of cases of Legionnaires' disease acquire their infection in the community (23). Residual disinfection of municipal drinking water with monochloramine seems an inexpensive and efficient way to prevent many of these cases. In addition, supplemental injection of monochloramine may become one of the preferred methods for control of *Legionella* and *Legionella*-like organisms in hospitals, hotels, and similar institutions.

## REFERENCES

1. **Adeleke, A., J. Pruckler, R. Benson, T. Rowbotham, M. Halablab, and B. Fields.** 1996. *Legionella*-like amebal pathogens: phylogenetic status and possible role in respiratory-disease. *Emerg. Infect. Dis.* **2:**225–230.
2. **Bartlett, J. G., R. F. Breiman, L. A. Mandell, and T. M. J. File.** 1998. Community-acquired pneumonia in adults: guidelines for management. The Infectious Diseases Society of America. *Clin. Infect. Dis.* **26:**811–838.
3. **Biurrun, A., L. Caballero, C. Pelaz, E. Leon, and A. Gago.** 1999. Treatment of a *Legionella pneumophila*-colonized water distribution system using copper-silver ionization and continuous chlorination. *Infect. Control Hosp. Epidemiol.* **20:**426–428.
4. **Centers for Disease Control and Prevention.** 1997. Guidelines for prevention of nosocomial pneumonia. *Morb. Mortal. Wkly. Rep.* **46:**1–79.
5. **Centers for Disease Control and Prevention.** 1997. Sustained transmission of nosocomial Legionnaires disease—Arizona and Ohio. *Morb. Mortal. Wkly Rep.* **46:**416–421.
6. **Chen, X., and P. S. Stewart.** 1996. Chlorine penetration into artificial biofilm is limited by a reaction-diffusion interaction. *Environ. Sci. Technol.* **30:**2078–2083.

7. **Dice, J.** 1985. Denver's seven decades of experience with chloramination. *J. Am. Water Works Assoc.* **77:**34.

8. **Environmental Protection Agency.** 1998. National primary drinking water regulations: disinfectants and disinfection byproducts; final rule. *Fed. Regist.* **63:**69389–69476.

9. **Fiore, A.E., J.C. Butler, T.G. Emori, and R. P. Gaynes.** 1999. A survey of methods used to detect nosocomial legionellosis among participants in the National Nosocomial Infections Surveillance System. *Infect. Control Hosp. Epidemiol.* **20:**412–416.

10. **Fiore, A. E., J. L. Kool, J. Carpenter, and J. C. Butler.** 1997. Eradicating *Legionella* from hospital water—reply. *JAMA* **278:**1404–1405.

11. **Helms, C. M., R. M. Massanari, R. P. Wenzel, M. A. Pfaller, N. P. Moyer, and N. Hall.** 1988. Legionnaires' disease associated with a hospital water system. A five-year progress report on continuous hyperchlorination. *JAMA* **259:**2423–2427.

12. **Hoebe, C. J., J. J. Cluitmans, and J. H. Wagenvoort.** 1998. Two fatal cases of nosocomial *Legionella pneumophila* pneumonia associated with a contaminated cold water supply. *Eur. J. Clin. Microbiol. Infect. Dis.* **17:**740.

13. **Kilvington, S., and J. Price.** 1990. Survival of *Legionella pneumophila* within cysts of *Acanthamoeba polyphaga* following chlorine exposure. *J. Appl. Bacteriol.* **68:**519–525.

14. **Kirmeyer, G. J., G. W. Foust, G. L. Pierson, J. J. Simmler, and M. W. LeChevallier.** 1993. *Optimizing Chloramine Treatment.* American Water Works Research Foundation, Denver, Colo.

15. **Kool, J. L.** 10 May, 2000. Preventing Legionnaires' disease. Ph.D. dissertation. University of Amsterdam, Amsterdam, The Netherlands.

16. **Kool, J. L., D. Bergmire-Sweat, J. C. Butler, E. W. Brown, D. J. Peabody, D. S. Massi, J. C. Carpenter, J. M. Pruckler, R. F. Benson, and B. S. Fields.** 1999. Hospital characteristics associated with colonization of water systems by *Legionella* and risk of nosocomial Legionnaires' disease: a cohort study of 15 hospitals. *Infect. Control Hosp. Epidemiol.* **20:**798–805.

17. **Kool, J. L., J. C. Carpenter, and B. S. Fields.** 1999. Effect of monochloramine disinfection of municipal drinking water on risk of nosocomial Legionnaires' disease. *Lancet* **353:**272–277.

18. **Kool, J. L., A. E. Fiore, C. M. Kioski, E. W. Brown, R. F. Benson, J. M. Pruckler, C.** Glasby, J. C. Butler, G. D. Cage, J. C. Carpenter, R. M. Mandel, B. England, and R. F. Breiman. 1998. More than 10 years of unrecognized nosocomial transmission of legionnaires' disease among transplant patients. *Infect. Control Hosp. Epidemiol.* **19:**898–904.

19. **Landeen, L. K., M. T. Yahya, and C. P. Gerba.** 1989. Efficacy of copper and silver ions and reduced levels of free chlorine in inactivation of *Legionella pneumophila*. *Appl. Environ. Microbiol.* **55:**3045–3050.

20. **LeChevallier, M. W., C. D. Cawthon, and R. G. Lee.** 1988. Inactivation of biofilm bacteria. *Appl. Environ. Microbiol.* **54:**2492.

21. **Lee, T. C., R. M. Vickers, V. L. Yu, and M. M. Wagener.** 1993. Growth of 28 *Legionella* species on selective culture media: a comparative study. *J. Clin. Microbiol.* **31:**2764–2768.

22. **Liu, Z., J. E. Stout, L. Tedesco, M. Boldin, C. Hwang, W. F. Diven, and V. L. Yu.** 1994. Controlled evaluation of copper-silver ionization in eradicating *Legionella pneumophila* from a hospital water distribution system. *J. Infect. Dis.* **169:**919–922.

23. **Marston, B. J., H. B. Lipman, and R. F. Breiman.** 1994. Surveillance for Legionnaires' disease. Risk factors for morbidity and mortality. *Arch. Intern. Med.* **154:**2417–2422.

24. **McNally, C., B. Hackman, B. S. Fields, and J. F. Plouffe.** 2000. Potential importance of legionella species as etiologies in community acquired pneumonia. *Diagn. Microbiol. Infect. Dis.* **38:**79–82.

25. **Nafziger, D. A.** 1997. Successful chlorination for *Legionella* at Henry Ford Hospital. *Infect. Dis. Clin. Pract.* **7:**118.

26. **Rohr, U., M. Senger, F. Selenka, R. Turley, and M. Wilhelm.** 1999. Four years of experience with silver-copper ionization for control of legionella in a German university hospital hot water plumbing system. *Clin. Infect. Dis.* **29:**1507–1511.

27. **Stout, J. E., Y. S. Lin, A. M. Goetz, and R. R. Muder.** 1998. Controlling *Legionella* in hospital water systems: experience with the superheat-and-flush method and copper-silver ionization. *Infect. Control. Hosp. Epidemiol.* **19:**911–914.

28. **Stout, J. E., V. L. Yu, P. Muraca, J. Joly, N. Troup, and L. S. Tompkins.** 1992. Potable water as a cause of sporadic cases of community-acquired legionnaires' disease. *N. Engl. J. Med.* **326:**151–155.

# EFFICACY OF COPPER-SILVER IONIZATION IN CONTROLLING *LEGIONELLA* IN A HOSPITAL HOT WATER DISTRIBUTION SYSTEM: A GERMAN EXPERIENCE

*Werner Mathys, Curro Palma Hohmann, and Elisabeth Junge-Mathys*

# 84

Hot water distribution systems of hospitals and other large buildings are well known to be frequently contaminated by *Legionella* bacteria. In many cases, the presence of *Legionella* in the hospital environment could be associated with the presence of nosocomial legionellosis, especially with high-risk patients (8). Thus numbers of *Legionella* in the main environmental source, the hot water distribution system, have to be controlled. As an alternative to permanently raising hot water temperatures to 60°C, copper-silver ionization is reported to be a useful tool to control growth of *Legionella* (2, 5, 6, 9). The objective of our study was thus an assessment of the efficacy of this technique and of possible side-effects within a complex high-volume hot water plumbing system in a German hospital.

## STUDY DESIGN

The object of this study was a building housing six surgical wards, one ICU, and one transplant unit. Due to refurbishment measures, hot water temperatures could not be raised above 50°C and were kept at 45 to 49°C during the whole study. The incoming municipal drinking water (calcium, 87 mg/liter; magnesium, 5.5 mg/liter; chlorides 49 mg/liter; sulfates 77 mg/liter; pH 7.7; conductivity, 609 $\mu$S/cm) was not chlorinated or otherwise treated. The hospital plumbing material consisted exclusively of copper, causing relatively high background levels of copper of about 1 mg/liter (Table 1). Copper-silver ionization was tested over a period of 1 year as the first step in a multiple-barrier system controlling *Legionella*. All water outlets in wards with high-risk patients are equipped with point-of-use sterile filters in addition to sanitation measures within the water-distribution system.

After getting a special and temporary permit to add copper to drinking water (highest permitted concentration, 2.0 mg/liter) and to exceed the German limit value of 10 $\mu$g of silver per liter (highest permitted concentration, 80 $\mu$g/liter), issued by the German Ministry of Health, the copper-silver ionization unit was installed in a bypass of the hot water circulating line near the outlet of the hot water storage tank (volume, 1,200 liters). The current of the unit was monitored and adjusted daily. Samples ($n = 539$) were taken from the central water supply, the recirculation lines, and the distal outlets (water faucets),

*Werner Mathys, Curro Palma Hohmann, and Elisabeth Junge-Mathys*   Institute for Hygiene, University of Münster, Münster, D-48129, Germany.

*Legionella*, Edited by Reinhard Marre et al.
© 2002 ASM Press, Washington, D.C.

**TABLE 1** Summary statistics of *Legionella* counts, silver, and copper levels in a German hospital's hot water system[a]

| Phase | *Legionella* (CFU/ml) | | | | Silver (μg/liter) | | | | Copper (mg/liter) | | | |
|---|---|---|---|---|---|---|---|---|---|---|---|---|
| | Avg | Median | Maximum | SD | Avg | Median | Maximum | SD | Avg | Median | Maximum | SD |
| 0 | 45 | 47 | 92 | 19.9 | <5 | <5 | <5 | 0.00 | 1.1 | 1.0 | 1.5 | 0.15 |
| 1 | 10 | 6 | 161 | 18.8 | 21.5 | 16.7 | 100.0 | 16.97 | 1.3 | 1.3 | 2.0 | 0.26 |
| 2 | 4 | 2 | 25 | 11.1 | 15.7 | 13.1 | 48.0 | 8.97 | 1.0 | 1.0 | 3.0 | 0.32 |
| 3 | 13 | 12 | 28 | 7.7 | 31.2 | 31.0 | 53.0 | 7.10 | 1.9 | 1.9 | 2.5 | 0.27 |
| 4 | 2 | 1 | 9 | 2.2 | 40.1 | 30.0 | 189.0 | 33.76 | 2.4 | 2.1 | 12.3 | 1.79 |
| 5 | 1 | 1 | 9 | 1.8 | 33.8 | 32.2 | 128.2 | 12.96 | 1.6 | 1.6 | 2.4 | 0.32 |
| 6 | 2 | 1 | 8 | 1.8 | 15.6 | 16.3 | 22.2 | 3.38 | 1.1 | 1.0 | 1.6 | 0.17 |

[a] Phase 0, period before installation of ionization unit; phase 1, period after starting silver-copper ionization; phase 2/3, period after first/second cleaning of electrodes; phase 4, period after feeding the unit with softened water; phase 5, after third cleaning of electrodes; phase 6, after deactivating and removing unit. SD, standard deviation.

first on a daily basis and later on a weekly basis after discarding 5 liters of tap water. Contents of copper and silver were analyzed by atomic absorption spectroscopy. *Legionella* was cultured by plating each time: 1 ml of tap water on two selective 0.1% α-ketoglutarate supplemented buffered charcoal-yeast extract agar plates (BCYE-α agar, Oxoid, Wesel, with anisomycin, polymyxin B, and vancomycin) and on one nonselective buffered charcoal-yeast agar plate.

## RESULTS

Baseline cultures showed that during the period of low hot water temperatures (48°C), legionellae had amplified to high counts (up to 92 CFU/ml) in the hot water distribution system of all wards. Serogrouping revealed *L. pneumophila* serogroup 1 and serogroup 6, and *Legionella dumoffii*.

After activating the electrodes, silver concentrations increased to 20 to 60 μg/liter and copper concentrations to 1.5 to 1.8 mg/liter within 2 days. During the same period, counts for *Legionella* decreased to about 10% in the recirculating line, but sporadically, very high counts occurred in the hot water of central and distal sampling sites. After about 5 weeks, buildup of deposits (mainly calcium carbonate) on the electrodes forced intensive maintenance and de-scaling procedures to guarantee sufficient levels of silver in the hot water. This procedure had to be repeated a second time 1 month later. To improve the performance of the unit and to increase silver levels in the hot water, we fed the unit with decalcified (softened) water from day 199 after starting the ionization. As a consequence, silver and copper concentrations increased significantly ($P < 0.05$ by analysis of variance) to average levels of >40 μg of silver per liter and >2.0 mg of copper per liter, respectively (Table 1, Fig. 1) with high variations. Maximum values of silver reached 189 μg/liter. Despite these relatively high concentrations of silver and copper, a complete eradication of *Legionella* could not be achieved. All sample sites remained positive with maximum values of 9 CFU/ml (Table 1, Fig. 2). Comparing ioni-

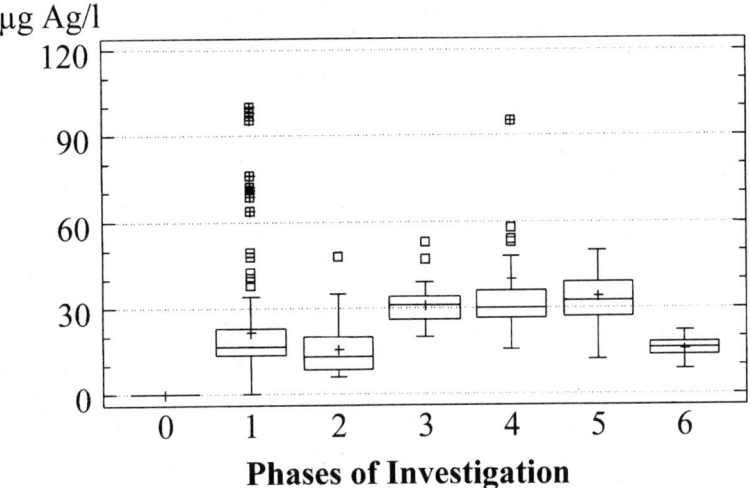

**FIGURE 1**  Effect of silver-copper ionization on silver concentrations in a German hospital's hot water system. Phase 0, period before installation of unit; phase 1, period after starting ionization; phase 2/3, period after first/second cleaning of electrodes; phase 4, period after feeding the unit with softened water; phase 5, after third cleaning of electrodes; phase 6, after deactivating and removing unit.

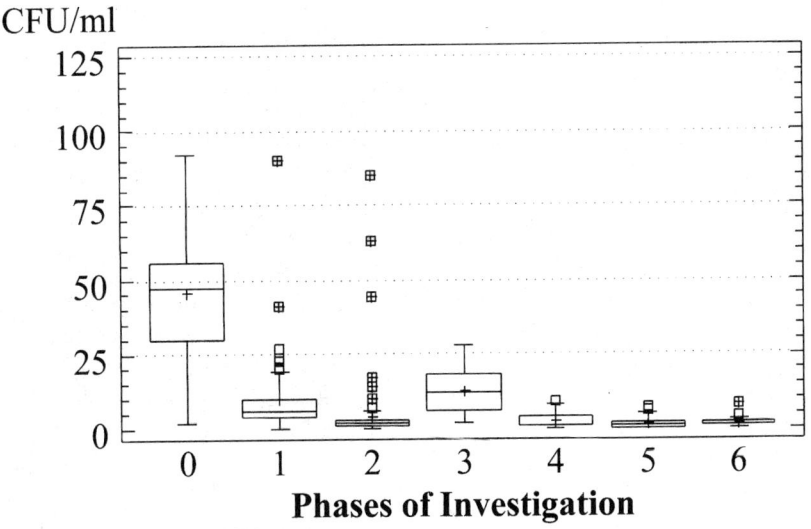

**FIGURE 2**  Effect of silver-copper ionization on *Legionella* counts in a German hospital's hot water system. Phase 0, period before installation of unit; phase 1, period after starting ionization; phase 2/3, period after first/second cleaning of electrodes; phase 4, period after feeding the unit with softened water; phase 5, after third cleaning of electrodes; phase 6, after deactivating and removing unit.

zation phases with high average concentrations of 36.4 $\mu$g of silver per liter and low average concentrations of 16.4 $\mu$g of silver per liter, levels of silver in the hot water revealed significant differences of copper concentrations (1.17 mg/liter versus 2.01 mg/liter copper) and of the efficacy of *Legionella* reduction ($P < 0.01$, Mann-Whitney-Wilcoxon-U test). Arithmetic means/medians for *Legionella* counts were 5.7/4.0 CFU/ml in the low silver phase and 3.3/2.0 CFU/ml in the high silver phase. After inactivating the ionization on day 364, silver concentrations dropped to 10 to 15 $\mu$g/liter and remained on this level for more than 3 months, indicating processes of resolution of silver from sediments and deposits. Copper levels decreased rapidly to background values of 1 mg/liter. *Legionella* counts continued to be between 1 and 8 CFU/ml. This long-term residual effect is undoubtedly one advantage of silver-copper ionization compared with other sanitation measures.

No change within the distribution of species, serogroups, or strains (performed by pulsed-field gel electrophoresis) could be observed during the whole investigation.

## ASSESSMENT OF BENEFITS AND DRAWBACKS OF COPPER-SILVER IONIZATION

Our investigation has clearly shown that the growth of *Legionella* could be reduced by copper-silver ionization, but *Legionella* could not be completely eradicated from the hot water system, even at silver concentrations above 30 $\mu$g/liter. All sampling sites remained positive. Results of other studies are contradictory. Biurrun et al. (1) also reported only an incomplete eradication of *Legionella*. Adjustments of silver levels and an additional continuous chlorination were necessary. Liu et al. (7) described a significant reduction of *Legionella* only when silver was added at values exceeding 40 $\mu$g/liter (with mean values of 163 $\mu$g/liter). Miuetzner et al. (9) used silver concentrations that in some cases remarkably exceeded 100 $\mu$g/liter. To control biofouling,

40 $\mu$g of silver per liter were reported to be necessary (12). Disinfection of swimming pools with silver/copper is reported to be efficacious (4) at silver concentrations of 40 $\mu$g/liter and in the presence of 0.4 mg of free chlorine per liter. Apparently bactericidal effects of silver are enhanced by the addition of free chlorine (1, 3, 11, 13), perhaps enabling a two-stage disinfection (11).

Higher silver levels and possible positive effects of water chlorination might be one explanation for the higher efficacy in *Legionella* reduction in some studies (2, 6, 7, 9) compared with our investigation. Because of other sampling procedures (swab sampling instead of water sampling) and missing data of, e.g., water temperature, water chemistry, and free chlorine levels, the results are generally difficult to compare.

Our findings show that reduction of *Legionella* is not as efficacious as in water systems, where the hot water temperature was permanently kept at about 60°C and more than 90% of all samples remained culture-negative for *Legionella* over long periods of time (8). The average reduction by silver-copper dosing was only 1.6 log. This reduction is nearly the same as in another German investigation reported by Rohr et al. (10), who added 30 $\mu$g of silver per liter.

Since copper and silver are released at a constant ratio, high silver values are always associated with copper values exceeding the permitted maximum concentrations of copper. Since electrolysis of copper and silver is not controlled by water consumption, heavy metal concentrations cannot be kept on a constant level. In stagnating water, a considerable buildup of silver and copper could be observed in this and other studies (7, 9). Concentrations of both metals vary depending on water flow, causing uncontrollable peak values of both silver and copper. Values exceeding national standards are reported by others as well (7, 9).

Water quality (electrolytes, especially calcium, chlorides, pH) influences the performance and effectiveness of the units dramatically. Frequent and time-consuming maintenance procedures are necessary (1, 7, 9, 11) and must be done regularly. High amounts of silver are precipitated into sludges and sediments of storage tanks. In areas with hard waters, a softening of the water feeding the electrodes is necessary (11) and may enhance the performance of the ionization process and maintenance intervals.

Development of resistance to silver, as discussed by Rohr (10) or Goetz and Yu (2), remains an unsolved question, but cannot be totally excluded at this time. Long-term effects of silver/copper have to be evaluated in the future, taking into account the whole ecosystem of the water-distribution system, including organisms of the biofilm and protozoa.

## CONCLUSIONS FOR THE USE OF COPPER-SILVER IONIZATION IN GERMANY

After assessing all data of our and other studies, our opinion is that silver-copper ionization cannot be generally recommended for German hospitals as an alternative measure to reduce *Legionella* counts in hot water systems and cases of legionellosis. The main reasons are summarized as follows:

In Germany, additions of silver and copper to drinking water need special approval of the Ministry of Health and are permitted only with substantial restrictions.

Measurable effects in *Legionella* reduction can be achieved only at silver concentrations significantly exceeding the German standard of 10 $\mu$g/liter.

Copper values exceeded national standards, preventing a short-term high dosing of silver. Concentrations of both metals vary depending on water flow. Silver cannot be analyzed directly within the system, causing a considerable feedback delay.

*Legionella* counts stayed above targeted values (working standard, *Legionella* counts <1 CFU/ml). Reduction is not as efficacious as in hot water systems maintaining about 60°C.

Long-term effects (e.g., development of heavy-metal resistance) of adding silver and copper have still to be evaluated.

## REFERENCES

1. **Biurrun, A., L. Caballero, C. Pelaz, E. Leon, and A. Gago.** 1999. Treatment of a *Legionella pneumophila*-colonized water distribution system using copper-silver ionization and continuous chlorination. *Infect. Control Hosp. Epidemiol.* **20:**426–428.
2. **Goetz, A., and V. L. Yu.** 1997. Copper-silver ionization: cautious optimism for *Legionella* disinfection and implications for environmental culturing. *Am. J. Infect. Control* **25:**449–451.
3. **Landeen, L. K., M. T. Yahya, S. M. Kutz, and C. P. Gerba.** 1989. Microbiological evaluation of copper:silver disinfection units for use in swimming pools. *Water Sci. Technol.* **21:**267–270.
4. **Landeen, L. K., M. T. Yahya, S. M. Kutz, and C. P. Gerba.** 1989. Efficacy of copper and silver ions and reduced levels of free chlorine in inactivation of *Legionella pneumophila*. *Applied Environ. Microbiol.* **55:**3045–3050.
5. **Lin, Y. E., J. E. Stout, V. L. Yu, and R. D. Vidic.** 1998. Disinfection of water distribution systems for *Legionella*. *Semin. Respir. Infect.* **13:**147–159.
6. **Lin, Z., J. E. Stout, L. Tedesco, M. Boldin, C. Hwang, W. F. Diven, and V. L. Yu.** 1994. Controlled evaluation of copper-silver ionization in eradicating *Legionella pneumophila* from a hospital water distribution system. *J. Infect. Dis.* **169:**919–922.
7. **Liu, Z., J. E. Stout, M. Boldin, J. Rugh, W. F. Diven, and V. L. Yu.** 1998. Intermittent use of copper-silver ionization for *Legionella* control in water distribution systems: a potential option in buildings housing individuals at low risk of infection. *Clin. Infect. Dis.* **26:**138–140.
8. **Mathys, W., M. C. Deng, J. Meyer, and E. Junge-Mathys.** 1999. Fatal nosocomial Legionnaires' disease after heart transplantation: clinical course, epidemiology and prevention strategies for the highly immunocompromized host. *J. Hosp. Infect.* **43:**239–248.
9. **Miuetzner, S., R. C. Schwille, A. Farley, E. R. Wald, J. H. Ge, S. J. States, T. Libert, and R. M. Wadowsky.** 1997. Efficacy of thermal treatment and copper-silver ionization for controlling *Legionella pneumophila* in high-volume hot water plumbing systems in hospitals. *Am. J. Infect. Control* **25:**452–457.
10. **Rohr, U., M. Senger, F. Selenka, R. Turley, and M. Wilhelm.** 1999. Four years of experi-

ence with silver-copper ionization for control of *Legionella* in a German university hospital hot water plumbing system. *Clin. Infect. Dis.* **29:**1507–1511.

11. **Thurman, R. B., and C. P. Gerba.** 1989. The molecular mechanisms of copper and silver ion disinfection of bacteria and viruses. *Crit. Rev. Environ. Control* **18:**295–315.

12. **Walker, J. T., A. A. West, M. Morales, S. Ives, and N. Pavey.** 1997. Controlling Legionella and biofouling using silver and copper ions: fact or fiction?, p. 279–286. *In* J. Wimpenny, P. Handley, P. Gilbert, H. Lappin-Scott, and M. Jones (ed.), *Biofilms. Community Interactions and Control.* British Biofilm Club, Cardiff, United Kingdom.

13. **Yahya, M. T., L. K. Landeen, S. M. Kutz, and C. P. Gerba**. 1989. Swimming pool disinfection. An evaluation of the efficacy of copper: silver ions. *J. Environ. Health* **51:**282–285.

# EDUCATIONAL PROGRAM FOR PREVENTION OF LEGIONELLOSIS IN THE TOURISM SECTOR

Sebastian Crespi and Juan Ferrer

# 85

Travelling and staying in hotels are a known risk factor of infections by *Legionella* (3). In Europe, it is known that more than 20% of all declared cases of legionellosis are associated with travelling. Nevertheless, in spite of the current regulations on the prevention of legionellosis, the existence of the European Surveillance Scheme for travel-associated Legionnaires' disease (TALD) and its rapid alarm system, the efforts of the health authorities in several countries in the Mediterranean area, and the high degree of awareness of this disease at every level of the European tourism industry, the number of TALD cases declared to the European health authorities has continued to grow over the last few years. In Spain, a country that receives 50 million tourists every year and which has one of the most important tourism industries in the world, the TALD cases have followed a parallel evolution (Fig. 1).

## PREVENTION IN THE TOURIST SECTOR

Fully aware of this problem, the European tourism industry has developed several initiatives in an endeavor to prevent TALD cases as much as possible (1). In addition, several tourism regions in southern Europe have implemented general preventive strategies based fundamentally on permanent chlorination of cold water and on maintaining high temperatures in hot water systems (2). But the epidemiological data from the tourist regions suggest that these strategies alone are not enough to reduce the incidence of TALD cases.

In addition, the existence of specific buildings, particularly hospitals, with endemic cases of legionellosis has been recognized (4). Similarly, epidemiological studies carried out in various tourist areas have also led to the detection of hotels repeatedly associated with cases (S. Crespi, M. Sabria, and J. Ferrer, *14th Meet. Eurp. Working Group on Legionella Infect.*, abstr. 10, 1999). It has also been suggested that these buildings require specific preventive treatment (S. Crespi and J. Ferrer, *13th Meet. Eurp. Working Group on Legionella Infect.*, abstr. 3, 1998).

We believe that given the specific characteristics of the tourism sector, an adequate

*Sebastian Crespi* Clinical Laboratory, Policlinica Miramar, Camino de la Vileta 30, 07014 Palma de Mallorca, Spain. *Juan Ferrer* HOSBEC, Via Emilio Ortuño 5, 1°-5ª, 03500 Benidorm, Spain.

*Legionella*, Edited by Reinhard Marre et al.
© 2002 ASM Press, Washington, D.C.

hygiene-health education of management and maintenance personnel in tourist accommodation establishments, combined with a strict vigilance of the buildings repeatedly associated with cases, could be a key to a significant reduction in the number of cases.

## A PILOT EDUCATIONAL SCHEME IN BENIDORM, SPAIN

A program of this nature has been implemented by the hotel industry in Benidorm, Spain, a region that receives more than 5 million tourists a year. A total of 130 hotels—with a combined total of more than 20 million bed-nights/year—took part in the program organized under the auspices of the Valencia Autonomous Government and carried out by the Benidorm Hotel Association (Hosbec).

In the context of this program, all the hotels were initially inspected by expert personnel, and numerous theoretical-practical courses were arranged for the management and maintenance staff of the hotels concerned. Strict and specific recommendations were made to certain hotels repeatedly associated with cases, the remainder being advised of the general preventive measures contained in the Spanish Guideline UNE-100-030-94 and in the official recommendations of the Spanish Health Authorities.

The program that has been in operation for 1 year (June 1999 to July 2000) is a pioneer of its kind in the European tourist sector.

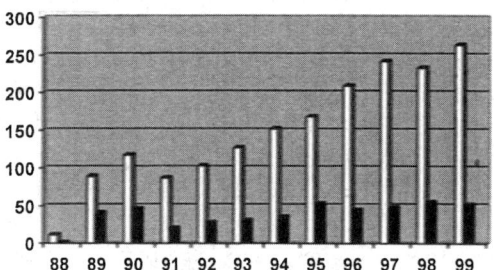

**FIGURE 1** Evolution of TALD cases in Europe and Spain from 1988–1999. White bars, Europe; black bars, Spain. (Source: European Working Group on *Legionella* Infections.)

We have christened the preventive methodology we followed with an easy-to-remember name—the e-micro method—an acronym composed of the initial letters of the key words and concepts on which the program is based: "education" for the personnel involved, adequate "maintenance" of the facilities, periodic "inspection" of the water system, periodic "control" of points of risk, "registration" of all measurements and operations effected, and the "obligation" to carry out every one of the preventive measures established.

## STATE OF HOTEL INSTALLATIONS AND THEIR OPERATION

The Hotel Inspection Programme—which also had the objective of providing a practical class for the maintenance staff—led to the detection of some generalized and very significant deficiencies (Table 1).

## PRIOR KNOWLEDGE OF PERSONNEL

Prior to the courses, an initial evaluation was made of the knowledge of the maintenance personnel concerned. The following conclusions may be drawn from this evaluation. (i) The majority of the maintenance personnel were aware that legionellosis is a serious disease and that infection can be spread through water cooling towers (84%) and showers (68%). (ii) Some 77% knew that Spanish standards oblige maintenance of hot water temperatures at above 50°C and that the jacuzzi baths (65%) require higher chlorination levels than swimming pools. (iii) About 30% erroneously believed that the pH of the water in the system is more important than chlorine in maintaining good hygiene. (iv) Some 60% did not know the water system chlorination levels required by current Spanish legislation. (v) About 20% believed—contrary to the official recommendations—that it is not necessary to read the chlorine level in the water every day, and 33% mistakenly believed that the most important water-treatment process from the hygiene point of view is decalcification.

**TABLE 1** Deficiencies detected in the water systems[a]

| Deficiencies in hotels | Standard required | % |
|---|---|---|
| Water tank deficiencies | Spanish guidelines (UNE-100-030-94) | 80 |
| Chlorination level in water | 0.2–0.8 ppm free residual chlorine | 65 |
| Deficiencies in control measures | Spanish Official Recommendations | 85 |
| Technical deficiencies in systems | Spanish guidelines (UNE-100-030-94) | 25 |
| Hot water temp | >51°C in outlets | 66 |
| Cooling towers | Adequate biocide treatment | 100 |

[a] The % indicates the hotels with deficiencies.

## PROGRAM EVALUATION

The educational program was evaluated by the organizers (the Benidorm Hotel Association) and by a governmental body (Agencia Valenciana de Turismo) through questionnaires issued to those taking part. The two evaluations produced very satisfactory results among both the maintenance personnel and the management staff. More than 80% of those taking part evaluated it positively (with the highest possible score) and more than 90% would like to continue receiving periodic training and information related to the prevention program.

## CONCLUSIONS

(i) The program adequately accomplished its original objective, basically the hygiene-health training of the management and maintenance staff of the hotels involved. Collaterally, it acted as a means of detecting certain generalized hygienic deficiencies in the water and air-conditioning systems of the hotels, and is likely to have had a positive influence on their being remedied.

(ii) The data derived from the evaluations that were made show that the program was very well received by those taking part and that, consequently, this experience may be used to advantage in other tourism areas in the Mediterranean.

(iii) Finally, and although it is early to venture conclusions on the epidemiological impact of the program, the data available to us from the first year of its application are very encouraging and suggest that the educational factor may play a key role in the prevention of legionellosis in the tourist sector.

## REFERENCES

1. **Cartwright, R.** 2000. How British tour operators contribute to prevention and control of travel associated legionnaire's disease in Europe. *Eurosurveillance Weekly* Issue 41, 12th Oct. 2000. http://www.eurosurv.org/
2. **Crespi, S.** 1992. Medidas preventivas generales, p. 11–18. *In* S. Crespi (ed.), *Legionella y Legionelosis: Normas Básicas de Prevención y Control en Instalaciones Hoteleras*. Fundación Barceló, Palma de Mallorca, Spain.
3. **World Health Organization.** Epidemiology, prevention and control of legionellosis: memorandum from a WHO meeting. *Bull. W. H. O.* **68:** 155–164.
4. **World Health Organization.** 1982. Legionnaire's disease: Report on a WHO Working Group. EURO Reports and Studies, 72. Regional Office for Europe. W. H. O. Copenhagen, Denmark.

# AUTHOR INDEX

# SUBJECT INDEX

ABI Prism 310 Genetic Analyzer, 244–247
*Acanthamoeba castellanii*
  Mip protein localization inside phagosomes, 49–51
  selection of signature-tagged *L. pneumophila* mutants in, 152–160
*Acanthamoeba polyphaga*
  mechanism of *Legionella* uptake, 174
  multiplicity of infection with *Legionella*, 171–172
  pore formation-mediated egress of *Legionella* from, 146–149
Acid phosphatase, 18–21
  mutants deficient in, 18–19
  secretion kinetics in different legionellae, 27–30
  tartrate-resistant, 19
  tartrate-sensitive, 19
Acid pretreatment, effect on recovery of *Legionella*, 281–282, 285–286, 288
Acid resistance, intracellular *L. pneumophila*, 80
*acn* gene, 252
Adaptive immunity, to *L. pneumophila*, 109–119
Adhesin, 168
Aerobactin synthetase, 34
Aerosol, ability to form stable aerosols, 54
AFLP analysis, *see* Amplified fragment length polymorphism analysis
Agglutination test, 286
*Agrobacterium*, plasmid transfer genes, 93–94
Air-conditioning system
  Australia, 353–355
  Germany, 387–389
  prevention and control of *Legionella*, 387–389
American Legion Convention (Philadelphia, 1976), 4–5, 9
American Society of Heating, Refrigerating and Air-Conditioning Engineers guidelines, *see* ASHRAE guideline 12–2000

Amoebae, *see also specific species*
  industrial waters, 288–290
  intracellular infection, CAMP-resistant *L. pneumophila*, 39–40
  intracellular multiplication of legionellae, 13, 82
  potting soil, 357, 359
  uptake of *L. pneumophila*, 165–169
Amoeba/*Legionella* coculture
  effect of exogenous bacteria, 170–175
  effect of *Tetrahymena*, 170–175
Amplified fragment length polymorphism (AFLP)
  analysis, 229–234, 251–253
  procedure
    adapter preparation, 243–244
    gel electrophoresis of AFLP fragments, 244–246
    PCR amplification, 244
    restriction and adapter ligation, 244
    separation of AFLP products, 244–247
  subtyping *L. pneumophila* serogroup 6, 243–247
  typing of *L. pneumophila*, 260–262
Amplifiers, ASHRAE guideline 12–2000, 378–382
Antibody response, to *Legionella* infection, 113–115
Antibody titer
  against legionellae in residential population, 325–329
  *Legionella* surveillance in Poland, 338–341
  patients in hospitals colonized with legionellae, 334–337
Antigens, *L. pneumophila*, 109–111
Antimicrobial agents, *see also specific drugs*
  concentrated within lysosomes, 184
  efficacy, 183
    in guinea pig model of *L. pneumophila* pneumonia, 185
  human studies, 185–186
  intracellular activities, 184–185